# Fertility Control

**Biologic and Behavioral Aspects**

Edited by

# Rochelle N. Shain, Ph.D.

Assistant Professor
Department of Obstetrics and Gynecology
University of Texas
Health Science Center at San Antonio
San Antonio, Texas
and

# Carl J. Pauerstein, M.D.

Professor and Chairman
Department of Obstetrics and Gynecology
University of Texas
Health Science Center at San Antonio
San Antonio, Texas

18 Contributors

# Fertility Control

**Biologic and Behavioral Aspects**

**HARPER & ROW, PUBLISHERS**

HAGERSTOWN

Cambridge
New York
Philadelphia
San Francisco

London
Mexico City
São Paulo
Sydney

*1817*

6  5  4  3  2  1

**Library of Congress Cataloging in Publication Data**
Main entry under title:
Fertility control, biologic and behavioral aspects.
   Includes index.
   1.   Birth control—Addresses, essays, lectures.
2.   Fertility, Human—Addresses, essays, lectures.
3.   Human reproduction—Addresses, essays, lectures.
I.   Shain, Rochelle N.   II.   Pauerstein, Carl J.
HQ766.F48         304.6'6         80-10120
ISBN 0-06-142376-9

The authors and publisher have exerted every effort to ensure
that drug selection and dosage set forth in this text are in ac-
cord with current recommendations and practice at the time of
publication. However, in view of ongoing research, changes in
government regulations, and the constant flow of information
relating to drug therapy and drug reactions, the reader is urged
to check the package insert for each drug for any change in
indications and dosage and for added warnings and precau-
tions. This is particularly important when the recommended
agent is a new or infrequently employed drug.

*We dedicate this book to the
memories of population scientists
Barrie J. Hodgson (1946–1977), reproductive biologist, and
Steven Polgar (1931–1978), anthropologist.
Their untimely deaths diminished mankind.
Their productive humanism continues to
inspire us to be more than we are.*

11-14-80

# Contents

# Contributors

**Mohammad M. Ahmad, M.D.**
*Associate Professor*
*Department of Obstetrics and Gynecology*
*The University of Texas Health Science Center*
*San Antonio, Texas*

**Andrzej Bartke, PH.D.**
*Associate Professor*
*Department of Obstetrics and Gynecology*
*The University of Texas Health Science Center*
*San Antonio, Texas*

**Harley L. Browning, PH.D.**
*Professor*
*Sociology and Research Associate*
*Population Research Center*
*University of Texas*
*Austin, Texas*

**Harold D. Dickson, PH.D.**
*Deputy Director*
*Health Services Research Institute*
*Division of Sociology*
*Department of Psychiatry*
*Department of Obstetrics and Gynecology*
*The University of Texas Health Science Center*
*San Antonio, Texas*

**Carlton A. Eddy, PH.D.**
*Associate Professor*
*Department of Obstetrics and Gynecology*
*The University of Texas Health Science Center*
*San Antonio, Texas*

**Richard Garcia**
*Administrative Associate Director*
*Department of Obstetrics and Gynecology*
*The University of Texas Health Science Center*
*San Antonio, Texas*

**C. E. Gibbs, M.D.**
*Professor*
*Department of Obstetrics and Gynecology*
*The University of Texas Health Science Center*
*San Antonio, Texas*

**Michael J. K. Harper, PH.D.**
*Associate Professor*
*Department of Obstetrics and Gynecology*
*The University of Texas Health Science Center*
*San Antonio, Texas*

**Margaret S. Hoppe, PH.D.**
*Associate Professor*
*Division of Sociology*
*Department of Psychiatry*
*University of Texas*
*San Antonio, Texas*

**Robert Jansen, M.D.**
*Assistant Professor*
*Department of Obstetrics and Gynecology*
*The University of Texas Health Science Center*
*San Antonio, Texas*

**Victoria H. Jennings, PH.D.**
*Administrative Director*
*Adolescent Medicine Program*
*Medical College of Virginia*
*Virginia Commonwealth University*
*Richmond, Virginia*

**Rebecca Lane, PH.D.**
*Postdoctoral Fellow*
*Department of Obstetrics and Gynecology*
*The University of Texas Health Science Center*
*San Antonio, Texas*

**Carl J. Pauerstein, M.D.**
*Professor and Chairman*
*Department of Obstetrics and Gynecology*
*The University of Texas Health Science Center*
*San Antonio, Texas*

**Dudley L. Poston, Jr., PH.D.**
*Associate Professor*
*Sociology and Research Associate*
*Population Research Center*
*University of Texas*
*Austin, Texas*

**Barbara A. Sanford, PH.D.**
*Associate Professor*
*Microbiology*
*Department of Obstetrics and Gynecology*
*The University of Texas Health Science Center*
*San Antonio, Texas*

**Rochelle N. Shain, PH.D**
*Assistant Professor*
*Department of Obstetrics and Gynecology*
*The University of Texas Health Science Center*
*San Antonio, Texas*

**Marguerite K. Shepard, M.D.**
*Associate Professor*
*Department of Obstetrics and Gynecology*
*The University of Texas Health Science Center*
*San Antonio, Texas*

**Paul C. Weinberg, M.D.**
*Professor*
*Department of Obstetrics and Gynecology*
*The University of Texas Health Science Center*
*San Antonio, Texas*

# Foreword

It is indeed a great pleasure to be asked to write the foreword to this important new volume. I was intimately involved with the conceptualization and early development of the core curriculum of the Center for Research and Training in Reproductive Biology, and it has been a rare privilege and a great source of personal satisfaction to observe the tremendous progress which the program has made since its inception. I therefore feel that it is most appropriate, and, in fact, essential, that the curriculum developed from this highly successful program be made available for use by others.

At the time that the center was established, simultaneous training in laboratory research, applied clinical medicine, and relevant social science methodology was being widely advocated. Whereas this concept was often articulated, it rarely, if ever, materialized into the formation of programs in which all parts of this trilogy received equal attention and were equally interesting to trainees. It is my belief that, for the first time in this program at the University of Texas Health Science Center, these three disciplines were successfully amalgamated into a single course of instruction in such a way that they were all highly relevant to students coming from widely diverse backgrounds and countries.

A decision was made to draw students from both the biomedical and social sciences and to provide them with training from both medical and social science staff members. The program had three major objectives. First, the students were to leave with a clear understanding of laboratory research, having completed their own projects and analyzed their results for publication. Second, they were to become skilled in all aspects of fertility regulation, the delivery of contraceptive services, and the problems involved in infertility. Finally, they were to receive training in social science aspects of the population field, including demography, anthropology, sociology, and general research methods. It was believed (and correctly so, it was later found) that only such a comprehensive course of instruction could prepare them for the multiple and complex problems they would face upon their return to their countries of origin.

Throughout the development of this training program, the initial courses were continually reexamined and refined. The students as well as the faculty made significant contributions to the development of the curriculum outlined in this volume. It is my belief that this dual input has led to a volume which will be of tremendous value to those attempting to deal with the multiple aspects of fertility regulation. It will be of help not only to those in the biomedical and public health fields, but also to individuals working in the demographic, anthropologic, and other social science disciplines. It has been so structured that medical students; graduate students in public health, medical anthropology and sociology, and population anthropology; population researchers; and administrative and medical staff members of public and private family planning programs and international organizations should all find the curriculum, either totally or in part, valuable in their own professional careers or training efforts.

The chapters on reproductive biology and its clinical application will increase the general understanding of the physical problems involved in population overgrowth and the medical means which are available to cope with them. The chapters on the behavioral aspects of population change will also be of value as people from many disciplines continue to try to understand and cope with the motivational components of fertility control.

In summary, it has been very satisfying to see this program grow from an abstract idea into a highly practical and successful entity. All of those involved in its development are to be congratulated. During its lifetime the activities of the center have enriched the students and faculty alike, as they worked together to develop a curriculum relevant to the diverse needs of many types of individuals and programs. The results of their combined expertise now stand ready to enrich those who, in the use of this volume, will be able to profit from their hard work, vast experience, and incisive presentation of a new and exciting approach to population problems.

*Elizabeth B. Connell,* M.D.
*Department of Obstetrics and Gynecology*
*Northwestern University Medical School*
*Chicago, Illinois*

# Preface

The training of population researchers and workers requires information contained within a variety of disciplines. To function effectively, population workers must understand and appreciate basic principles of demography, sociology, anthropology, and biostatistics, as well as the anatomy, physiology, and biochemistry of reproduction. Thus, to offer an optimal learning environment, training centers must bring together multidisciplinary materials and educators with diverse professional backgrounds.

Based on this conviction, the Center for Research and Training in Reproductive Biology was established within the Department of Obstetrics and Gynecology at the University of Texas Health Science Center at San Antonio in 1974, funded by a Rockefeller Foundation grant to Carl J. Pauerstein. The center's postdoctoral program consists of a six-month core curriculum of didactic instruction in social science, reproductive biology, and clinical procedures, followed by individual specialization in one of these areas. Its objective is to provide comprehensive training to physicians and scientists from the United States and abroad in the hope that they will then make contributions in the laboratory, in the establishment and direction of family planning clinics, and/or in social science research.

Because of the varying national, ethnic, and academic backgrounds of the fellows, the core curriculum is taught with the aid of written instructional units. This volume is a product of continued evaluation and revision of the instructional materials. The contributors are program instructors or fellows. Because of the potentially wide audience that this book hopes to reach, we have attempted to make the material sufficiently sophisticated to be useful to specialists, but have written in language designed (with the aid of a glossary) to be comprehensible to nonspecialists. The resulting monograph is a multidisciplinary effort which strives to minimize the language barrier which often renders technical matter incomprehensible to individuals outside a given specialty.

Part One, "Reproductive Biology," considers embryology, maturation, and anatomy of the reproductive system; reproductive endocrinology; physiology of preimplantation and implantation phenomena (sperm and ovum transport, fertilization, and implantation); and human sexuality. A thorough understanding of this material will make the material in Part Two, "Clinical Applications of Reproductive and Behavioral Science," more meaningful. For example, identifying the sequence of events from gametogenesis to implantation facilitates a more thorough understanding of current contraceptive methods and potential innovations in this technology.

Part Three, "Demographic Aspects of Population Change," is basic to understanding fertility from the social science perspective. These chapters provide the necessary concepts and tools to allow the biomedical scientist to communicate with the social scientist. Many chapters in Part Four, "Anthropological and Sociological Perspectives," are outgrowths of, or responses to, demographic theory. These chapters consider different types of data, usually more broadly based, and offer interpretations or perspectives of fertility control different from that of traditional demography.

Part Five, "Social Science Methodology," attempts to demystify and clarify social science research design, including the statistical concepts and techniques useful to the administrator, researcher, or teacher in the population field.

*Carl J. Pauerstein*, M.D.
*Rochelle N. Shain*, PH.D.

# Fertility Control

## Biologic and Behavioral Aspects

# Reproductive
# Biology

I

Part One provides an overview of genetic, hormonal, and physiological aspects of sexual maturation and reproductive function. Its primary purpose is to provide the reader with an understanding of those aspects of reproduction that might be vulnerable to contraceptive interference. Specifically, Chapter 1 describes the anatomical development of male and female reproductive systems; reproductive endocrinology is addressed in Chapter 2. Chapter 3 summarizes what is currently known about conception, including sperm transport, ovum pickup, fertilization, nature and transport of the preimplantation embryo, and implantation. Chapter 4 considers various aspects of sex typing, including gender, legal sex, gender identity and gender role, and describes human sexual response.

# 1

# Embryology, Maturation, and Anatomy of the Reproductive System

Carl J. Pauerstein
Andrzej Bartke

## EMBRYOLOGY

The sex of an individual is determined at conception by the chromosomal contributions of the maternal and paternal gametes (ova and spermatozoa). In the majority of mammals, including man, all female gametes (*ova;* sing., *ovum*) contain identical sex chromosomes, termed *X,* while only half of the male gametes (*spermatozoa;* sing., *spermatozoon*) contain an X chromosome. The remainder of spermatozoa carry a morphologically distinguishable sex chromosome, termed *Y.* The mechanisms by which genetic factors control sex differentiation remain undefined, but involvement of the H-Y antigen is strongly suggested by recent observations (14). The gonads and the internal and external genitalia develop along female lines unless induced toward male differentiation by the Y chromosome, which may exert its influence directly, or by modifying the activity of other genes.

Although the sex genotype is determined at fertilization, sex differentiation of the gonads and internal and external genitalia is not completed until after about 12 weeks of embryonic life in the female and 14 weeks in the male. Just as the genotype determines the direction in which the gonads will differentiate, so the gonads determine the differentiation of the internal ducts and the external genitalia.

## GONADS

The ovaries and testes develop from an undifferentiated gonadal primordium (embryonic precursor). This primordium, called the genital ridge, is visible in the 5-week embryo.

The germ cells (precursors of ova and spermatozoa), which arise in the yolk sac or gut endoderm, migrate to and become incorporated into the urogenital ridge to form the sexually undifferentiated gonad, which has two major components, the cortex and medulla. It is usually stated that the medullary element is capable only of becoming a testis and the cortical element is capable only of development as an ovary, but some new findings challenge this concept (11).

In the female, the gonad differentiates into an ovary during the 7th week of embryonic life. One can then distinguish connective tissue and epithelial tissue, in the form of medullary cords. These cords contain primordial germ cells (oogonia), as well as primitive granulosa cells. After reaching the genital ridge, the germ cells are designated *oogonia.* Early generations of oogonia degenerate. Later generations of oogonia differentiate into *oocytes.*

Late in embryonic life, the fetal ovary contains many primary follicles, each characterized by an oocyte surrounded by a single layer

**3**

of flattened granulosa cells. Each follicle is surrounded by connective tissue. These changes define the gonad as an ovary.

In male embryos, testes become distinguishable during the 7th week of embryonic life. The indifferent gonad is divided into cords by septa (partitions). These cords are then segregated from the surface epithelium by a sheet of connective tissue, which will become the *tunica albuginea* (testicular capsule). The primordial germ cells become incorporated into the testicular cords, which are lined by several layers of supporting ("nursing") cells, the Sertoli cells. The incorporated germ cells are called *spermatogonia.* At about 60 days, Leydig cells (androgen-producing cells) are seen in the interstitial tissues near the tunica albuginea. These cells reach their

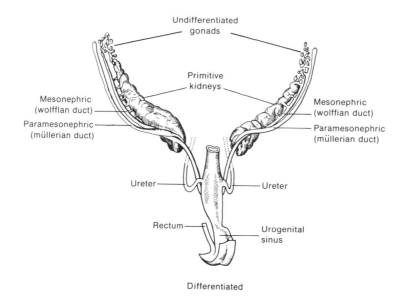

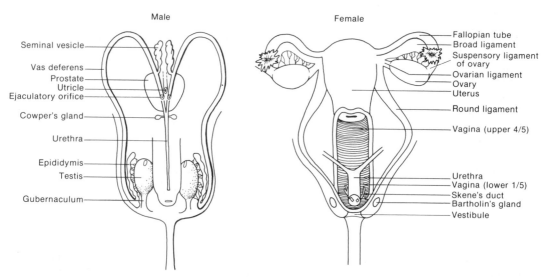

**FIG. 1–1.** (*Top*) Reconstruction of the urogenital system during the indifferent stage. Note the relationships of the wolffian and müllerian ducts to each other and to the mesonephros. (*Bottom right*) Adult form of internal ducts in embryo that had undergone female differentiation. The wolffian ducts have regressed and the müllerian ducts have come together in the midline to form the uterus. The cephalad portions remain unfused to form the fallopian tubes. (*Bottom left*) Adult form of internal ducts after male differentiation. See text for details.

maximum number during the 3rd and 4th months of fetal life, and begin to decrease during the 4th month. The fetal testes produce androgens, which influence the development of the internal ducts and the external genitalia. A nonsteroidal substance produced by the testes causes degeneration of the female (müllerian) ducts (12).

## INTERNAL DUCTS

During the indifferent stage, the embryo possesses both mesonephric (male, wolffian) and paramesonephric (female, müllerian) ducts (Fig. 1–1). If embryos are castrated at the indifferent stage, the mesonephric ducts regress, and the paramesonephric ducts develop. Local implantation of a testosterone crystal in a female fetus prevents mesonephric regression, but does not induce paramesonephric regression. In contrast, local implantation of a testis both supports the mesonephric ducts and induces paramesonephric regression. The embryonic testis thus has two organizing functions, only one of which can be replaced by testosterone. In the absence of testes, the internal ducts always develop along female lines, whether or not the ovaries are present.

By the end of the 3rd month, the mesonephric ducts in the female have largely disappeared. The right and left müllerian ducts fuse for most of their course, resulting in a single tube, with two lumens (channels)—the future uterus. The unfused portions of the müllerian ducts are the precursors of the fallopian tubes. The medial septum (partition) then disappears, completing the creation of the uterus (Fig. 1–1).

In male embryos, the paramesonephric ducts begin to regress during the 9th week. Their remnants persist near the testes as the appendix testes and prostatic utricle (sac). Subsequent male development involves the formation of the *epididymides* (sing., *epididymis*), *vasa deferentia* (sing., *vas deferens*), seminal vesicles, and prostate gland (Fig. 1–1). Development of all of these structures is androgen-dependent.

## EXTERNAL GENITALIA

During the undifferentiated stage, the external genitalia are bordered laterally by the labioscrotal folds (genital swelling) and medially by the urethral groove. Just lateral to the urethral groove on each side, the urethral folds are interposed between the urethral groove and the genital swellings. The urethral groove is bounded anteriorly by the genital tubercle (eminence, precursor to penis or clitoris) (Fig. 1–2). The urogenital sinus (cavity) opens into the urethral groove.

The caudal extremity of the fused müllerian duct ends against the urogenital sinus. In female differentiation the vaginal cord, which is derived from the blind ends of the müllerian ducts, is interposed between the latter and the urogenital sinus. The vagina, formed at about 5 months, is contributed to both by the müllerian ducts and by the urogenital sinus (Fig. 1–1).

In female differentiation, the urethral groove becomes the vestibule, the urethral folds become the labia minora, and the genital swellings form the labia majora. The genital tubercle becomes the clitoris (Fig. 1–2).

Development of male external genitalia occurs in genetic males in response to androgen secreted by the embryonic testes. Male genital development may also occur in genetic females exposed to androgens. Because testosterone is necessary for the development of male genitalia, genetic males with defective testes have female genitalia. The changes establishing the male genitalia involve expansion of the genital tubercle, genital swellings, and urogenital folds, and fusion of the urogenital folds. The genital tubercle forms the glans penis. The urogenital folds fuse to convert the urogenital groove into the penile urethra along the shaft of the penis. The labioscrotal folds fuse to form the scrotum (Fig. 1–2).

The active secretion of androgens by the fetal testis is followed by a period of relative testicular quiescence which continues until shortly before the onset of puberty (1).

## MATURATION

At puberty, the gonads manufacture sex hormones in sufficient quantity to cause rapid growth of the genitalia, development of the secondary sex characteristics, and skeletal growth and maturation.

### THE FEMALE

The mean age of onset of pubertal changes in girls is 8 years (the range is 7 to 10 years). The sequence begins with uterine and ovarian growth. Two years later (about age ten), the

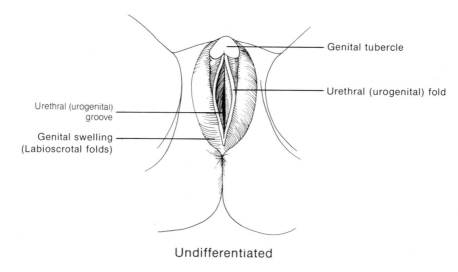

Undifferentiated

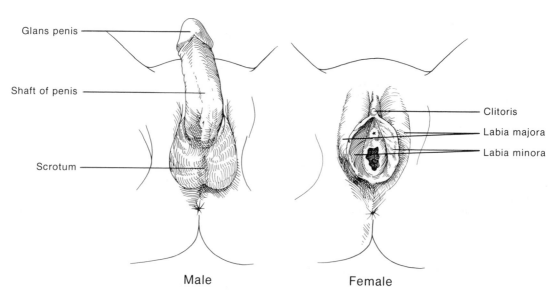

Male                    Female

**FIG. 1–2.** Diagrammatic representation of the development of the external genitalia. (*Top*) The indifferent stage; (*bottom left*) male differentiation; (*bottom right*) female differentiation. (Pauerstein CJ. In Huff RW, Pauerstein CJ (eds): Physiology and Pathophysiology of Reproduction. New York. Copyright © 1979, John Wiley & Sons, Inc. Reprinted by permission.)

first clinical manifestation of the pubertal sequence appears as an increase in diameter of the breast areola to form a small mound. This occurs in approximately half of the girls. In the other half, appearance of pubic hair is the first change noted. At first, lightly pigmented hair is present on the labia only. As estrogen output increases, the uterus and ovaries continue to enlarge. During the 11th year, other anatomic changes begin. The bony pelvis widens, and

deposition of fat begins on the hips, buttocks, and over the pubis. The pubic hair becomes coarser, curlier, and begins to grow over the mons pubis. The breast enters a second stage of development in which the breast bud enlarges. The vaginal mucosa thickens. At this point, gonadotrophins become detectable, and cyclic secretion of estrogen begins (see Chap. 2 for a detailed discussion of ovulation).

At about age twelve, girls begin the premenarcheal growth spurt. Breast changes continue, as the nipple and areola project to form the secondary breast mound. Axillary hair appears (adrenarche). In most youngsters, the first episode of menstrual bleeding (menarche) occurs within 6 months of the development of axillary hair. The first menstrual episodes may be anovulatory.

Menarche is the single event that can be accurately documented. At menarche the pubic hair has assumed the adult pattern, with a sharp superior border. The nipples project from the breast mound. This projection is more noticeable because of recession of the areola to the breast contour. The uterus weighs 18 g. and the ovaries about 8 g. The premenarcheal growth spurt now decelerates. Most women will grow only 6 in. over the next three years. At puberty (the first ovulation), pubic hair begins to grow toward the intercrural folds. The breasts have assumed their contours, and the nipples point laterally. Three, or three-and-a-half years beyond menarche, skeletal growth ceases. The ovaries are at the adult weight of 10 g. and the uterus weighs 30 to 40 g. The girl has now become an adult.

## THE MALE

The onset of puberty in boys occurs at an average age of 14 years. Interestingly, the hormonal events that occur at male puberty are most probably the result of patterns imprinted upon the embryonic central nervous system by the fetal testis. The early "masculinizing" effect of androgens on the brain is responsible for the male pattern of release of pituitary hormones, as well as for the appearance of masculine sexual and aggressive behaviors later in life, in response to the pubertal increase in androgen production. On the basis of these observations, it is also suspected that spontaneous, or drug-induced changes in the hormonal balance of the mother during early pregnancy may influence sexual orientation and behavior of her child in adulthood, and may perhaps account for at least some cases of homosexuality. These concepts represent application of data obtained in animals to man, but they have gained some support from behavioral observations in female rhesus monkeys exposed to exogenous androgens during their fetal development (7).

In the male, major maturational changes are manifested in the testes themselves, and, consequently, in the secondary sex characteristics of the body.

The testis is composed of seminiferous tubules, which occupy most of its volume, and interstitial tissue. During development, the seminiferous cords present in the fetal testis increase in length and diameter to give rise to seminiferous tubules. The tubules contain germinal cells which divide and differentiate to form spermatozoa.

### SPERMATOGENESIS

The process of producing spermatozoa from the stem cells (spermatogonia) is termed *spermatogenesis*. Spermatogonia give rise to primary spermatocytes after a series of mitotic divisions. The spermatocytes then undergo meiosis (reduction division), which consists of two cell divisions following each other in relatively rapid sequence. As the result, each diploid (having a full set of chromosomes) primary spermatocyte gives rise, first, to two secondary spermatocytes (which are haploid, that is, have a single set of chromosomes), and then to four spermatids (precursors of spermatozoa). The spermatids then undergo morphologic and functional differentiation into spermatozoa. The nucleus moves toward the periphery of the cell and becomes flattened and elongated, the flagellum (whiplike appendage) is formed, and eventually most of the cytoplasm is lost (Fig. 1-3). The nucleus, together with the acrosome (caplike structure), forms the head of the spermatozoon, whereas the flagellum becomes the tail. The acrosome contains enzymes which are required for the dissolution of the ovum's covering layers and its subsequent penetration (17). The spermatids become separate cells, rather than components of a syncytium (multinuclear aggregate of cells) only after their release from the germinal epithelium (cellular lining) into the tubular lumen. The duration of each step of spermatogenesis is rigidly fixed and characteristic for the species. In the human, the duration of complete spermatogenesis is 74 days (10). The differentiation of neighboring spermatogonia into more advanced cells is synchronized by an unknown mechanism. In each region of the seminiferous (semen-producing) epithelium, new cohorts of spermatogonia begin to differentiate at regular intervals. This, together with the fixed rate

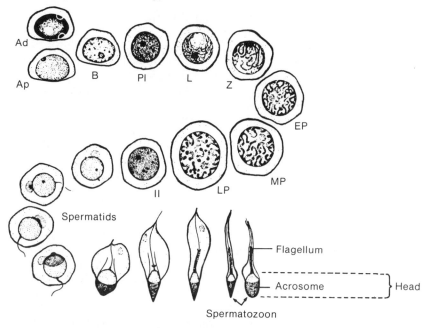

**FIG. 1–3.** Germinal cells of the human testis. Spermatogenesis begins with the spermatogonia (*top left*) and terminates with a spermatozoon (*bottom right*). Ad, Ap, B—different types (subsequent generations) of spermatogonia; P1, L, Z, EP, MP, LP—primary spermatocytes in various stages of preparation for the first meiotic division; II—secondary spermatocyte; also shown are various steps of spermatid differentiation, and spermatozoa viewed in two different planes (lateral and frontal aspects). (Adapted from Clermont Y. In Rosemberg E, Paulsen CA, (eds): The Human Testis. New York, Plenum Press, 1970, p. 49)

of progression through the various stages of spermatogenesis, is responsible for the occurrence of characteristic associations of germinal cells at different stages of their development (3). These associations of different types of germinal cells are called *stages of the cycle of the seminiferous epithelium* (Fig. 1–4).

In contrast to the constant rate of spermatogenesis, its efficiency varies considerably. This reflects differences in the proportion of germinal cells surviving various stages of spermatogenesis. The survival of dividing and differentiating germinal cells depends on hormonal balance, temperature, and the age of an individual. It can be modified by drugs, chemicals, ionizing radiation, and a host of environmental influences. The number of spermatozoa produced by the testis reflects the proportion of the survival of germ cells during various stages of spermatogenesis.

Throughout their development, the germinal cells are intimately associated with nurturing elements of the seminiferous epithe-lium, the Sertoli cells. The nuclei of the Sertoli cells are located near the outer perimeter of the seminiferous tubules, but the cytoplasm of Sertoli cells extends all the way to the tubular lumen and envelops the spermatocytes and spermatids. Adjacent Sertoli cells are connected to each other in areas where their cell membranes come into intimate contact. These occluding junctions form a barrier to the transfer of large organic molecules between the outer (basal) and the more central (adluminal) compartments of the seminiferous tubule (4). This barrier prevents the entry of various substances from the blood to spermatocytes, spermatids, and the tubular lumen, and is called the *blood-testis barrier* (Fig. 1–5). The spermatogonia begin development outside the barrier (in the basal compartment) but their daughter cells (cells following division) move toward the lumen of the tubule and enter the adluminal compartment, as the Sertoli cells form new occluding junctions peripheral to differentiating spermatocytes. The

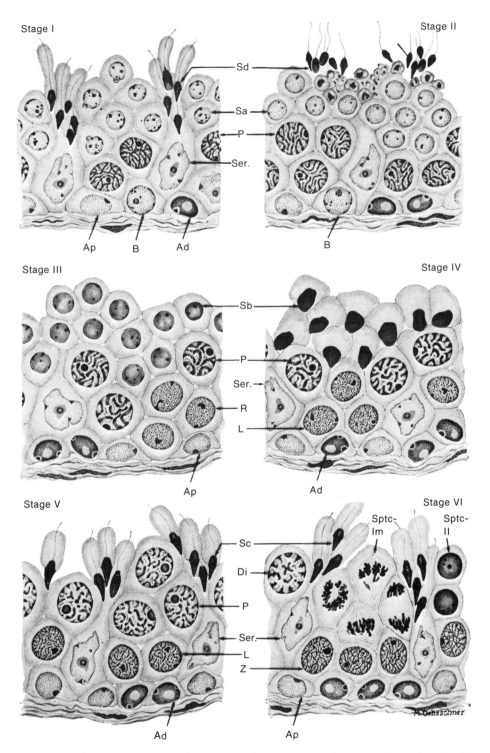

**FIG. 1–4.** Cellular composition of six stages of spermatogenesis in man. Ser—Sertoli-cells nuclei; Ap, Ad, B—subsequent generations of spermatogonia; R, L, Z, P, Di—different stages of development of primary spermatocytes; Sptc-Im—primary spermatocytes in division; Sptc-II—secondary spermatocytes; Sa, Sb, Sc, Sd—spermatids at various steps of their differentiation; Sz—spermatozoa. (Clermont Y: Am J Anat 112:35, 1963)

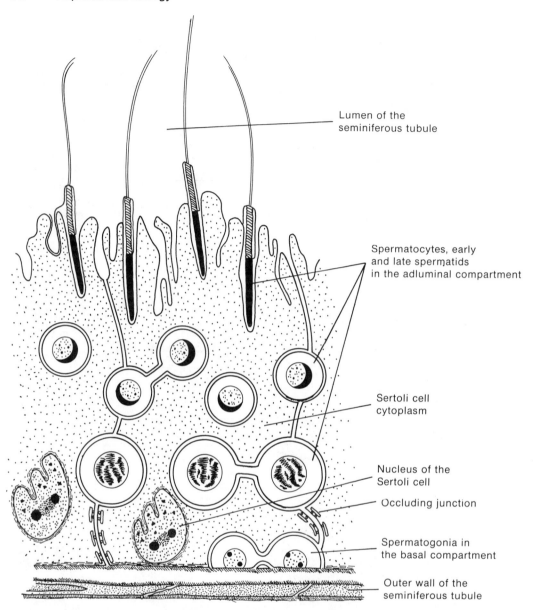

Lumen of the
seminiferous tubule

Spermatocytes, early
and late spermatids
in the adluminal compartment

Sertoli cell
cytoplasm

Nucleus of the
Sertoli cell

Occluding junction

Spermatogonia in
the basal compartment

Outer wall of the
seminiferous tubule

**FIG. 1–5.** The fine structure of Sertoli cells, and the occluding junctions between the adjacent Sertoli cells within a seminiferous tubule. These junctions subdivide the seminiferous tubule epithelium into basal and adluminal compartments. (Dym M, Fawcett DW: Biol Reprod 3:308, 1970)

observation that the surface components of the more advanced germinal cells can be antigenic (see Chap. 7) is consistent with the effective separation of these cells from the circulation by the blood-testis barrier. Testicular injury or leakage of the sperm from the ruptured epididymis or vas deferens may result in formation of antibodies to a male's own spermatozoa (autoimmune reaction). This is pre-

sumably a fairly common sequel of vasectomy (2), but the significance, if any, of the circulating antisperm antibodies to the health, longevity, or testicular function of the vasectomized male, or to the prospects for restoration of fertility after surgical reversal of vasectomy, remain speculative (see Chap. 8).

Sertoli cells appear to provide the environment necessary for the development and differentiation of germinal cells and to mediate the effects of hormones, temperature, and other factors on spermatogenesis (9).

### SECONDARY SEX CHARACTERISTICS

Changes in the secondary sex characteristics are mediated by androgens produced by the testis. The testicular interstitium (tissue in the spaces between the seminiferous tubules) contains Leydig cells, which produce the androgens (13). The Leydig cells possess typical morphologic characteristics of steroid-producing cells. The proper functioning of the Leydig cells depends on stimulation by anterior pituitary hormones, primarily luteinizing hormone (LH; also called interstitial cell-stimulating hormone, ICSH). The steroidal hormones elaborated by the Leydig cells, of which testosterone is the most important, exert a variety of effects at different sites involved in the reproductive process. Testosterone, acting directly or by giving rise to other steroids (dihydrotestosterone and estradiol) is responsible for the maintenance of spermatogenesis; the growth and functioning of accessory reproductive glands; for some aspects of epididymal function and sperm maturation; for the pubertal appearance and subsequent maintenance of the familiar, external secondary sexual characteristics, such as masculine distribution of facial and body hair, deepening of the voice, and increase in muscularity; for fetal differentiation and pubertal growth of the external genitalia; and for libido and potency. In other words, both the morphological differentiation and the reproductive potential of the male depend on the secretory function of the Leydig cells. Under androgen influence, the penis grows in width and length. The skin of the scrotum becomes pigmented and rugose (wrinkled). Changes in the internal genitals include enlargement of the seminal vesicles, the prostate gland, and the bulbourethral glands.

The general body conformation changes, as the shoulders broaden and muscles enlarge. General body hair increases, the male hair pattern appears in the pubic region, and hair grows in the axillae (armpits), on the chest, and around the anus. A beard appears, and some recession of the hair of the scalp is noted in the region of the temples, bilaterally. Acne may develop, due to increased sebaceous gland secretion. The voice deepens, as the lar-

ynx enlarges and the vocal cords become larger and thicker.

The levels of total (free, plus protein-bound) androgens in the circulation remain essentially unchanged until the 7th or 8th decade of life. Although there may be a reduction of androgen synthesis by the testes with age, there is a proportional decrease in metabolic clearance of male sex hormones. Thus the aging process in the male is probably not directly related to diminished total blood levels of male sex hormones. However, the amount of free (and presumably biologically active) testosterone in the blood decreases after the 4th or 5th decade.

## ANATOMY

In this section, the anatomy of the adult pertinent to reproduction and contraception is discussed.

## THE FEMALE REPRODUCTIVE SYSTEM

The adnexa (the uterine appendages), uterus, cervix, vagina, vulva, and the supporting structures of the pelvic floor are described below. The ovary is described in the context of female reproductive endocrinology in Chapter 12.

### THE ADNEXA

The uterine adnexa are composed of the ovaries, fallopian tubes, and their mesenteries (membranes) (Fig. 1–6). Each fallopian tube is approximately 12 cm. in length and extends from the endometrial cavity to the ovaries. Four distinct areas of the tube are recognized: *1)* the intramural, or uterine, portion extends from the endometrial cavity (uterine mucous membrane) through the myometrium (uterine muscle). *2)* The isthmus is 2 to 3 cm. in length and contains a heavy muscular wall. The lumen (channel) of the tube is narrowest in the isthmus. *3)* The ampulla is adjacent to the isthmus, and the ampullary-isthmic junction (AIJ) can be detected by palpating the tube and noting the change in consistency. The ampulla is 5 to 8 cm. in length, and its lumen varies from 1 mm. in diameter near the AIJ to a centimeter or more near the infundibulum. *4)* The infundibulum is the trumpet-shaped, distal portion of the tube which terminates in the fingerlike fimbria which delineate the abdominal ostium (cavity). See Chapter 8 for a detailed discussion of tubal sterilization.

The tube is enclosed in the leaves of the broad ligament, and this portion of the broad ligament is termed the mesosalpinx. This mesentery blends into the infundibulopelvic ligament which encloses the ovarian vessels. The blood supply is from the ovarian and uterine arteries. The venous drainage follows the arterial supply (Fig. 1–6A).

The mucous membrane of the tube consists of a single layer of columnar (pillarlike) cells. Some cells are secretory, others have cilia (hairlike structures) beating toward the uterus, and some cells seem to be exhausted secretory cells (called "peg cells"). The mucous membrane is located on extensive longitudinal folds which decrease in height and complexity when examined from the ampulla to the intramural portion of the tube. There is some change in the appearance of the epithelium during different phases of the ovarian cycle. Tubal fluid is actively secreted, as well as transudated (diffused) into the lumen.

The muscular coat of the tube consists of two or three layers, depending upon the region. The intramural portion of the tube has an inner longitudinal layer which virtually disappears in the isthmus, leaving only a circular layer and an outer longitudinal layer for the remainder of the tube.

## THE UTERUS

The uterus is a muscular organ located between the bladder and the rectum. Its posterior wall is covered by peritoneum (inner lining of the abdominal cavity). The upper portion of the anterior wall is also covered by peritoneum, the lower portion of which is loosely attached to the posterior surface of the bladder. The uterus is composed of three layers: an outer serosal surface (peritoneal), a layer of smooth muscle (myometrium), and a mucosal layer (endometrium). The uterus of an adult nulliparous woman (one who has never borne children) weights 45 to 70 g., whereas the uterus of a parous woman weighs 80 g. or more. In the nonpregnant state, the smooth muscle fibers of the uterus are approximately $50\mu$ in length. The smooth muscle bundles are arranged in layers, but are not sharply defined.

The uterus is mobile and is supported by several ligaments. Peritoneal sheets, called the broad ligaments, sweep from either side of the uterus to the pelvic walls. They provide little support, but enclose vascular and lymphatic vessels, the fallopian tubes, and the round ligaments. The round ligaments extend from the upper lateral aspects of the uterus to the inguinal canals (of the groin) and provide some support to the uterus. The main supports of the uterus are the cardinal, or transverse, cervical ligaments located in the base of the broad ligaments. They are condensations of pelvic fascia (connective tissue) and anchor the uterine cervix to the pelvic side walls. They also enclose the uterine arteries and ureters. The uterosacral ligaments are the other main support of the uterus. These condensations of the pelvic fascia anchor the upper portion of the uterine cervix posteriorly to the sacrum (Fig. 1–6B).

The endometrium is responsive to changes in the concentrations of ovarian hormones. It varies in thickness from 0.5 mm. at the end of a menstrual period to as much as 5 mm. or more just prior to menstruation. Its blood is supplied via two sets of arterioles (minute arterial branches) which enter it at right angles. Straight arterioles serve a nutritive function and supply the basal layer of endometrium, an area not shed during menstruation, from which the endometrium regenerates after menstruation. Coiled or spiral arterioles supply the outer functional area of the endometrium. This area is composed of a compact zone, which includes the surface epithelium and stroma (supporting tissue), and a spongy zone, which contains endometrial glands. Spiral arterioles, because of their ability to respond to the ovarian hormones, are instrumental in producing cyclic sloughing of the functional layer of the endometrium at menstruation.

## THE CERVIX

The cervix is that portion of the uterus which is adjacent to the vagina (Fig. 1-6). It lies below the internal os (mouth); the lowermost portion, which contains the external os of the cervix, projects into the vagina. The stroma of the cervix contains little smooth muscle and is mostly composed of connective tissue. The endocervical (endo denotes "within") canal runs between the internal and external os and contains an epithelium composed of a single layer of tall, mucus-secreting columnar cells.

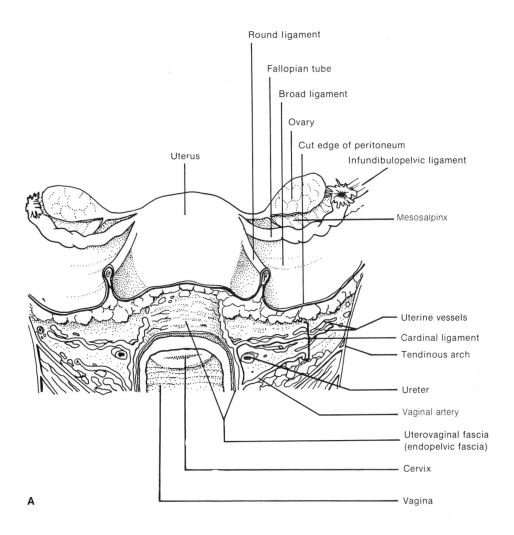

A

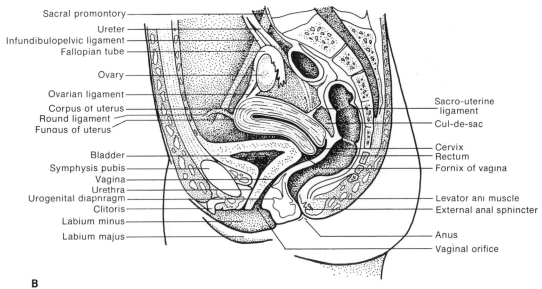

B

**FIG. 1–6.** Adult female genital tract and related structures. See text for explanation.

Within the endocervical canal is an intricate system of ridges, tunnels, and clefts. The epithelium of the endocervix also responds to the concentrations of sex hormones. At mid-cycle, when high levels of estrogen and low levels of progesterone are produced, the mucus is thin, watery, and clear, and can be stretched for several centimeters. When progesterone is present in high concentrations, the mucus becomes viscid (sticky) and tenacious—this is seen after ovulation or during pregnancy.

The intravaginal portion of the cervix is covered with a stratified (arranged in several layers) epithelium. The point where the columnar and stratified epithelia meet is referred to as the *squamo-columnar junction* (SCJ), or transition zone. The anatomic location of the SCJ may vary from the lower endocervical canal to the outer part of the cervix.

### THE VAGINA

The vagina is a muscular, tubular structure lined by a mucous membrane. It extends from the vulva to the lower portion of the uterus. It lies between the bladder and urethra, anteriorly, and the rectum, posteriorly (Fig. 1-6). In the usual state, the vagina is collapsed, and its anterior and posterior walls are in contact. There is some free space at its lateral margins, so that in cross section the vagina is shaped like the letter *H*.

The vaginal mucous membrane contains no glands and is loosely attached to the underlying connective tissue. The connective tissue is dense and contains elastic fibers, lymphoid nodules, and blood vessels.

The muscular coat of the vagina has two layers which are not sharply defined. There is an inner, circular layer and an outer, longitudinal layer. Closure of the vagina is mainly accomplished by the levator ani muscles (Fig. 1-7).

The anterior and posterior walls of the vagina contain prominent longitudinal ridges, or columns, from which transverse ridges, or rugae, extend at right angles. The rugae give the vagina a corrugated appearance in nulliparous women. After repeated births, the rugae become less prominent, and after the

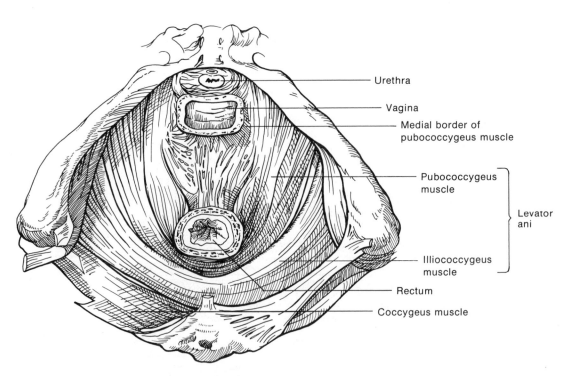

**FIG. 1–7.** Muscles of the female pelvic floor. Note relationships to urethra, vagina, and rectum. See text for explanation. (Pauerstein CJ. In Huff RW, Pauerstein CJ (eds): Physiology and Pathophysiology of Reproduction. New York. Copyright © 1979, John Wiley & Sons, Inc. Reprinted by permission.)

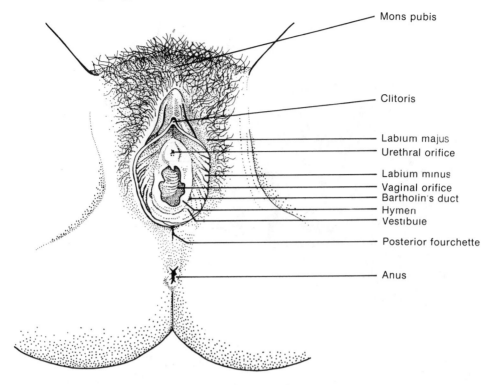

**FIG. 1–8.** Vulva of adult woman. See text for description of structures.

menopause they disappear, and the vagina becomes smooth.

The vagina is separated from the bladder, urethra, and rectum by connective tissue. The upper part of the posterior vagina is not adjacent to the rectum, but rather to the cul-de-sac, and is covered with peritoneum (Fig. 1–6).

### THE VULVA

The vulva is comprised of skin and its appendages (Fig. 1–8). The mons pubis is a fatty cushion covering the junction of the pubic bones. The skin of the mons contains hair follicles, sebaceous glands, and sweat glands. The labia majora are longitudinal folds of skin blending into the mons. They acquire pigmentation and fatty tissue at puberty. The skin of the labia majora contains usual skin appendages, including apocrine sweat glands, which secrete in response to stress or stimulation. These secretions are sterile and odorless. Apocrine gland function is considered a secondary sex characteristic.

The labia minora are small, firm, vascular folds of skin medial to the labia majora. They fuse anteriorly over the clitoris and blend to-

gether posteriorly. The skin of the labia minora contains no hair follicles, and its sebaceous glands secrete directly onto the skin surface.

The clitoris is a midline structure of vascular erectile tissue homologous to the penis in the male. It is richly supplied with nerve endings but contains no urethra. The urethral orifice opens in the vulva between the labia minora, about 1.5 cm. below the clitoris.

The hymen or its remnants, which partially occlude the vaginal opening, consist of a double layer of stratified squamous epithelium covering vascular connective tissue.

Bartholin's glands open on either side of the vulva, just outside the hymen, approximately one-third of the distance from the fourchette (see Fig. 1–8) to the clitoris. The glands are located deep beneath the fascia. The ducts of the glands are lined with squamous epithelium at the orifice.

### THE PELVIC FLOOR

In the adult woman the pelvic floor, or pelvic diaphragm, is formed by the levator ani and coccygeus muscles, which meet in the midline.

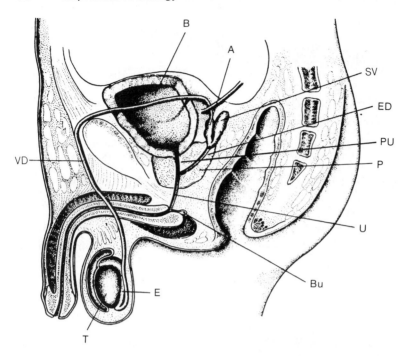

**FIG. 1–9.** The human male reproductive tract. A—ampulla; B—bladder; Bu—bulbo-urethral (Cowper's) glands; E—epididymis; ED—ejaculatory duct; P—prostate; PU—prostatic urethra; SV—seminal vesicle; T—testis; U—urethra; VD—vas deferens. (Austin CR. In Austin CR, Short RV (eds): Reproduction in Mammals. Cambridge Univ. Press, 1972, p. 110)

It is covered by endopelvic fascia. Viewed from above, it appears as a broad hammock of muscle sweeping down from the pelvic brim to surround the urethra, vagina, and rectum (Fig. 1–7). There are two gaps in the muscular diaphragm. The anterior gap is bridged by the urogenital diaphragm and transmits the urethra and vagina. The posterior gap transmits the rectum and the anal canal.

The levator ani muscles, composed of the pubococcygeus and the iliococcygeus muscles, form the major part of the pelvic diaphragm. The coccygeus muscle completes the pelvic diaphragm posteriorly.

The pelvic floor has inherent tone and responds to changes in intraabdominal pressure. The pubococcygeus muscle is traversed by the urethra, vagina, and rectum, and supports the vagina, the uterus (indirectly), and the bladder, urethra, and rectum.

## THE MALE REPRODUCTIVE SYSTEM

In this section, the testes, the efferent ducts, the *epididymides* (sing., *epididymis*), the deferent ducts, and the accessory reproductive glands (particularly the seminal vesicles and the prostate) are discussed (Fig. 1–9).

**THE PENIS**

The penis is composed of three cylinders of erectile tissue, the paired corpora cavernosa and a single corpus spongiosum, enclosed within a fibrous capsule—the tunica albuginia—and covered by fascia.

The urethra extends the length of the penis, from the external urethral meatus (opening) to the internal orifice of the bladder. Three anatomic portions of the urethra are recognized: the penile urethra, which extends from the meatus to the distal leaf of the urogenital diaphragm; the membranous urethra, which lies within the urogenital diaphragm; and the prostatic urethra, which extends from the proximal aspect of the urogenital diaphragm to the vesical (of the bladder) neck. This portion contains the ejaculatory duct and prostatic duct openings.

### THE PROSTATE AND THE SEMINAL VESICLES

The prostate surrounds the proximal urethra. It is enclosed in a thick fibrous capsule derived from the pelvic fascia. The seminal vesicles are paired lobulated structures 5 to 7 cm. in length, which lie between the bladder and the rectum. Their anterior surfaces are immediately adjacent to the wall of the bladder, and their posterior surfaces lie against the rectum, separated by connective tissue. Each seminal vesicle, at its anterior extremity, narrows into a straight duct which joins its corresponding duct to form the ejaculatory duct. The ejaculatory ducts end in tiny slitlike openings in the prostatic urethra.

### THE TESTIS AND ITS DUCTS

The testis lies in a thin membranous sac, the tunica vaginalis, formed by the peritoneum during the descent of the testes. The tunic covers the testicle anteriorly, but posteriorly the tunica vaginalis is lacking where the testis is capped by the epididymis (Fig. 1-9). Each testis is covered by a thick fibroelastic capsule,

the tunica albuginea. This tunica sends numerous septa through the organ, which divide the testes into pyramidal lobules, which, in turn, contain the glandular elements of the testis. Each lobule is filled with convoluted seminiferous tubules. Both ends of each seminiferous tubule open into a branched reservoir, the rete testis (Fig. 1-10). Spermatozoa liberated from the germinal epithelium are immotile, and are carried toward the rete testis by fluid secreted by the Sertoli cells—the "tubular fluid," which differs from blood serum in its composition (16). The movement of fluid toward the rete is facilitated by peristaltic contractions of the seminiferous tubules and by the contractile activity of the testicular capsule.

Near the upper pole of the testis, the tunica albuginea is pierced by the efferent ducts, which originate in the rete testis (Fig. 1-10). The efferent ducts carry spermatozoa from the rete testis to the epididymis. The epididymis consists of a single long, coiled duct and supporting connective tissue elements. Spermatozoa enter the epididymis in a fairly dilute suspension (rete testis fluid) which un-

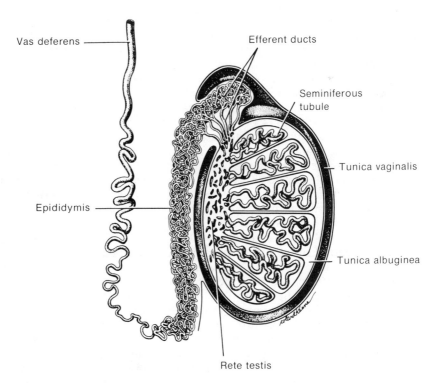

**FIG. 1-10.** The seminiferous tubules and the duct system of the human testis. (Dym M. In Weiss L, Greep RO (eds): Histology, 4th ed. New York, McGraw-Hill, 1977, p. 981)

dergoes concentration in the head of the epididymis. Various substances are added to the contents of the epididymal duct as they move toward the tail of the epididymis (8). The ability to fertilize and the capacity for forward swimming movement are acquired by spermatozoa as they are transported through the epididymis.

Passage through the long epididymal duct provides the time necessary for the sperms to mature, and exerts some as yet unidentified effects on the spermatozoa (15). The spermatozoa which reach the tail of the epididymis are tightly packed in the relatively wide duct of this region, and are fully mature. Since the only known physiological function of the epididymis is transporting the spermatozoa and providing the environment necessary for their maturation, reversible suppression of epididymal function would provide a very satisfactory male contraceptive.

The epididymis covers the posterior border of the testes. Its tail is attached to the base of the scrotum by the genito-inguinal ligament. In man, and most mammals, the testes and the epididymides are located in the scrotal sac. This extraabdominal location ensures testicular and epididymal temperatures several degrees below body temperature (18). Maintenance of the testes at their normal (scrotal) temperature is necessary for sperm production and fertility. Failure of the testes to descend into the scrotum during development (cryptorchidism) results in sterility. The possibility of heating the scrotum at regular intervals as a means of fertility control is being explored.

The primary artery to the testes is the internal spermatic branch of the aorta, which arises just below the renal arteries. Two other blood supplies to the testes exist: the artery of the vas deferens, and the external spermatic artery. Venous drainage from the testis and epididymis forms a network of vessels. This network consists of eight or ten veins which constitute a part of the spermatic cord. With the cord, the veins enter the inguinal canal and form two main trunks near the internal inguinal ring. Higher up, these two trunks unite to form a single spermatic vein. The right spermatic vein drains into the inferior vena cava. The left spermatic vein enters the left renal vein. The architecture of the testicular blood supply helps maintain the temperature gradient between the scrotum and the abdominal cavity. The passage of arterial blood through a long and coiled artery surrounded by a basketlike venous network allows dissipation of heat from the blood before it reaches the testis. The proximity of the testicular artery to the network which drains the blood from the epididymis and the testis also provides an anatomical basis for direct transfer of testosterone (and perhaps also other substances produced by the testis) from venous to arterial blood. This counter-current mechanism is responsible for a significant elevation of testosterone levels in the testicular artery, as compared to peripheral vessels (6). It is, however, unclear whether the direct transfer of substances from the venous to the arterial vasculature of the testis has any physiological significance.

From the epididymides, the spermatozoa pass into the vasa deferentia, long tubes with thick muscular walls (Fig. 1–9 and 1–10). During ejaculation, peristaltic contractions of the vasa move spermatozoa to the ampullae (distended distal portions of the vasa), and into the urethra, a single duct located in the penis (Fig. 1–9). Before entering the urethra, spermatozoa are suspended in the secretions of accessory reproductive glands, the seminal vesicles and the prostate.

Surgical transsection of the vas deferens (vasectomy) results in ejaculates devoid of spermatozoa and, consequently, in sterility. This method of fertility control can sometimes be reversed. Data on the consequences of vasectomy in man are surprisingly scarce, but the endocrine activity of the testis and the libido appear to remain unaffected (see Chap. 7).

During ejaculation, contraction of the musculature of the prostate and the seminal vesicles cause partial emptying of these glands to provide much of the volume of the ejaculate. The spermatozoa become suspended in the secretions of the accessory glands, but mixing of vasal contents, prostatic secretions and seminal vesicle secretions is not complete. Analysis of the composition of the initial and the subsequent portions of the ejaculate (the split-ejaculate technique) reveals considerable differences in sperm density and predominance of prostatic or seminal vesicle secretions in seminal fluid emitted at different times during the ejaculation (5). The secretions of the prostate and the seminal vesicle provide the bulk of the ejaculate and nearly all of the seminal plasma. The suggested functions of the seminal plasma also include altering the pH of the vagina, exerting an antibacterial effect, and modulating the contractions of the female reproductive tract. However, the physiological importance of the secretions of accessory reproductive glands is not completely understood.

Whereas areas for contraceptive intervention in the female are well recognized, considerably less is known regarding the male. For contraceptive intervention in the male, the epididymis and the vas deferens are the most logical sites. Maturation and transport of spermatozoa are the only known functions of these organs. The transport of spermatozoa can be readily interrupted by surgical resection of the vas (vasectomy). Methods for reversible vasectomy and for selective inhibition of epididymal function are being actively sought. (See Chap. 7 for a detailed discussion on male contraceptive intervention.)

# REFERENCES

1. Albert A: The mammalian testis. In Young WC (ed): Sex and Internal Secretions, Vol I, 3rd ed. Baltimore, Williams & Wilkins, 1961, p 305
2. Alexander NJ, Wilson BJ, Patterson GD: Vasectomy: immunologic effects in rhesus monkeys and men. Fertil Steril 25:149, 1974
3. Clermont Y: The cycle of the seminiferous epithelium in man. Am J Anat 112:35, 1963
4. Dym M, Fawcett DW: The blood-testis barrier in the rat and the physiological compartmentation of the seminiferous epithelium. Biol Reprod 3:308, 1970
5. Eliasson R, Lindholmer C: Distribution and properties of spermatozoa in different fractions of split ejaculates. Fertil Steril 23:252, 1972
6. Free MJ, Jaffe RA: Dynamics of venous-arterial testosterone transfer in the pampiniform plexus of the rat. Endocrinology 97:169, 1975
7. Goy RW, Resko JA: Gonadal hormones and behavior of normal and pseudohermaphroditic nonhuman female primates. In Astwood EB (ed): Recent Progress in Hormone Research, Vol 28. New York, Academic Press, 1972, p 707
8. Hamilton DW, Olson GE, Beeuwkes R III: Epididymal physiology and sperm maturation. In Hubinont PO, L'Hermite M, Schwers J (eds): Sperm Action. Basel, Karger, 1976, p 62
9. Hansson V, Weddington SC, Naess O, Attramadal A: Testicular androgen binding protein (ABP)—a parameter of Sertoli cell secretory function. In French FS, Hansson V, Ritzen EM, Nayfeh SN (eds): Hormonal Regulation of Spermatogenesis. New York, Plenum Press, 1975, p 323
10. Heller CG, Clermont Y: Kinetics of the germinal epithelium in man. In Pincus G (ed): Recent Progress in Hormone Research, Vol 20. New York, Academic Press, 1964, p 545
11. Jost A, Magre S, Cressent M: Sertoli cells and early testicular differentiation. In Mancini RE, Martini L (eds): Male Fertility and Sterility. New York, Academic Press, 1974, p 1
12. Jost A, Vigier B, Prepin J, Perchellet JP: Studies on sex differentiation in mammals. In Greep RO (ed): Recent Progress in Hormone Research, Vol 29. New York, Academic Press, 1973, p 1
13. Neaves WB: Cytologic correlates of testosterone production. In Spilman CH, Lobl TJ, Kirton KT (eds): Regulatory Mechanisms of Male Reproductive Physiology. Amsterdam, Excerpta Medica, 1976, p 35
14. Ohno S, Christian LC, Wachtel SS, Koo GC: Hormone-like role of H-Y antigen in bovine free martin gonad. Nature 261:597, 1976
15. Orgebin-Crist M-C, Danzo BJ, Davies J: Endocrine control of the development and maintenance of sperm fertilizing ability in the epididymis. In Am Physiol Soc: Handbook of Physiology. Hamilton DW, Greep RO (eds): Endocrinology, Section 7, Male Reproductive System—Male, Vol 5. Baltimore, Williams & Wilkins, 1975, p 319
16. Setchell BP: The secretion of fluid by the testes of rats, rams and goats, with some observations on the effects of age, cryptorchidism and hypophysectomy. J Reprod Fertil 23:79, 1970
17. Stambaugh R, Smith M: Sperm enzymes and their role in fertilization. In Hubinont PO, L'Hermite M, Schwers J (eds): Sperm Action. Basel, Karger, 1976, p 222
18. Waites GMH: Temperature regulation of the testis. In Johnson AD, Gomes WR, Vandemark NL (eds): The Testis, Vol 1. New York, Academic Press, 1970, p 241

# 2

# Endocrinology of the Reproductive Cycle

Carl J. Pauerstein
Michael J. K. Harper

The normal human menstrual cycle is dependent upon a complex system containing several components, including higher brain centers, the hypothalamus, the pituitary gland (hypophysis), the ovaries, and the uterus. The cohesive function of these components is integrated by positive and negative feedback signals, and comprises the endocrine system in the female (Fig. 2–1).

In the male the same system operates, only the testes take the place of the ovaries as the major steroid-hormone–secreting organs. Briefly, the reproductive endocrine system functions as an integrated unit in which a releasing hormone (known as gonadotropin releasing hormone [GnRH], or luteinizing hormone releasing hormone or factor [LRF or LHRH]) is produced and released by the hypothalamus under the stimulatory influence (positive feedback) of steroid hormones produced by the target organs (ovaries and testes). LRF then stimulates the anterior pituitary gland to release the gonadotropic hormones—follicle-stimulating hormone (FSH) and/or luteinizing hormone (LH)—which stimulate production of steroidal hormones from the target organs. In the case where steroid hormones inhibit release of hypothalamic releasing hormone, this is known as negative feedback (see the section on Integration).

Recent technological advances which have facilitated the measurement of hormones in biologic fluids, coupled with advances in the study of the interaction between hormones and target organs, have opened the way to a better understanding of the regulatory systems. We now enjoy a reasonably complete understanding of the endocrinology of the menstrual cycle. This chapter will first discuss the individual components of the system, then their integrated function, and finally the effects of the hormones on their target organs. Discussion of the male system is limited because of its previous coverage in Chapter 1.

## THE COMPONENTS

### THE CENTRAL NERVOUS SYSTEM

Although there are conflicting data and hypotheses, the majority of evidence suggests that transmitter substances such as dopamine and norepinephrine, in the brain (particularly in the hypothalamus) affect the specialized nerve cells which contain the hormone-releasing and inhibiting factors (13). Current data support the existence of a dual system: dopamine inhibits, and norepinephrine stimulates, gonadotropin releasing factor secretion. The cell bodies of the neurons containing norepinephrine are largely located in the medulla and pons, whereas those containing dopamine are found in highest concentration in the arcuate and periventricular nucleii (15). This type of neuronal activity is largely regulated directly by changes in the circulating levels of the steroid hormones—estrogen and progesterone.

The hypothalamus secretes a releasing factor for each of the tropic hormones produced

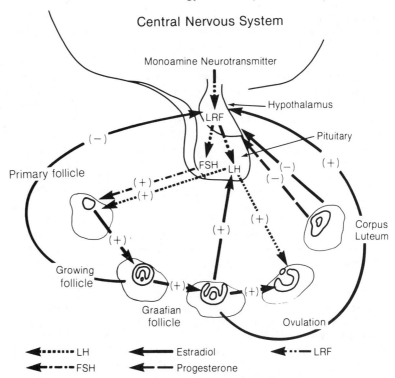

**FIG. 2–1.** Positive (+) and negative (−) feedback (long-loop) pathways in the central nervous system and the ovary. Arrows point in direction of feedback. See text for explanation of the pathways.

by the anterior pituitary gland except the gonadotropins, which are probably regulated by a single releasing hormone. The structures of two of these hypothalamic releasing hormones, thyrotropin releasing factor or hormone (TRF or TRH) and gonadotropin releasing factor or hormone (LRF, GnRh, or LHRH), have been elucidated. Thyrotropin releasing factor is a tripeptide that causes release of thyroid-stimulating hormone (TSH), as well as prolactin (PRL)—another trophic hormone which has a major action on the mammary gland. However, it may not be the primary prolactin releasing factor. Gonadotropin releasing factor is a decapeptide. Although it causes synthesis and secretion of both follicle-stimulating hormone (FSH) and luteinizing hormone (LH), it is a much more potent stimulator of the latter.

In addition to its inhibitory action on release of gonadotropin releasing factor, dopamine has an inhibitory effect on the synthesis and release of prolactin, probably through synthesis of an as yet uncharacterized prolactin inhibiting factor (PIF).

The LRF neuronal system has been described in the monkey (20) and in the human (2). The cell bodies of LRF-containing neurons are found in the anterior hypothalamus and in the tuberal hypothalamus. LRF is synthesized in these neurosecretory cells of the hypothalamus, and then released into the hypothalamic-hypophyseal portal system, in which they are transported to the anterior pituitary. At this site, they stimulate synthesis and release of LH and FSH.

## THE PITUITARY

Three gonadotropic hormones of the anterior pituitary have been identified: follicle-stimulating hormone (FSH), luteinizing hormone (LH), and prolactin (PRL).

FSH and LH are glycoprotein hormones containing alpha ($\alpha$) and beta ($\beta$) subunits. They are closely related, structurally and chemically. The $\alpha$ subunits of these hormones are essentially identical. The immunologic specificity of FSH and LH is invested in the $\beta$ subunit. FSH and LH are synthesized in basophilic cells, called *gonadotropes*, which are scattered throughout the anterior pituitary.

There has been debate about the source of FSH and LH. The critical question was whether both hormones are made in the same gonadotropes, or whether there are two separate populations of gonadotropes, one for LH synthesis and one for FSH synthesis. This question remains incompletely settled, but recent evidence strongly supports the contention that FSH and LH are located in the same gonadotropes in the human pituitary (19). LRF seems to control both FSH and LH synthesis and release.

The third hormone produced by the pituitary, prolactin, is a single-chain polypeptide composed of 198 amino acid residues. It is synthesized and released by acidophilic cells of the anterior pituitary. The role of PRL in the normal human menstrual cycle has been less precisely defined than the roles of FSH and LH. Recently Vekemans and his coworkers reported a midcycle PRL peak, with continued elevated levels during the luteal phase (21). However, other investigators have found no cyclic variation in PRL. Current opinion holds that prolactin is necessary for ovarian and testicular steroidogenesis (14).

FSH and LH exert two types of influence on the reproductive cycle. Their primary effect is stimulation of target cells in the gonad. Although there may be some overlap of activity, because of the structural similarities of the two hormones, each gonadotropin has a specific role in the regulation of gonadal function. FSH stimulates follicular growth and maturation in the female, and initiates spermatogenesis in the male. In addition, FSH catalyses the aromatization of testosterone to estradiol in both sexes. LH stimulates the conversion of cholesterol to pregnenolone in the gonads of both sexes. LH stimulation is indispensable to the complete maturation of germ cells in male and female gonads. However, steroidogenesis proceeds to functional levels under the stimulation of relatively low levels of LH. FSH alone produces neither complete germ cell maturation nor complete steroidogenesis. Thus it appears that LH, even if FSH is present only at very low levels, can induce steroidogenesis, but that both trophic hormones must be present in adequate amounts, in order for reproduction to be normal. Thus the gonadotropins are ultimately responsible for the production of the ovarian hormones, which, in

turn, control LRF release through the "long-loop" positive or negative feedback system (see Fig. 2–1).

In addition to their primary effects on the gonads, the pituitary gonadotropins exert a negative feedback effect on the hypothalamus, through a retrograde "short-loop" vascular system connecting the pituitary and the hypothalamus. Recent animal experiments have demonstrated a neurohypophyseal capillary network common to the median eminence and the infundibular stalk and neural lobe of the pituitary. Three vascular routes have been demonstrated: fenestrated portal vessels to the anterior lobe of the pituitary; capillary connections to the medial basal hypothalamus, with orientation of the capillary loop toward the arcuate nucleus; and an internal plexus to the ependyma of the median eminence (3, 4, 17). Additional data have been reported demonstrating retrograde transport to the hypothalamus of LH and prolactin, in the rat (16). Thus, there is strong evidence for short-loop feedback of the gonadotropins to the hypothalamus.

## THE OVARY

The human menstrual cycle is under ovarian control, in the sense that the ovarian steroids profoundly influence the entire complex. For clarity of exposition, it is convenient to begin with a description of the hormonal events of the menstrual cycle.

The average length of the menstrual cycle is 28 days. By convention, the day of initiation of bleeding is designated day 1. The new follicle for a given cycle starts to develop during the luteal phase of the preceding cycle. Just before and during menses, the cells of the developing follicles proliferate (the follicular phase), and the follicles increase in size, soon to exceed 1 mm. in diameter. Many do not attain this size, but become atretic. The follicle that is most sensitive to FSH stimulation gets a lead that it never relinquishes. The rising FSH stimulates the follicle to grow, by inducing mitotic proliferation of the granulosa cells and formation of the theca. The early follicular phase ends when a definite rise in plasma estrogen is noted (Fig. 2–2).

The locally produced estrogen also stimulates the follicle to grow, so that the mature follicle, i.e., the Graafian follicle, reaches a diameter of 6 mm. The next largest follicles be-

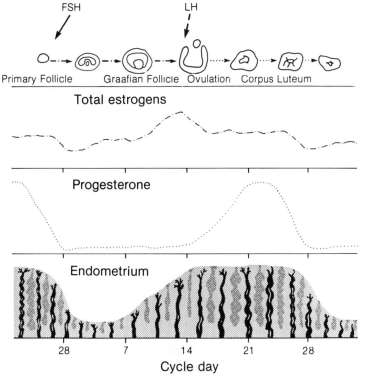

**FIG. 2–2.** Relationships among pre- and post-ovulatory changes in the ovary, plasma levels of estrogen and progesterone, and endometrial response.

come atretic at a size of 1 to 3 mm. The concentrations of estradiol (the major biologically active estrogen) in the general circulation rise from 50 pg./ml. on day 1 to about 75 pg./ml. on day 6 of the cycle. Estradiol concentrations increase more sharply to reach levels of about 150 pg./ml. on day 9. A sharp rise, usually called a "surge," then occurs, to reach a peak of about 350 pg./ml. on day 11. Estradiol levels decline rapidly, to values of about 250 pg./ml. on day 14. The estradiol concentration then gradually rises again (Fig. 2–3).

The central nervous system–hypothalamic-pituitary axis becomes increasingly sensitive to the positive feedback action of estradiol as the concentration of estradiol in the bloodstream increases during follicular development. An acute surge of LH and FSH at midcycle is induced by estradiol. This positive feedback requires a circulating level of estradiol of 100 to 200 pg./ml., which is sustained for 36 to 42 hours (8, 9, 23, 26, 29). Current evidence suggests that estradiol is required for the initiation, but not for the maintainence, of

the LH surge. In primates, including man, the interval between the estrogen peak and the LH peak is 14 to 27 hours. Ovulation follows the LH peak within 11 to 24 hours (18).

Shortly before ovulation, plasma levels of 17-hydroxyprogesterone, produced by the ovary, increase. Just after the onset of the LH surge, levels of progesterone, coming from the ovary, also begin to rise (29).

Around the time of ovulation, the granulosa cells luteinize. Luteinization is initiated by LH. For the first three postovulatory days (cycle days 15 to 17) the granulosa cells proliferate, and the corpus luteum reaches a size of 1 cm. During postovulatory days 4 to 9 (cycle days 18 to 23) capillaries, previously found only in the thecal cells, grow to reach the granulosa, and peak vascularization begins. After day 23, regression begins. The highest levels of plasma progesterone are reached on cycle days 18 to 23.

To summarize, the following endocrinologic events are hallmarks of the normal menstrual cycle (Fig. 2–3): *1*) The estrogen peak

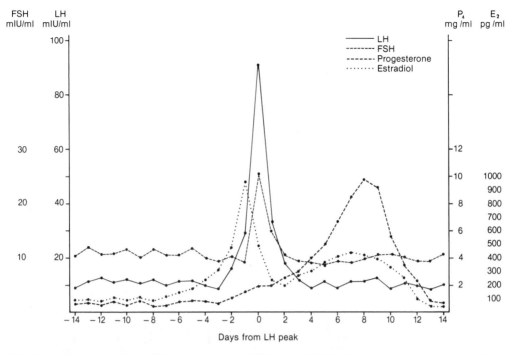

**FIG. 2–3.** Patterns of estradiol, progesterone, LH, and FSH in the normal menstrual cycle. See text for explanation.

precedes the LH peak; *2)* estrogen secretion attains appropriate levels; *3)* the LH peak occurs at least 13 days prior to the onset of menses; *4)* initial rises in plasma 17-hydroxyprogesterone and progesterone levels occur, coincident with the LH rise; *5)* a second rise in plasma 17-hydroxyprogesterone occurs later, coincident with the marked rise in plasma progesterone; *6)* plasma progesterone begins to rise with the LH surge, and reaches a maximum 6 to 8 days after the LH peak.

## THE ENDOMETRIUM

The cyclic changes in the ovary elaborating first estrogen, and then estrogen and progesterone, induce, in the endometrium, first, proliferation, and then differentiation. These changes are reflected in the endometrial morphology, and the functional state of the ovaries can be inferred with reasonable accuracy from the histologic appearance of the endometrium (Fig. 2–2).

During the first half of the cycle, endometrial glandular and stromal cells undergo replication. The endometrium thickens, and the glands begin to elongate. The epithelial cells become taller, and mitotic activity is seen in glands and stroma (Fig. 2–4). The first morphologic change after ovulation is the formation of subnuclear vacuoles in the glandular epithelium. This is first seen on the 15th to 16th day of a 28-day cycle. The vacuoles are caused by the accumulation of glycogen, which on the 19th or 20th day is deposited in the glandular lumen. From the 19th to the 23rd day, no mitoses are seen in either the glands or the stroma, suggesting that progesterone causes cessation of hyperplastic growth. The earliest stromal change seen under progesterone influence is progessive loosening of the stroma, with accumulation of fluid between the cells. This is due to a change in the ground substance, presumably related to preparation for implantation. At about the 23rd day, evidence that progesterone causes hypertrophic growth and differentiation can be inferred from the appearance of changes in the stromal cells surrounding the blood vessels which will allow for implantation. These decidual changes progress over the next few days, until the stroma has undergone generalized decidual transformation. If pregnancy does not occur, the stroma becomes infiltrated with inflammatory cells.

The premenstrual endometrium consists of

thousands of tiny units composed of large numbers of stromal cells and exhausted glands surrounding markedly coiled arterioles. The first event in menstruation is vasoconstriction of these arterioles. The resulting ischemia results in dissolution of the architecture of the endometrium. Foci of swelling and distortion appear, the stromal cells begin to clump, hemorrhage occurs within the stroma, and the endometrium is shed as the menstrual discharge or flow. The raw, denuded surface of the endometrium is rapidly covered by epithelium, so that within three days healing is complete.

Thus, the changes caused by progesterone in a nonfertile cycle are peak secretion, followed by peak edema in the endometrium, followed by decidual formation. If conception occurs, instead of each of these endometrial changes peaking and waning in sequence, all continue and peak together. This lends a char-acteristic appearance to the endometrium, which has been described as "gestational hyperplasia."

## INTEGRATION

Integration of the components of the endocrine system is controlled by the hormones described in the first section of this chapter. The same hormones are synthesized by both men and women, but the patterns of secretion are different in the two sexes.

The gonadotropins are secreted in pulses, at intervals of about 90 minutes. Pulse amplitude is greater for LH than for FSH. In males, the pulses are maintained in a tonic pattern, whereas in females the cyclic gonadotropic peak that occurs before ovulation is superimposed upon the tonic pulsatile pattern.

Tonic secretion of LH and FSH is regulated

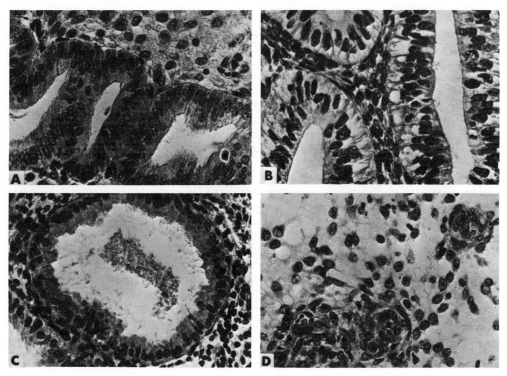

**FIG. 2–4.** Endometrial histology at different times in the normal menstrual cycle. A. Proliferative endometrium. Note pseudostratification of glandular nuclei and presence of mitotic figures in glands—an example of the effect of estrogen on the endometrium. B. Secretory endometrium, early. Note that the glandular nuclei have moved toward the luminal borders of the cells; subnuclear vacuoles have formed in many of the gland cells. C. Secretory endometrium, about mid-luteal phase. The nuclei have returned to the base of the glandular cells, and prominent secretion is seen in the gland lumen. D. Stromal cells surrounding the capillaries are enlarged, in both nuclear and cytoplasmic volume, demonstrating a predecidual reaction. (Modified from Noyes RW, Hertig AT, Rock J: Dating the endometrial biopsy. Fertil Steril 1:3–25, 1950)

by a feedback loop involving central nervous system components (i.e., dopamine, norepinephrine, and LRF), ovarian steroids, and the gonadotropins. Estradiol is the most potent gonadotropic inhibitor. A quantitative relationship between the negative feedback action of ovarian steroids and gonadotropin release can be demonstrated by interrupting the negative feedback loop by withdrawing estradiol through ovariectomy; this results in significant increases in circulating LH and FSH concentrations. The rise in gonadotropins continues until a plateau is attained at approximately ten times preoperative levels about 3 weeks after the operation (26). The increase is greater for FSH than for LH. This differential effect may reflect preferential inhibition of FSH by estradiol (25, 27, 28) and, possibly, by follicular inhibin (6).

There is some evidence that inhibin, a nonsteroidal gonadal factor, is involved in the feedback control of gonadotropic secretion. A protein which inhibits FSH secretion has been identified in the testes and in testicular secretions (1, 7, 11). Because the increase in FSH levels in menopausal women is disproportionate to the increase in LH levels, an inhibin factor has also been postulated to be present in women. Some evidence for the presence of inhibin in ovarian follicles has been obtained in animals (6, 12, 22). Although incomplete, the inhibin story may prove to be an exciting breakthrough, because the presence of a specific inhibitor of FSH secretion and release would explain the differential levels of FSH and LH observed under certain circumstances.

Other observations provide further evidence of the feedback effects of estradiol on gonadotropin output: *1*) during the first week after ovariectomy, a greater rise in LH and FSH is seen in women operated upon during the follicular phase of the cycle than in those operated upon during the luteal phase (26); *2*) withdrawal of estradiol results in elevated secretion of hypothalamic LRF and thus of pituitary gonadotropins (5, 10); *3*) there is also a rapid decline of circulating gonadotropin levels in response to estradiol administration to ovariectomized and postmenopausal women (27).

Moderate levels of estradiol, as seen in the early follicular phase of the menstrual cycle, maximally inhibit gonadotropin output. In the normal menstrual cycle, a change in es-

tradiol levels in either direction reduces inhibition and stimulates the hypothalamic-hypophyseal axis (24). As mentioned above, when the hypothalamic-pituitary axis is maximally stimulated through ovariectomy or the menopause, then the action of estradiol will be solely inhibitory. The negative and positive feedback actions are not interrupted phenomena, but rather a continuum. The positive feedback effect of estrogen on gonadotropin release is always preceded by a phase of negative feedback.

To summarize, in response to a nadir in circulating levels of estrogen, gonadotropin releasing hormone is secreted by the hypothalamus. The pituitary, in turn, releases FSH, which stimulates follicular growth. LH, secreted by the pituitary in basal amounts, stimulates synthesis of estradiol by the theca interna of the developing follicles. Estradiol synthesized by the Graafian follicle has a local trophic effect on the follicle and an inhibitory effect on pituitary release of FSH. As FSH declines, the remaining follicles regress and become atretic. Estradiol synthesis in the ovulatory follicle increases dramatically. Peak levels of estradiol are reached approximately 2 days prior to ovulation. In response to the sustained estradiol peak, a surge of stored LH is released from the anterior pituitary, presumably due to increased secretion of gonadotropin releasing factor by the hypothalamus. A smaller increase in FSH concentration is noted at the same time. Thus estradiol inhibits the hypothalamus in the follicular phase, but stimulates the hypothalamus at mid-cycle.

After ovulation, the granulosa cells become vascularized as the corpus luteum forms. Basal levels of LH stimulate secretion of estradiol and progesterone by the corpus luteum. In combination, these steroids are potent inhibitors of the synthesis of gonadotropin releasing factors. Progesterone may also inhibit further follicular maturation. In the absence of a luteotrophic factor (hCG), the corpus luteum ceases to function after 12 to 14 days. The cells of the corpus luteum show evidence of degeneration. Although the yellow color is maintained for months, the structure becomes smaller and is eventually replaced by hyaline tissue. The resultant structure is called a corpus albicans.

In response to falling levels of estradiol and progesterone, FSH secretion increases, and a new crop of follicles begins to grow and synthesize estradiol, thus perpetuating the cyclic pattern. The nadir of steroid synthesis occurs approximately 2 days before the onset of menses. The rise in FSH begins shortly before this nadir is reached.

Variations in cycle length are generally considered to take place at the expense of the follicular phase. Thus, in normally ovulating women, the length of the postovulatory phase was thought to remain constant from cycle to cycle, whereas the duration of the preovulatory phase was thought to be variable. However, recent data suggest that the luteal phase may also vary in duration. These variations may be a reflection of very fine adjustments between FSH secretion and follicular response which take place until one follicle becomes large enough to assume major estradiol synthesis. Once this critical size has been achieved, only modest amounts of FSH and LH are required for continued growth of the follicle.

## THE TARGET ORGANS

### THE TESTIS

The fetal testis differentiates earlier than the fetal ovary and secretes testosterone and dihydrotestosterone by the end of the first trimester of pregnancy, at which time differentiation of the external genitalia also occurs. Fetal gonadal steroidogenesis is thought to occur in response to hCG secreted by the placenta. This mechanism is substantiated by the identification of Leydig cells in the fetal testis from the end of the first trimester. They revert to mesenchymal cells shortly after birth.

From birth until shortly before puberty, the testis is inactive. The germinal epithelium, although present, displays no active spermatogenesis. Levels of FSH and LH rise perceptibly as puberty approaches and induce increased testosterone synthesis and spermatogenesis.

As adult males reach middle age, dihydrotestosterone levels may increase, testosterone levels decrease, androgen-binding globulin levels increase, and spermatogenesis becomes less efficient. However, there is no sudden cessation of reproductive function in the male such as occurs in the female.

Medullary elements dominate in the adult testis. Each testis is composed of specialized cell lines, the Sertoli cells, which nourish and support spermatogenesis, and the germinal epithelium, from which the spermatozoa develop. Scattered about the stroma surrounding the seminiferous tubules are interstitial (Leydig) cells which synthesize and release testosterone. The seminiferous tubules converge into a secondary collecting tubular system called the rete testis, and from there merge into a single long convoluted tubule, the epididymis, in which spermatozoa complete maturation and are stored. Testosterone secreted by the Leydig cells diffuses directly to the Sertoli cells. It does not become absorbed into the bloodstream until it reaches the region of the rete testis. An effective blood-testes barrier appears to exist up until this point.

FSH is necessary for the initiation of spermatogenesis, and testosterone is required for the later steps in spermatogenesis. Both FSH and testosterone stimulate Sertoli cells to elaborate androgen-binding protein (ABP). The exact role of this protein in spermatogenesis is uncertain. Sertoli cells also convert testosterone to 5α-dihydrotestosterone and estradiol. Testosterone, rather than 5α-dihydrotestosterone, appears to be important in spermatogenesis. Estradiol may be the primary mediator of feedback inhibition from the testis to the hypothalamus. However, as noted with respect to the ovary, inhibin may, either alone or in concert with estradiol, be the mediator of testicular negative feedback.

The spermatogenic cycle in man takes 74 ± 6 days. All stages of spermatogenesis can be observed simultaneously in the same seminiferous tubule. Spermatogenesis involves production of haploid germ cells (spermatids) from diploid stem cells (spermatogonia). Spermiogenesis is the process by which the spermatids mature into cells which are capable of independent motility and transport (spermatozoa).

The spermatogonia are divided into two groups: those which constantly divide to maintain the stem cell population and those which undergo growth preparatory to meiotic division, producing two secondary spermatocytes. Each secondary spermatocyte, in turn, undergoes reduction division to produce two spermatids. Development of head, midpiece, and tail then occurs, resulting in mature spermatozoa. (See Chap. 1 for a more detailed discussion of spermatogenesis.)

Spermatozoa are released into the lumen of the seminiferous tubules and transported to the epididymis, where they undergo further maturation and storage. At ejaculation, they are propelled as a bolus through the vas deferens. Seminal plasma secreted by the seminal vesicles and prostate is added to the bolus of sperm as it traverses the prostatic urethra, thus completing the composition of the ejaculate.

As noted above, the testis produces testosterone and other androgens, which are secreted in pulsatile fashion. The testis also produces estrogen, which may be involved in the feedback mechanisms at the hypothalamic and pituitary levels.

Thus FSH is important for spermatogenesis and LH for production of testosterone. The regulation of the components of the hypothalamic-pituitary-testis system is similar to that in the female, with testosterone and testicular inhibin playing major roles in the long-loop feedback system. The short-loop system of pituitary tropic hormones (FSH and LH) feeding back on the hypothalamus and its releasing hormone (LRF) is also probably operative. Since the production of LH in the male is only tonic, and not both tonic and cyclic as in the female, the regulatory system is simpler and less susceptible to disruption.

Testosterone has two major roles in the male. It stimulates development of male secondary sex characteristics, such as enlargement of the genitalia, increase in laryngeal size with concomitant deepening of the voice, increase in muscle mass, and growth of body hair. It also is indispensable to normal spermatogenesis. The effects of androgens on other tissues and organs are discussed later in this chapter.

## THE OVARY

The fetal ovary does not demonstrate the hormonal activity seen in the fetal testis. Ovarian steroid synthesis is not necessary for differentiation of female external or internal genitalia. However, the fetal ovary actively produces germ cells. The full complement of ova is achieved by 20 weeks of intrauterine life, and the process of follicular maturation and regression is evident by the third trimester of pregnancy.

The ovary is composed of numerous follicles, in varying stages of maturation, surrounded by stromal cells. Follicular units consist of an ovum surrounded by a layer of granulosa cells, and internal and external layers of thecal cells. The maximum number of follicles (millions) is reached at approximately 20 weeks of intrauterine life. From this time, follicles become involved in an inexorable cycle of partial maturation followed by atresia. Most follicles become atretic; only about 500 develop to the stage of ovulation in a lifetime.

Gonadotropin levels in females are low in infancy and rise gradually as puberty approaches. Levels of FSH are slightly higher than those of LH, but the ratio is nearly one to one. In contrast, during reproductive life LH is always higher than FSH, except early in the follicular phase of the cycle, when growth of a new crop of follicles is stimulated.

The rising gonadotropin levels of late childhood stimulate estrogen synthesis in the ovarian stroma. The secreted estrogen causes maturation of the external genitalia and stimulates growth of the breasts. Eventually, when there has been sufficient estrogen stimulation of the endometrium, uterine bleeding occurs. The first episode of bleeding is called the menarche. The initial endometrial shedding probably occurs in response to a drop in circulating levels of estrogen. The first several "menstrual" episodes may occur at irregular intervals because ovulation has not yet been initiated. Once an ovulatory pattern has been established, it recurs with consistent periodicity in an individual woman. Toward the end of the reproductive age, ovulation and menstrual cycles again become irregular. At menopause, estradiol synthesis decreases drastically, and gonadotropin levels become markedly elevated.

The pattern of ovarian steroid secretion fluctuates throughout the menstrual cycle. The ovulatory follicle and corpus luteum are the major sources of estradiol synthesis and secretion. Average production rates range from 0.07 mg./day in the early follicular phase to 0.8 mg./day at the time of the preovulatory peak. Estrone is also secreted by the ovary, but most of the circulating estrone is derived from peripheral conversion of androstenedione. About half of circulating androstenedione is of ovarian origin and half is of adrenal origin; it is secreted by the ovary in a cyclic pattern which parallels that of estradiol and estrone. Mean testosterone levels in the normal woman are about 40 ng./ml. of serum. Approximately half is secreted by the ovary and the remainder by peripheral conversion of androstenedione and of dehydroepiandrosterone, an androgen mostly produced (in normal circumstances) in the adrenal gland.

About 50 per cent of the estrone and estradiol secreted daily undergoes 16-hydroxylation to form estriol. Estriol is then conjugated with sulfate or glucuronide to facilitate excretion.

Progesterone and 17-hydroxyprogesterone are predominantly secreted by the corpus luteum during the luteal phase of the cycle. Low levels of progesterone found in the follicular phase of the cycle are presumably of adrenal origin. As noted earlier, ovarian progesterone and 17-hydroxyprogesterone secretion become detectable in the periovulatory period concomitant with the LH surge. Peak secretion of progesterone and 17-hydroxyprogesterone in the mid-luteal phase is about 24 mg./24 hours and 4 mg./24 hours, respectively. Progesterone gradually rises, beginning in the periovulatory period, whereas 17-hydroxyprogesterone rises sharply before ovulation, and again during the mid-luteal phase.

## MECHANISMS OF HORMONE ACTION

Gonadotropins and steroids select their target cells because of the presence of specific receptors on, or in, these cells. The mechanism of hormone receptor interaction differs for each class of hormones.

The protein hormones, FSH and LH, attach to receptors located on the plasma membrane. The resulting membrane receptor-hormone complex, in turn, activates a membrane-bound enzyme, adenylcyclase. In the presence of intracellular magnesium, adenylcyclase acts on ATP to produce cyclic AMP. Cyclic AMP then activates protein kinases, which mediate the biologic responses of the cell. In the case of LH, steroidogenesis is initiated, and in the case of FSH, specific proteins are elaborated which affect germ cell growth and development.

In contrast, steroid hormones combine with specific receptors in the cytoplasm of target cells and are carried by these receptors to the nucleus of the cells, where they interact with specific sequences of DNA to effect messenger RNA synthesis and protein synthesis.

Steroids secreted by the gonads are transported to target tissues in the bloodstream in free and bound forms. Testosterone and es-

tradiol bind to a specific binding globulin known as TEBG (testosterone-estradiol binding globulin), or sex steroid binding globulin. Progesterone has no specific binding globulin of its own but appears to bind preferentially to corticosteroid binding globulin (CBG). Only free steroids are biologically active in target organs and in the feedback mechanisms.

In addition to feedback relationships with the hypothalamus and pituitary, gonadal steroids affect a variety of target organs including the skin and its appendages, subcutaneous fat, muscle, breast, larynx, uterus, cervix, vaginal mucosa, external genitalia, and the gonad itself.

Androgens exert their primary tropic effect on skin, muscle, laryngeal tissue, and male external genitalia. Androgens are responsible for the laryngeal enlargement which produces the deep male voice and for the increased muscle mass characteristic of the male. Androgens stimulate penile and testicular growth and are responsible for rugations of the scrotum. They stimulate growth of body hair and secretory activity of sebaceous glands and, paradoxically, are also responsible for the temporal recession of the hair line seen in males. At the peripheral level, the active androgen is 5α-dihydrotestosterone, which is usually derived by peripheral conversion of testosterone through an irreversible reaction mediated by 5α-reductase.

Estrogens are responsible for growth of the breast and development of the ductile system, and for the deposition of fat in the breasts, abdomen, hips, and thighs which produces the characteristic female body habitus. Estrogens also induce hyperplastic growth of the endometrium, increased production of cervical mucus, and thickening and rugation of the vaginal mucosa. Estrogen induces the growth of estrogen and progesterone receptors in target tissues, whereas progesterone eliminates these receptors.

Progesterone is a complement, as well as an antagonist, to estrogen. In the breast, progesterone induces growth of the lobule-alveolar complexes after estrogen-induced growth of the ductile system has taken place. Estrogen causes increased water content of cervical mucus, resulting in a copious, clear mucoid secretion, and progesterone induces increased viscosity and production of an opaque, gummy mucoid material.

The endometrium is probably the single

most important tissue that is responsive to the effects of both estrogen and progesterone. Estrogen induces mitotic growth of the endometrial glands and stroma, and increased endometrial blood flow. Progesterone halts proliferation of endometrial tissue and induces hypertrophic growth and differentiation of the existing tissues. The interaction of these two steroids is finally responsible for the cyclic bleeding referred to as "menstrual periods."

Gonadal steroids also affect target tissues that are not related to sexual or reproductive function. The anabolic action of testosterone results in positive nitrogen balance and retention of potassium, phosphorus, and calcium. Testosterone also stimulates hemoglobin synthesis. Both testosterone and estradiol are vasoactive and abrupt depletion, as experienced in loss of gonadal function, produces vasomotor instability, with accompanying "hot flashes."

Estradiol increases serum levels of triglycerides and hormone binding globulins, including those for sex steroids, cortisol, progesterone, and thyroxine. Estrogen increases insulin response to carbohydrate and causes sodium retention, through interaction with the renin-angiotensin system; it also affects the ability of the liver to secrete substances such as bromosulfophthalein. Progesterone induces natriuriesis, probably by competing with estradiol.

All three major sex steroids may cause changes in mood. Estradiol and testosterone are alleged to enhance libido and contribute to a feeling of optimism and well-being. Progesterone is said to contribute to depression. Evidence for these effects is largely inferential, and requires further documentation.

## REFERENCES

1. Baker HWG, Bremner WJ, Burger HG, De Kretser DM, Dulmanis A, Eddie LW, Hudson B, Keogh EJ, Lee VWK, Rennie GC: Testicular control of follicle-stimulating hormone secretion. Recent Prog Horm Res 32:429, 1976
2. Barry J: Characterization and topography of LH-RH neurons in the human brain. Neurosci Lett 3:287, 1976
3. Bergland RM, Davis SL, Page RB: Pituitary secretes to brain. Experiments in sheep. Lancet II:276, 1977
4. Bergland RM, Page RB: Can the pituitary secrete directly to the brain? (Affirmative anatomical evidence). Endocrinology 102:1325, 1978
5. Carmel PW, Araki S, Ferin M: Pituitary stalk portal blood collection in rhesus monkeys: Evidence for pulsatile release of gonadotropin-releasing hormone (Gn-RH). Endocrinology 99:243, 1976
6. DeJong FH, Sharpe RM: Evidence for inhibin-like activity in bovine follicular fluid. Nature 263:71, 1976
7. Franchimont P, Chari S, Hazee-Hagelstein MT, Debruche ML, Duraiswami S: Evidence for existence of inhibin. In Troen P, Nankin HR (eds): The Testis in Normal and Infertile Men. New York, Raven Press, 1977, pp. 253–270
8. Keye WR Jr, Jaffe RB: Strength-duration characteristics of estrogen effect on gonadotropin response to gonadotropin-releasing hormone in women. I. Effects of varying duration of estradiol administration. J Clin Endocrinol Metab 41:1003, 1975
9. Knobil E: On the control of gonadotropin secretion in the rhesus monkey. Recent Prog Horm Rest 30:1, 1974
10. Kobayashi RM, Lu KH, Moore RY, Yen SSC: Regional distribution of hypothalamic luteinizing hormone-releasing hormone in proestrous rats: effects of ovariectomy and estrogen replacement. Endocrinology 102:98, 1978
11. Lee VWK, Keogh EJ, Burger HG, Hudson B, De Kretser DM: Studies on the relationship between FSH and germ cells: evidence for selective suppression of FSH by testicular extracts. J Reprod Fertil [Suppl] 24:1, 1976
12. Marder ML, Channing CP, Schwartz NB: Suppression of serum follicle stimulating hormone in intact and acutely ovariectomized rats by porcine follicular fluid. Endocrinology 101:1639, 1977
13. McCann SM, Moss RL: Putative neurotransmitters involved in discharging gonadotropin-releasing neurohormones and the action of LH-releasing hormone on the CNS. Life Sci 16:833, 1975
14. McNatty KP, Sawer RS, McNeilly AS: A possible role for prolactin in control of steroid secretion by the human Graafian follicle. Nature 250:653, 1974
15. Moore RY, Bloom FE: Central catecholamine neuron systems: Anatomy and physiology of the dopamine systems. Annu Rev Neurosci 1:129, 1978
16. Oliver C, Mical RS, Porter JC: Hypothalamic-pituitary vasculature: Evidence for retrograde blood flow in the pituitary stalk. Endocrinology 101:598, 1977
17. Page RB, Leure-duPree AE, Bergland RM: The neurohypophyseal capillary bed. II. Specializations within median eminence. Am J Anat 153:33, 1978
18. Pauerstein CJ, Eddy CA, Croxatto HD, Hess R, Siler-Khodr TM, Croxatto HB: Temporal relationships of estrogen, progesterone, and luteinizing hormone levels to ovulation in women and infrahuman primates. Am J Obstet Gynecol 130:876, 1978
19. Phifer RF, Midgley AR, Spicer SS: Immunohistologic and histologic evidence that follicle-stimulating hormone and luteinizing hormone are present in the same cell type in the human pars distalis. J Clin Endocrinol Metab 36:125, 1973
20. Silverman AJ, Antunes JL, Ferin M, Zimmerman

EA: The distribution of luteinizing hormone-releasing hormone (LHRH) in the hypothalamus of the rhesus monkey. Light microscopic studies using immunoperoxidase technique. Endocrinology 101:134, 1977

21. Vekemans M, Delvoye P, L'Hermite M, Robyn C: Serum prolactin levels during the menstrual cycle. J Clin Endocrinol Metab 44:989, 1977

22. Welschen R, Hermans WP, Dullaart J, DeJong FH: Effects of an inhibin-like factor present in bovine and porcine follicular fluid on gonadotrophin levels in ovariectomized rats. J Reprod Fertil 50:129, 1977

23. Yen SSC, Lasley BL, Wang CF, Leblanc H, Siler TM: The operating characteristics of the hypothalamic-pituitary system during the menstrual cycle and observations of biological action of somatostatin. Recent Prog Horm Res 31:321, 1975

24. Yen SSC, Lein A: The apparent paradox of the negative and positive feedback control system on gonadotropin secretion. Am J Obstet Gynecol 126:942, 1976

25. Yen SSC, Llerena LA, Pearson OH, Littell AS: Disappearance rates of endogenous follicle-stimulating hormone in serum following surgical hypophysectomy in man. J Clin Endocrinol 30:325, 1970

26. Yen, SSC, Tsai CC: The effect of ovariectomy on gonadotropin release. J Clin Invest 50:1149, 1971

27. Yen SSC, Tsai CC, Naftolin F, VandenBerg G, Ajabor L: Pulsatile patterns of gonadotropin release in subjects with and without ovarian function. J Clin Endocrinol Metab 34:671, 1972

28. Yen SSC, Tsai CC, VandenBerg G, Rebar R: Gonadotropin dynamics in patients with gonadal dysgenesis: a model for the study of gonadotropin regulation. J Clin Endocrinol Metab 35:897, 1972

29. Yen SSC, Vela P, Rankin J, Littell AS: Hormonal relationships during the menstrual cycle. JAMA 211:1513, 1970

# 3

# Gamete Transport, Fertilization, and Implantation

Carlton A. Eddy
Michael J. K. Harper

Conception, the creation of a new individual through union of sperm and ovum, is a complex process which embraces a variety of physiologic phenomena. The fertilizing sperm must gain entrance into the female reproductive tract, be transported to the vicinity of the ovum, and undergo changes rendering it capable of penetrating and combining its genetic material with that of the ovum.

Concurrently the newly ovulated ovum must be transported from the ovary to the oviduct, where fertilization occurs. Following fertilization, the developing embryo must be transported to the uterus, where it will implant, establish intimate contact with the maternal organism, and develop into a new individual.

## SPERM TRANSPORT

### SPERMATOZOA AT THE TIME OF EJACULATION

In some species—for example, rodents, ferrets, and pigs—spermatozoa ejaculated at coitus are deposited directly into the uterine lumen. This is not the case in primates, where spermatozoa are deposited in the vagina, close to the external cervical os. The pH of the vagina is acid, about 5.7 in normal women: the acidity is maintained by the presence of lactic acid formed by the action of *Doederlein bacilli* on the secretions of the vaginal mucosa. By contrast, the pH of semen is basic, between 7.2 and 7.8,

reflecting the relative contributions of the acidic prostatic fluid and alkaline seminal-vesicular secretion. These fluids are secreted into the ejaculate and are its primary constituents; 30 per cent of the ejaculate is derived from the prostate, 60 per cent from the seminal vesicles, and the remainder from the epididymis, ampullae, and bulbourethral and urethral glands (45). Because of the differences in pH, the spermatozoa find the vagina a relatively hostile environment. Those that fail to pass into the cervical canal die and are voided to the exterior.

The concentration of sperm in a normal ejaculate varies, but between 40 to 250 million spermatozoa per ml. is considered "normal." However, new reports indicate that sperm counts above 10 million per ml. (or total sperm counts above 25 million per ejaculate) may occur with equal frequency among fertile and infertile males (50). Zuckerman and his co-workers (64) suggested that "unless other parameters are found to be abnormal, sperm counts above 10 million per ml. and 25 million per ejaculate, respectively, cannot be considered major factors in a couple's infertility." It should be noted that pregnancies have been achieved by men whose ejaculates contained less than 10 million spermatozoa per ml., so that these values should only be considered guidelines.

The usual volume of the ejaculate is between 2 and 6 ml. in the fertile male. The majority of ejaculated spermatozoa are morphologically normal and viable. The presence of many abnormal forms or many immotile and/or dead spermatozoa is commonly associated with male infertility. In the vagina, ejaculated semen coagulates within 1 min. and then liquifies, partially or completely, within the next 30 min. Full motility of sperm is not achieved until liquefaction of the coagulated ejaculate occurs. Failure of liquefaction to occur has been reported as a cause of infertility.

## SPERM TRANSPORT THROUGH THE CERVIX

Spermatozoa are probably transported from the vagina into the cervical canal by contractions of the vaginal wall. Despite this, seminal plasma per se does not enter the uterine cavity, except, perhaps, in very small quantities.

Sperm are most readily transported into the uterus at the time of ovulation. A major determinant of sperm transport is the physical nature of the mucus filling the cervical canal.

The mucus which is secreted from the complex cervical crypts lining the canal is comprised of two main components—cervical mucin and soluble components (32). The mucin is a glycoprotein rich in carbohydrates (more than 40 per cent) with a fibrillar (chain) system of glycoproteins linked, either directly, by disulphide bonds, or through cross-linking polypeptides. The soluble components of mucus include inorganic salts, mainly sodium chloride, and organic compounds of low molecular weight such as glucose, maltose, mannose, amino acids, peptides, proteins and lipids. The soluble proteins are dispersed throughout the aqueous phase of the cervical mucus gel. The consistency of the cervical mucus (hydrogel) changes in relation to the changes in gonadal steroidal hormones. At mid-cycle, under estrogenic dominance, the mucus is thin and watery and is composed of macromolecular fibrils arranged to form parallel chains, or micelles, with spaces between the micelles large enough to permit passage of spermatozoa. In contrast, under progesterone dominance, during the luteal phase of the menstrual cycle, or if the woman is taking progesterone for oral contraception, cervical mucus contains less water, is thicker, and lacks a micellar structure, which renders the mucus unfavorable for sperm migration.

Four major factors appear to be involved in sperm passage through the cervix: *1*) sperm motility; *2*) muscular activity of the reproductive tract; *3*) the structure of the cervical mucus at the time of ovulation, and; *4*) cervical crypts which permit sperm storage and subsequent release to the upper reproductive tract.

Following ejaculation, a pool of seminal plasma collects in the upper vagina, into which the external opening of the cervix is immersed. If intercourse has taken place at mid-cycle (when ovulation occurs), the cervical mucus will be receptive to sperm passage. Entrance of sperm into the cervix is the result of both intrinsic motility of sperm and contractile activity of the female reproductive tract. There are three phases of sperm transport through the female reproductive tract: an initial, rapid phase, immediately after intercourse, in which relatively few sperm enter the oviduct, followed by a colonization phase, in which large numbers of sperm enter the cervical crypts (glands) to form a reservoir, and a final slow, prolonged phase, in which sperm are released from storage sites in the cervical crypts. The sperm which fertilizes the ovum is thought to be derived from this last phase of transport.

Prolonged survival of spermatozoa in cervical crypts is assisted by the fact that mucus is a favorable medium for sperm survival and protects them from phagocytic attack. In vitro, spermatozoa migrate through mid-cycle cervical mucus at a rate of 0.1–3.0 mm. per min., and this speed alone could not cause appearance of sperm in the oviduct within 5 min. of insemination, as has been observed, strongly suggesting contractile activity of the reproductive tract as a mechanism for rapid transport. Following the initial rapid phase of spermatozoa transport, sampling of cervical mucus from the upper and lower cervical canals at increasing lengths of time after intercourse shows an orderly increase of sperm concentration in the upper part of the cervix (22). However, only a small percentage of ejaculated spermatozoa actually enter the uterine cavity.

## SPERM TRANSPORT THROUGH THE UTERUS

Sperm transport through the uterus in women has been little studied. The pattern of distribution of sperm throughout the uterine lumen following ejaculation is not known. By analogy with other species, notably rodents and rabbits, it seems likely that spermatozoa invade the endometrial crypts, but whether this process creates a reservoir of sperm, as in the cervix, which can continue to release sperm for further transportation to the oviduct over a period of many hours, is not clear. It is well established from studies on the appearance of spermatozoa in the oviduct, in relation to insemination (58), that sperm transport through the uterus is very rapid and cannot be due to intrinsic motility of the spermatozoa. It has been suggested that motility of the uterine smooth muscle (myometrium) is responsible for the rapid transit of the sperm from the internal cervical os to the uterotubal junction. Myometrial activity may be stimulated by the presence of prostaglandins in the ejaculate. However, it seems unlikely that much, if any, seminal plasma enters the uterus, and many of the prostaglandins in the semen are 19-hydroxylated compounds with minimal biological activity (14). Little or no prostaglandins F (15) but substantial quantities of prostaglandins E (14) have been found in human semen samples. A relationship between lowered fertility and low levels of prostaglandins E in seminal plasma has been claimed (14), but more recent studies (59) have confirmed that, although there are substantial amounts of prostaglandins E and 19-hydroxylated prostaglandins E in semen of fertile men, the concentrations are so variable that meaningful correlation with fertility is not possible. Oxytocin has also been implicated as a potential myometrial stimulant, since oxytocin levels are elevated in peripheral blood immediately after orgasm (34). However, nonpregnant human myometrium is not particularly sensitive to oxytocin (44). Measurements of intrauterine pressure during intercourse showed minimal changes during male orgasm, but a substantial increase during female orgasm, followed by a sharp fall after orgasm to a negative pressure (35).

**PHAGOCYTOSIS OF SPERM**

Studies in the rabbit indicate that active phagocytosis of sperm starts within 6 to 8 hours of sperm entry into the uterus. The exact timing of this reaction in the human is not known, but it seems likely to be similar. This is one mechanism by which dead, immotile, or damaged sperm are removed from the reproductive tract. Rubinstein and his coworkers (57) reported consistently finding uterine sperm up to 24 hours after insemination, and few thereafter. Examination of uteri for presence of sperm between 25 to 41 hours after coitus (a period when many sperm were still present in cervical mucus) revealed very few sperm in the uterine cavity (49). These data indicate a preferential destruction or removal of uterine sperm.

**CAPACITATION**

Freshly ejaculated sperm, or those surgically removed from the male tract, are incapable of fertilizing an ovum. During their brief stay in the uterus and/or oviduct, spermatozoa, in most species, undergo a process known as capacitation, which renders them capable of accomplishing fertilization. Capacitation involves a destabilization of the plasma membrane of the sperm head, without any visible morphological changes. The necessity for capacitation of human sperm has been debated because fertilization of human ova has been achieved in vitro (11, 30, 31) in defined media containing follicular fluid or human blood serum. Capacitation, in many species, requires sequential exposure to both uterine and oviductal environments; however, in others, capacitation can easily be achieved in vitro. It is possible either that human spermatozoa do not require capacitation, or that they are quickly capacitated in in vitro incubations. In either event, it would seem that only minimal exposure to the uterine environment is a prerequisite to achievement of fertilizing capacity.

## SPERM TRANSPORT TO THE OVIDUCT

Previous studies have generally concluded that sperm are not found in the oviducts (fallopian tubes) sooner than 30 min. after insemination (57). A more recent study found no motile sperm in the oviducts sooner than 2 hours after insemination (2). By contrast, Settlage and her coworkers (58) found spermatozoa in the oviducts of women within 5 min. of insemination. Sperm numbers varied between 4 per oviduct and 53 per oviduct, within the period from 5 to 45 min. after insemination. Such data strongly implicate motility of the reproductive smooth muscle in ensuring such rapid sperm transport to the site of fertilization. It is noteworthy that despite rapid sperm transport, the first sperm to arrive in the oviduct often do not achieve fertilization, since this depends on time of ovulation. Settlage and her coworkers (58) concluded that sperm do not remain in the ampulla until fertilization occurs, but pass into the peritoneal cavity. This conclusion is supported by the presence of spermatozoa in peritoneal washings following coitus, found by other investigators (3, 4). Studies in other species have confirmed this concept and have also shown that many sperm are retained in the isthmic portion of the oviduct and pass to the site of fertilization at about the time of ovulation (41). It is not known whether this is also true for the human. Ahlgren (2) observed not more than 171 sperm per oviduct in women with nonoccluded tubes, whereas in women with occluded oviducts, thousands of sperm were found, presumably owing to their failure to pass continuously into the peritoneal cavity. In the studies of Croxatto et al. (19), in which oviducts were flushed for sperm at 8 to 15 hours after coitus, larger numbers of sperm (ranging from 8 to 2184 per oviduct, but generally numbering in the hundreds) were recovered. Ahlgren and his coworkers (3) also found

similar numbers, from 10 to 35 hours after coitus. All available data indicate that only a very small proportion of ejaculated spermatozoa enter the oviducts (about 0.05%).

Various factors have been implicated in the transport of sperm from the uterotubal junction to the site of fertilization; among these are activity of the myosalpinx, ciliary activity, motility of the sperm, oviductal secretions, and a chemical message from the ovum. The relative contribution of each is not known, but it is thought that muscular contractions of the enclosing oviductal walls are primarily responsible. The contractile activity of the isthmic region (except for the proximal portion, which is relatively quiescent) is random in nature. These contractions tend to mix the contents of the oviduct, thereby distributing sperm throughout the tube. It is in the quiescent portion (close to the uterotubal junction) that sperm may remain for many hours. In view of this muscular activity and the speed of sperm transport, it seems unlikely that sperm motility plays any role in transport in the oviduct, although it is clearly important for the process of fertilization. The role of cilia is obscure and is probably not a major factor in

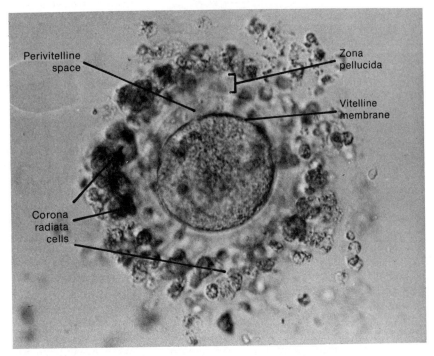

**FIG. 3-1.** Nonhuman primate ovum recovered from the ampulla of the oviduct 48 hours after ovulation (Eddy CA et al: Obstet Gynecol 47:658, 1976)

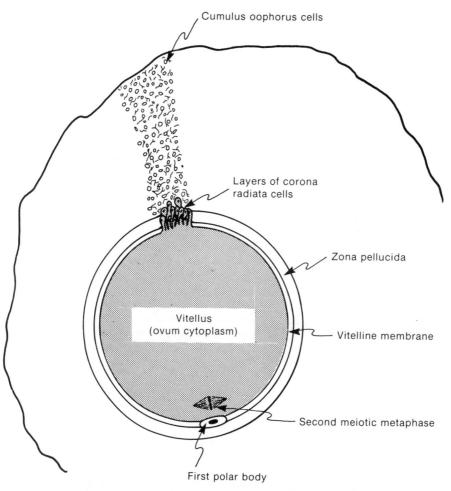

**FIG. 3–2.** Diagrammatic representation of a freshly ovulated ovum with its cellular investments.

sperm transport. In most species, cilia beat toward the uterus and would thus tend to inhibit sperm migration to the site of fertilization. At present there is no good evidence that the ovum does produce a chemical signal which attracts sperm over any great distance, since obviously any such substance would be quickly diluted by oviductal fluid. There is some evidence, however, that in the immediate vicinity of the ovum, sperm may be oriented toward the ovum surface by the radial arrangement of the cellular layers surrounding the ovum (Figs. 3–1 and 3–2).

There has been much debate about the length of time that spermatozoa can remain motile in the human reproductive tract. Ahlgren and his coworkers (3) have reported that motile progressive spermatozoa could be recovered from human oviducts up until 85 hours after coitus, but it is not known whether such aged sperm can still fertilize an ovum. In general, fertilizing ability is lost before motility.

Following capacitation, (assuming that this occurs) sperm undergo the acrosome reaction—an unmasking of enzymes contained in the sperm head which dissolve the coverings surrounding the ovum. Unlike capacitation, which may take place in the uterus and/or oviduct, the acrosome reaction usually occurs only in the oviduct and in close proximity to the ovum. This reaction involves the progressive breakdown and fusion between the sperm plasma membrane and the outer acrosomal membrane, which contracts and wrinkles to form a series of round bodies, or vesicles. These vesicles are loosely located around the anterior portion of the sperm head, and the acrosomal contents are released through these vesiculated pores. The complex formed by the vesiculation between the plasma and outer acrosomal membranes is always lost from the sperm head before penetration by the sperm through the zona pellucida; however, sperm adhering to the surface of the zona pellucida can be found which retain vesiculated acrosomal remnants. If degeneration of a spermatozoon occurs, the acrosome is always lost intact, and vesiculation does not occur.

## OVUM TRANSPORT

### STRUCTURE OF THE OVIDUCT

Although the oviduct has been described in Chapter 1, a more comprehensive presentation is included here because of the central role played by that organ in ovum transport. The oviduct is a muscular, tubular organ lined with secretory and ciliated cells. It may be described in four anatomic segments, each with distinct structural features (Fig. 3-3).

That portion of the oviduct which passes through the uterine wall is called the *intramural*

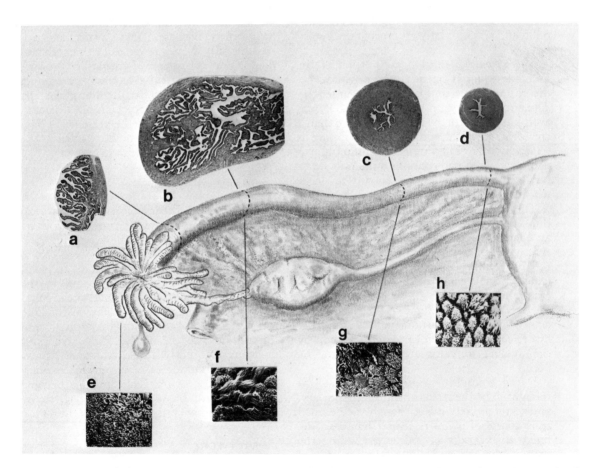

**FIG. 3-3.** Anatomy and morphology of the human oviduct. a–d. Light microscopy photomicrographs depicting cross sections taken at the level of the distal and mid-ampulla, distal and proximal isthmus. e–h. Scanning electron microscopy photomicrographs depicting surface ultrastructure of the oviduct lumen at the level of the fimbriae, mid-ampulla, distal and proximal isthmus. (Eddy CA, Pauerstein CJ: Tubal reproduction and the development of reversible sterilization techniques. In Sciarra JJ, Zatuchni GI, Spiedel JJ (eds): Reversal of Sterilization. Hagerstown, Harper & Row, 1978)

or *interstitial* segment. It extends from the uterine cavity to the external surface of the uterus. It is 1 to 2 cm. long, with a luminal diameter of 0.1 to 1.0 mm.

The *isthmus* begins at the junction between the uterus and oviduct (uterotubal junction) and extends distally for 2 to 3 cm., ending at the ampullary isthmic junction. It contains the heaviest musculature of any portion of the extrauterine oviduct. The isthmus also contains the narrowest lumen of any segment, the diameter averaging 0.4 mm. The isthmus meets one of the anatomic criteria of a sphincter, namely, that the musculature is better developed in this region than in adjacent ones, and appears to be a major determinant in regulating final passage of ova into the uterus. The lumen is less densely ciliated than the ampulla and contains large numbers of secretory cells.

The *ampulla* is the longest portion of the human oviduct. It extends from the isthmus to the infundibulum and is 5 to 8 cm. in length. The ampullary lumen varies from 1 to 2 mm. at its junction with the isthmus to more than 1 cm. near its distal end. The musculature is relatively thin. The lining of the ampulla is densely ciliated and contains numerous secretory cells. Fertilization is thought to occur within this portion of the oviduct.

The *infundibulum* is the trumpet-shaped, thin-walled, outermost portion which ends in an opening to the abdominal cavity, the *tubal ostium,* which is surrounded by densely ciliated, petallike structures, termed *fimbriae* (sing., *fimbria*). The fimbriae are partially attached to the ovaries, thus helping to retain the ovary and the abdominal tubal ostium in close proximity; this arrangement assures that ova released from the ovary are picked up by the oviduct for ultimate transport to the uterus.

Ovum transport through the oviduct is thought to be the result of contractile, ciliary, and secretory activity. Although the detailed time course of ovum transport has been defined in a variety of species, including the human, the role and relative importance of each of these components remains incompletely defined. With few exceptions, the overall time course of ovum transport appears to be remarkably similar in all mammalian species examined: 3 to 4 days are required for ova to travel from the ovary to the uterus.

## THEORIES OF OVUM PICKUP

Ovum transport begins when the ovum, released from the ovary, enters the oviduct. Theories of the mechanism of ovum pickup may be considered in three categories: suction, mechanical, and cilial.

### SUCTION THEORY

It has been speculated that a region of negative pressure caused by tubal peristalsis exists at the tubal ostium, causing the newly released ovum to be sucked into the oviduct (60). Negative pressures within the oviduct, following contractions, have been detected by intraluminal catheters placed in the human oviduct (46). The significance of this finding is difficult to interpret, because a suction mechanism is possible only in the presence of a pressure gradient, and a sustained negative pressure within a nonrigid tube such as the oviduct would probably cause it to collapse. In any event, normal ovum pickup has been demonstrated in rabbits despite the presence of ligatures placed around the oviduct close to the fimbriated abdominal ostium (17).

### MECHANICAL THEORY

The mechanical theory of ovum pickup proposes integrated contractions of the oviduct, its accessory membranes, the tubal fimbriae, and the ovary itself. Movements of these structures at ovulation have been described in laboratory species (24, 37, 38) and in the human (23). The smooth muscle of the tubal and ovarian ligaments contracts, so that the fimbriated end of the oviduct is brought into apposition with the ovary. These structures contract, vigorously and rhythmically, moving the fimbriae across the surface of the ovary to contact the ovum. The fimbriae become engorged with blood and exhibit rhythmic contractile activity, thus picking up the ovum.

### CILIARY THEORY

The surfaces of the folds of the tubal fimbriae and ampulla are covered with cilia, which beat in the direction of the oviductal ostium. Current evidence suggests that direct ciliary contact with the cumulus cells surrounding the newly ovulated egg is critical to ovum pickup (6).

In rabbits, ovum pickup seems to be accomplished by a combination of mechanical and ciliary actions. Species variations in the anatomy of the ovary-infundibulum region may accompany differences in ovum-reception mechanisms. In rats and mice, in which the ovary and infundibulum are enclosed in an ovarian sac, ovum pickup may be dependent upon the flow of fluid secretions within that sac (43).

In primates, ovum pickup is probably similar to that in the rabbit. The few observations made in women seem to indicate that the fimbriae and oviductal ostium are brought into contact with the ovary. However, transperitoneal migration of ova has been shown to occur in women with one ovary and only the contralateral oviduct (33).

Ovum pickup is completed shortly after ovulation. If coitus has taken place, fertilization probably occurs soon after ovum pickup, while the ovum is in the tubal ampulla (see the following discussion for details).

## FERTILIZATION

### PENETRATION OF THE OVUM

At ovulation, the ovum is enclosed within an acellular mucopolysaccharide layer, the zona pellucida, and is surrounded by cumulus cells, four to eight cells in thickness, those immediately adjacent to the zona being termed the corona radiata (Figs. 3–1 and 2–2). The sperm head contains several enzymes located on the outer or inner acrosomal membranes which are thought to be important in the fertilization process. Among these the most important are hyaluronidase, acrosin (a trypsinlike enzyme), and a corona-dispersing enzyme. Hyaluronidase is thought to be located on the outer acrosomal membrane and to be responsible for the removal of the cumulus cells which surround the ovum at the time of ovulation (Fig. 3–2). Acrosin and the corona-dispersing enzyme are thought to be located on the inner acrosomal membrane and are thus released only very close to the ovum surface. These enzymes assist in the removal of the corona cell layer, which is tightly adherent to the zona pellucida at ovulation, and in sperm penetration through the zona pellucida (11).

Embryologically, fertilization involves activation of the ovum by a sperm. The human ovum does not normally cleave without this stimulus. Genetically, fertilization involves introduction into the ovum of hereditary material from the father. Thus it is possible for genetic characteristics arising far apart in time and space actually to be combined in a single individual. The importance of this process for natural and artificial selection cannot be overemphasized. The current belief is that the essential hereditary material is chromosomal DNA in the sperm nucleus. Fertilization begins with sperm penetration of the vitelline membrane (cell wall) and ends with syngamy (combination of male and female pronuclei). The combination of the male and female pronuclei during fertilization is thought of as the central process.

### CELL DIVISION

The two gametes possess an haploid number of chromosomes at the time of fertilization, since they have undergone meiotic (reduction) divisions. The spermatozoon has undergone two meiotic divisions during spermatogenesis before extrusion from the seminiferous tubule. (Meiosis is the process by which the normal complement of chromosomes (diploid) is reduced to half the original number (haploid) so that combination of two haploid gametes (an ovum and a sperm) will give rise to a new embryo with a normal chromosome complement.) The ovum, by contrast, has only undergone one complete meiotic division and is at the metaphase stage of the second meiotic division at the moment of ovulation. At the completion of each meiotic division of the female gamete, a polar body is extruded, and thus at ovulation the ovum has one polar body, which is not extruded until after penetration of the ovum by a spermatozoon; penetration activates the completion of the second meiotic division. Some photographs of different stages of fertilization, in vitro, of human ova have been published (5, 30, 47, 51), but no detailed series of photographs of fertilization in vivo of human ova are available. Consequently, the various stages are demonstrated here by photographs of rabbit ova undergoing fertilization (Fig. 3–4) (40).

The sequence of events is very similar in human and rabbit. The exact time required for fertilization of human ova is not clearly defined, although Edwards (29) records finding 50 per cent of ova penetrated within 7.0 to 10.5 hours of in vitro insemination, and pro-

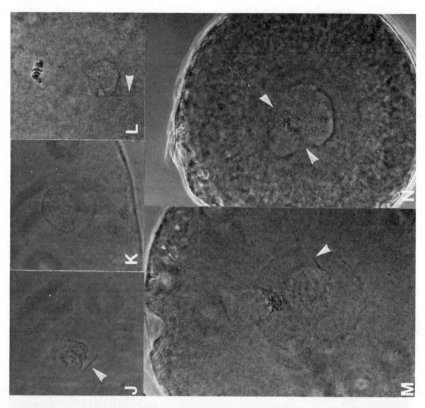

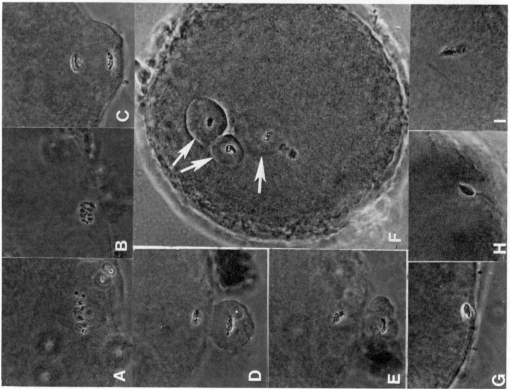

nuclear ova within 11 hours. However, more data are available for the rabbit. In vitro, Brackett and his coworkers (11) report that sperm penetration takes 2 to 3 hours, second polar body formation 2 to 5 hours, and pronuclear formation 4 to 9 hours. In vivo experiments in rabbits, in which ova were placed in the oviduct containing capacitated spermatozoa, have shown that these events can occur more rapidly. Within 1 hour, 15 per cent of ova are penetrated and of these, 8 per cent have the second polar body extruded. By 2 hours, 44 per cent are penetrated and 64 per cent of these have a second polar body (39).

Soon after entry of the fertilizing sperm, the sperm head begins to swell; gradually, nucleoli appear within the surrounding nuclear envelope, and the sperm head becomes converted into a male pronucleus. At the same time, the second polar body is extruded from the ovum, and the group of chromosomes remaining within the vitellus migrates to the center of the ovum and becomes converted into a female pronucleus. The pronuclei increase progressively in volume until they reach about 20 times their original size and move together, in close contact, in the center of the ovum. Then, quite suddenly, they shrink in volume, and only the two groups of chromosomes remain. The chromosomes move to form a single group, representing the prophase of the first cleavage (mitotic) division. Syngamy is the stage extending from contact of the pronuclei to chromosomal union, and signals the end of fertilization. The fertilizable life span of the human ovum is not known, but by analogy with other species, is not thought to persist for more than 24 hours.

### BLOCK OF POLYSPERMY

Immediately following fertilization, reactions occur at the zonal surface and at the vitelline membrane. Called, respectively, the zona and vitelline reactions, they prevent further sperm entry into the ova. These changes, which result from the breakdown of cortical granules located just underneath the vitelline surface, are known as the *block of polyspermy*. This is a defense reaction by the ovum to prevent more than one sperm penetrating the cytoplasm and causing abnormal development, owing to the presence of double the normal complement of male nuclear material (a condition known as polyspermy). If an ovum becomes unfertilizable owing to aging, then cortical granule breakdown does not occur—an indication that some other unknown factor is responsible for preventing sperm penetration in this situation.

### TRANSPORT

Despite the similarity in the overall time course of tubal ovum transport in different species, major differences exist in the detailed

---

**FIG. 3–4.** Rabbit eggs mounted *in toto*. All figures were photographed under a phase-contrast microscope after fixation in acetic alcohol and staining with lacmoid. A. Second meiotic metaphase spindle in an unpenetrated egg with sperm in the perivitelline space. B. Anaphase of the second meiotic division in a penetrated egg, shortly after penetration by the fertilizing sperm. C. Telophase of the second meiotic division in a penetrated egg and beginning of the formation of the second polar body. D. & E. Later stages in the formation of the second polar body, with its complete abstriction from the ooplasm. F. An egg shortly after penetration by a fertilizing sperm. Division of the first polar body (PB1) has occurred, and the formation of the second polar body (PB2) can be seen. G. The fertilizing sperm, shortly after penetration through the vitelline membrane, showing slight swelling. H. The fertilizing sperm showing increased swelling and some curvature. I. Separation of the sperm tail from the head, and breakdown of the outer membrane of the sperm head. The nuclear material of the sperm head still stains darkly. J. Early male pronucleus. The nuclear material of the sperm head no longer stains darkly. The sperm tail is shown by the arrow. K. Male pronucleus at a slightly later stage than in J. The pronucleus has now become rounded. L. Migration of the male pronucleus (tail:*arrow*, out of focus), which still stains only lightly, and the female pronucleus (less distinct boundary), which stains darkly, to the center of the ooplasm. Note similarity of stage of development of male pronucleus with that in K. M. Male pronucleus (large, lighter staining, and with a portion of the sperm tail—*arrow*—still visible) and female pronucleus (smaller, and chromatin darkly staining) come together at the center of the ooplasm. N. Syngamy—fusion of the nuclear material of male and female pronuclei, shown by band (*arrow*) of darkly staining material between the two pronuclei. (Harper MJK: J Exp Zool 174:141, 1970) (Magnification × 500)

pattern of transport through various portions of the oviduct. These differences probably reflect anatomical and endocrinological differences between species.

The detailed time course of ovum transport has been examined in two species of primates in which ovulation was accurately timed—the rhesus monkey (27), and the baboon (28). It was concluded that transport in the rhesus monkey required approximately 3 days, during most of which time ova resided in the ampulla, and then passed through the isthmus into the uterus. Similar studies, in which ova were recovered from the oviducts and uteri of women at known intervals after ovulation, have been performed (16, 20, 21). Ovum transport in women is characterized by retention in the ampulla for approximately 72 hours, followed by rapid transit through the isthmus. Ova are delivered to the uterus approximately 80 hours after release from the ovarian follicle (Fig. 3–5). Thus, the detailed time course of ovum transport in women and rhesus monkeys is virtually identical. Both differ dramatically from the rabbit, in which ova traverse the ampulla in minutes and are then retained at the ampullary isthmic junction for up to 48 hours before slowly traversing the isthmus and entering the uterus, 66 to 72 hours after ovulation (52).

Although the detailed time course of ovum transport is now known for various species, including the human, little is known of the mechanisms responsible for ovum transport. Knowledge of these mechanisms is important to the development of contraceptive technology, and to the evaluation and treatment of infertility.

## ROLE OF THE TUBAL MUSCULATURE

Although it seems obvious that contractions of the oviduct are important in gamete and embryo transport, the relationship between contractility and transport is unknown. Compounds which increase .or decrease tubal contractility have virtually uniformly failed to alter transport consistently. It appears that motility of the oviduct, unlike that of the gut, does not propagate in a given direction for long distances. Instead, contractions appear to be random. In the rabbit, tubal contractions propagate for extremely short distances both toward the ovary and toward the uterus, imparting a to-and-fro movement to the ovum. Over the 3-day period of transport, a net directional bias toward the uterus is thought to develop, which results in final entrance of the ovum (or embryo, if fertilization has occurred) into the uterus (42, 56). What creates this bias is not presently known.

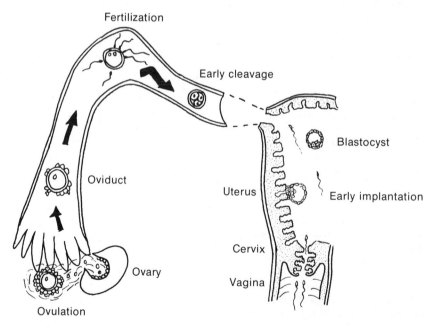

**FIG. 3–5.** Ovum transport and early embryo development in the human reproductive tract, from ovulation to early implantation.

## ROLE OF TUBAL INNERVATION

The dense innervation of the oviductal isthmus, together with its prominent muscle layer, suggest that this segment of the oviduct functions as a sphincter to regulate passage of the ovum or embryo through the oviduct into the uterus. However, destruction of the nerve supply to the oviduct does not disrupt normal ovum transport (8, 25, 53, 54, 55). Autotransplantation of the oviduct and ovary, a procedure which leads to denervation, has been shown to be consistent with normal pregnancy in the rabbit (63) and in the ewe (18), which casts further doubt on the importance of tubal innervation in ovum transport.

## ROLE OF SECRETORY AND CILIATED CELLS

In spite of much speculation, there are no hard data which demonstrate a role for tubal secretions in ovum transport. Although such secretions may supply nutrients to the developing embryo, the necessity of secretory cells for normal reproduction has not been proved. Because tubal ectopic pregnancy often occurs in oviducts that have been previously damaged by infectious agents, it is unlikely that a normal complement of secretory cells is necessary for the survival of the human embryo.

In contrast it has been shown that the cilia are involved in ovum pickup and transport through the ampulla of the rabbit oviduct. Inhibition of tubal muscular activity banishes the to-and-fro movement of ova within the ampulla, but does not affect the net transport time (37). Microsurgical reversal of short segments of rabbit ampulla prevents ovum transport and pregnancy, due to the presence of cilia within the reversed segment beating toward the ovary, thereby actively impeding transport toward the uterus (26).

The role of the cilia in human ovum transport and fertility is much more difficult to appraise. Although a correlation has been made between the percentage of ciliated cells present on the fimbriae and fertility (13), recent reports have demonstrated normal fertility in several women suffering from the so-called immotile cilia syndrome, in which cilia throughout the body are nonfunctional (1, 7). Not surprisingly, men suffering this syndrome are infertile, due to the resultant immotility of their spermatozoa.

## THE PREIMPLANTATION EMBRYO

The fertilized ovum begins to cleave while being transported through the tube toward the uterine cavity.

The first four cleavages produce 2, 4, 8, and then 16 cells of similar size which cluster together to form a solid ball, the morula, still inside the zona pellucida. At about the time the embryo enters the uterine cavity, it has been transformed, through continuing cleavage, into a hollow, fluid-filled sphere called a blastula or blastocyst (Fig. 3–5). By this time, cellular differentiation has occurred, so that certain cells of the blastocyst, the "inner cell mass," are destined to become the embryo, while the remaining mantle of cells, the trophoblast, will form the extraembryonic tissues, or placenta.

Between ovulation and implantation, a period of approximately a week, the developing embryo exists in a "free-living" state, and must obtain its metabolic support from the tubal and uterine surroundings. The fluids of the reproductive tract provide the nutrients during the preimplantation period.

Unlike the embryos of lower forms, such as those of invertebrates or amphibians, which rely on the availability of considerable amounts of stored nutrients to allow them to develop in relatively neutral or hostile surroundings, the mammalian embryo is dependent on a continuing supply of energy from the maternal environment.

In order to develop and undergo cleavage, the fertilized ovum (zygote) requires both a source of energy and a source of biosynthetic precursors. At ovulation, the ovum contains a wide variety of enzymes capable of catalyzing the necessary metabolic reactions in support of embryonic development. The types, amounts, and activities of these enzymes reflect the progressive changes in metabolic activities of the developing embryo.

Growth-factor requirements vary with the stage of development. Early embryos are much more fastidious in their requirements than embryos in later stages of development. The two-cell mouse embryo, for example, is capable of utilizing a limited number of growth factors. Pyruvate, lactate, oxaloacetate, and phosphoenolpyruvate are the only compounds which will support development of the two-cell embryo to a blastocyst (12, 61, 62).

Amino acids and proteins are also required. Most developing embryos will die before reaching the eight-cell state in the absence of amino acids or protein, although there appears to be no specific requirement of the amino nitrogen source.

During the preimplantation period, the endometrial glands, under the influence of ovarian estrogen and progesterone, begin to secrete glycogen, a convenient energy source for the preimplantation embryo. The increasing size, complexity, and metabolic requirements of the developing blastocyst, coupled with the inadequate exchange of nutrients possible through simple mechanisms of diffusion, ultimately mandate a more complex and intimate interaction between blastocyst and maternal organism. This is accomplished through implantation.

## IMPLANTATION

### TRANSPORT WITHIN THE UTERUS

Transportation of the blastocyst to the site at which it implants is primarily a result of the muscular activity of the uterus. In the human, implantation occurs most often on the surface of the mid-portion of the posterior wall of the uterus. The regularity of this positioning strongly suggests a discrete mechanism. Ciliated cells in the luminal epithelium which might contribute to the orientation of the blastocyst within the endometrial cavity have been described in the human, but have not been shown to have this function.

In the rabbit, after the blastocyst enlarges to several millimeters in diameter, it acts as the focal point for the initiation of waves of muscular contraction. This interaction results in spacing of the blastocysts a uniform distance apart in each of the uterine horns (9). It is likely that uterine contractile activity of either spontaneous or blastocyst-induced origin results in the transport of the blastocyst to the usual area of implantation in the human, as well (10).

### ORIENTATION

Prior to contact with the endometrial epithelium, the blastocyst, which exhibits polarity (in that the inner cell mass which gives rise to the embryo is located at one end, or pole, of the spherical blastocyst), must be oriented so that the inner cell mass faces the endometrial surface (Fig. 3–6A). Such directional implantation has been suggested as being the reason for the eventual central position of the umbilical cord on the placenta, and "upside-down" implantation has been thought to be a possible reason for abnormal development of the placenta and fetus. It is most probable that it is the blastocyst which orients itself in the appropriate position for implantation, perhaps with the aid of contractile elements within the uterine epithelial cells. The apposition of the blastocyst to the endometrium is very important, since it is a necessary prerequisite for the initiation of adhesion (48).

## ADHESION

Adhesion fixes the trophoblast in relation to the uterine epithelium and precedes deeper penetration. Prior to implantation, the zona pellucida is shed from the blastocyst, exposing the trophoblastic cells surrounding the inner cell mass. The denuded blastocyst is sticky. The simplest current hypothesis explaining this is that there is a progressive addition of materials to the trophoblast surface which causes it to become more adhesive (36). The uterine surface simultaneously undergoes changes in its cellular membrane to serve as a focus of adhesion. Adhesion between trophoblast and uterine epithelium initially involves the free surfaces of cells, with interdigitation of the numerous protrusions present on the surface of the cells.

## FUSION AND PENETRATION

As adhesion progresses, the trophoblast penetrates into the uterine luminal epithelium (Fig. 3–6B), and, in subsequent stages, during which maternal and endometrial glands are surrounded by trophoblastic tissue, an association between the trophoblast and maternal epithelial cells is established through junctional connections between adjacent cells. The trophoblast uses maternal cells as an anchorage during invasion of the endometrium. The outer layer trophoblast (syncytiotrophoblast) overlying the inner cell mass hypertrophies and becomes a syncytium, that is, it loses its individual cell membranes and coalesces to form an aggregate, which penetrates into the endometrial stroma. As implantation progresses, more and more syncytiotrophoblast forms from the original thin trophoblastic shell of the blastocyst and penetrates into the

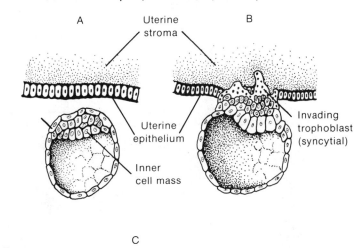

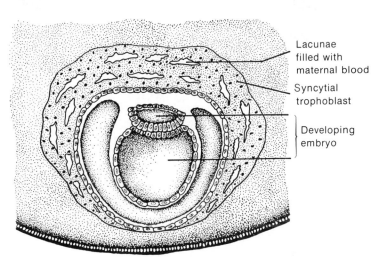

**FIG. 3–6.** Implantation, in the human. A. Free-floating blastocyst prior to adhesion to uterine lining. Note orientation of inner cell mass toward uterine surface. B. Attachment and early invasion of the uterine lining by trophoblast. C. Complete penetration of the uterine lining by invading blastocyst. (Tuchmann-Duplessis H, David G, Haegel P: Illustrated Human Embryology, Vol 1. New York, Springer-Verlag, 1971)

endometrium, which is edematous and highly glandular.

Within 3 days, the blastocyst is completely implanted beneath the surface epithelium (Fig. 3–6C). The syncytiotrophoblast, derived from the inner, less-differentiated cytotrophoblast, forms the outer invasive margins of implantation. The invading trophoblast digests the walls of maternal capillaries near the implanting embryo. Maternal blood fills the resulting intercellular spaces (lacunae) with sluggishly flowing blood. At this stage, the rudiment of a placenta has been formed.

Chorionic gonadotropin, a hormone necessary to promote and maintain pregnancy, is secreted by the trophoblast at this time, reaching the maternal blood in sufficient amounts to prolong the function of the corpus luteum, thus increasing and sustaining progesterone production to support the pregnancy.

The advancing columns of trophoblast constitute the primary villi which branch to form secondary villi, and later branch again to form tertiary villi (Fig. 3–7). These become the major surfaces for fetal-maternal exchange throughout the period of pregnancy.

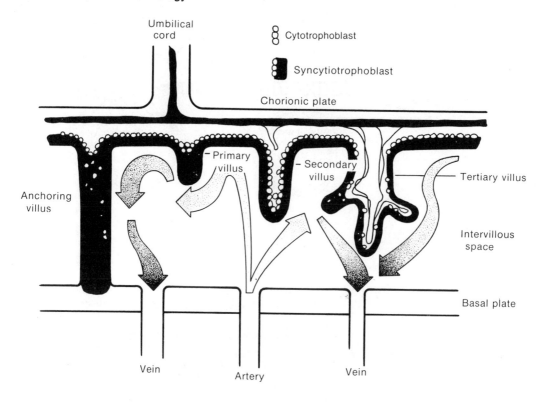

**FIG. 3–7.** Schematic cross section of the human placenta. Note the various types of villi and the pattern of maternal blood-flow between uterus and placenta, and fetal blood-flow through tertiary villi.

## REFERENCES

1. Afzelius BA, Camner P, Mossberg B: On the function of cilia in the female reproductive tract. Fertil Steril 29:72, 1978
2. Ahlgren M: Migration of spermatozoa to the Fallopian tubes and the abdominal cavity in women including some immunological aspects. Lund, Sweden, Studentliteratur 1969, 139 pp
3. Ahlgren M, Bostrom K, Malmqvist R: Sperm transport and survival in women with special reference to the Fallopian tube. In Hafez ESE, Thibault CG (eds): The Biology of Spermatozoa. Basel, Karger, 1973, p 63
4. Asch RH: Laparoscopic recovery of sperm from peritoneal fluid in patients with negative or poor Sims Huhner test. Fertil Steril 27:1111, 1976
5. Bavister BD, Edwards RG, Steptoe PC: Identification of the midpiece and tail of the spermatozoon during fertilization of eggs *in vitro*. J Reprod Fertil 20:159, 1969
6. Blandau RJ, Verdugo P: An overview of gamete transport—comparative aspects. In Harper MJK, Pauerstein CJ, Adams CE, Coutinho EM, Croxatto HB, Paton DM (eds): Ovum Transport and Fertility Regulation. WHO Symposium, Copenhagen, Scriptor, 1976, p 138
7. Bleau G, Richer CL, Bousquet D: Absence of dynein arms in cilia of endocervical cells in a fertile woman. Fertil Steril 30:362, 1978
8. Bodkhe RR, Harper MJK: Changes in the amount of adrenergic neurotransmitter in the genital tract of untreated rabbits, and rabbits given reserpine or iproniazid during the time of egg transport. Biol Reprod 6:288, 1972
9. Boving BG: Rabbit blastocyst distribution. Am J Anat 98:403, 1956
10. Boving BG: Implantation mechanisms. In Hartman CG (ed): Mechanisms Concerned with Conception. New York, Pergamon Press, 1963, p 321
11. Brackett BG, Seitz HM Jr, Rocha G, Mastroianni L Jr: The mammalian fertilization process. In Moghissi KS, Hafez ESE (eds): Biology of Mammalian Fertilization and Implantation. Springfield, IL, CC Thomas, 1972, p 165

12. Brinster RL: Studies on the development of mouse embryos *in vitro*. I. Effect of energy source. J Exp Zool 158:59, 1965
13. Brosens IA, Vasquez G: Fimbrial microbiopsy. J Reprod Med 16:171, 1976
14. Bygdeman M, Fredericsson B, Svanborg K, Samuelsson B: The relation between fertility and prostaglandin content of seminal fluid in man. Fertil Steril 21:622, 1970
15. Bygdeman M, Samuelsson B: Analyses of prostaglandins in human semen. Prostaglandins and related factors. Clin Chim Acta 13:465, 1966
16. Cheviakoff S, Diaz S, Carril M, Patritti N, Croxatto HD, Llados C, Ortiz ME, Croxatto HB: Ovum transport in women. In Harper MJK, Pauerstein CJ, Adams CE, Coutinho EM, Croxatto HB, Paton DM (eds): Ovum Transport and Fertility Regulation. WHO Symposium, Copenhagen, Scriptor, 1976, p 416
17. Clewe TH, Mastroianni L, Jr.: Mechanisms of ovum pickup. I. Functional capacity of rabbit oviducts ligated near the fimbriae. Fertil Steril 9:13, 1958
18. Cohen BM, Morgenthal JC, Davey DAD, Van Niekerk CH, Uys CJ, Botha MC, Dutoit E, Harrison VC, Hickman R, Lotter F, Poole DMJ: Completed pregnancy following vascularized heterotopic autotransplantation of the fallopian tube of the ewe. Int J Fertil 21:153, 1976
19. Croxatto HB, Faundes A, Medel M, Avendaño S, Croxatto HD, Vera C, Anselmo J, Pastene L: Studies on sperm migration in the human female genital tract. In Hafez ESE, Thibault CG (eds): The Biology of Spermatozoa. Basel, Karger, 1973, p 56
20. Croxatto HB, Ortiz MES: Egg transport in the Fallopian tube. Gynecol Invest 6:215, 1975
21. Croxatto HB, Ortiz MES, Diaz S, Hess R, Balmaceda J, Croxatto HD: Studies on the duration of egg transport by the human oviduct. II. Ovum location at various intervals following LH peak. Am J Obstet Gynecol 132:629, 1978
22. Davajan V, Kunitake GM: Fractional *in vivo* and *in vitro* examination of postcoital cervical mucus in the human. Fertil Steril 20:197, 1969
23. Doyle JB: Ovulation and effects of selected uterotubal denervation: direct observations by culdotomy. Fertil Steril 5:105, 1954
24. Dukelow RW: The morphology of follicular development and ovulation in nonhuman primates. J Reprod Fertil [Suppl] 22:23, 1975
25. Eddy CA, Black DL: Ovum transport through rabbit oviducts perfused with 6-hydroxydopamine. J Reprod Fertil 38:189, 1974
26. Eddy CA, Flores JJ, Archer DR, Pauerstein CJ: The role of cilia in fertility: an evaluation by selective microsurgical modification of the rabbit oviduct. Am J Obstet Gynecol 132:814, 1978
27. Eddy CA, Garcia RG, Kraemer DC, Pauerstein CJ: Detailed time course of ovum transport in the rhesus monkey (Macaca mulatta). Biol Reprod 13:363, 1975
28. Eddy CA, Turner TT, Kraemer DC, Pauerstein CJ: Pattern and duration of ovum transport in the baboon (Papio anubis). Obstet Gynecol 47:658, 1976
29. Edwards RG: Fertilization and cleavage *in vitro* of human ova. In Moghissi KS, Hafez ESE (eds): Biology of Mammalian Fertilization and Implantation. Springfield, IL, CC Thomas, 1972, p 263
30. Edwards RG, Bavister BD, Steptoe PC: Early stages of fertilization *in vitro* of human oocytes matured *in vitro*. Nature 221:632, 1969
31. Edwards RG, Steptoe PC, Purdy JM: Fertilization and cleavage *in vitro* of preovulatory human oocytes. Nature 227:1307, 1970
32. Elstein M, Moghissi KS, Borth R (eds): Cervical Mucus in Human Reproduction. Copenhagen, Scriptor, 1973, 163 pp
33. First A: Transperitoneal migration of ovum or spermatozoon. Obstet Gynecol 4:431, 1954
34. Fox CA, Knaggs GS: Milk ejection activity (oxytocin) in peripheral venous blood in man during lactation and in association with coitus. J Endocrinol 45:145, 1969
35. Fox CA, Wolff HS, Baker JA: Measurement of intra-vaginal and intra-uterine pressures during human coitus by radio-telemetry. J Reprod Fertil 22:243, 1970
36. Fridhandler L: Gametogenesis to implantation. In Assali NS (ed): Biology of Gestation, Vol I, The Maternal Organism. New York, Academic Press, 1968, p 67
37. Halbert SA, Tam PY, Adams RJ, Blandau RJ: An analysis of the mechanisms of egg transport in the ampulla of the rabbit oviduct. Gynecol Invest 7:306, 1976
38. Halbert SA, Tam PY, Blandau RJ: Egg transport in the rabbit oviduct. Science 191:1052, 1976
39. Harper MJK: Factors influencing sperm penetration of rabbit eggs *in vivo*. J Exp Zool 173:47, 1970
40. Harper MJK: Cytological observations on sperm penetration of rabbit eggs. J Exp Zool 174:141, 1970
41. Harper MJK: Relationship between sperm transport and penetration of eggs in the rabbit oviduct. Biol Reprod 8:441, 1973
42. Hodgson BJ, Talo A, Pauerstein CJ: Oviductal ovum surrogate movement: interrelation with muscular activity. Biol Reprod 16:394, 1977
43. Humphrey KW: Observations on transport of ova in the oviduct of the mouse. J. Endocrinol 40:267, 1968
44. Kumar D: Hormonal regulation of myometrial activity: clinical implications. In Wynn RM (ed): Cellular Biology of the Uterus. New York, Appleton-Century-Crofts, 1967, p 449
45. Lundquist F: Aspects of the biochemistry of human semen. Acta Physiol Scand 19 [Suppl 66], 1949, 108 pp
46. Maia H, Coutinho EM: Peristalsis and antiperistalsis of the human Fallopian tube during the menstrual cycle. Biol Reprod 2:305, 1970
47. McMaster R, Yanagimachi R, Lopata A: Penetration of human eggs by human spermatozoa *in vitro*. Biol Reprod 19:212, 1978
48. Mossman HW: Orientation and site of attachment of the blastocyst: a comparative study. In Blandau RJ (ed): The Biology of the Blastocyst. Chicago, University of Chicago Press, 1971, p 49
49. Moyer DL, Rimdusit S, Mishell DR: Sperm distribution and degradation in the human female

reproductive tract. Am J Obstet Gynecol 35:831, 1970

50. Nelson CMK, Bunge RG: Semen analysis: evidence for changing parameters of male fertility potential. Fertil Steril 25:503 1974
51. Overstreet JW, Hembree WC: Penetration of the zona pellucida of nonliving human oocytes by human spermatozoa *in vitro*. Fertil Steril 27:815, 1976
52. Pauerstein CJ, Anderson V, Chatkoff ML, Hodgson BJ: Effect of estrogen and progesterone on the time course of tubal ovum transport in rabbits. Am J Obstet Gynecol 120:299, 1974
53. Pauerstein CJ, Hodgson BJ, Fremming BD, Martin JE: Effects of sympathetic denervation of the rabbit oviduct on normal ovum transport and on transport modified by estrogen and progesterone. Gynecol Invest 5:121, 1974
54. Polidoro JP, Heilman RD, Culver RM, Reo RR: Effects of adrenergic drugs or denervation on ovum transport in rabbits. In Harper MJK, Pauerstein, CJ, Adams CE, Coutinho EM, Croxatto HB, Paton DM (eds): Ovum Transport and Fertility Regulation. WHO Symposium, Copenhagen, Scriptor, 1976, p 331
55. Polidoro JP, Howe GR, Black DL: The effects of adrenergic drugs on ovum transport through the rabbit oviduct. J Reprod Fertil 35:331, 1973
56. Portnow J, Talo A, Hodgson BJ: A random walk model of ovum transport. Bull Math Biol 39:349, 1977
57. Rubenstein B, Strauss H, Lazarus ML, Hankin H: Sperm survival in women. Motile sperm in the fundus and tubes of surgical cases. Fertil Steril 2:15, 1951
58. Settlage DSF, Motoshima M, Tredway DR: Sperm transport from the external cervical os to the Fallopian tubes in women: a time and quantitation study. Fertil Steril 24:655, 1973
59. Templeton AA, Cooper I, Kelly RW: Prostaglandin concentrations in the semen of fertile men. J Reprod Fertil 52:147, 1978
60. Westman A: Investigations into the transit of ova in man. Br J Obstet Gynaecol 44:821, 1937
61. Whitten WK: Culture of tubal mouse ova. Nature 177:96, 1956
62. Whitten WK: Culture of tubal ova. Nature 179:1081, 1957
63. Winston RML, McClure-Browne JC: Pregnancy following autograft transplantation of Fallopian tube and ovary in the rabbit. Lancet 2:494, 1974
64. Zuckerman Z, Rodriguez Rigau LJ, Smith KD, Steinberger E: Frequency distribution of sperm counts in fertile and infertile males. Fertil Steril 28:1310, 1977

# 4

# Human Sexuality

**Paul C. Weinberg**

Anatomy, embryology, and maturation have been considered in previous chapters. This chapter discusses developmental aspects of human sexuality. These complex aspects can be considered in linear sequence over the life cycle. Each level has an impact upon the following one, and upon future development (4).

## GENDER AND LEGAL SEX

Fertilization results in the encoding of genetic sex. The sperm's genetic component determines the fetal genotype: if it carries an X chromosome, the fetus is genotypically 46XX, a female, whereas if it contains a Y chromosome, the fetus is genotypically 46XY, a male. This is the primary determinant of future development.

The genotype (XX or XY) influences gonadal development in the embryo. If XX, the cortex becomes dominant in the gonad; if XY, medullary dominance ensues. The XY medullary dominance causes the testis to develop an internal gametal transport system. In the XY gonad (the ovary) in which the cortex dominates, the gametal transport system will be external (fallopian tube).

The gonad also develops a characteristic hormonal output. In the presence of an ovary, the embryonic müllerian system persists, forming the internal genitalia—the tubes, uterus, and upper portion of the vagina. The male gonad is more active in its coding. It secretes androgen, and a müllerian regression factor. The result is almost complete regression of the müllerian ductal system. The wolffian system persists, to form the tubal system which later transports the sperm and seminal fluid from the prostate and seminal vesicles into the urethra.

Gonadal hormones also determine the structure of the external genitalia. In the male, fusion produces an external phallus and scrotum, whereas in the presence of an ovary, no fusion occurs; the genital ridges form the labia and vaginal vestibule. The clitoris forms, but does not incorporate the urethra, and the urogenital sinus invaginates to join the upper vagina, forming the vaginal canal.

The structure of the external genitalia assumes particular significance because their form determines whether a newborn is labeled as male or female. Nursery, and legal, sex identity are decided in the delivery room. The nursery tag identifies the child as boy or girl, and the birth certificate which establishes legal sex is recorded with a specific gender, based upon the conformation of the external genitals, since the body is otherwise asexual in character.

## GENDER IDENTITY AND GENDER ROLE

With the establishment of gender and legal sex, psychologic mechanisms begin to play a significant role in the child's sexual development. Nursery and legal-sex determinants have been communicated to the parents. They respond in a socioculturally conditioned fashion. In Western civilization the child is dressed in blue or pink, toys are usually dolls, for girls, or trucks for boys, and children may be handled differently—a boy bounced and jostled, a girl cuddled more closely. The infant responds, over time, by developing a *gender identity* and a *gender role*. Gender identity is that gender declared in the nursery and on the birth certificate. This is the gender to which the parents and environment respond in their relationship with the infant. The gender role represents the growing child's response to what are perceived as environmental expectations of social conduct for boys and girls, including ways of interacting with same and opposite-sexed parents and other family members. Through this interaction, the child ultimately learns adult male and female roles.

Gender identity is firmly established approximately between the ages of two-and-a-half and three. This is of clinical importance in dealing with genital ambiguity, since clinical experience has shown that beyond this age, reassignment of gender identity is fraught with serious emotional problems. In cases of ambiguous genitalia, a sex of rearing must be decided upon prior to this age, even though corrective surgery may not take place until a later time (6).

Gender role evolves from gender identity. From approximately age three through the first decade of life, the child remains sexually undifferentiated, except for the genitalia. However, psychoanalytic theory holds that many unconscious and preconscious conceptions of sexuality are developed before the child reaches age five. From age five to nine, the child enters what, psychoanalytically, is considered the period of latent sexuality. However, behavioral scientists have suggested that this period is, in fact, quite dynamic. Environmental inputs concerning the proper roles for men and women come from family, peers, teachers, and religious figures. Verbal and nonverbal expressions of values and expectations suggest, and indeed often dictate, modes of expected behavior. Gender role thus becomes the social expression of previous gender identity, the foundation of intra- and inter-personal relationships. Differences between males and females at this stage affect personality and emotional makeup, and choices concerning the gender of close friends, preferences in dress, athletic endeavors, and hobbies. Much of this behavior is being investigated at both a sociocultural and biomedical (hormonal) level. Research has not yet determined the respective influence of social conditioning and innate biological propensities.

## PUBERTY

During the 9th or 10th year, the changes of the pubertal sequence begin. These first alterations are not clinically apparent. Serial laboratory determinations, however, show elevation of the gonadotrophins common to both male and female (FSH and LH) and, later, the appearance of ovarian estrogens and testicular androgens. The first physical change noted in the male is beginning growth of pubic hair whereas, in the female, either pubic hair growth or breast-budding may be the first evidence of puberty. Once begun, the development of secondary sexual characteristics follows a predictable pattern over the next 4 to 5 years. After a growth spurt in the early teens, full statural growth is achieved in the late teens. The gonadal hormones and growth hormone are crucial in the control of these somatic changes (see Chap. 1).

The male evolves a muscular body form. Body-hair growth increases, with growth of a beard, chest hair, and a broader distribution of pubic hair. The larynx widens, and the voice deepens. Penile and testicular growth occurs, and ejaculatory capability is seen, with masturbatory activity or nocturnal emission.

The female develops a more rounded body habitus, especially over the hips, buttocks, and mons pubis. Growth of body hair is more localized to the pubic area than in the male. Adrenarche, the growth of axillary hair, is of clinical interest, since menarche usually follows within 6 months. The average age at first menses is 12.5 years, in the United States. The pattern of menstrual flow may be irregular at first, but usually within 6 months it becomes cyclic, denoting ovulation.

The differences in gonadotrophin and hypothalamic hormone patterns may be the primary biologic difference between males and females. The male pattern of gonadotrophin output is tonic, whereas the female pattern is cyclic. The cyclic quality in the female continues through the reproductive years. The site of this difference is probably hypothalamic, and is considered to be of genetic origin.

By the mid-teens, the individual has achieved physical sexual maturity and is capable of sexual function and procreation. This is a period of rapid physical and emotional change. The adolescent has experienced the emotional complexities of choosing between dependence and independence, passivity and aggressiveness, marked change in his or her interpersonal relationships with peers and family, and has begun to establish his or her individuality and self-image.

One of the most interesting models of emotional development in children is described in Erik Erikson's *Childhood and Society*. Erikson divides psychologic growth into stages of basic trust, autonomy, and initiative (in childhood) and finally (in adolescence)—identity. The identity stage is defined as that period in which the attitudes of the individual are differentiated from the beliefs and value systems of the parents (2). This process should not be confused with earlier gender identity.

By the late teens, the majority of individuals have experienced erotic impulses which may be acted out in autoerotic masturbatory or coital episodes (over 50% by age 19).

## SEXUAL MATURITY

The work of Masters and Johnson has furnished basic understanding of the physiology of human arousal and orgasm. According to their research, arousal is divided into an excitement and plateau phase. The arousal state is characterized by increasing sexual tension, manifested by heightened muscular tension (myotonia) and venous filling (vasocongestion) of the genital area. Tension rises to its highest level with orgasm, and then falls with orgasmic relief. A resolution phase follows, where altered psychic and bodily states return to their normal prearousal condition.

These changes are characterized in Figure 4–1, for the male, and Figure 4–2, for the female. The male response is less varied than that of the female. After orgasm, the male must pass through a refractory phase, returning to lower levels of excitement, before being able to experience arousal and orgasm again.

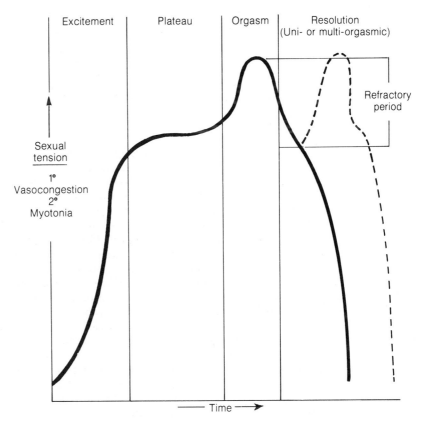

**FIG. 4–1.** Curves of typical male coital response (variations usually in duration). (After: Masters & Johnson)

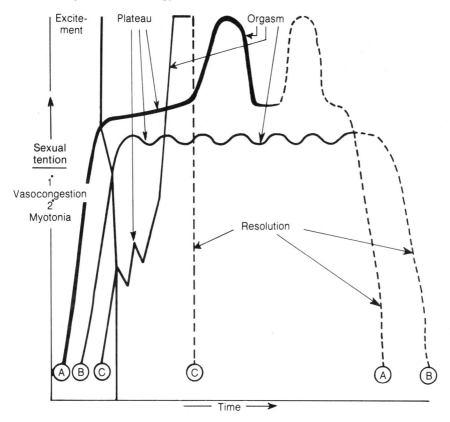

**FIG. 4–2.** Curves of typical female coital response (variations in both duration and intensity. No true refractory period). (After: Masters & Johnson)

This period may be quite short, but lengthens with aging and may require several days, in the older age group.

Figure 4–2 depicts three typical curves of sexual tension for the female. Curve *A* is very similar to that of the male; however, the female does not seem to require a refractory period, and can be multiorgasmic over short periods of time. Unfortunately, the description of such possibilities can lead to sexual dissatisfaction in some people who then expect to achieve multiple orgasms, but cannot. Multiple orgasms are not the only normal female response. Curve *B* depicts a response which the female may perceive in two very disparate ways: positively, as multiple orgasms of diminished intensity, or negatively, as anorgasmia. Curve *C* represents very rapid arousal to peak orgasm, with very rapid resolution. One individual may, in different sexual encounters, experience these variant patterns of orgasm;

others may experience a single pattern. All such patterns are normative.

Sexual pleasure and gratification depend on more than physiology—expectation also plays a role. Many males and females enjoy sexuality even if it does not culminate in coitus or orgasm. Others expect great "highs" of tension and release. Each must define individual goals, and these are generally attainable, unless there is organic or psychologic dysfunction. On occasion, the alleviation of dissatisfaction requires education, counseling, or, in more serious cases, psychotherapy.

In the detailed physiologic responses catalogued by Masters and Johnson, during orgasm, the uterus elevates out of the true pelvis and exhibits a contractile pattern. These contractions are of low amplitude and pose no threat of miscarriage in the normally pregnant woman. However, caution might dictate avoiding orgasm in the woman with a repeated history of spontaneous abortion or premature labor.

Vaginal changes include lubrication, as a result of transudation from the vaginal mucosa. This lubrication allows penile intromission without discomfort or trauma to the tissues. Congestion affects the outer third of the vagina, causing a narrowing of the vaginal barrel. This "orgasmic platform" contracts rhythmically with orgasm, analogous to the perineal contractions of ejaculation in the male.

Concomitant changes are noted in the external genitalia. The labia become congested and enlarged, and separate from the midline. The clitoris elongates and enlarges, and retracts under the arch of the bony pelvis. Clitorial stimulation after this retraction occurs through tension on neighboring structures. Although at this time direct clitoral stimulation is not necessary, and may even be painful for some women, for others it is a necessary prerequisite of orgasm. Orgasm achieved by clitoral stimulation, intromission, or even fantasy is physiologically similar. This finding refutes the Freudian concept of vaginal orgasm as being superior to other forms of orgasmic release (5).

The clitoral changes are analogous to erection in the penis. In erection, there is increased inflow of blood into the penis, with obstruction of its outflow, so that the penis enlarges in length and diameter. During the plateau phase, the vasocongestion and myotonia of excitement continue in the male as in the female.

With orgasm, the seminal fluid that has collected in the posterior urethra is propelled into the urethra and out of the urethral meatus as the ejaculate, by rhythmic contractions of the perineal musculature analogous to the rhythmic contractions of the orgasmic platform in the female.

Extragenital responses also occur. In both male and female there is an increase in pulse, blood pressure, and respiratory rate. There is a transient "rash" over the anterior chest, the sex flush. In the female, the breasts swell and the nipples become turgid and erectile. After orgasm, the tissues return to normal within 10 to 15 minutes, unless further erotic stimulation ensues.

These alterations are subject to individual variation. It is folly for partners to take "observer" roles to determine if these precisely defined changes occur. Pleasurable sexual relations take place only in an environment of willingness, spontaneity, and trust.

## SEXUAL ORIENTATION

The majority of individuals achieve adulthood having chosen a heterosexual orientation. They are then faced with the developmental "crises" of that orientation. Most choose marriage. Many then face the crises of parenthood, which are shared by both male and female. The experiences of pregnancy, delivery, and breastfeeding are uniquely female. However, they are increasingly being shared by male partners, to the extent of the male's presence, interest, and support. These shared experiences have been enhanced by prepared childbirth and educational efforts concerning parenthood.

Although the majority of individuals in the United States choose persons of the opposite gender as sexual partners (heterosexuality), a minority of 5 per cent to 10 per cent develop a preference for selection of partners of the same sex (homosexuality). In contemporary American society, more homosexual relationships are now overt, allowing more thorough research, and, thus, better estimates of incidence than in the past (1). It appears that homosexuality and heterosexuality do not represent exclusive choices. A given orientation may be followed throughout the life cycle; however, it is often a dynamic and changing choice. The ability of many to change orientation over time, while remaining quite functional, supports the hypothesis that none of these orientations, in themselves, connote psychopathology (1). In fact, some individuals engage in sexual activity with both sexes (bisexuality). Homosexual and heterosexual orientations evolve, for the most part, into dyadic pairing, whereas bisexuality is most frequently triadic. Scientifically, little is known about these relationships; however, anecdotal reports appear in the media relating the sexual experiences and preferences of renowned individuals who openly report their life styles. The media approach is of value, especially in terms of understanding individual experience (anecdotal), until it can be analyzed behaviorly or biomedically.

Still other individuals elect not to relate at all sexually, at least overtly (asexuality).

Asexuality may be dictated by religious mandate, as it is with priests and nuns, or can be chosen by some who have other over-riding interests, such as careers, which absorb most of their energies.

Sexual interrelationships in today's society involve much experimentation. Examples include communes of the 1960s, with group sexual relationships and "swinging," and "key clubs," representing partner exchange. There is little sociobehavioral data as to the "success" of these relationships. They seem a part of the "sexual revolution," and only the future will shed light upon the durability of such sexual choices.

## SEXUALITY IN LATER YEARS

Young people have a tendency to "neuter" older adults, especially their parents. Recently, it has become apparent that the perception of old age as asexual is erroneous. Though the aging process may physiologically alter sexual function, a significant number of individuals continue coital activities into the later years. Coital frequency may diminish, the male may ejaculate less frequently, and arousal time may lengthen. If the physiologic

changes of aging are explained to older couples, their anxiety about performance may be minimized, and many of them may find sexual experiences different from those of their youth, but still very fulfilling.

Considered in its overarching context, sexuality developes from varied biomedical and behavioral inputs. We are evolving more openness about sexuality, and sexual behavior seems to be changing. More precise understanding—biologic and behavioral—can only enhance the positive force which sexuality brings to bear upon our civilization.

## REFERENCES

1. Bell AP, Weinberg MS: Homosexualities. New York, Simon & Schuster, 1978
2. Erickson E: Childhood and Society, 2nd ed. New York, Norton, 1963
3. Kantner J, Zelnick M: Sexual experience of young unmarried women in the U.S. Fam Plann Perspect 4:9, 1972
4. Katchadourian HA, Lunde DP: Fundamentals of Human Sexuality. New York, Holt, Rinehart & Winston, 1972
5. Masters W, Johnson V: Human Sexual Response. Boston, Little, Brown, 1966
6. Money J, Erhardt AA: Man and Woman, Boy and Girl. Baltimore, Johns Hopkins University Press, 1972

# Clinical
# Applications
# of Reproductive
# and Behavioral
# Science

# II

Part Two focuses upon the applied use of biologic and behavioral science in clinical practice, contraceptive development, and family planning programs. Chapter 5 discusses the incidence, etiology, evaluation, and treatment of male and female infertility, drawing on information presented in Chapters 1 and 2. Chapter 6 describes in detail available contraceptives, including their mechanisms of action, efficacy, advantages, disadvantages, and side effects; Chapter 7 describes contraceptive methods in the developmental phase, including vaccines; intrauterine, cervical, and vaginal devices; long-term injectables; prostaglandins; and male contraceptive agents. A review of immunology is also presented to maximize understanding of contraceptive vaccines. Sterilization is the topic of Chapter 8, in which the complications and sequelae of vasectomy, fallopian-tube occlusion, and hysterectomy are

considered. Choice of procedure and reversibility are also discussed. Procedures of pregnancy termination and the legal, ethical, demographic, and psychosocial considerations surrounding such events are summarized in Chapter 9.

The administration of family planning programs—from patient recruitment to funding sources, types of services provided, and differences between hospital-based and free-standing outpatient projects—are considered in Chapter 10. Methods of evaluating the effectiveness and efficiency of family planning programs follow, in Chapter 11. Attention is directed to overall program evaluation, including design of records with this purpose in mind, and to quality-care assessment of the medical services provided. The measurement of costs and benefits of family planning programs is addressed in Chapter 12.

# 5

## Infertility

**Marguerite K. Shepard**

In a society increasingly conscious of individual rights and the quality of life, infertility is beginning to assume an importance approaching that of excess fertility. The thrust of family planning services has been changed from that of population control to that of achieving ideal family size. To this end, infertility services are now being offered by the same agencies which formerly offered only contraception and sterilization services.

As a result of the combined forces of more liberal contraception and pregnancy-termination policies, and more liberal attitudes toward the rearing of out-of-wedlock children, the number of children available for adoption has decreased sharply. Thus, the proper diagnosis and management of fertility problems have become more crucial if every couple is to be permitted the option of child-rearing.

### INCIDENCE

Infertility occurs as either a primary complaint or as an incidental finding in approximately 15 per cent of couples having unprotected coitus for 1 year. Most studies indicate that about 65 per cent of couples will achieve conception within 3 months of regular unprotected coitus, another 10 per cent within 6 months, and a final 5 per cent at the end of 1 year. Another 5 per cent will achieve conception within the 2nd year of exposure (13, 21).

As strictly defined, infertility is the inability of a couple to achieve a pregnancy after 1 year of unprotected coitus. The condition is referred to as *primary* if there has been no history of a previous pregnancy, and *secondary* if there has been a previous pregnancy. For practical purposes, infertility could also be defined as the inability to carry a pregnancy to the stage of fetal viability, or repeated loss of viable infants in the perinatal or neonatal period.

In evaluating the infertile couple, it is most important that the condition be viewed as a joint, rather than an individual process. Although texts (32a) sometimes state that the female partner is "at fault" in 60 per cent of cases and the male in 40 per cent, there are many instances in which several small abnormal findings in each partner add up to an infertile state that might not exist if each were married to another, more fertile, individual.

The causes and treatment of infertility disorders in the individual will be discussed in anatomic and functional order, moving from the central to peripheral organs. This approach permits discussion of disorders in *1*) approximate order of occurrence, moving from the most to the least common, and *2*) in order of relative importance—for example, a basic function such as ovulation or spermatogenesis will be discussed first, since if it does not occur, the state of the rest of the reproductive tract is relatively unimportant.

Evaluation will be discussed from the standpoint of cyclic function, because cyclicity or tonicity determines, to a large extent, the timing of various tests.

### CAUSES

The most obvious cause of infertility is failure of the couple to have frequent successful intercourse. The definitions of the terms *frequent* and *successful,* as applied to infertility, have little to do with sexual satisfaction and gratification. The concern is rather with the likelihood that the couple's sexual practices will insure the presence of an adequate population of sperm in the female reproductive tract at the time of ovulation, thus permitting fertilization to occur. The available data suggests that couples who have at least two well-spaced episodes of coitus per week should demonstrate normal fertility, if no abnormalities are present. However, the speed with which conception occurs may be directly related to frequency of coitus (17). The "success" of the coital act refers to the likelihood that sperm will be deposited in the vagina in the vicinity of the cervix with each coital episode. Although pregnancies have been reported when ejaculation has occurred at the opening of, but not inside, the vagina, this practice (known as *premature ejaculation,* if it occurs prior to attempted penetration) is generally associated with infertility. Very infrequently, couples present for evaluation who do not realize that coitus is necessary in order for conception to occur (7). Such a situation arises rarely in these days of sexual enlightenment, but the possibility must never be overlooked. Thus, obtaining an adequate sexual history is an important part of the evaluation.

## THE FEMALE

Factors which may result in female infertility include: failure to ovulate on a regular basis, if at all; obstruction of the fallopian tubes, preventing conception; abnormalities of the uterine cavity or cervix, preventing satisfactory implantation and/or maintenance of pregnancy to the point of fetal viability; abnormal cervical mucus, preventing penetration by sperm; and various major anomalies involving absence of the ovaries, uterus, cervix, or vagina. Patients in this latter category generally have absence of menses as a presenting complaint long before their fertility status comes into question.

### ABSENCE OF REGULAR OVULATION

Absence of regular ovulation may accompany a variety of conditions. Emotional stress, such as that related to a change in environment, crisis in an interpersonal relationship, or pressure to assume a role for which the individual is unprepared, may often result in cessation of ovulation and regular menses. Rapid loss or gain in weight is also related to anovulation. Since a change in dietary habits is often stress-induced, it is difficult to say whether the

stress, or the actual weight change, effects the loss of cyclic ovarian function. Commonly, menses cease when the trend toward gain or loss has been established, but before a stable weight has been reached (28).

Persistent anovulation following the use of oral contraceptives is encountered with increasing frequency in infertility clinics because of the widespread use of these medications. The actual percentage of women who remain anovulatory after stopping birth control pills is quite small, less than 2.5 per cent. There also appears to be no relationship between the strength and type of pill used, or the duration of use and the occurrence of postpill anovulation. At least 30 per cent of women with amenorrhea following the cessation of pill use will report irregular menses prior to starting the pill, so that the failure to ovulate in these cases probably represents a preexisting condition (6, 10).

Most patients in the groups just discussed are not totally lacking in ovarian activity. The ovary secretes estrogen, or its precursors, but the cyclic relationships which result in orderly maturation of follicles and release of ova are interrupted. Generally, the degree of ovarian function is established by administering what is referred to as *progestin challenge.* If the ovary has been secreting estrogen, the uterine lining, or endometrium, will undergo growth. If a synthetic or natural progestin is administered, the lining will undergo orderly maturation, and slough after the effect of the hormone is withdrawn. This event is referred to as *progestin-withdrawal bleeding,* and those patients who demonstrate this phenomenon are referred to as *estrogen-primed.*

Some women who are not ovulating may have polycystic ovary disease. This disorder is characterized by a hormonal pattern of low levels of follicle-stimulating hormone (FSH), elevated levels of luteinizing hormone (LH), and relatively elevated levels of estrogen. The estrogen inhibits FSH secretion, thus preventing proper growth of a follicle to the point of ovulation. Instead, the ovary contains multiple cystic follicles. LH stimulates the ovarian stroma to make estrogen or its precursors, and thus a vicious cycle is established.

Evidence for ovarian function can be seen in estrogen-responsive tissues, especially the cervix and the vaginal mucosa. The former will produce clear, watery mucus and the latter will be pale pink, thick, and well-lubricated. Absence of estrogen stimulation is generally characterized by scanty cervical mucus and very thin, red vaginal mucosa. Patients exhibiting these findings will often complain of painful intercourse and lack of libido.

Patients who are anovulatory and fail to demonstrate estrogen stimulation generally have a much more serious disturbance than lack of ovarian cycling. Lack of estrogen is the result of inability of the ovary to respond to the usual stimuli for hormone synthesis (*ovarian failure*), or lack of the usual stimuli to hormone synthesis (*hypothalamic-pituitary* failure).

Ovarian failure occurs normally at menopause. The term *premature menopause* is applied to cases in which ovarian failure occurs before the age of forty (9). Failure to respond to pituitary stimulation occurs because the ovary has exhausted its supply of ova, or, at least, its supply of responsive ovum-bearing follicles. Other causes of ovarian failure are high doses of radiation, or chemical agents used to treat malignancies. These agents eradicate the population of responsive follicles. Patients with ovarian failure are not amenable to treatment with current methods.

Hypothalamic-pituitary failure may occur as the result of a tumor, use of oral contraceptives, certain inherited disorders, and severe blood loss following delivery. Patients in the last category present with secondary infertility.

### FALLOPIAN-TUBE OBSTRUCTION

Fallopian-tube obstruction generally results from tubal infection, especially from gonorrhea (36). Some degree of obstruction may be caused by a condition known as *endometriosis.* In this disorder, implants of tissue which normally constitutes the uterine lining are found growing throughout the pelvis. If the tubes become adherent to such a growth, normal ovum-transport patterns are altered. Nonreproductive-tract abdominal infections, such as appendicitis with rupture, can also cause tubal obstruction. A third category of patients with tubal obstruction are women who have undergone voluntary tubal occlusive surgery for sterilization, and subsequently seek restoration of fertility.

### ABNORMALITIES OF THE UTERINE CAVITY AND CERVIX

Uterine problems which may result in some degree of infertility include: fibroid tumors which project into the uterine cavity; scarring from previous uterine surgery, such as dilatation and curettage for therapeutic, or criminal, abortion; and fusion anomalies of the uterus, forming septa (partitions) of varying lengths down the center of the cavity. Cervical incompetence may result in inability to carry a pregnancy to the point of fetal viability. In this condition, the fibers of the cervix have become weakened, usually by previous trauma, so that dilatation, or opening, occurs when the uterine contents become heavy enough to exert pressure.

### ABNORMAL CERVICAL MUCUS

Cervical mucus is an essential factor in normal sperm transport. Its consistency may be altered by chronic infection, or by lack of response of the glands to usual hormonal stimulation. In either case the mucus may be impenetrable to sperm during the periovulatory period, and thus a cause of infertility.

### THE MALE

Causes of infertility in the male have superficial parallels to those in the female, but there are significant differences related to the basic differences in germ-cell maturation and hormonal function in the testis and ovary.

Development of ova is a slow but continuous process of maturation and regression of small cohorts of follicles, which actually begins in the female fetus in utero, about halfway through pregnancy (27). Actual release of ova from the ovary does not begin until after the onset of menses. The hormonal function of the ovary is intimately dependent on the presence of responsive follicles. Because the process of ovum development is such a slow one, the population of ova is relatively resistant to destruction by such agents as infection, chemotherapeutic drugs, and low doses of radiation. If the fallopian tubes become blocked, either from infection or from intentional sterilization, the ovary continues to function normally, as far as ovulation is concerned. The ova are simply released into the peritoneal cavity.

In the male, spermatogenesis begins only at puberty, but is a continuous, active, dynamic process. New spermatozoa are formed daily. However, the hormonal function of the testis is not dependent on normal spermatogenesis. Thus, if the entire germinal epithelium (sperm-producing tissue) is destroyed, normal hormonal function continues, even though the individual is infertile.

Because spermatogenesis is a dynamic process, the germinal epithelium is relatively easily destroyed, either partially or totally, by infections, irradiation, and chemotherapeutic agents. Because sperm are produced in great numbers and have no egress from the testis other than through the ductile system, obstruction of the ejaculatory ducts can eventually result in partial or total destruction of the germinal epithelium (31).

### FAILURE TO PRODUCE SPERM

As in the case of the ovary, failure of the testis to produce sperm may result from failure of the pituitary gland to appropriately stimulate the testis, or from inability of the testis to respond to pituitary stimulation, because of absence of the germinal epithelium.

Pituitary failure in the male may be caused by congenital absence of the tissues in the hypothalamus and/or pituitary which secrete the gonad-stimulating hormones. Such conditions can be hereditary, or sporadic. As in the female, pituitary failure can also be caused by tumors (34).

Absence of germinal epithelium occurs in some congenital disorders, such as Klinefelter's syndrome and the Sertoli-cell-only syndrome. Destruction of the germinal epithelium can be caused by mumps, severe gonococcal infections, irradiation, cancer chemotherapy, and injury to the testis, with compromise of the blood supply (2).

Retention of the testis in the abdominal cavity (*cryptorchidism*) past early childhood can also cause total, permanent destruction of the germinal epithelium. As normal spermatogenesis in the human takes place only at temperatures that are several degrees lower than body temperature, it is presumed that the elevated temperature of the abdominal cavity causes the damage.

### PRODUCTION OF ABNORMAL SPERM

Production of abnormal sperm can also result from infection, irradiation, chemotherapy, and trauma, if the insult has been only of moderate severity. Testicular tumors also result in abnormal spermatogenesis, on both the affected and the normal side. A common cause

of production of abnormal sperm is *varicocele* (varicosities of the veins draining the scrotum). This condition is felt by some to elevate scrotal temperature and by others to permit backflow of adrenal hormones into the testis, with a resulting toxic effect on spermatogenesis (2).

Tight clothing, such as "jockey" shorts and tight jeans, have been cited as a cause of abnormal sperm production because they may elevate scrotal temperature. However, these factors must be looked upon as relative. They may make a difference in the individual who has a borderline sperm count, but probably have little effect in the normal population.

### LOW SPERM COUNT

*Oligospermia* (low sperm count) may result from partial destruction of the germinal epithelium, or from inadequate hormonal stimulation by the pituitary gland (2). Some cases of oligospermia may also be caused by hypothyroidism. Although hormonal function of the testis can continue in the absence of spermatogenesis, the converse is not true. Testosterone is especially important in normal sperm maturation. If levels are low, oligosperma may result. Normal hormonal function of the testis, with constant oligospermia, may also result from chronic liver disease. Since the liver is an important metabolic deactivating site for steroid hormones, liver damage results in relative suppression of the gonadotropin-secreting cells in the pituitary, because gonadal hormone levels in the blood remain elevated.

### OBSTRUCTION OF THE OUTFLOW TRACT

Obstruction of the epididymis or vas deferens may be congenital, or acquired secondary to infection or vas ligation. Congenital absence of the ejaculatory ducts is rare. It is more commonly partial than total, but even in the latter circumstance there is often insufficient tissue to permit the surgeon to effect repair. The most common infectious cause of vas or epididymal obstruction is gonorrhea. The intended obstruction of vasectomy may cause a secondary obstruction in the epididymis because of pressure-induced rupture, followed by scarring (31) (see Chap. 8). As mentioned previously, the pressure can cause eventual destruction of the germinal epithelium.

## ALTERATIONS IN THE INNERVATION OF THE PELVIS

The nerve supply of the male pelvis is such that the processes of erection and orgasm require different innervation than those involved in ejaculation. For this reason, such events as spinal cord injury, prostate surgery, aortic lymph node dissection (with attendant neurologic damage), and the use of certain medications, may have differing effects on male reproductive capacity (14, 15).

Erection and orgasm without ejaculation of sperm or seminal plasma occurs commonly in men who have had para-aortic lymph node dissection for lymphoma, and in men taking guanethidine for control of hypertension. In these instances the nerve supply to the vasa deferentia, the prostate, and the seminal vesicles have been interrupted (14, 15).

In some spinal cord injuries, and in neurologic disease such as multiple sclerosis, erection and orgasm are impaired, but ejaculation can be accomplished by masturbation.

Retrograde ejaculation (ejaculation into the bladder) may occur after prostatic surgery and following spinal cord injury. In such cases sperm may be found in the urine following orgasm or masturbation.

### ABNORMAL SEMINAL PLASMA, AND SPERM ANTIBODIES

Abnormal seminal plasma is a common concomitant of prostate infection. Such infections may often be subacute or chronic, and thus asymptomatic. These infections tend to be nonspecific in nature—that is, they can be caused by a number of different organisms. They usually do not have a deleterious effect on the individual's general health, but the presence of the infection in the seminal plasma may impair sperm viability.

Sperm antibodies have been the subject of much investigation in recent years (29). The antibodies thus far described may cause either agglutination (clumping together) or immobilization of the spermatozoa, presumably interfering with the movement of sperm to the upper reaches of the female reproductive tract, so that they are unable to reach the ovum. They may be found in the serum of both men and women. Sperm antibodies are frequently found in males following vasectomy (see Chaps. 2 and 8). Antibodies to sperm have also been found at varying sites along the female reproductive tract. These antibodies appear to represent a local, rather than a systemic response to foreign protein. Their relative importance as a cause of infertility is unclear at this time (5).

## EVALUATION

The purpose of the infertility evaluation is to determine, by the taking of a history, physical examination, and appropriate testing, which of the known causes can be implicated or exculpated in the case under study. As a general principle, all major possibilities are considered, regardless of their probability, in order to eliminate unsuspected factors.

Under ideal circumstances, both members of the couple seeking infertility evaluation would undergo initial history and physical examination together. In actuality, such an event happens rarely, since the male and female partners seldom appear for treatment at the same time. Usually the female partner seeks evaluation because she is the symptomatic member of the couple—that is, she has not become pregnant. Occasionally the male will seek evaluation first because of some suspicion that he may be infertile. He may, for example, have experienced an episode of venereal disease or testicular trauma, or may have failed to impregnate any of several partners, in spite of inadequate contraception. Since a person who is fertile (infertile) within one relationship may be infertile (fertile) with another partner, it is important to emphasize that all statements regarding fertility are only valid within the context of the couple under study, and that evaluation of a single individual can only provide qualified answers.

### HISTORY

An adequate history is the cornerstone of fertility evaluation. For the couple as a unit, this includes information about the duration of infertility, both planned and unplanned (for example, a couple may have been desirous of pregnancy for 1 year, but may have been practicing inadequate contraception for the preceding 5 years, thus making the actual duration of infertility 6 years), and sexual habits, including frequency of intercourse, probability of satisfactory sperm deposition, and use of lubricants.

For the female, adequate history includes

age at onset of menses, cycle length, duration of menses, previous contraceptive use, history of pelvic infection or surgery, presence or absence of pain during menses and/or intercourse, abnormal menstrual patterns, reproductive history, and chronic illness.

For the male, points of importance in the history include childhood infection with possible testicular involvement (most commonly, mumps); postnatal descent of the testes; age at puberty; previous genital infection, such as orchitis, epididymitis, prostatitis, or urethritis; previous testicular trauma; chronic use of tight trousers; periods of impotence or failure to ejaculate, with or without orgasm; and chronic illness.

## PHYSICAL EXAMINATION

A complete physical examination should be carried out in each partner. In both sexes particular attention is paid to general body habitus—distribution of hair, body fat, and muscle mass—as there are characteristic patterns of distribution related to sex. Particular attention is paid to development of secondary sex characteristics, such as breasts.

Careful examination of the internal and external genitalia is mandatory. In the female, particular attention is paid to clitoral size; possible abnormalities of the hymenal opening; presence or absence of vagina, uterus, and tubes; appropriateness of the cervical mucus in relation to the time of the menstrual cycle; size, shape, consistency, mobility, and position of the uterus; and presence or absence of abnormalities of the ovaries and tubes. A rectovaginal examination is included, to evaluate the lowermost portion of the pelvis, which lies between the vagina and rectum, and may be important as a reservoir for sperm and as a site of ovum pickup.

In the male, testicular size is of greater importance than penile size, but the penis must be examined carefully for abnormal placement of the urethral meatus and possible adherence of the foreskin, in uncircumsized men. The scrotum must be examined for abnormalities of venous drainage (varicocele) and the testes evaluated for size, shape, consistency, and presence or absence of masses. A rectal examination is also mandatory in the male to evaluate the size and consistency of the prostate.

The information obtained from both his-

tory and physical examination is used to formulate a working diagnosis. Appropriate laboratory tests are then selected to confirm this diagnosis. Certain examinations are considered standard, regardless of the presumptive diagnosis. However, many of the more expensive and specialized examinations need not be regarded as routine, but are employed only in certain cases.

## TESTING

### THE FEMALE

Routine evaluation for the female includes testing for patency of the fallopian tubes, evaluation of the cervical mucus just before ovulation (to determine its favorability for sperm transport), and confirmation that ovulation routinely occurs. In the normally menstruating woman, these tests must be conducted at specific times during the menstrual cycle, in order for the data to be valid.

**Tubal Patency Tests.** Evaluation of tubal patency (that is, of whether the tubes are open) is carried out after the menses have ceased, but before the presumed time of ovulation. This segment of the cycle is chosen to avoid the dual hazards of forcing menstrual fragments back through the tube during examination, which could cause endometriosis or interference with ovum transport, causing tubal or abdominal pregnancy.

The three major techniques available for the evaluation of tubal patency are the Rubin test, hysterosalpingography and endoscopy. The Rubin test involves injection of $CO_2$ through the cervix into the uterine cavity and measurement of the passage of the gas through the tubes and into the abdominal cavity with pressure gauge. This evaluation can be carried out in the physician's office. It is the simplest of the techniques to perform, but also the least accurate.

Hysterosalpingography is a more accurate technique than the Rubin test. This study involves injection of radiopaque dye through the cervical canal into the uterus. It provides considerably more information than the Rubin test, but requires the use of x-ray. Although both of these examinations indicate whether the tube is patent, neither will identify peritubal adhesions around the tube with any degree of accuracy.

Endoscopy, or direct visualization of the pelvis with a fiberoptic telescope, is the best method available for the evaluation of tubal patency and mobility. The pelvis may be visualized via a puncture incision through the posterior portion of the vagina (*culdoscopy*), or via an infraumbilical incision (*laparoscopy*). The former technique may be performed satisfactorily under local anesthesia, but provides only a limited view of the pelvis, and may not be performed if there are adhesions present. The latter technique requires general anesthesia, but permits a panoramic view of the entire pelvis, as well as close visualization of adhesions around the fallopian tube, and between the tube and the ovary, which may interfere with ovum pickup and transport. Endoscopy is usually not performed until all other testing has been completed. It is generally reserved for those cases in which tubal disease is strongly suspected or those cases in which no factor has been identified in either partner.

**Postcoital Test.** The Huhner-Sims, or postcoital test, is the name given to the evaluation of cervical mucus. This examination is performed within several hours of intercourse in the period immediately before ovulation, since that is the time when cervical mucus is most favorable for sperm transport. The mucus is evaluated for certain physical and chemical properties, in addition to being observed for numbers of motile sperm. The glands which secrete cervical mucus are responsive to the hormonal output of the ovary. The secretion of estrogen by a developing ovarian follicle causes the mucus to increase in water content and to decrease in cell content. At the mid-cycle, just at the time of ovulation, the mucus bears a strong physical resemblance to egg white. It is clear, copious, and watery. If drawn out in a syringe, it forms a long thread (Spinnbarkeit) and, if permitted to dry on a glass slide, the salts in the mucus form a distinctive, fernlike pattern. The mucus is alkaline, to a degree similar to that of seminal plasma. In optimal mid-cycle mucus, at least 6 to 12 actively motile sperm should be seen in each high-power microscopic field within 2 hours of intercourse.

Once ovulation has occurred, the secretion of progesterone by the corpus luteum causes the mucus to become cloudy, thick, and gummy in consistency, thus impeding sperm transport. Poor cervical mucus may be thick, cloudy, and full of white blood cells (suggesting infection) or clear but scanty, with poor Spinnbarkeit, and filled with epithelial cells (suggesting poor response of the glands to estrogen, or perhaps suboptimal estrogen stimulation).

**Confirmation of Presumptive Ovulation.** The positive confirmation of ovulation requires either visualization of the ovulation process, recovery of an ovum, or pregnancy. Since the two former techniques are impractical on a routine basis, and the latter has generally eluded the couple under study, the examiner is left with the presumptive establishment of ovulation by indirect means. There are four techniques for ascertaining presumptive ovulation, all of which depend on the fact that the corpus luteum secretes progesterone following ovulation. The most common, and simplest technique is observation of a rise in the basal body temperature (first morning temperature), which occurs 18 to 24 hours after ovulation and persists until 1 or 2 days prior to the onset of menses. In point of fact, it requires less progesterone to raise the basal body temperature than that which is secreted by the normal corpus luteum. Paradoxically, it has been estimated that fully 20 per cent of women who ovulate do not show a biphasic basal body temperature curve (20).

Another technique for detecting progesterone secretion is vaginal cytology. Cells are scraped from the vaginal wall with a spatula similar to that used for obtaining a pap smear. They are spread on a slide fixed, stained, and then evaluated for degree of maturation. The type of cells shed by the vaginal mucosa will reflect the amount of estrogen in, or the estrogen-progesterone balance of, the environment. Unfortunately this technique is only reliable if performed on a daily basis, and consequently is not practical in the usual infertility evaluation.

The most commonly used technique for confirmation of presumptive ovulation is the endometrial biopsy. This is ideally performed about 9 to 12 days after the presumed time of ovulation. The objective is to observe changes in the structure of the uterine lining or endometrium which normally occur in response to progesterone. This technique involves introducing a 4-mm. diameter hollow curette through the cervix into the uterine cavity. Near the uterine end of the curette, there is an opening surrounded by serrations. Negative pressure is applied to the other end to pull a small amount of tissue into the opening in the uterine end of the curette. The tissue is then pulled away by a swift, scraping motion. This technique is a simple one which may be performed in the physician's office, but it may be accompanied by severe cramping.

The simplest, and probably most reliable method of confirmation of presumptive ovulation is determination of the level of progesterone in the patient's blood. This test is ideally performed 5 to 9 days after the presumed time of ovulation, when progesterone levels are the highest. In spite of its accuracy, it is not yet in general use. Many commercial laboratories do not perform the test, and those which do tend to charge exhorbitant prices, discouraging use by the average practitioner.

In women who are anovulatory, all of the tests mentioned already are conducted to identify possible additional factors which could contribute to infertility. Because these patients are acyclic, it is possible to conduct all of the necessary fertility tests at the same visit. Many of these patients are in a constant state of estrogen stimulation, unopposed by progesterone. For this reason, the cervical mucus should almost always be favorable for sperm transport. Since these patients do not ovulate, interference with ovum transport is not a consideration. Thus, a Rubin test for tubal patency may be carried out with impunity. Finally, even though confirmation of ovulation is not a consideration, the endometrium should always be sampled. Patients who are subject to constant unopposed estrogen are at risk for uncontrolled growth of the endometrium (hyperplasia), which may be a precursor of endometrial cancer.

The proper sequence for performing the various fertility tests when they are planned for a single visit is as follows: *1*) postcoital test, before the mucus is disturbed by probing the uterus, *2*) tubal patency test, and, finally, *3*) endometrial biopsy, because bleeding and fragmentation of tissue will result from this procedure.

**THE MALE**

**Semen Analysis.** Evaluation of the male begins with semen analysis. If all values are normal, further evaluation is deferred until all testing of the female has been completed. If the analysis is abnormal, a repeat is requested, usually after a lapse of 1 or 2 months. This lapse is related to the cycle of spermatogenesis. The maturation time from the most immature to the most mature state, is 70 to 76 days (35a) (see Chap. 1 for further details). Incidents such as trauma or a viral illness may affect spermatogenesis temporarily, and a lapse of at least 1 month must be expected before any change can be anticipated. If two analyses are abnormal, further investigation of the male is initiated. If one is abnormal and one is normal, a third sample is usually collected to ascertain the modal pattern.

The normal values for a semen analysis, or (stated another way) the criteria for a fertile ejaculate have been the subject of much debate in recent years. Standards are usually ascertained by examining prevasectomy ejaculates from men of proven fertility (16, 22, 38).

The ejaculate is evaluated for volume, sperm concentration, total sperm count, pH (degree of acidity or alkalinity), motility and morphology of the sperm, liquefaction time, and presence or absence of red and white blood cells. Specific patterns do not always correlate with a specific disease process, but they will indicate the appropriate direction for further study.

Some currently accepted values for fertile ejaculates are discussed in Chapter 3.

**Hormone Evaluation.** Evaluation of the individual's hormonal status is indicated if azoospermia (absence of sperm) or oligospermia (low sperm count) is detected on repeated semen analyses. If hypothyroidism is suspected on the basis of clinical findings, evaluation of thyroid function by thyroid-stimulating hormone (TSH) or $T_3T_4$ is indicated to establish the diagnosis. If thyroid function is normal, the function of the hypothalamic-pituitary-testicular axis may be evaluated by obtaining follicle-stimulating hormone (FSH) and testosterone levels. FSH stimulates the germinal epithelium (19). The germinal epithelium, in turn, controls FSH secretion by secretion of a protein hormone called inhibin (4). If the germinal epithelium has been partially or totally destroyed, inhibin secretion will be severely curtailed, and FSH levels may be elevated. On the other hand, if FSH levels are very low, spermatogenesis may be poor, because of lack of appropriate stimulation of the germinal epithelium. Finally, testosterone is important for sperm maturation. If testosterone levels are abnormally low, the sperm count may also be low, with a large number of immature forms (4).

**Testicular Biopsy.** Although more data is accumulating that the hormonal pattern in the blood correlates well with the histologic findings in the testis, there is still enough disagreement to justify the use of testicular biopsy in the diagnosis of oligospermia and azoospermia (1). The biopsy is an office procedure which can be performed under local anesthesia, utilizing a special hollow needle. The biopsy is evaluated to determine presence or absence of the germinal epithelium, Sertoli cells, and Leydig cells.

**Vasogram.** A vasogram is a dye-contrast x-ray study of the ejaculatory ducts which is carried out if obstruction or congenital absence of the vas is suspected. It is generally performed if the patient has repeated azoospermic ejaculates but normal spermatogenesis on biopsy.

## TREATMENT

Treatment of infertility has greatly increased in sophistication during the last several years. One of the by-products of contraceptive research has been a greater understanding of the causes and treatment of infertility.

## THE FEMALE

### ANOVULATION

If the female does not ovulate, it must be ascertained whether or not her ovary is capable of responding if appropriately stimulated. The patient with ovarian failure is hopelessly infertile because there are no ova remaining.

There are two medications available for treatment of anovulation in which the cause is lack of cyclic stimulation of the ovary, or hypothalamic-pituitary failure. The first of these is a tablet medication called clomiphene citrate.

Patients who are in a state of constant estrogen stimulation have a block in the feedback mechanism which normally causes release of follicle-stimulating hormone from the pituitary. The exact mechanism of action of clomiphene is unknown, but it does compete with estrogen for receptor sites. Because it is a weak estrogen, it does not inhibit FSH release to the extent that estrogen does, and therefore follicular growth is stimulated, followed by ovulation. Patients who are anovulatory, but not estrogen-primed, presumably do not have an estrogen block in the feedback mechanism as the cause of their anovulation. As would be expected, clomiphene therapy is less successful in this group of patients than in those who are estrogen-primed. Clomiphene is of no use in patients who suffer from congenital or disease-related absence of pituitary function.

Clomiphene is administered according to a graduated treatment regimen, starting with one 50-mg. tablet daily for 5 days, working up to a maximum of five tablets. The customary course of treatment is prescribed for about 5 days each month. The dose is increased with each treatment cycle until ovulation results. Although approximately 70 per cent of patients who are given medication can be expected to ovulate, only about 50 per cent will conceive (3).

The multiple-pregnancy rate with clomiphene is approximately 10 per cent, and most of these are twin pregnancies. The spontaneous abortion or miscarriage rate is about 20 per cent. The incidence of birth defects in clomiphene-induced pregnancies is no greater than that in the general population (3).

Patients who do not respond to clomiphene are candidates for treatment with human menopausal gonadotrophin (HMG). This medication consists of the two pituitary hormones, follicle-stimulating hormone (FSH), and luteinizing hormone (LH), which are responsible for stimulation of follicular growth and of hormone synthesis in the ovary. The medication is a naturally occurring substance which is extracted from the urine of postmenopausal women.

HMG is an injectable medication. It has a greater potential for the causing of harmful side effects, such as hyperstimulation of the ovary and multiple pregnancy, than does clomiphene. HMG acts directly on the ovary, and thus bypasses the usual system of checks and balances that exists in the woman with a normal cycle to prevent maturation of more than one follicle per cycle.

In spontaneously ovulating women, or women who ovulate in response to clomiphene, the entire process of follicular development is controlled by a sensitive feedback system in which the amount of estrogen secreted by the developing follicle influences the amount of stimulating hormone secreted by the hypothalamus and pituitary. When an estrogen level is reached which corresponds to the output of an imminently preovulatory follicle, the secretion of stimulating hormone is automatically decreased, thus depriving other, less developed, follicles of the hormone necessary for further growth. In this way, the human reproductive system ensures that only one follicle will ovulate per cycle under ordinary circumstances. Patients who are given HMG generally require it because the hypothalamic-pituitary portion of the axis is incapable of responding properly. Thus the physician administering the drug must take over the fail-safe role ordinarily assumed by the hypothalamus.

The dose must be adjusted to each patient's individual response. This response must be measured daily to prevent overdosing. The most satisfactory way to gauge response is by measuring the blood estrogen level. This fact necessarily limits use of HMG to centers where such an assay is available daily at low cost. Estrogen-related changes in cervical mucus and ovarian size are measured daily. Even with careful monitoring, multiple pregnancies do occur. The multiple-pregnancy rate is as high as 30 per cent, in some studies (24). However, the incidence of congenital anomalies is no greater than that in the general population.

The pregnancy rate with HMG-therapy is approximately 30 per cent. However, because the medication is very expensive, many patients abandon therapy before an adequate trial has been given. Thus, the quoted success rate may be spuriously low.

**OBSTRUCTION AND RECONSTRUCTION OF THE FALLOPIAN TUBES**

Pregnancy rates with tubal reconstruction are no better than those for ovulation induction, and in many cases are worse.

The prognosis depends to a great extent on the degree of distortion which must be corrected, and on the realization that patency is but a part of normal tubal function.

Tubal disease is generally divided into four major categories, depending on the area of involvement of each tube. The simplest disorder to correct is that involving fine adhesions which may alter tubal mobility without actually occluding the tube, or which may sur-

round the opening of the tube, keeping it physically separated from the ovary and thus interfere with ovum transport. When lysis of such adhesions is the only surgery required, pregnancy rates in the range of 60 per cent may be achieved (12).

Distal tubal obstruction, or fimbrial occlusion, represents a more severe disease with a much poorer prognosis. In such cases, the fimbriae, which are very specialized appendages of the tube, designed for ovum pickup, are totally or partially destroyed. Reopening of the tube does not replace the fimbriae, and thus pregnancy rates usually do not exceed 25 per cent (11, 34).

Reconstruction of the isthmic, or mid-portion, of the fallopian tube is usually required only in women who have undergone previous tubal sterilization, since most disease processes involving the fallopian tube do not limit themselves to the isthmic portion. Success rates as high as 50 per cent have been reported with conventional surgery, probably because the tissue is otherwise healthy (30).

The cornual area, or uterotubal junction, is the fourth area in which tubal obstruction commonly occurs. Such obstruction is often the sequel of an intrauterine infection, and thus does not usually involve the other portions of the tube. The usual approach to repair involves creation of a new intramural canal, followed by reimplantation of the patent portion of the tube in the canal. Success rates as high as 50 per cent have been reported with this procedure (25).

The need for using rather coarse instruments and materials on very delicate tissue has always been a major problem in tubal surgery. With the development of the operating microscope, tubal microsurgery (using extremely fine materials) has been perfected. Although it is too early to say, initial reports indicate that higher pregnancy rates will be obtainable with these techniques (10). Since the new techniques require very specialized training, it appears that tubal surgery will gradually become the province of the superspecialist, and not part of the average gynecologic surgeon's repertoire.

**UTERINE ABNORMALITIES**

Uterine surgery for infertility is performed much less commonly than tubal surgery. Anomalies of the uterus, such as septa or blind horns, are not corrected unless they prevent delivery of a viable infant. Repeated premature deliveries do not warrant a repair procedure unless the infants are too immature to survive. Repair procedures usually require a large incision in the uterus, going through the entire thickness in order to remove a septum or a tumor. Such incisions may weaken the wall of the uterus, so that rupture could conceivably occur during pregnancy or labor. Many obstetricians feel that a woman should be limited to no more than two pregnancies after such a procedure, and that delivery should be accomplished by cesarean section (8).

Surgery for postabortal intrauterine adhesions is performed via the vagina and cervix and does not carry the same risk as that for correcting fusion anomalies or for removal of tumors. The most satisfactory approach to correction is to remove the adhesions under direct vision, using an instrument called the hysteroscope (18). This condition may be increasing in incidence because of liberalized abortion policies. The underlying process which leads to the formation of adhesions is destruction of the basal layer of the uterine lining by overly vigorous curettage, or by infection. If the basal layer of the endometrium is destroyed, the myometrium, or muscular layer of the uterus, is exposed. Because the anterior and posterior uterine walls lie in apposition, the exposed muscle layers will become adherent to one another if the protective endometrial layer is absent.

Ordinarily, cyclic regeneration of the lining after sloughing begins from the basal layer. Once the adhesions are removed, it is necessary to place some object in the cavity temporarily, to prevent adhesions from reforming. A catheter or an intrauterine device is generally employed for this purpose (18). In addition, the patient is placed on rather high doses of estrogen, as this hormone stimulates growth of the endometrial tissue. This is done on the premise that small islands of basal tissue still remain, which were prevented from coalescing and lining the uterine cavity while adhesions were present. The subsequent pregnancy rate following this procedure is approximately 50 per cent, but varies from report to report (18).

## REPAIR OF INCOMPETENT CERVIX

Cervical incompetence may be treated with a variety of procedures, all of which are variations on the same theme. Since the basic anatomic defect lies at the level of the internal cervical opening, or os, some type of natural or synthetic supporting material is tied around the cervix at this point. Usually, this material is partially, or totally, buried beneath the mucosal covering of the cervix. The suture-ligature (or tie) may be placed early in the second trimester of pregnancy, after fetal viability is established, or prior to conception, if it is anticipated that placement of the ligature will be particularly difficult. Method of delivery depends on the intended permanence of the suture. Most sutures are utilized for a single pregnancy, and are replaced with each subsequent pregnancy. The suture is cut at the onset of labor to permit vaginal delivery without tearing the cervix. Some sutures are intended to be permanent, because satisfactory placement is difficult. Such patients require delivery by cesarean section.

## ABNORMAL CERVICAL MUCUS

Hostile cervical mucus may be treated either with antibiotics, if infection appears to be the cause, or with estrogen, if the cause appears to be estrogen-deficiency. Infection is indicated by the persistent appearance of white blood cells in the mucus in the preovulatory phase of the cycle; these cells normally appear in the cervical mucus after ovulation. Attempts to culture the offending organism are usually not very successful. In the past, it was common practice to cauterize the cervix, if infection persisted. This procedure tends to be counterproductive, as the mucus-secreting glands may be destroyed, leaving no mucus for transport.

If the mucus is continually unfavorable and there is no sign of infection, the patient may benefit from estrogen therapy. A low dose of estrogen is given by mouth for 5 to 10 days prior to, and including, the presumed time of ovulation. The exogenous estrogen may have the effect of decreasing the amount of follicle-stimulating hormone secreted by the pituitary, thus delaying the follicular maturation process. As a result, some women will experience a delay in ovulation of several days while on this therapy.

## THE MALE

Male infertility is far more difficult to treat than female infertility. Far less is known about the hormonal relationships involved in normal spermatogenesis than those which affect normal ovulation. There are a few conditions for which there is well-recognized treatment, but in many cases treatment is almost empiric.

### VARICOCELE LIGATION

Varicocele ligation is one of the most commonly performed surgical procedures for correction of male infertility. Men who suffer from a varicocele (varicose veins of the scrotum) have an ejaculate that is characterized by a low count, poor motility, and a moderate percentage of abnormal forms, especially spermatozoa with tapered heads. With ligation (tying off) of the varicocele, scrotal temperature returns to normal. After this procedure, the pregnancy rate is about 50 per cent (2). However, not all men with a varicocele are infertile, and many men with a spermogram typical for varicocele have no identifiable venous abnormality of the scrotum.

### HORMONAL MEDICATION

Many men are treated empirically with thyroid medication to improve spermatogenesis, but few have demonstrable thyroid hypofunction.

Clomiphene and HMG, used to treat anovulation, have been used in the treatment of abnormal spermatogenesis, with variable success. Again, this method of treatment is somewhat empiric, as the exact mechanism of action of these agents in the male is poorly understood. Success rates are far lower than those achieved with the same drugs in treatment of female infertility.

When the problem is an isolated one, of low count with normal motility and morphology, artificial insemination of the female, using a concentrate of the male partner's semen, is quite successful. Concentration is achieved by having the male collect a split ejaculate, that is, an ejaculate collected in two different portions. Since most of the sperm are expelled in the very first portion of the ejaculate (2), an attempt is made to collect this portion separately from the rest. The concentrated semen is then injected through a syringe and a plastic catheter directly into the cervical canal of the female.

Because the degree of concentration of sperm in the seminal plasma, and not total volume of ejaculate, determines fertility, this same effect can be achieved through the practice of coitus interruptus, or withdrawal. With this method withdrawal is performed immediately following the first ejaculatory surge, depositing only the sperm-rich portion of the ejaculate in the vagina. Success rates as high as 50 per cent have been reported (2).

### CORRECTION OF VAS OBSTRUCTION

Treatment of vas obstruction, whether it is congenital, caused by inflammation, or the result of sterilization, is less successful. As is the case with tubal-obstruction disease in women, mere patency is not the total answer. Many men will have alterations in spermatogenesis after an obstructive process. Animal experimentation in primates has demonstrated that rupture and subsequent inflammation, with obstruction, in the vas deferens and/or epididymis, will be caused by the backup of sperm between the testis and the initial point of obstruction, especially following vasectomy (31). Thus there may be multiple sites of obstruction, making repair difficult.

### INFECTIONS AND NEUROLOGIC DISEASE

Acute or chronic prostatitis, or inflammation of the prostate gland, may be a cause of male infertility. As is the case with cervicitis, an organism may not always be identified, but the condition usually responds to empiric use of broad-spectrum antibiotics.

Inability to achieve or maintain an erection, or to ejaculate, may be either a transient or a permanent phenomenon. As previously mentioned, alterations in the innervation of the pelvis may interfere with erection or ejaculation. Situational stress, medication, alcoholism, and some neurologic disorders may predispose the individual to temporary loss of these functions, while severe diabetes, spinal cord injury, and radical pelvic surgery commonly result in their permanent loss.

### ARTIFICIAL INSEMINATION

Individuals who are azospermic (without sperm), as demonstrated by testicular biopsy, cannot be made fertile. In such situations, donor insemination performed during the fertile period of the woman's cycle may be offered. Donor-insemination practices differ from state to state, and from institution to institution. Either fresh or frozen semen may be used. Frozen semen offers convenience, and the opportunity to screen for venereal disease before use, and is less expensive than fresh semen. However, motility tends to decrease with the freezing and thawing process. On the average, one more cycle is required to achieve conception with frozen semen than with fresh (33). Some physicians mix semen from the male partner with that of the donor, in order to leave open the possibility that conception resulted from the partner's sperm. This practice should be discouraged, because agents in the partner's seminal plasma may cause abnormal motility of the donor sperm, thus defeating the purpose of artificial insemination (26).

### SPERM ANTIBODIES

Couples who demonstrate sperm antibodies generally have a fair to poor prognosis. If the female demonstrates antibodies, use of condom contraception for 6 months to temporarily remove the antigenic stimulus has been reported to have a success rate of 50 per cent (33). If the male partner produces antibodies to his own sperm, the prognosis is much worse. Some success has been reported with the use of cortisone and its derivatives, but a success rate of 20 per cent hardly appears to justify the possible side effects of such therapy (29).

## UNEXPLAINED INFERTILITY

Finally, there are some couples in whom no abnormality can be demonstrated. Such couples cannot be considered normal, but one can only surmise that subtle factors are operating which cannot be identified by currently available techniques. In such cases, one must be wary of embarking on an extensive course of costly medications without a real indication of need. Patients with a fertility problem are often desperate enough to agree to any plan proposed, and it is up to the physician to exercise sound judgement.

## REFERENCES

1. Aafjes JH, van der Vijver JCM, Docter R, Schenck PE: Serum gonadotrophins, testosterone, and spermatogenesis in subfertile men. Acta Endocrinol (Kbh) 86:651, 1977
2. Amelar RD, Dubin L: Male infertility: current diagnosis and treatment. Urology 1:1, 1973
3. Asch RH, Greenblatt RB: Update on the safety and efficacy of clomiphene citrate as a therapeutic agent. J Reprod Med 17:175, 1976
4. Baker HWG, Bremner WJ, Burger HG, de Kretser DM, Dulmanis A, Eddie LW, Hudson B, Keogh EJ, Lee VWK, Rennie GC: Testicular control of follicle stimulating hormone secretion. Recent Prog Horm Res 32:429, 1976
5. Beer AM, Neaves WB: Antigenic status of semen from the viewpoints of the female and male. Fertil Steril 29:3, 1978
6. Buttram VC, Vanderheyden JD, Besch PK, Acosta AA: Post "pill" amenorrhea. Int J Fertil 19:37, 1974
7. Friedman LJ: Virgin Wives. Springfield, Il, CC Thomas, 1962, p 130
8. Gibbs CE: Diagnosis and treatment of uterine conditions that may cause infertility. Clin Obstet Gynecol 16:159, 1973
9. Gold JJ (ed): Textbook of Gynecologic Endocrinology. New York, Hoeber Medical Division, Harper & Row, 1968, p 243
10. Gomel V: Tubal reanastosnosis by microsurgery. Fertil Steril 28:415, 1978
11. Gomel V: Salpingostomy by microsurgery. Fertil Steril 29:380, 1978
12. Horne HW Jr, Clyman M, Debrovner C, Griggs G, Kistner R, Kosasa J, Stevenson CS, Taymor M: The prevention of postoperative pelvic adhesions following conservative treatment for human infertility. Int J Fertil 18:109, 1973
13. Israel SL (ed): Diagnosis and Treatment of Menstrual Disorders and Sterility, 5th ed. Hoeber Medical Division, Harper & Row, 1967, p 410
14. Kedia K, Markland C: The effect of pharmacological agents on ejaculation. J Urol 114:569, 1975
15. Kedia KR, Markland C, Fraley EE: Sexual function following high retroperitoneal lymphadenectomy. J Urol 114:237, 1975
16. MacLeod J: Human male infertility. Obstet Gynecol Surv 16:335, 1971
17. MacLeod J, Gold RZ: The male factor in fertility and infertility. Fertil Steril 4:10, 1953
18. March CM, Israel R, March AD: Hysteroscopic management of intrauterine adhesions. Am J Obstet Gynecol 130:653, 1978
19. Means AR, Fakunding JL, Huckins C, Tindall DJ, Vitale R: Follicle stimulating hormone, the sertoli cell and spermatogenesis. Recent Prog Horm Res 32:477, 1976
20. Moghissi KS: Accuracy of basal body temperature for ovulation detection. Fertil Steril 27:1415, 1976
21. Moghissi KS, Evans TN: Infertility. In Danforth DN (ed): Obstetrics and Gynecology. Hagerstown, Harper & Row, 1977, p 812
22. Nelson CMR, Bunge RG: Semen analysis: evidence for changing parameters. Fertil Steril 25:503, 1974
23. O'Brien JR, Arronet GH, Eduljee SY: Operative treatment of fallopian tube pathology in human infertility. Am J Obstet Gynecol 103:520, 1969
24. Oelsner G, Serr DM, Mashiach S, Blankstein J, Snyder M, Lunenfeld B: The study of induction of ovulation with menotrophins: analysis of the results of 1879 treatment cycles. Fertil Steril 30:538, 1978
25. Peterson EP, Musich JR, Behrman SJ: Uterotu-

bal implantation and obstetric outcome after previous sterilization. Am J Obstet Gynecol 128:662, 1977

26. Quinlivan WLG, Sullivan H: Effect on donor semen of husband's seminal plasma during artificial insemination (abstr). Fertil Steril 27:212, 1976

27. Ross GT: Gonadotrophins and preantral follicular maturation in women. Fertil Steril 25:522, 1974

28. Russell GFM: Psychological and nutritional factors in disturbances of menstrual function and ovulation. Postgrad Med J 48:10, 1972

29. Shulman S: Immunologic barriers to fertility. Obstet Gynecol Surv 27:553, 1972

30. Siegler AM, Perez RJ: Reconstruction of the fallopain tubes in previously sterilized patients. Fertil Steril 26:383, 1975

31. Silber SJ: Vasectomy and vasectomy reversal. Fertil Steril 29:125, 1978

32a,b. Speroff L, Glass RH, Kase NG: Clinical Gynecologic Endocrinology and Infertility, 2nd ed. Baltimore, Williams & Wilkins, 1978. a, p 317; b, p 329

33. Steinberger E, Smith KD: Artificial insemination with fresh or frozen semen. JAMA 223:778, 1973

34. Swolin K. Electromicrosurgery and salpingostomy. Long term results. Am J Obstet Gynecol 121:418, 1975

35a,b. Williams RH (ed): Textbook of Endocrinology. Philadelphia, WB Saunders, 1974, a, p 325, b, p 409

36. Woodruff JD, Pauerstein CJ: The Fallopian Tube. Baltimore, Williams & Wilkins, 1969, p 183

37. Young PE, Egan JE, Barlow JJ, Mulligan WJ: Reconstructive surgery for infertility at the Boston Hospital for Women. Am J Obstet Gynecol 108:1092, 1970

38. Zukerman Z, Rodriguez-Rigan LJ, Smith KD, Steinberger E: Frequency distribution of sperm counts in fertile and infertile males. Fertil Steril 28:1310, 1977

# 6

# Nonsurgical Methods of Contraception

## Marguerite K. Shepard

Fertility control has been practiced for centuries, but only within the last several decades has it become publicly acceptable. As recently as the early 1960s, two states had statutes making the prescription or sale of contraceptive devices a felony.

Three factors have revolutionized the attitudes of society toward contraception: *1*) the threat of a rapidly expanding population, *2*) the desire for increased personal freedom, and *3*) the development of oral contraceptives.

The change in attitudes toward, and acceptability of contraception is reflected in the terminology that has come into common usage. The term *contraception* literally refers to prevention of conception. In actuality, "contraceptive" practices may embrace any technique or method purposefully employed to prevent the birth of a viable infant. Thus, abortion has been used as a contraceptive since the beginning of recorded history (see Chap. 18). Other synonyms and euphemisms employed to express the concept of fertility control are *family planning, family size limitation,* and *birth control.* All are vaguely reminiscent of some type of numbers game. The terms *planned parenthood* and *child spacing,* on the other hand, tend to emphasize the individual experience of each pregnancy rather than the achievement of a particular number of offspring. Proponents of this terminology tend to emphasize the importance of contraception in permitting readiness for child-rearing before embarking on pregnancy.

The following discussion considers factors influencing successful use of contraception, and includes detailed descriptions of individual methods, including mechanism of action, efficacy, advantages, disadvantages, side effects, and recommendations for contraceptive choice for healthy individuals with no medical contraindications toward use of any method.

## FACTORS INFLUENCING SUCCESSFUL USE

Successful use of contraception depends on a variety of factors, including effectiveness, aesthetic acceptability, ease of use, and religious or cultural prohibitions.

### EFFECTIVENESS

The effectiveness of a contraceptive technique is generally discussed in relationship to theoretical rather than to use effectiveness. The former refers to the success rate that could be expected with appropriate use of the method, as described by the developer or manufacturer. The latter refers to the actual success rate that can be expected, taking into account improper application of the technique or failure to use it with each coital episode. Table 6–1 lists the theoretical and use effectiveness of commonly practiced methods. The accepted convention for expressing effectiveness states the number of pregnancies per hundred "women years" (HWY) of use, or 1200 months of total exposure on the part of many women using a given method. Statistical bias is easily introduced into this type of calculation because no allowance is made for dropouts. A life

**Table 6-1. Theoretical Versus Use Effectiveness of Various Methods, Expressed as Pregnancies per Hundred Women Years**

| Method | Theoretical | Range of use effectiveness |
|---|---|---|
| Rhythm | 3.0 | 14–32 |
| Condom | 3.0 | 7–15 |
| Foam | 3–5.0 | 10–40 |
| Diaphragm | 2.5 | 11–29 |
| IUD | 2.0 | 3–8 |
| Pill | 0.1 | 1–3 |
| Mini-pill | 2–4.0 | Unknown |

(Adapted from: Peel J, Potts M: Textbook of Contraceptive Practice. Cambridge, England, Cambridge University Press, 1970)

table method (see Chap. 14) would be preferable, in that it would account for the different months of exposure experienced by cohorts of users; however, it has never gained favor.

### ACCEPTABILITY

The acceptability of a method is determined by a variety of factors which generally relate to a person's comfort in touching his or her own and/or the partner's genitalia, openness about sexual activity, and response to the use of medication and mechanical devices (see Chap. 23 for a cross-cultural perspective).

A woman who refuses to wear tampons because she is reluctant to insert anything into the vagina will be an ineffective user of female-directed barrier methods. Males may object to using condoms, because they may believe that sexual pleasure is decreased if there is no direct penile contact with the vaginal mucous membranes. Event-relatedness (requirement for application of a device just prior to coitus—often after arousal) is considered by many to jeopardize the successful consummation of intercourse. Women who are hesitant to take medication of any kind may refuse to take oral contraceptives. Those who fear the semipermanent presence of a foreign object within the body reject the use of intrauterine devices.

### EASE OF USE

Ease of use influences the acceptability of a method, and, in turn, is strongly influenced by the circumstances under which coitus occurs. Teenagers may not be motivated to take a birth control pill daily, and the back seat of a car is not the optimal location in which to insert a diaphragm. Under such circumstances,

even foam may be too cumbersome to insert properly. Thus, the intrauterine device (IUD) may be most suitable for teenagers and other women who have neither an established home nor a settled lifestyle. Either the IUD or oral contraceptive is recommended for individuals not sufficiently motivated to use coitus-related methods, or who lack access to sufficient privacy to conveniently do so.

## INDIVIDUAL METHODS

Contraceptive techniques are commonly classified as couple-controlled, male-controlled, or female-controlled. The designation is generally determined by which partner's body is most affected by the device's use. Thus, the condom is a male-controlled method, and oral contraceptives a female-controlled method. However, the condom can become a female-controlled method if it is obtained and applied by the woman, and "the pill" a male-controlled method if the male oversees its administration (8). Even the IUD is not sacred, in that many men have threatened to remove it from their partners. Individuals may share contraceptive responsibility to varying degrees; however, the average individual usually considers contraception only as it affects his or her own body. Thus, when a woman of low parity and long marital duration is asked what she has used for contraception, she may answer, "nothing," because her husband has always used condoms. In actuality, she has also been using the condom for the duration of their relationship.

All methods currently employed as conventional contraceptives, except the IUD, are intended to prevent conception. The IUD is intended to prevent implantation. Conception may be thwarted by abstinence, modification of coital techniques, placing of a mechanical or chemical barrier between the ejaculate and the cervix, or inhibition of germ-cell release. The IUD presumably does not affect conception, but some information suggests that sperm-transport patterns may be altered in IUD wearers (14).

### TIMED ABSTINENCE

#### DETAILS OF METHOD AND MECHANISM OF ACTION

Timed abstinence, or rhythm, involves the avoidance of coitus during the periovulatory period, when the female is fertile. The periovulatory period may be determined by one of three methods: calendar rhythm, temperature rhythm, and the Billings technique. All are based on the premise that the ovum is potentially fertilizable only for the first 24 to 48 hours after ovulation. A major limitation of the rhythm method is that the duration of the survival of sperm and of their fertilizing capability in the female reproductive tract are unknown. Current available evidence indicates that this period probably lasts at least 72 hours (13). Based on these observations, the couple attempts to abstain from coitus for at least 3 days before, on the day of, and 2 days after, presumed ovulation.

**Calendar Rhythm.** To practice calendar rhythm, the woman should record menstrual-cycle length for at least 1 year. Based on the observation that the postovulatory period is generally of a standard length (12 to 16 days, but generally of consistent length for the individual woman), she calculates the presumed time of ovulation for the longest and shortest cycles which she has experienced in the previous year. Her appropriate period of abstinence for each cycle will then extend from 3 days before presumed ovulation in the shortest cycle through 2 days after presumed ovulation in her longest cycle.

**Temperature Rhythm.** Temperature rhythm is based on the assumption that the lowest point (thermal nadir) before a sustained rise in basal body temperature represents the time of ovulation. In fact, this may be true in only 80 per cent of women (29). The couple is instructed to abstain from coitus from the onset of menses through the 2nd day following the thermal nadir.

**The Billings Method.** The Billings method was developed in an attempt to determine the presumed time of ovulation in each cycle prospectively, thus obviating the need for prolonged periods of abstinence (3). This technique is based on the observation that the vaginal mucosa becomes more moist and the cervical secretions more watery as the preovulatory estrogen peak approaches. The woman is instructed to slip her finger into the vagina daily to check for moistness of the vaginal mucosa and consistency of the cervical secretions. When the moistness increases and the consistency of the mucus changes from sticky to slimy or watery, she is to abstain from

coitus. When the cervical mucus again becomes thick and sticky, she is presumed to be at least 2 days beyond ovulation, and coitus may be resumed.

### EFFICACY

It has been estimated that properly practiced rhythm techniques are effective in deferring pregnancy for 2-year intervals. The unknown duration of sperm viability, and occasional early or late ovulation in the normally cycling woman, are most commonly responsible for method failure. However, the primary source of failure is nonobservance of the appropriate periods of abstinence.

### ADVANTAGES, DISADVANTAGES, AND SIDE EFFECTS

The major advantage of the timed abstinence techniques is their grudging acceptance by the Roman Catholic hierarchy. A minor advantage is that physical and physiologic side effects are essentially nil, because no mechanical or chemical agents are involved.

The disadvantages rest primarily in the need for abstinence. If a couple abstains from coitus during the woman's menstrual period in addition to the timed abstinence period, they may spend more time abstaining than participating. Recent evidence indicates that women have a peak of sexual desire coincident with the preovulatory estrogen peak (1). Thus abstinence at this time requires more control on the woman's part than merely saying "no" to her partner.

The major complication, aside from recurrent sexual frustration, may involve an increased risk of abnormal offspring and pregnancy wastage if the method fails. German (15) has suggested that the increase in mongoloid infants in older women may be related to infrequent coitus and the fertilization of an ovum more than 48 hours after ovulation. Guerrero and Rojas (17) report an increased incidence of spontaneous abortion in couples experiencing a rhythm failure when the responsible insemination occurred more than 3 days before, or 2 days after, the presumed time of ovulation. Jongloet and Van Erkelens-Zwets (21) even suggest that the increased incidence of anencephaly (failure of the skull to form properly) and spina bifida (failure of the spinal column to fuse) in infants in areas with a high Roman Catholic population may be related to rhythm failure, with fertilization of aging gametes. Although more extensive studies are needed to substantiate this suggestion, strong consideration must be given to this explanation.

## MODIFICATION OF COITAL TECHNIQUES AND USE OF ALTERNATE METHODS OF SEXUAL GRATIFICATION

### DETAILS OF METHOD AND MECHANISM OF ACTION

Techniques involving other than penile-vaginal coitus beyond the point of ejaculation may be practiced consistently or only during the presumed fertile period, as a modification of timed abstinence.

**Coitus Interruptus.** The modified technique most commonly practiced for contraceptive purposes is coitus interruptus, or withdrawal. This method has been credited with effecting the decline in birth rate in France during the nineteenth century and has been cited by some as the most commonly practiced contraceptive technique in the world (see Chap. 18). Successful performance requires withdrawal of the penis from the vagina prior to ejaculation.

**Nongenital Coitus.** Other techniques that may be practiced for contraceptive purposes, but also for variation in obtaining sexual gratification, are penile-anal coitus, penile-oral coitus, cunnilingus, mutual oral-genital coitus, and mutual masturbation.

### EFFICACY

There are no real data available regarding the efficacy of nongenital techniques as contraceptive methods. Since they are practiced as a modification of rhythm, they probably have similar failure rates.

The greatest controversy over efficacy of coitus interruptus relates to the sperm content of different portions of the ejaculate. It has been assumed that the very first few drops of seminal plasma that seep out before forceful ejaculation contain a high concentration of sperm. However, Eliasson and his coworkers (10) have shown that the highest sperm concentration in normal volunteers is in the second of a six-portion ejaculate. Consequently, most

failures appear to result from failure to withdraw prior to ejaculation.

### ADVANTAGES, DISADVANTAGES, AND COMPLICATIONS

The major advantages of these techniques are that they do not involve expense, or the insertion, application, or ingestion of a mechanical or chemical agent. The major disadvantage of coitus interruptus is the need for ejaculation to occur outside the vagina. Dissatisfaction on the part of both partners is cited as a major cause for its lack of popularity in the United States. The fact that the technique is so widely practiced elsewhere suggests that the individual's or couple's expectations of the coital experience may materially influence satisfaction.

The major disadvantage of penile-anal coitus are possible penile infection, for the male, and hemorrhoid or fissure-development for the female. Complications of oral-genital coitus may include the introduction of oral flora into the genital organs. The greatest disadvantage of either method is lack of satisfaction, in that neither was the most desired method of sexual gratification. None of these methods is approved by Roman Catholic doctrine.

## BARRIER METHODS

### DETAILS OF METHOD AND MECHANISM OF ACTION

The barrier methods consist of condoms (rubbers, prophylactics); spermicidal creams, jellies, foams, suppositories; and the diaphragm-spermicide combination. Of these, the condom has been used longest and most extensively.

**Condoms.** Condoms were first used in the sixteenth century. They were initially made of linen, and then of animal intestine. They were originally developed to prevent transmission of venereal disease, and still serve that function (34a). Most condoms are now made of rubber or synthetic elastic material. They are generally fashioned with a small reservoir at the tip to contain the ejaculate and the inner surface may be coated with a spermicidal agent. The condom must be applied after an erection has been achieved. For maximum effectiveness, it should be applied prior to intromission, but it may be applied any time after erection and before ejaculation, if thrusting can be interrupted long enough for its application. For maximum effectiveness, the penis should be withdrawn from the vagina before it becomes flaccid, so that no leakage of the ejaculate from the condom occurs.

**Vaginal Spermicides.** The vaginal spermicides are modifications of one chemical agent, nonoxynol-9, incorporated in a variety of vehicles. All should be inserted several minutes prior to coitus, and all depend on adequate coverage of the vaginal mucosa and cervix for maximum effectiveness. Reapplication is required prior to each episode of coitus. The jellies, creams, and foam require use of an applicator for proper insertion. The newest suppository is designed to be inserted manually.

Jelly and cream have been judged to be poorer in overall effectiveness than foam because of uneven distribution of these agents over the vaginal mucosa. The aerosol component of the foam causes even spreading (20). However, the container of foam is substantially larger than the tube of jelly or cream and requires a larger applicator, making it more cumbersome to carry around. Two new suppositories have been developed, in an attempt to combine the advantages of all the other vaginal spermicidal formulations. They are small, and therefore easily transported and/or concealed. They require no inserter. One foams on contact with the vaginal mucosa, while the other does not (37). The suppositories are best kept in the refrigerator; although they can be carried around in a pocket, they may melt in hot weather. There is also some indication that they are not effective unless placed high in the vagina (11).

**Diaphragm-Spermicide.** The diaphragm, in its current form, was first developed in the late nineteenth century (34b). It became popular in the early twentieth century through the efforts of Margaret Sanger. With the advent of non-event-related methods, such as the IUD and oral contraceptives, the diaphragm lost favor. There has been a resurgence of diaphragm usage, especially among educated segments of the population, because of the recently reported serious side effects of birth control pills and the IUD.

Unlike the other barrier methods, the diaphragm requires an office visit to a physician, and prescription, because size requirements vary. Available diaphragms range in size from 60 mm. to 90 mm. in diameter, with intervening sizes available in 5 mm. increments. The required size depends to a certain extent on the size of the pelvic area, but more directly on the strength of the supporting vaginal tissue. Thus, required diaphragm size tends to increase after vaginal delivery, because the supporting tissue is stretched by passage of the fetal head and never regains its original tone.

The diaphragm is made of rubber or a synthetic elastic material. It consists of an almost hemispherical cup, with a circular, spring-type rim that may be one of three designs—flat, coiled, or arcing. The device is designed to hold spermicidal cream or jelly against the cervix. The diaphragm is fitted so that the posterior rim fits in the posterior vaginal fornix (the area of the vagina behind the cervix) and the anterior rim locks in place behind the pubic bone. If a diaphragm has been properly fitted, the wearer should not be able to feel it.

The diaphragm may be inserted any time from 1 to 2 hours to immediately prior to intromission. It should be left in place for at least 6 to 8 hours after coitus for the spermicide to have maximal effect. If another episode of coitus occurs within 6 hours of the initial one, the diaphragm should not be removed, but one or two applications of spermicide should be made intravaginally, outside the diaphragm. The diaphragm retention period then extends for 6 hours from the most recent coital episode. To ensure appropriate placement and effective use, the diaphragm's position should be checked immediately after insertion.

The diaphragm is most satisfactory, from an anatomic point of view, in the woman of low parity with good vaginal support. Masters and Johnson have shown it most effective in the female supine position, and readily dislodged in either the female superior and lateral coital positions, or with episodes of multiple mounting (20).

**EFFICACY**

Failure rates for barrier methods vary widely and are lowest in highly motivated upper-middle-class groups. Most failures stem from nonuse, rather than from improper use. Several studies (22) indicate that youthful and lower socioeconomic populations use the diaphragm very successfully, if properly instructed and well motivated.

In addition to nonuse, condom failures may result from breakage or leakage because of delayed withdrawal. Manufacturers' quality-control specifications accept a breakage rate of 2.5:1000 condoms (39).

Chemical barriers fail primarily because of improper application. However, in a small number of instances the spermicide may not be effective.

### ADVANTAGES, DISADVANTAGES, AND SIDE EFFECTS

The greatest advantage of the barrier methods is their relatively high efficacy with low incidence of side effects. No period of abstinence is required, and there is no need to utilize the method at times other than just before, during, and after coitus. The condom and the vaginal spermicides used without the diaphragm have the further advantage of being readily available, without the need for an office visit to a physician or a prescription.

The greatest disadvantage of the barrier methods is their event-relatedness; many complain that the need for application at the time of coitus destroys the mood and makes the experience less than satisfactory. However, the diaphragm can be inserted an hour or two prior to intercourse. Some women complain of the expense of this type of preparation, in that the spermicidal agent is used needlessly if coitus does not eventuate as anticipated. Other disadvantages cited for barrier methods are messiness of the spermicides, and need for manipulation of the genitalia, carrying around of cumbersome equipment, and the problem of finding a convenient place to apply the device or agent.

Side effects for all methods are few. Occasionally either the male or female develops an allergy or chemical sensitivity to the rubber or spermicide. The incidence of these side effects is very low, however.

## INTRAUTERINE DEVICES

The invention of the intrauterine device has been attributed to Bedouins, who noted that a pebble placed in a camel's uterus would prevent pregnancy on long trips over the desert. The Romans used gold rings in the uterus as contraceptives (38).

The intrauterine device enjoyed brief popularity in the 1920s and early 1930s in the form of the Gräfenberg ring, a stainless steel device developed in Germany. The ring fell out of favor because of an unacceptably high incidence of infections (12).

With the development of inert plastic devices in the 1950s, and the availability of effective antibiotics, the intrauterine device again gained popularity with both patients and physicians. Metal IUDs were also introduced at this time but have since fallen into disuse because of problems with infection and perforation. Currently available IUDs are either inert plastic, inert platsic impregnated with or wrapped with copper, and inert plastic impregnated with progesterone. All have strings attached that protrude through the cervix for easy location of the device (see Fig. 6–1).

### DETAILS OF METHOD AND MECHANISM OF ACTION

The exact mechanism of action of the IUD is unknown, but it appears to be dependent on the development of a sterile inflammatory response within the uterine cavity which hampers implantation and alters sperm-transport patterns (31).

Intrauterine devices come in various shapes and sizes, most of which are intended for the parous uterus; however, some have been specifically designed for the nulliparous one. The device must be inserted, and removed by a physician or trained health professional. For maximum efficacy the device must be placed high in the uterine fundus, as this is the most common site of implantation.

Ideally, the device should be inserted and removed during a menstrual period. At this time the cervical os may be slightly dilated, the tract lubricated with menstrual blood, and the woman is, almost always, not pregnant. Insertion is generally accompanied by some cramping, which may range from very mild to sufficiently severe to cause syncope (loss of consciousness). For the latter reason some physicians inject a local anesthetic in the cervix prior to insertion. Some uterine cramping and excessive bleeding may characterize the first two or three postinsertion cycles.

There is some difference of opinion regarding the length of time an inert plastic IUD may be retained. Some physicians arbitrarily change the device every 2 years. Others will

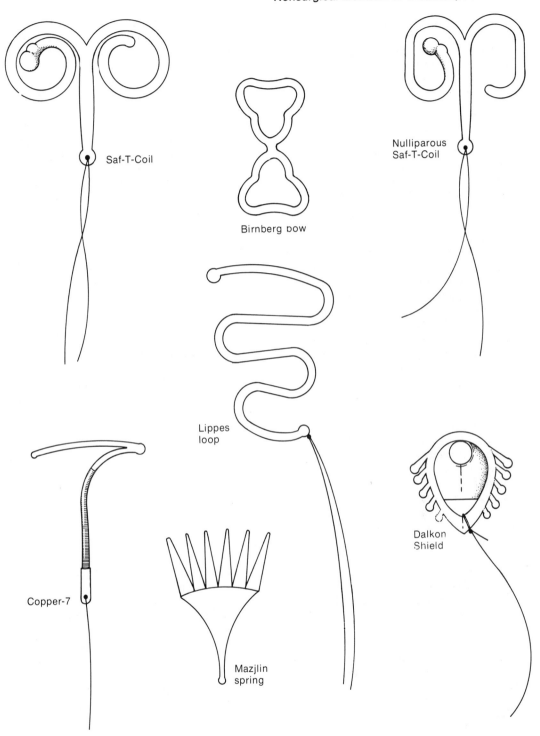

**FIG. 6–1.** Types of intrauterine devices. (The Birnberg bow, Mazjlin spring, and Dalkon shield have been withdrawn from the market).

leave it in place until adverse symptoms, such as pain, increased menses, or intermenstrual bleeding occur. The copper IUD is considered effective for 3 years, whereas the progesterone-impregnated IUD must be replaced yearly to retain its effectiveness.

### EFFICACY

The IUD is the single method for which theoretical and use effectiveness are almost identical (See Table 6-1). Occasionally a patient expels the device and is not aware of its loss. For this reason, IUD-wearers are instructed to check the position of the string after each menstrual episode, since expulsion is most likely to occur during menses. Some IUD-wearers may check string position before and after coitus. The in situ pregnancy rate for IUDs has been estimated at between 1 per cent and 2 per cent (7). Lehfeldt and his coworkers suggest that the IUD is 99 per cent effective in preventing intrauterine pregnancy, 95 per cent effective in preventing tubal pregnancy, and ineffective in preventing ovarian pregnancy (23).

### ADVANTAGES, DISADVANTAGES, AND SIDE EFFECTS

The greatest advantages of the IUD are that its use is not related to coitus, and that only one volitional act, that of having the device inserted, is required for effective use.

Its disadvantage is that the uterus is exposed constantly to a foreign body. Women who normally experience cramping and heavy flow with menses tend to note accentuation of these symptoms. Most women experience an increase in the duration of menses (28).

Undesirable side effects include infection, perforation, and an increased risk of tubal pregnancy in the event of failure.

**Infection.** Several investigators, including Eschenbach (12) in the United States and Westrom (43) in Sweden have reported a significant increase in pelvic inflammatory disease, especially the nongonococcal variety, in IUD-wearers. The increase is especially evident in nulliparous women and in those of upper socioeconomic classes. In addition, Christian (4) and others have reported the alarming occurrence of severe, often fatal, asymptomatic uterine infections in women who become pregnant with the IUD in situ

and retain the device, rather than having it removed. These infections were allegedly common with the shield-shaped intrauterine device, with protruding teeth, which is no longer available. Many of these infections eventuate in loss of fertility, either through hysterectomy, to control infection, or through irreparable infectious damage to the fallopian tubes. Although infections have been treated successfully with the IUD in situ in nonpregnant patients, current practice recommends removal, after institution of proper antibiotic therapy. Removal of the IUD, accompanied by pregnancy termination, is recommended in all pregnancy-related IUD infections.

**Perforation.** Perforation of the uterine wall by the IUD occurs most commonly at the time of insertion. Some of the now discontinued steel devices, especially the Mazjlin spring, would gradually erode through the uterine wall into the peritoneal cavity or vagina, but this occurs less often with the plastic devices. The most common sites of perforation are the posterior cervix, at the junction with the uterus, and the dome of the fundus. Neither site is excessively vascular, and the perforation may go unnoticed until weeks later, when the woman or physician can no longer locate the string. When closed-ring IUDs were available, the intraperitoneal IUD was a source of intestinal obstruction, because a loop of small bowel could slip into the ring and become trapped. There is difference of opinion over whether currently available models need to be removed from the peritoneal cavity upon diagnosis of perforation.

**Tubal Pregnancy.** Most available data indicates that the incidence of both intrauterine and tubal pregnancies is substantially lower among IUD-wearers than in the unprotected population (1% and 5% respectively). However, in IUD failures, the ratio of tubal to intrauterine pregnancies is significantly higher than that for the unprotected population. Therefore, the patient with an IUD failure must be evaluated carefully for possible tubal pregnancy.

## ORAL CONTRACEPTIVES

Oral contraceptives were first field-tested in Puerto Rico and Latin America in the 1950s and became available for clinical use in 1960.

This medication is now the most commonly used temporary contraceptive technique for women (42).

## DETAILS OF METHOD

The formulation of oral contraceptives has undergone several changes since their introduction. The original pills consisted of a combination of a synthetic estrogen and a synthetic progestin, in relatively high doses. It soon became evident from clinical trials that substantially lower doses of medication were effective and did not have the high incidence of annoying side effects, such as nausea, vomiting, breast tenderness, fluid retention, weight gain, and copious vaginal discharge. Because the normal female does not secrete a fixed combination of estrogen and progesterone throughout the menstrual cycle, sequential preparations were introduced, in an attempt to make oral contraceptives mimic the body's normal physiology. These preparations consisted of pills containing estrogen alone, for the first two-thirds or three-quarters of the treatment cycle, and an estrogen-progestin combination for the remainder. In the wake of reports of debilitating and fatal side effects of oral contraceptives related to the estrogen component, pills containing small doses of estrogen, or progestin only, were developed.

The original formulations consisted of 20 pills per pack. Current formulations, except for the progestin-only pills, contain 21 or 28 tablets per package. Originally, pills were to be taken daily, beginning with the 5th day of the menstrual cycle. After completing the pack, the patient was instructed to await the onset of menses, and begin the next pack on the 5th day of the following cycle. This practice was revised to make it easier for the user to remember when to begin each pill pack. The American woman has been conditioned to expect a 28-day menstrual cycle, and with the 20-day pack and fifth-day starting regimen, most women were having 26-day menstrual cycles. With the 21-day regimen, the woman takes pills for 21 days, then takes none for 1 week, during which she has a menstrual period. She resumes medication at the end of a week, regardless of when her menses begin. The 28-day preparations consist of 21 active, and 7 inert pills which are of different colors. With this regimen, she begins the next pack the day after she takes the last inert pill in the previous pack. Menses occurs while she is taking the inert tablets.

Another important reason for fixing the regimen to ensure 28-day pill cycles was that some women were experiencing delayed onset of menses after each pack. With the 5th-day starting regimen, a period of more than 7 days elapsed between pill packs. Some women were ovulating and becoming pregnant, because of the long time interval without suppressive medication.

Although oral contraceptive preparations have been marketed in tablet form in Western countries, an alternate preparation in the form of a hormone-impregnated edible cellulose sheet, known as the paper pill, has been developed and widely used in China. The package resembles a book of postage stamps. Each perforated square contains the same amount of contraceptive hormone as a tablet of the corresponding type. The squares are numbered with the appropriate cycle day. The sheets are intended to be dissolved on the tongue instead of swallowed. For purposes of mass distribution, the paper pill has the advantage of being easier to package, transport, and store than the conventional tablet. Studies by Morris and his coworkers (30) from the United Kingdom indicate that paper and tablet formulations of the same oral contraceptive are equally effective in preventing pregnancy.

Damm and his coworkers (6) recently compared the acceptance of the paper pill and the tablet among a group of Mexican women who had not previously used oral contraceptives. Each woman had an opportunity to use both forms. Although the paper pill was found to be quite acceptable by most of the women, the tablet was preferred. Eighty-five per cent needed some water to swallow it, and 28 per cent complained of the taste, whereas no one complained of the taste of the pill. However, the authors felt that if the paper pill were substantially cheaper than the tablet, its acceptance rate would be high.

The progestin-only pills are designed to be taken daily, without stopping. Menstrual intervals vary according to patient and cycle. The package complement of pills generally reflects the manufacturer's educated guess regarding the average cycle length for the particular preparation, and ranges anywhere from 35 to 42 pills.

## MECHANISM OF ACTION

Oral contraceptives have several mechanisms of action which prevent pregnancy. The combined and sequential pills prevent ovulation by ablation of the mid-cycle peak of luteinizing hormone. In addition, the progestational agent has an antagonistic effect on endometrial proliferation which makes the endometrium suboptimal for implantation and may also alter ovum-transport patterns. The progestin also produces thick, gummy cervical mucus which is essentially impenetrable to sperm (9). This last effect is probably the major mechanism of action of the pure progestin pills; it has been shown that 30 per cent of women taking this preparation ovulate.

## COMPONENTS OF ORAL CONTRACEPTIVES

Available combination oral contraceptives contain one of two synthetic estrogens, and one of five synthetic progestins. The estrogens are derivatives of estradiol, the most potent of the 18-carbon steroids. Both have been altered to make them orally active, since native estradiol is rapidly inactivated in the liver. The more widely used of the two is ethinyl estradiol. Mestranol, which is a 3-methyl ether of ethinyl estradiol, was the first of the two to be used. It is slightly less potent and acts more slowly, because it must be demethylated by the liver before it becomes biologically active. Gual and his coworkers (16) have estimated that 50μg. of ethinyl estradiol have the same potency as 80μg. of mestranol. Mestranol is the synthetic estrogen in these brand-name preparations: Enovid-E, Ovulen, Ortho Novum-Norinyl 1/80, and Ortho Novum and Norinyl 1/50. All other preparations, including those containing less than 50μg of estrogen, contain ethinyl estradiol.

The five synthetic progestins are norethynodrel, ethynodiol diacetate, norethindrone, norethindrone acetate, and norgestrel. They are all derivatives of the 19-carbon androstane nucleus and are thus called progestins or progestagens, because they share some of the biologic activities of progesterone without being direct progesterone derivatives. They can all be metabolized to estrogen to some extent, and thus may be referred to as "weak" or "strong" progestins. With the exception of norethynodrel, they all have mild, to moderate, masculinizing potential.

The concept of weak and strong progestins is an important one: the potency of the preparation on a per-milligram basis may be as, if not more, important than the milligram amount of progestin, when trying to gauge its effect in combination with the synthetic estrogen. For example, Enovid-E, which contains 2.5 mg. per tablet of norethynodrel, has less progesterone effect than Ovral, which contains 0.5 mg. of norgestrel, because norgestrel is approximately ten to twenty times more potent a progestin than norethynodrel. These relationships must be considered when a change in birth control pills is contemplated, to avoid undesirable side effects, such as amenorrhea, or breakthrough bleeding.

## ADVANTAGES, DISADVANTAGES, AND SIDE EFFECTS

The overwhelming advantage of oral contraceptives is their efficacy. If the medication is taken properly, the failure rate is probably about 1:1000 users for the estrogen-progestin combination pills. The progestin-only pills have a significantly higher failure rate, roughly 3 per cent. A second advantage is non-event-relatedness. Use of the medication is totally independent of coital activity. Thirdly, manipulation of the genitalia is not required.

The greatest disadvantage is the need for daily ingestion of a pill, regardless of coital frequency. A daily volitional act is required which may not be suited to the life-style and habits of some individuals.

From the medical point of view, there are distinct disadvantages to oral contraceptives, in the form of minor and major systemic side effects.

**Minor Side Effects.** Minor side effects include nausea, vomiting, breast tenderness, weight gain (secondary to fluid retention), anabolic weight gain (increase in muscle mass), acne, recurrent vaginitis (usually attributable to yeast), hair loss, scanty to absent menses, breakthrough bleeding, and depression. Many of these side effects are dose-dependent and can be eliminated by change of medication. However, there is no "right pill" for every patient. In a small percentage of patients, one or more side effects persists, regardless of which preparation is used. These women will opt for another contraceptive method.

**Major Side Effects.** Major side effects include fatal and nonfatal myocardial infarctions, strokes, pulmonary embolism (development of blood clots which break off and lodge in the circulation of the lungs), hypertension, optic neuritis, retinal thrombosis, benign liver tumors, and endometrial cancer (with sequential pills only).

The first reports of increased risk of thromboembolic disorders emanated from Great Britain. In 1968, Inman and Vessey (18) reported the results of their case-control studies of thromboembolic phenomena in women taking oral contraceptives. Their studies, and others, indicated a two- to eleven-fold increased risk for various thrombotic vascular accidents in users of oral contraceptives, as opposed to nonusers. These studies were confirmed by Sartwell and his coworkers (35) in the United States, who also determined that the incidence was related to the dose of estrogen in the particular preparation. Their data suggested that the risk was substantially decreased for women taking pills containing 50µg. of estrogen. These findings led to the development of a whole series of "micro"-dose estrogen preparations containing 20µg. to 35µg. of estrogen, on the assumption that with the reduced dose, the incidence of harmful side effects would also decrease.

In 1973 the Collaborative Stroke Project published data which indicated a nine-fold risk of thrombotic stroke in women using oral contraceptives over a control population drawn from the same hospital and the same neighborhood as the stroke patients (5). In 1975 Mann and his coworkers (26, 27) published the results of retrospective case-control studies indicating an increased risk of fatal, and nonfatal myocardial infarction in oral contraceptive users, as opposed to nonusers. These findings were confirmed by prospective studies of the Royal College of General Practitioners (2) and of the Oxford University Family Planning Association (41). The risk was shown to increase with age, cigarette smoking, and possibly duration of pill use for more than 5 years. Data from the Royal College of Family Practitioners study also indicated for the first time that the risk of death from pill use was greater than the risk of death from pregnancy in the control group. In the past, one of the strongest arguments for pill use, despite significant side effects, was that it was safer to be using the pill than to be pregnant. This argument is now questioned.

Recently Tietze (40) has questioned the validity of applying the risk estimates derived from the British studies to American populations. His question is based on the observation that there has been a decline in death from cardiovascular disease in all age groups in the United States from 1950 until the present, and that the decline has been greater for women than it has been for men, in spite of use of oral contraceptives. He does not dispute the British findings that pill use may increase the risk of mortality from cardiovascular disease, but only the British estimates of the level of risk, because they were derived from relatively small numbers. He feels that large-scale prospective studies carried out in the United States are needed.

A different approach was taken in a recent issue of *Population Reports* (33), especially in respect to the benefit-risk ratio of pill use versus pregnancy. The authors concluded that in developing nations the risk of death from childbirth was clearly greater than the risk of death from pill use. However, in developed countries, especially among affluent populations, the situation might be less clear. Not only is maternal mortality substantially lower in developed than in developing countries, but there is also a higher incidence of conditions that might contribute to pill-related cardiovascular disease, such as obesity, hypertension, diabetes, and cigarette smoking.

Cigarette smoking itself increases the risk of myocardial infarction in women. The combination of cigarette smoking and pill use has a synergistic effect. The risk of myocardial infarction in pill users who smoke is substantially higher than for either pill use or cigarette smoking alone (19).

Oral contraceptives may cause hypertension in users with previously normal blood pressure and may significantly increase blood pressure in women with preexisting hypertension. Blood pressure tends to revert to "pre-pill" levels when oral contraceptives are discontinued, but the patient is at risk for severe side effects of hypertension while taking them. Consequently, oral contraceptives should not be prescribed for women with hypertension and should be discontinued promptly in women who develop hypertension while on the pill.

In 1975 Nissen and his coworkers (32) reported an increased incidence of hepatomas (benign liver tumors) in women taking oral contraceptives, particularly those containing mestranol. Although the incidence of this condition is low, a marked increase is evident which appears to be specifically related to pill use. The relationship to mestranol-containing pills may be real, resulting from a deficiency in enzymes necessary for demethylation, or it may be spurious, resulting from the fact that pills containing mestranol have been marketed for 8 years longer than pills containing ethinyl estradiol. There appears to be a temporal relationship, in that the majority of reported cases have occurred in women who have used the pill for 4 years or longer. The greatest risk of these tumors is hemorrhage within the tumor, with subsequent rupture of the liver. The tumors tend to regress when oral contraceptives are discontinued, but may enlarge with subsequent pregnancy.

Several studies (25, 36) indicate an increased incidence of endometrial cancer, and possibly of breast cancer, in women taking exogenous estrogens, primarily after the menopause. To date, the only evidence linking oral contraceptives to an increased incidence of cancer are reports implicating sequential contraceptives in the development of endometrial carcinoma. These agents generally contained $100\mu g$. of estrogen per tablet and consisted of estrogen, unopposed by a progestin, for at least 15 days of each pill cycle. The medications were withdrawn by the manufacturers before extensive studies could be conducted.

Other reported side effects of oral contraceptives include the ocular changes mentioned previously, relative or absolute glucose intolerance (diabetic state), and continued hypothalamic suppression, with failure to ovulate after discontinuing the medication (see Chap. 5).

Galactorrhea (abnormal production of breast milk) may result from oral-contraceptive therapy itself, from postpill hypothalamic suppression, or from stimulation of previously existing microscopic pituitary tumors. These side effects are rare and are not fatal.

Thus there are substantial risks related to oral-contraceptive use. Certain disease states, or preexisting conditions, should be considered absolute, or relative, contraindications to pill use, despite the pills' contraceptive efficacy. Absolute contraindications include hypertension; history of previous thromboembolic episodes, including stroke, myocardial infarct, and pulmonary embolism; history of

deep venous thrombophlebitis, without embolism; age of 35 or over; and cigarette smoking. The latter is subject to some dispute. Relative contraindications include diabetes; vascular headaches, such as severe recurrent migraines; and a history of hepatitis (for mestranol-containing pills).

## RECOMMENDATIONS FOR CONTRACEPTIVE CHOICES

It behooves the health care professional to be familiar with the relative merits of the various contraceptive techniques, in order to best fulfill the needs of patients. There are some individuals who desire sexual freedom without pregnancy, but who will not accept abortion, and find fault with all available methods. There are others who prefer to use abortion as their routine method of contraception (24). The medical disadvantages of this approach are discussed in Chapter 5.

The attitude which the health care professional expresses toward a given method greatly influences its successful use. A positive attitude will contribute markedly to the patient's acceptance of a method which was not her first choice when there are medical contraindications to the one which she originally preferred.

In the normal, healthy individual with no specific health problems, such factors as age, parity, habits, lifestyle, coital frequency, and circumstances of coitus should be considered. Available data indicate that risks of harmful side effects of oral contraceptives are increased substantially in women over thirty-five. On the other hand, there is some concern that adolescents are more susceptible than adults to the development of postpill amenorrhea. It is evident that women with grossly irregular menses have a greater risk of developing postpill amenorrhea than women with regular menses.

Women who tend to have irregular work hours, or to be forgetful or somewhat irresponsible, will comply poorly with oral contraceptive methods and will fare better with an intrauterine device, or possibly even with an event-related barrier method. The reported increased frequency of IUD-related infections in nulliparous women must be weighed against the risk of an unwanted pregnancy in a sexually active adolescent. The same can be said regarding the risk of pill use in adolescents with irregular menses.

Nonprescription barrier methods may be the best choice for teenagers who have difficulty in obtaining medical advice or who are having coitus under suboptimal conditions, and do not have access to pills or the IUD.

Barrier methods would seem to be ideal for highly motivated individuals having infrequent coitus, since the risks of the IUD and the pill are not justifiable if coitus is occurring less frequently than once a week. Barrier methods should also be encouraged for individuals having more frequent coitus who fear the side effects of the pill or IUD. In such circumstances, the diaphragm is an excellent choice.

The most difficult decision for the health care professional is how to handle the patient who insists on a particular method to which there exists a strong contraindication. The 35-year-old cigarette smoker who insists on pills is the best example. If no other medical contraindication exists, the only choice may be prescription, with ample warning and close surveillance.

## REFERENCES

1. Adams DB, Gold AR, Burt A: Rise in female sexual activity at ovulation blocked by oral contraceptives. N Engl J Med 299:1145, 1978
2. Beral V, Kay CR: Mortality among oral contraceptive users. Royal College of General Practitioners Oral Contraceptive Study. Lancet (8041): 729, 1977
3. Billings J: Natural Family Planning: The Ovulation Method. Collegeville, MN, Liturgical Press, 1972
4. Christian CD: Maternal deaths associated with an intrauterine device. Am J Obstet Gynecol 119:441, 1974
5. Collaborative Group for the Study of Stroke in Young Women. Oral contraception and increased risk of cerebral ischemia or thrombosis. N Engl J Med 288:871, 1973
6. Damm RR, Huerta HA, Valenzuela, FL, de Mier MA, de Monarrez GC, Cisneros EO, Zaldivar MH, Perkin GW: Use and acceptance of the "paper pill": A novel approach to oral contraception. Contraception 19:273, 1979
7. Davis HJ: Intrauterine contraceptive devices: present status and future prospects. Am J Obstet Gynecol 114:134, 1972
8. Deys CM, Potts M: Factors affecting patient motivation. In Sciarra J, Markland C, Speidel JJ (eds): Control of Male Fertility. Hagerstown, Harper & Row, 1975, p 210
9. Diczfalusy E: Mode of action of contraceptive drugs. Am J Obstet Gynecol 100:136, 1968
10. Eliasson R, Lindholmer C: Distribution and properties of spermatozoa in different fractions of split ejaculates. Fertil Steril 23:252, 1972
11. Encare oval, the Med Letts 20:29, 1978
12. Eschenbach DA. IUD-associated acute pelvic inflammatory disease. In Sciarra JJ, Zatuchni GI, Speidel JJ (eds): Risks, Benefits and Controversies in Fertility Control. Hagerstown, Harper & Row, 1977, p 413
13. Ferin J, Thomas K, Johanson EDB: Ovulation detection. In Hafez ESE, Evans T (eds): Human Reproduction: Conception and Contraception. New York, Harper & Row, 1973, p 261
14. Fordney DS: Personal communication.
15. German J: Mongolism, delayed fertilization, and human sexual behavior. Nature 217:516, 1968
16. Gual C, Becerra C, Rice-Wray E, Goldzieher JW: Inhibition of ovulation by estrogens. Am J Obstet Gynecol 97:443, 1967
17. Guerrero R, Rojas OJ: Spontaneous abortion and aging of human spermatozoa. N Engl J Med 293:573, 1975
18. Inman WH, Vessey MP: Investigation of deaths from pulmonary, coronary and cerebral thrombosis and embolism in women of child-bearing age. Br Med J 2:193, 1968
19. Jain AK: Cigarette smoking, use of oral contraceptives and myocardial infarction. Am J Obstet Gynecol 126:301, 1976
20. Johnson VE, Masters WH, Lewis KC: The physiology of intravaginal contraceptive failure. In Calderone ML (ed): Manual of Family Planning and Contraceptive Practice, 2nd ed. Baltimore, Williams & Wilkins, 1970, p 232
21. Jongbloet PH, van Erkelens-Zwets JHJ: Rhythm methods: are there risks to the progeny. In Sciarra JJ, Zatuchni GI, Speidel JJ (eds): Risks, Benefits and Controversies in Fertility Control. Hagerstown, Harper & Row, 1977, p 520
22. Lane ME: Benefits and risks of diaphragm and condom use. In Sciarra JJ, Zatuchni GI, Speidel JJ (eds): Risks, Benefits and Controversies in Fertility Control. Hagerstown, Harper and Row, 1977, p 547
23. Lehfeldt H, Tietze C, Gorstein F: Ovarian pregnancy and the intrauterine device. Am J Obstet Gynecol 108:1005, 1970
24. Luker K: Taking Chances: Abortion and The Decision Not to Contracept. Berkeley, University of California Press, 1975
25. Lyon FA: The development of adeno-carcinoma of the endometrium in young women receiving long-term sequential oral contraceptives. Am J Obstet Gynecol 123:299, 1975
26. Mann JI, Inman WH: Oral contraceptives and death from myocardial infarction. Br Med J 2:245, 1975
27. Mann JI, Vessey MP, Thorogood M, Doll R: Myocardial infarction in young women with special reference to oral contraceptive practice. Br med J 2:241, 1975
28. Mishell DR, Jr: Pregnancy-related complications and bleeding problems with IUD's. In Sciarra JJ, Zatuchni GJ, Speidel JJ (eds): Hagerstown, Harper & Row, 1977, p 428
29. Morris NM, Underwood LE, Easterling W Jr: Temporal relationship between basal body temperature nadir and luteinizing hormone surge in normal women. Fertil Steril 27:780, 1976
30. Morris SE, Scarisbrick JJ, Cameron EHD, Groom GV, Buickingham MS, Everitt J, Elstein M: Comparison of plasma hormone changes using a

"conventional" and a "paper" pill formulation of a low-dose oral contraceptive. Fertil Steril 29:296, 1978

31. Moyer DL, Mishell DR Jr: Reactions of human endometrium to the intrauterine foreign body. II. Long-term effects on the endometrial histology and cytology. Am J Obstet Gynecol 111:66, 1971

32. Nissen ED, Kent DR: Liver tumors and oral contraceptives. Obstet Gynecol 46:460, 1975

33. Oral Contraceptives: Population Reports Series A, No. 5, January, 1979

34a, b. Peel J, Potts M: Textbook of Contraceptive Practice. Cambridge, University Press, 1970, a, p 52; b, p 62

35. Sartwell PE, Masi AT, Arthes FG, Greene GR, Smith HE: Thromboembolism and oral contraceptives: an epidemiologic case-control study. Am J Epidemiol 90:365, 1969

36. Silverberg S, Makowski E: Endometrial carcinoma in young women taking oral contraceptive agents. Obstet Gynecol 46:503, 1975

37. Squirre JJ, Berger GS, Keith L: A retrospective clinical study of a vaginal contraceptive suppository. J Repro Med 22:319, 1979

38. Tatum H: Intrauterine contraception. Am J Obstet Gynecol 112:1000, 1972

39. Tietze C: The condom. In Calderone ML (ed): Manual of Family Planning and Contraceptive Practice 2nd ed. Baltimore, Williams & Wilkins, 1970, p 232

40. Tietze C: The pill and mortality from cardiovascular disease: another look. Inter Fam Plann Perspect 5:8, 1979

41. Vessey MP, McPherson K, Johnson B: Mortality among women participating in the Oxford Family Planning Association contraceptive study. Lancet 2:731, 1977

42. Westoff CF, Jones EF: Contraception and sterilization in the United States, 1965–1975. Fam Plann Perspect 9:153, 1977

43. Westrom L, Bengtsson LP, Mardh PA: The risk of pelvic inflammatory disease in women using intrauterine contraceptive devices as compared to non-users. Lancet 2:221, 1976

# 7

# Innovative Approaches in Contraceptive Research

**Michael J. K. Harper**
**Barbara A. Sanford**

Many useful and effective methods of contraception are presently in use. However, for a variety of reasons—technical, medical, cultural, and ethical—methods suitable for all women are not available. Hence in the last decade there has been great interest in the development of new forms and methods of contraception, and in the improvement of existing ones. In this chapter, only new methods of contraception still under development will be discussed. (Modifications and improvement of existing methods have been discussed in the previous chapter.)

## VACCINES

One of the most significant advances in the field of contraception concerns the development of contraceptive vaccines. To understand the theoretical and practical bases of such an approach, it is necessary to be familiar with certain fundamental immunological principles, which are described in the following section.

## BASICS OF IMMUNOLOGY

### GENERAL PRINCIPLES

The science of immunity is introduced to most people in a very practical way during the first year of life. During this time babies are started on a program of vaccination intended to induce immunity against certain infectious diseases. After introduction into the body of a foreign substance (*antigen*), in the form of a vaccine, the cells of the immune system (*lymphocytes*) and cells of the reticuloendothelial system (*macrophages*) interact with the antigen. As a consequence of this interaction, plasma cells appear, which synthesize and secrete *immunoglobulins* (the primary products of *humoral immunity*), and *sensitized T lymphocytes* appear, which effect *cell-mediated* immunity (Fig. 7–1). The ultimate purpose of any immune response is to cause elimination of foreign antigens from the body.

B and T lymphocytes both arise from lymphoid stem cells; B cells mature in the microenvironment of the bone marrow and spleen, while T cells mature under the influence of the thymus. B and T cells are genetically programmed to recognize and react with specific chemical moieties (*antigenic determinants*) on the surface of antigens. An immune response can occur in a host only if lymphocytes which recognize that particular antigen are present. A major consequence of any immune response is that the products of the immune response (immunoglobulins and/or sensitized T cells) can later react only with the antigen which caused their production; they cannot react with a dissimilar antigen. This is why vaccination with polio virus promotes specific resistance against polio, but not against measles or mumps, which are caused by totally different viruses.

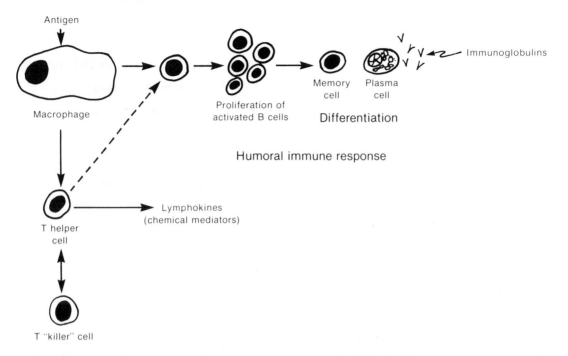

**FIG. 7–1.** The dual immune response.

Lymphocytes, which comprise both the cellular and humoral immune system, are widely distributed throughout the body—in bone marrow, blood, the spleen, lymph nodes, the gut-associated lymphoid tissues (tonsils, Peyer's patches, and appendix), and beneath the mucous membranes lining the respiratory and genitourinary tracts. This wide distribution enhances the chance that lymphocytes will come into contact with their respective antigens.

Ordinarily, the cells of the immune system react against foreign invaders, not against the body's own constituents; the body has a natural immunological tolerance which allows it to recognize its own ("self") antigens and distinguish them from foreign ones. The molecules which are recognized as "self" are called *histocompatibility antigens,* and they give the tissues and cells of each individual their own chemical identity. In the case of organ transplants, these antigens allow recognition that a transplanted organ from another individual is foreign.

There are, however, antigens within the body which appear to be hidden from cells of the immune system, and the body does not develop tolerance to these antigens. The sperm is an example of this type of antigen; a man inoculated with his own sperm can produce an immune response against them. Another exception to natural tolerance is seen in people with *autoimmune disease;* people with this problem lose their tolerance to certain natural antigens present in their own bodies and react against them as if they were foreign. A third exception to natural tolerance involves "self" antigens which become altered and no longer recognizable as "self." One example of this is a hypersensitivity response following the injection of penicillin. When penicillin is broken down by the body, some of the breakdown products may act as *haptens* and bind to the patient's own red blood cells or skin proteins, altering them enough to be recognized as foreign by the body. A hapten, by definition, is a substance of very low molecular weight, which is not antigenic unless it is bound to a carrier substance either before or after its introduction into the body. When coupled to a large carrier, the hapten acts as an antigenic determinant.

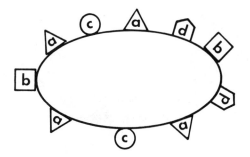

**FIG. 7–2.** A large antigen with multiple antigenic determinants.

Figure 7–2 represents a general, "all-purpose" antigen; it could be a whole cell, or perhaps a large protein molecule. This antigen has four different antigenic determinant groups on its surface. An immune response may be directed against any one, or a combination of several of these determinants. Immune reactants induced against the antigen can react specifically with the antigen, both in the body and in a test tube. These specific immune reactants may also cross-react with antigens which are similar but not identical, physically and chemically, to the antigenic determinants which elicited their production.

### THE HUMORAL IMMUNE RESPONSE

A paradox which has annoyed and fascinated scientists is immunoglobulin (antibody) specificity. How is the body able to respond to thousands of antigens by producing antibodies which are capable of reacting specifically, with the antigens that induced their production? The answer to this question lies in the structure of the antibody molecule (Fig. 7–3). A molecule of antibody is a glycoprotein which has two light chains and two heavy chains of polypeptides, held together by disulfide bonds (shown in Fig. 7–3 as black dots). The antibody consists of three fragments— two "Fab" fragments and one "Fc" fragment. The Fc fragment determines all of the physiochemical characteristics of the antibody—the class of the antibody, how fast it is catabolized in the body, whether or not it can cross the placenta from the mother's circulation to the fetus, and whether or not it can attach to mast cells, phagocytic cells, and other cell types in the body. The Fab fragments determine with what antigen the antibody can react. The amino acid sequence in the constant region of light and heavy chains may be the same in antibodies of the same class, but the sequence in the variable region differs, depending on the antigen-binding specificity of the antibody; thus an antibody molecule has two identical antigen-binding sites (see Fig. 7–3) where it can "recognize" and react with an antigenic determinant. The interaction of an antigenic determinant with the antigen-binding site of a specific antibody can be envisioned as putting together two complementary pieces of an interlocking puzzle. The amino acid sequence in

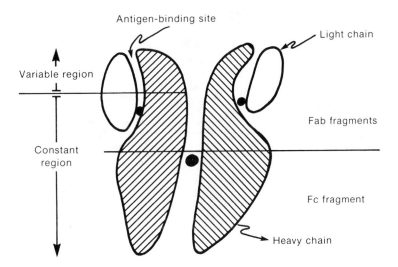

**FIG. 7–3.** Component parts of one molecule of antibody.

the region of the antigen-binding site determines the shape or configuration of one piece of the puzzle, and how well it "fits" with the antigenic determinant.

There are five classes of immunoglobulins—IgG, IgA, IgM, IgE, and IgD. IgG is the predominant antibody in man. This antibody is about equally distributed in the blood and extravascular body fluids. IgG is the only antibody possessing the ability to cross the placenta. Polymorphonuclear leukocytes and macrophages carry receptors for the Fc portion of IgG. Thus, after IgG combines with antigen, the Fc portion of the antibody reacts with the surface of polymorphonuclear leukocytes and/or macrophages; this interaction results in the ingestion (*phagocytosis*) of the antigen-antibody complexes. Once inside these phagocytic cells, the antigen is usually degraded, and is subsequently eliminated from the body.

Two types of IgA are present in the body: serum IgA and secretory IgA. From a functional standpoint, secretory IgA is the most important form of IgA (Fig. 7–4). The structure of secretory IgA differs from IgG; secretory IgA consists of two monomers joined by a J-chain and carrying a secretory component. As the name suggests, secretory IgA has 100

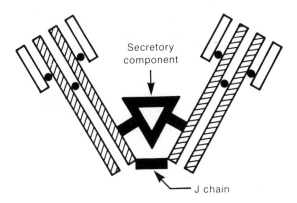

**FIG. 7–4.** One molecule of secretory IgA.

per cent distribution in the external body secretions, including saliva, colostrum (the "first milk," consisting mainly of serum and white blood cells, produced by the mother post partum), nasal secretions, bronchial secretions, intestinal-tract secretions, urine, tears, and prostatic and vaginal secretions. Secretory IgA is not the only antibody found in external secretions, but it is the major antibody in the secretions compared to IgG, IgM, and IgE, which may also be present. As Figure 7–5 shows, IgA is synthesized in plasma cells; a secretory component is produced in epithelial

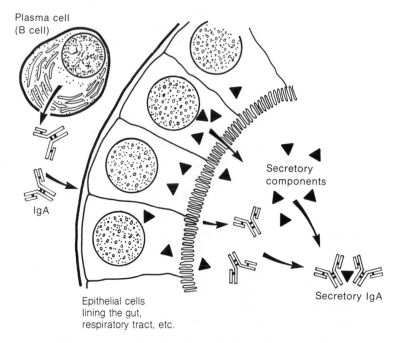

**FIG. 7–5.** Local antibody production of secretory IgA.

cells. The IgA molecules link up with one secretory component and enter the secretory fluid as a dimeric IgA–secretory-component complex.

The peculiar constant association of secretory component with IgA suggests that an important biological adaptation has evolved to enhance the activity of IgA, which must function on secretory surfaces. Two differences are apparent in comparing the activity of secretory IgA and antibody in the serum and internal body secretions. One is the ability of secretory IgA to adhere to the surface of mucous membranes (to become "antiseptic paint"), despite persistalsis. The other is its ability to resist proteolytic digestion, particularly in the gut. It has been postulated that secretory component offers a selective advantage to secretory IgA by promoting its adherence to mucous membranes and its resistance against enzyme degradation.

IgM is a large pentamer which is located primarily in the blood. One property of IgM seems to be its ability to respond early to an antigenic stimulus. Upon the first exposure to an antigen, the host responds by first producing IgM. This is called a *primary response,* and it is usually a weak response, which does not persist. After a primary response, the body has expanded clones of memory cells available to react when the antigen is reintroduced into the host. Thus, in a *secondary response,* antibodies (mostly IgG) appear sooner, they increase in amount faster, and are substantially more numerous, and they persist in the body for longer periods of time. In any vaccination program the basis for booster injections is to enhance the antibody response. Besides giving multiple injections of an antigen, another way of enhancing an immune response is to mix the antigen with an *adjuvant,* which nonspecifically enhances the immune response (humoral and/or cell-mediated). The adjuvant may act as a depot, holding the antigen in the body longer and allowing it to be released over a longer period of time; it may also act by increasing the numbers of immune cells in the area of antigen localization.

IgD and IgM appear to be the primary membrane-bound receptors on the surface of B cells. The presence of these antibodies on B cells allows the B cell to recognize and react with specific antigens, which, in turn, induces the B cell to differentiate into antibody-secreting plasma cells.

## ANTIGEN-ANTIBODY REACTIONS

In the development and testing of contraceptive vaccines, it is necessary to determine whether an immune response can be induced against specific antigens, and, in most cases, to determine the strength and persistence of the response; this will vary from antigen to antigen. A variety of immunological tests can be used to monitor an immune response. These tests make use of our ability to detect and quantitate the interactions of antigens and antibodies.

Antigen-antibody reactions are used as research and diagnostic tools in many disciplines outside of immunology. The most attractive characteristic of these reactions is their specificity, and, in some cases, their exquisite sensitivity. Some of the more commonly used tests include immunofluorescence, radioimmunoassay, precipitation, agglutination, and complement lysis. In the immunofluorescence test, a fluorescent dye is conjugated to antibody. When the dye-tagged antibody conjugant comes in contact with its antigen, an antigen-antibody reaction takes place. That a reaction has taken place can be visualized using a fluorescent microscope; the presence of the dye attached to antibody appears as an apple-green fluorescent color. If no reaction has taken place, the antibody with its bound dye is not present, and neither is the apple-green fluorescence. In radioimmunoassay, the antibody is tagged with a radioisotope, for example, $^{125}$I. In one form of the test a bead or microtiter well is coated with antigen. The bound antigen is then permitted to react with a serum which may or may not contain the specific antibody against the test antigen. If antibody is present, an antigen-antibody reaction takes place. A tagged anti-antibody is then added to the well. This anti-antibody will react with the antibody bound to antigen. The beads, or wells, are placed in tubes and counted in a gamma or liquid scintillation counter to detect the presence of the radioisotope, which indicates that the serum did contain specific antibody against the test antigen. The anti-antibody used in this test is produced by immunizing an animal (rabbit, sheep, goat) with human serum which contains all five classes of antibodies. The animal responds by producing antibodies against human serum proteins, including antibodies. Thus, the serum from this animal, referred to as *antiserum,* contains antibodies against human antibodies, or "anti-antibodies." By labeling the anti-antibodies with a radioisotope, it becomes possible to use this single reagent to test an infinite number of different sera for the presence of specific antibody.

The principle of the precipitation reaction is seen in Figure 7–6. In a precipitation reaction, the antigen is always soluble. Antibody is added, and if enough small antigen-antibody complexes interact, they form a lattice of larger aggregates; at a critical point the aggregates fall out of solution, or precipitate (tube B). The reaction does not take place if excess antibody (tube A) or excess antigen (tube C) is present. A variation of the precipitation reaction can be used employing agar gel (Fig. 7–7). Plate A illustrates double diffusion, in which the two reactants are allowed to diffuse toward each other; in the zone of equivalence, a line of precipitate is formed which represents the area of maximum interaction between the antigen and antibody. Plate B illustrates single diffusion, in which antibody is incorporated into the agar, and antigen diffuses out of the well; at equivalence, a ring of precipitate forms.

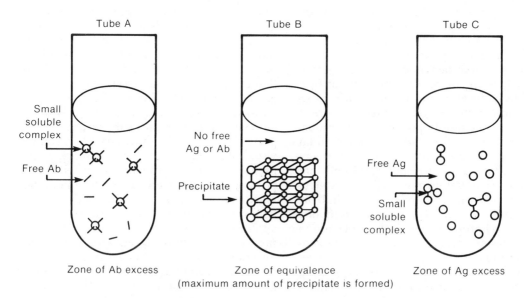

**FIG. 7–6.** The precipitation test.

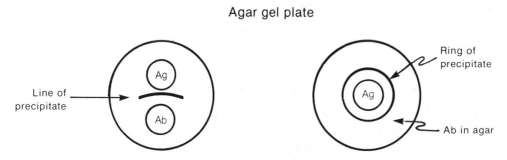

**FIG. 7–7.** The precipitation reaction in agar gel.

In an agglutination reaction, the antigen is a whole cell or large particle. When an antigen-antibody reaction occurs, a lattice is formed, and appears as large clumps of cells or particles; this reaction is more sensitive than the precipitation reaction. The relative amount of specific antibody present in sera or secretions can be determined by titration. When a constant amount of test antigen is reacted in a test tube with different dilutions of a serum or secretion, the highest dilution (lowest concentration) of antibody giving a positive reaction is the end-point of the titration. The antibody titer is expressed as the reciprocal of the end-point—e.g., an end-point of 1:512 is equal to a titer of 512.

*Complement* is an enzyme system of serum proteins that can be activated by many antigen-antibody reactions. The serum of all animal species contains varying quantities of complement. The activity of the complement system depends upon the operation of nine protein components (C1 through C9) acting in sequence. When the first component is activated by an antigen-antibody immune complex, it acquires the ability to activate several molecules of the next component, and so on, producing a cascade effect, with amplification. In this way, the activation of one molecule of C1 can lead to the activation of thousands of molecules of the other components. At each stage, activation is accompanied by the appearance of a new enzymatic activity, and since one enzyme molecule can process several substrate molecules, each complement factor can cause the processing or activation of many molecules of the next component in the sequence. The terminal components of the complement cascade have the ability to punch a "functional hole" through the cell membrane on which they are fixed. Thus, through this sequential amplification process, the activation of one C1 molecule can lead to a macroscopic event, namely, the lysis of a cell.

The effect of antibody and antigen upon the complement system may be used to measure an antigen-antibody reaction. Only two classes of antibody—IgM and IgG—can activate the first component of complement.

### IMMEDIATE HYPERSENSITIVITY

Some diseases result from the excessive action of the immune system. Antibody-mediated reactions which are harmful to the body are referred to as *immediate hypersensitivity reactions.* There are three types of immediate hypersensitivity responses. (There is also one type of delayed hypersensitivity response—Type IV—which is not considered here.)

**Type I.** Platelets, basophils in the blood, and *mast cells* in the tissues all contain receptor sites on their surfaces which are specific for the

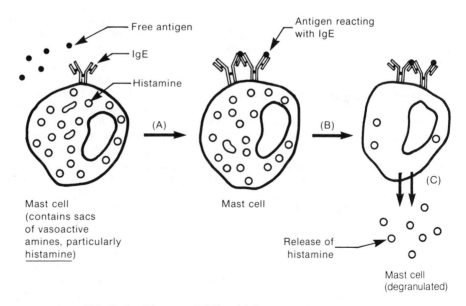

**FIG. 7–8.** The type I (allergic) hypersensitivity reaction.

Fc portion of IgE. Since the antibody is attached by the Fc portion, this leaves the combining sites in the Fab portions free to react with antigen. In an "allergic" individual, IgE attaches to mast cells by the Fc piece. When exposed to specific antigen (*allergen*) an antigen-antibody reaction takes place (Fig. 7–8). This antigen-antibody reaction near the cell surface triggers the release of pharmacologically active mediators (e.g., histamine) stored in cytoplasmic granules. These mediators then act on host tissues, causing the symptoms seen in an allergic individual. In an exquisitely sensitive individual, the reaction can lead to shock and death.

TYPE II. Complement-fixing antibodies (IgM or IgG) may be formed against: *1*) "self"-antigenic determinants on the surface of cells, or *2*) nonself haptens which may be attached to certain cells of the body. An antigen-antibody reaction which occurs on the cell surface leads to activation of the complement system, which results in lysis of the cells involved.

Type III. Antigen-antibody complexes formed in the circulation activate the complement system. Complement components then act to increase vascular permeability which, in turn, facilitates deposition of immune complexes on membranes of glomeruli, lungs, or in the walls of blood vessels. Factors generated by complement activation attract polymorphonuclear leukocytes to the area of reaction; the polymorphonuclear leukocytes phagocytize the immune complexes, but they also release degradative enzymes into the surrounding area, resulting in tissue destruction.

### THE CELL-MEDIATED IMMUNE RESPONSE

Cell-mediated immune reactions are those immunologic responses mediated by sensitized T lymphocytes, rather than circulating antibodies. The interaction of T cells with specific antigen causes activation of the T cells and release of lymphokines from the cells. The lymphokines are chemical mediators which affect other lymphocytes, as well as macrophages and polymorphonuclear leukocytes. Soluble lymphokines attract these three types of cells to the area of reaction. Once in the area, the macrophages become modified by lymphokines into "angry killer cells"; their phagocytic activity and their ability to degrade ingested foreign antigen are increased. Some specific T effector cells are also "killer" cells and appear to kill target antigens by direct contact. A delayed hypersensitivity (Type IV) reaction can be elicited by the subcutaneous injection of antigen. Twenty-four to forty-eight hours after antigen challenge, the site of injection becomes infiltrated with lymphocytes and macrophages, and edema and induration become apparent. The skin test can be used to determine if a subject has become sensitized to a particular antigen.

In summary, vaccination with a foreign antigen may induce a humoral and/or a cell-mediated immune response. The immune reactants produced—antibodies and sensitized lymphocytes—can react with the foreign antigen present in the body. This specific immune reaction usually leads to the elimination of the antigen. (It should be noted, however, that under certain circumstances vaccination may give rise to a detrimental hypersensitivity immune response.) If antibodies could be directed solely against an antigen associated only with the process of pregnancy, theoretically it should be possible to use this reaction as a very specific method of preventing a pregnancy without, for example, disrupting normal physiological processes in other tissues such as cell division or protein synthesis.

## CONTRACEPTIVE VACCINES

A comprehensive assessment of the immunological response of the female reproductive tract and of the status of programs in contraceptive vaccine development has recently been published (7). The concept of a contraceptive vaccine is to utilize a pregnancy-specific, or at least a reproductive-specific antigen to produce active immunization and antibody production in women. When pregnancy occurs, or the reproductive-specific antigen is subsequently detected by the body, the circulating antibodies will combine with the antigen and not only inhibit it immunologically but also neutralize its biological action. The ideal antigen should be organ-specific, and the immune response elicited should be inhibitory and reversible, rather than destructive, and should, as far as possible, be free of side effects.

The antigens that are being investigated fall into two broad categories—female-derived and male-derived. Antibodies to these antigens might interfere with sperm transport, capacitation, fertilization, ovum development, or implantation. The female antigens consist of placental hormones, other placental proteins, and zona pellucida proteins, while the male antigens are all derived from spermatozoa. This should not be construed to mean that the male-derived antigens will be used in the male, since antibodies against spermatozoa would almost certainly cause an irreversible destruction of the spermatogonia which are responsible for initiating each new wave of spermatogenesis. Thus the end result would be sterility—not a reversible means of contraception. Owing to the continuous nature of spermatogenesis, it is much more difficult to attack this process selectively and reversibly, whereas in the female, pregnancy is an episodic process. Hence all of the antigens considered to date have been conceived for immunization of women, rather than men. These sperm antigens will be used in the female to produce antibodies which might hopefully interfere with the process of sperm transport and/or fertilization.

## PLACENTAL HORMONES

### hCS

One placental hormone that has been examined experimentally is human placental lactogen (also known as human chorionic somatomammotropin, hCS). Experiments in which eight baboons were immunized with a highly purified baboon CS, altered by hapten coupling, showed that while antibodies reacting strongly with baboon CS were produced, two of three animals mated became pregnant. It was not clear whether the failure was due to saturation of circulating antibodies by the placental hormone or to retained biological activity in the antigen-antibody complex (33). In any event, hCS would be unlikely to prove useful as an antigen in a fertility control vaccine.

### hCG

Much more promising results have been obtained using portions of the placental hormone, human chorionic gonadotropin (hCG). This substance is synthesized by the trophoblast during early pregnancy from around the time of implantation (27) and is thought to be important in the maintenance of early pregnancy. It has been suggested that antibodies directed against hCG might prevent luteal maintenance or exert a direct cytotoxic effect on the developing blastocyst, and thus have a contraceptive effect (31). Human chorionic gonadotropin and the pituitary hormones—thyroid stimulating hormone, follicle stimulating hormone, and luteinizing hormone—have a similar chemical structure comprised of an alpha- and a beta-subunit chain of amino acids. Human chorionic gonadotropin has a common beta subunit with these pituitary hormones, and to avoid cross-reactivity of the antibodies against hCG with these other pituitary hormones, most experiments to date have been done using the beta subunit of hCG by itself. The beta subunit of these hormones provides the biological specificity, and hence antibodies directed to this portion of the structure alone should still neutralize the biological activity of the whole hormone (i.e., alpha and beta subunits combined). Indeed a high degree of antibody specificity to hCG from immunizations of experimental animals with purified beta-hCG has been achieved.

However, apart from 30 additional amino acids at the carboxyl terminus of beta-hCG, the subunits of hCG and human luteinizing hormone (hLH) are similar. Hence it seems impossible to produce antibodies to even very highly purified beta-hCG that will not cross-react, at least to some extent, with hLH (26, 32). Cross-reactive antibodies could be potentially damaging, in that they could induce autoimmune tissue damage in the pituitary, cause a hypofunctional state of target organs, e.g., hypoestrogenism, and form circulating immune complexes, resulting in glomerulonephritis (39).

Despite this, some women, previously sterilized or using other forms of contraception, have been immunized with highly purified beta-hCG conjugated to tetanus toxoid; menstruation and ovulation continued normally without any adverse reactions being observed. Whether such treatment would have been contraceptive was not examined in these experiments (8, 17, 22). The only definitive data in this regard come from immunization experiments with species of primates, in which antibodies to beta-hCG cross-react with their own CG, i.e., where beta-hCG behaves like an homologous antigen. Chimpanzees would be suitable (13), but are too scarce and expensive. Baboons are also suitable, although less so, because the cross-reaction is weaker (31). Because of lack of cross-reactivity between antibodies to hCG and the native CG, experiments using rhesus monkeys and marmosets are not relevant, since here beta-hCG acts as an heterologous antigen. Female baboons have been immunized with unaltered beta-hCG in Freund's's complete adjuvant, or hapten-coupled or conjugated beta-hCG in oil vehicle. Significant antibody titers were obtained in all animals, but, not surprisingly, immunization using Freund's adjuvant achieved the best response (31). The antisera produced reacted strongly with hCG, baboon CG, and hLH, but only weakly with baboon LH. Since there was little cross-reaction with baboon LH, ovulation occurred normally in 28 out of 30 cycles studied in 10 baboons. These 10 females had been proven fertile prior to immunization, and yet after immunization, and 3 matings each (30 total), no pregnancies ensued. These experiments clearly demonstrate the feasibility of this approach to development of a contraceptive vaccine.

The major disadvantage to the use of the whole beta subunit is the detectable but variable degree of cross-reactivity to LH. To obviate this, attention has been directed to the portion of beta-hCG which does not appear in beta-LH. Both synthetic and natural peptides derived from the carboxyl terminus of beta-hCG have been studied (34). Peptides comprised of as few as 20 amino acids have been tested, but lack of antigenicity in such small molecules has been a problem. Some success was achieved with a synthetic 35 amino acid sequence and a natural 38 amino acid peptide. Antibodies raised in baboons to these peptides cross-reacted with hCG, beta-hCG, and the peptides, but not with hLH (33). Thus this approach is feasible, but many questions remain as to the long-term risks of such therapy, and information is still needed regarding the optimal conjugates and adjuvants to give good antibody titers.

### OTHER PLACENTAL PROTEINS

Of the various proteins which have been claimed to be specific to the placenta, only two appear to be promising candidates as antigens for a fertility control vaccine. These are $SP_1$ (a pregnancy-specific beta-glycoprotein) and $PP_5$ (a placental glycoprotein) (1–4). $SP_1$ is a glycoprotein with a molecular weight of 90,000 daltons, and is 28 per cent carbohydrate. It is present in the placenta (30 mg. per placenta) and in pregnancy serum (5–30 mg. per 100 ml.). $PP_5$ has a molecular weight of 50,000 daltons and is only 10 per cent carbohydrate. There are only about 2 mg. per placenta, and very little in pregnancy serum (0.1 mg. per 100 ml.).

Antibodies to human $SP_1$ cross-react with placental extracts from chimpanzee, baboon, and *Macaca mulatta* and *Macaca fasicularis*, while $PP_5$ appears identical in various primates (5). While preliminary experiments in cynomolgus monkeys both passively (injected with antiserum from other animals) and actively (injected with antigen to develop their own antibodies) immunized with hapten-coupled human-$SP_1$ showed that abortion could ensue, these were generally late abortions and thus probably not acceptable as a method of fertility control. Additional studies in rhesus monkeys and baboons immunized with rhesus $SP_1$ were unsuccessful, and further work has been abandoned (43).

$PP_5$ remains at low concentrations throughout pregnancy and is localized in and on the cells of the syncytiotrophoblast. Preliminary experiments showed a marked reduction in fertility in cynomolgus monkeys immunized with human $PP_5$. Further work was planned with this antigen (43), but since only trace amounts of rhesus $PP_5$ could be recovered, isolation of sufficient material for antifertility studies was impossible, and work has been abandoned (44).

### SPERM ANTIGENS

Various antigens of spermatozoa have been isolated and purified. These antigens included carbohydrate antigens, T-antigen, acrosin, and hyaluronidase—these latter two are enzymes thought to be important in the fertilization process. However, tests of the fertility of animals actively immunized with such antigens showed little or no antifertility effect. It seems unlikely that they will be of any use as the basis for an antifertility vaccine.

Two other sperm antigens showed greater promise. One of these is lactate dehydrogenase-X (LDH-X). There is good evidence that this enzyme is specific to the sperm, and it is located in the mid-piece, but its exact function with regard to motility or fertilizing capacity is not known (11). Active immunization of rabbits with mouse LDH-X caused a significant reduction in fertility, and passive immunization of mice was similarly effective. At present, studies are being undertaken in baboons actively immunized with purified human LDH-X. Preliminary results have shown a reduction in conception rate. Further support for the importance of this enzyme for the functionality of sperm can be adduced from the fact that sera from 6 out of 76 infertile patients had antibodies against human LDH-X.

The other antigen with potential promise is the so-called sperm-immobilizing antigen (SIA). This antigen appears to be a testis-specific antigen common to man, rhesus monkey, baboon, and chimpanzee (18). Female rhesus monkeys immunized with human SIA developed sperm agglutinating and immobilizing activity in sera and vaginal washings, but fertility was apparently not affected. The search for other sperm-specific antigens, such as cell-membrane antigens, which might prove more fruitful for fertility control, is being continued. At this stage of development, however, the sperm antigens appear much less promising than the placental hormone approach.

## ZONA PELLUCIDA ANTIGENS

Active or passive immunization of several rodent species with ovarian homogenates caused a reduction in fertility. It was found that one or more specific antigens were located in the zona pellucida and that exposure of ova to the antibody to these antigens caused formation of a precipitate on the outer zona surface which prevented sperm penetration, and in fertilized ova blastocysts hatching from the zona pellucida, thus preventing implantation (29). Zona antigens have been identified in ova of many species and are present from the early stages of zona pellucida development in the follicle. It has been found that antibodies to pig zona antigens react with zonae of several nonhuman primates and of humans. Conversely, antibodies to human zonae cross-react with zonae of pigs. This means that pig zonae, which can be easily collected from ovaries at slaughterhouses, can provide a good source of starting-material for isolating and purifying zona antigens (24). Furthermore, $F(ab^1)_{2\alpha}$ immunoglobulin fractions prepared from several antisera which contained antizona activity reacted equally as much with zona as with

their whole-serum counterparts. This confirms that antizona binding and formation of a precipitation layer or the zona is the result of a specific antigen-antibody reaction (25).

Seven out of thirty-three sera from infertile women have shown presence of auto-antibodies to zone pellucida, but it should be noted that two of these seven women subsequently became pregnant (43). Thus at this time it is not clear what role antibodies to zonae play in human infertility. These findings may only indicate the reversibility of the reaction. Reversibility is, of course, a question of major importance: if the antizona antibodies react with follicular ova, there is a strong possibility of producing sterility, or at the very least a long period of infertility. For the moment, the answer to this question is not available. However, like beta-hCG peptides, zona antigens appear to show promise as the basis for a contraceptive vaccine.

## SAFETY EVALUATIONS

If contraceptive vaccines are to be successful, it will ultimately have to be shown that they are effective, and that their action is reversible and safe. Unlike other forms of immunization, this therapy is not designed to combat a life-threatening disease, and consequently, modest risks acceptable in other circumstances will not be so here. It will be necessary to answer the following questions: What type of antibody response—humoral, cellular, or both—is produced? Do hypersensitivities occur? Do antibodies cross-react with other tissues? Are immune complexes formed, and if so, will they give rise to glomerulonephritis? Many of these areas are still uncharted as far as contraceptive vaccines are concerned, and so progress to a usable vaccine will be slow. Guidelines for such safety studies have been published (45).

## DEVICE DEVELOPMENT

## INTRAUTERINE DEVICES

Although intrauterine devices have long been used for contraceptive purposes, they have only become popular during the last 40 years, after the work of Graefenberg and Ota. Until very recently these devices were fabricated from inert materials of various types. Of the inert devices, the one that has become the model against which all others have been measured is the Lippes Loop.

One of the major reasons for the development of the newer medicated intrauterine devices has been the necessity of improving continuation rates. With most inert devices, continuation rates at the end of 1 year, in controlled clinical trials, may be below 80 per cent, and, in family planning programs, less than 70 per cent; after 2 years, the rate may be less than 60 per cent (14).

Within the last few years, a variety of newer intrauterine devices have been developed which release chemicals, either copper or hormones (14). The two main types of copper-releasing devices are known as the Copper T and the Copper Seven. Of the devices with the T-configuration, the T Cu 200, with 200 sq. mm. of copper wire wound around both the vertical and horizontal arms, has proved the most satisfactory (38). This device has proved to be more acceptable than the Lippes Loop D (a polyethylene IUD) in terms of pain, bleeding, and expulsions, and as effective for contraception (35). Since the copper eventually becomes exhausted, it is recommended that such devices be replaced every 3 years. Studies are in progress with other configurations using, for example, multiple copper sleeves, rather than copper wire, which might be expected to increase the useful life-span (36). In addition, a device containing more copper, i.e., the T Cu 380A, has also been tested, and in preliminary studies, at least, has lower pregnancy, expulsion, and removal rates (38).

The Copper Seven seems somewhat similar. Copper wire is wound around the long stem of a copolymer of polypropylene and polyethylene shaped like a seven, to give an area of 200 sq. mm. of copper. Results from clinical trials suggest that there is little difference between the Copper T or Copper Seven and that both are at least equal, and probably superior in performance to the Lippes Loop (37). There is also some evidence that the Copper Seven device may be effective for more than 4 years, without need for removal and replacement (48). There may be some risk that the copper released in the uterus may accumulate in other organs of the body, but this has not been demonstrated yet.

Concurrently with the work on copper-releasing devices, devices releasing progesterone are being developed. It is known that a correct balance between estrogen and progesterone is required for normal endometrial development, which will permit implantation and decidualization. Consequently, it was suggested that intrauterine administration of minute doses of progesterone might prevent implantation, without producing systemic effects (28). Following successful preliminary trials, a T-configuration was selected. This system consisted of a biocompatible barrier polymer and an internal matrix which acted as a reservoir and rate-controlling membrane for releasing progesterone (16). The final configuration released approximately $50\mu g.$ per day with a zero-order (constant daily) release rate. It was found to have a low pregnancy, expulsion, and removal rate (21). Large-scale studies have confirmed the initial promise of this device. One significant advantage of the progesterone-releasing IUD (Progestasert) over other types of devices, particularly for women at risk from anemia, is the reduced blood loss at menstruation associated with its use. One disadvantage is the short life-span of the present generation of devices, only 12 to 18 months.

Efforts are now under way to prolong the life-span of the present devices, and to develop new ones loaded with synthetic progestins, such as norethisterone or levonorgestrel. Since these drugs are more active than progesterone, less would be required to produce the same effect on endometrial morphology. Thus the life-span of the device would be extended. A device releasing $2\mu g.$ of levonorgestrel per day has now been developed and fabricated, and is undergoing toxicological testing prior to Phase II clinical trials (44).

Most of the recent efforts to improve intrauterine devices have been directed to increasing their acceptability, rather than their contraceptive efficacy. In general, nearly all intrauterine devices have been contraceptively effective, provided they remained in situ and were not dislodged downward into the cervical canal. Therefore, improvement of their contraceptive efficacy would have only a very marginal effect on their utility and acceptability. Reducing the amount of menstrual bleeding, pain, and number of expulsions would, on the other hand, have a very great impact on their wider acceptance. As noted above, continuation rates are poor. Moreover, once a device has been expelled or removed, for whatever reason, the chances of the woman asking for a reinsertion are greatly diminished. Various studies are being made to determine the reasons for increased bleeding and pain following insertion of an intrauterine device. This research is also testing the ability of various chemicals to inhibit fibrinolysis (destruction of fibrinogen) and proteolysis (breakdown of protein), or increased uterine contractility, and thus diminish these side effects.

## INTRACERVICAL DEVICES

Interest has been aroused in recent years by the idea of developing an intracervical device which would release either hormones that would make cervical mucus impenetrable to sperm or other chemicals which would kill sperm. The attraction of such a device, as with the medicated intrauterine devices, is that the drugs would be released constantly in very small amounts and thus, theoretically, exert only a local effect. The problem of designing an intracervical device is that it is frequently expelled, especially in multiparous women. One way to circumvent this is to extend the device into the lower segment of the uterus, with small hooks around the inner cervical os. To date, a thoroughly satisfactory configuration for the device has not been designed, but some progress has been made in identifying the chemicals which would be released from the devices. The drugs chosen for initial study are quinine sulfate and levonorgestrel. Preliminary chemical studies appear promising (44). The first compound affects sperm viability, while the latter changes cervical mucus consistency. Many questions still remain to be answered concerning this approach—especially concerning the toxicity to the cervical mucosa of constant exposure to such compounds. A significant disadvantage of the intracervical device is that, like the intrauterine device, it would not easily be self-inserted by the woman, thus reducing its potential applicability in many countries.

## INTRAVAGINAL DEVICES

Unlike the intrauterine and intracervical devices, an intravaginal device can easily be self-inserted and, except in those cultures with taboos regarding genital manipulation, would appear to be widely acceptable. Furthermore, its insertion need not be coitally related, because the device can be left in situ for prolonged periods of time.

Two types of devices are under development. The basic design for all devices is a ring

configuration, and it is envisaged that, as with the intracervical devices, either steroids or spermicidal agents could be released. Steroids can be released in doses that will have a systemic effect and inhibit ovulation (thus working in a similar fashion to oral contraceptive pills) or at lower doses only affecting cervical mucus and sperm-penetration locally.

Initial trials centered on the use of medroxyprogesterone acetate (20) and chlormadinone acetate (12), two $17\alpha$-acetoxy progestins. The doses of medroxyprogesterone acetate used ensured inhibition of ovulation, and the results appeared sufficiently favorable for continued developmental work. Following the withdrawal of the $17\alpha$-acetoxy progestins from clinical trials, because of presumed toxicological hazards, work was switched to studies of 19-nortestosterone derivatives (19). Of the derivatives tested, it appeared that norgestrel was the most satisfactory, although not as effective as medroxyprogesterone acetate. Further developmental work was done on the devices to ensure a more constant release of drug, and this was achieved with an inner steroid-free core, covered with a thin layer of Silastic impregnated with racemic norgestrel (42). Although ovulation was inhibited, there was still a high incidence of breakthrough bleeding, and this continues to be a major problem with these high-dose devices.

Similar devices have been tested with lower levels of steroid hormones, progesterone, norethisterone, and norgestrel (43). When ovulation was inhibited, side effects of irregular cycles, spotting, and amenorrhea occurred, but when the doses were reduced so that ovulation was not inhibited, spotting or breakthrough bleeding was significantly reduced. However, these doses were still able to inhibit sperm-penetration through cervical mucus. The women in these trials found the devices acceptable. Determinations of blood hormones showed constant levels, indicating a zero-order release rate.

The favorable results from these studies permitted larger-scale trials to be started, using devices releasing $50\mu g$. per day of norethisterone or $20\mu g$. per day of levonorgestrel. It seems likely that such rings can be effective for 6 to 12 months. Unlike the devices that inhibit ovulation, these low-dose devices do not need to be removed monthly to permit menstruation, since its normal occurrence should be unaffected.

A comparative clinical trial of three types of

steroid-loaded devices is to be carried out by the World Health Organization's (WHO) network of Collaborating Centers for Clinical Research. The devices developed by the Population Council contain norgestrel in doses that inhibit ovulation; those developed by the Wyeth Pharmaceutical Company contain norgestrel and ethinyl estradiol in doses that inhibit ovulation; and those developed by WHO contain norgestrel, but in doses that do not inhibit ovulation. The results from such a trial will determine which approach is most promising, and test the acceptability of this type of device.

Spermicide-loaded intravaginal devices are also under development. The compounds being studied are nonoxynol-9 and quinine.

Of all the intracervical and the intravaginal devices presently under development, the intravaginal ones containing steroids offer more promise for widespread use. They are inexpensive, are easily inserted and removed, and have a reasonably long life-span. They also appear to be acceptable. Whether or not those with a tolerable level of side effects will be satisfactory contraceptives remains to be determined.

## LONG-TERM INJECTABLE CONTRACEPTIVES

Of all the available synthetic progestational agents, only two have been found suitable for use in long-term injectable preparations. Clinical trials have shown that depot-medroxyprogesterone acetate can be injected at a dose of 150 mg. once every 12 weeks and provide reliable contraception by suppressing ovulation. The disadvantage of this compound is that very few women using it experience normal menstrual cycles, and a high proportion become amenorrheic. There may also be reduced fertility following cessation of treatment. Norethisterone oenanthate, at a dose of 200 mg., does not provide effective ovulation inhibition when given once every 12 weeks, but does so when given once every 8 weeks. This preparation causes significantly less amenorrhea than medroxyprogesterone acetate, and because of toxicity problems with 17α-acetoxy progestins, remains an attractive compound. Preliminary results of large-scale clinical comparisons between depot-medroxyprogesterone acetate (every 3 months) and norethisterone oenanthate (every 2 months for 6 months, and then every 3 months) indicate

that both regimes provide effective contraception (44). There seems to be, however, a greater incidence of amenorrhea with the 8-week schedule of norethisterone oenanthate than with the 12-week regimen (43, 44).

Studies with monthly injectable preparations—depot medroxy-progesterone acetate (25 mg.) and estradiol cypionate (5 mg.), and norethisterone oenanthate (50 mg.) and estradiol valerate (5 mg.)—are also under way (43).

Another potentially attractive approach to long-term injectable contraception is development of biodegradable polymers that disappear as the steroid is released. With such systems it is much easier to ensure a zero-order release rate and, therefore, constant blood levels of the contraceptive steroid. This improves efficacy and reduces side effects.

Initial studies by WHO have concentrated on micronized norethisterone in a polymeric matrix (Chronomer TM) which will last 3 months. Longer-term devices may be developed, using norgestrel because of its greater potency. Phase I clinical trials are only just commencing on this system. Another system under development utilizes a polylactide device containing northisterone, but there appear to be variations among batches of the polylactide carrier which affect the consistency of the release rate.

The Contraceptive Development Branch of the Center for Population Research at the National Institute of Child Health and Human Development has also supported work in this field. An up-to-date report of the activities of their contractors has recently been published (10). Most work is still concentrated on development of a system that can give zero-order release rates. Those under investigation include glutamic acid/leucine copolymers and polymers of glycolide, DL-lactide, L(-)lactide, ε-caprolactone, and DL-3-caprolactone. At the time of publication, none of these systems has proved entirely satisfactory.

Thus, although the concept of a device employing a biodegradable matrix containing a contraceptive steroid is attractive, it seems to be some considerable way from practical implementation.

## PROSTAGLANDINS (PGs)

Since 1970, great interest has been shown in the potential of prostaglandins as contraceptive agents. Prostaglandins are long-chain fatty acids with a variety of physiological and pharmacological effects. They appear to be produced in most cells of the body, to a greater or lesser extent. The so-called primary, or (perhaps more properly) "classical" prostaglandins are those of the F, E, and D series. Most work has been done with these compounds and their effects on reproduction, because it appears that $PGF_{2\alpha}$ may be the normal substance produced in the uterus which controls the life-span of the corpus luteum in nonprimate species. This is not the case in primates. At this writing, it is not clear whether the life-span of the nonpregnant primate corpus luteum is controlled by a luteolytic substance, perhaps a PG, produced in the ovary, or whether the corpus luteum has an inherent "destruct mechanism," inhibited only by production of hCG by the trophoblast. In any event, it has not proved possible to demonstrate unequivocally that $PGF_{2\alpha}$ or its analogs can exert a luteolytic effect in humans. The general consensus is that failure of corpus-luteum function and progesterone secretion upon administration of either PGEs or PGFs is secondary to increased uterine contractility and disruption of the embryo's attachment to the endometrium.

Whether the newer prostanoid structures, such as Thromboxane $A_2$ or $PGI_2$ (prostacyclin), play any role in normal reproduction or exert pharmacological actions on pregnancy, is not known. However, it is known that the uterus produces large quantities of 6-keto-$PGF_{1\alpha}$, the major metabolite of $PGI_2$ (9).

Even though $PGF_{2\alpha}$ and $PGE_2$ are not luteolytic in humans and are metabolized very rapidly in vivo, initial studies using intravenous infusion or intra- or extra-amniotic injection showed that these compounds could produce abortion during the first and second trimesters of pregnancy (23). However, there remained difficulties with the stability of the PGE compounds and the rapid metabolism of both Es and Fs, so that repeated administration was often necessary to achieve the desired effect.

Once the first generation of PG analogs, especially the 15-methyl-$PGF_{2\alpha}$ and its methyl ester, and the 16, 16-dimethyl $PGE_2$ were available, more satisfactory results were achieved. These compounds were much more resistant to metabolism and hence could exert an effect over a longer period; smaller doses could be used, and this often meant that side effects—nausea, vomiting, and diarrhea—were also reduced. Various large-scale clinical

trials showed that 15-methyl $PGF_{2\alpha}$ could induce abortion satisfactorily during the second trimester of pregnancy, whether given intra-amniotically or extra-amniotically. The results were, moreover, just as satisfactory as those achieved with intraamniotic saline (46, 47).

For successful use as contraceptives, however, it was thought necessary to develop a system permitting vaginal self-insertion of a PG shortly after a missed menstrual period. One multicenter study compared administration of vaginal suppositories containing 1 mg. or 1.5 mg. of 15-methyl $PGF_{2\alpha}$ methyl ester every third hour, on four occasions, to patients between the 5th and 8th weeks of gestation. The overall success rate for complete abortion was 82 per cent and 84 per cent respectively, but varied between 70 per cent and 100 per cent in different centers (43). Some vomiting and diarrhea was observed, but duration of bleeding was similar to that seen after a vacuum aspiration. A single vaginal administration of a 3-mg. suppository containing 15-methyl $PGF_{2\alpha}$ methyl ester is also being evaluated. Initial studies indicate as good, or greater, efficacy than repeated administration, and similar levels of side effects—94.5 per cent complete abortion in patients through the 8th week of pregnancy (44).

In a randomized comparison of vacuum aspiration and repeated vaginal administration of 16, 16-dimethyl $PGE_2$ during the 5th to 8th week of gestation performed on an outpatient basis on 77 women, it was found that abortion occurred in all cases, except in one of vacuum aspiration. Frequency of complete abortion was over 90 per cent for both methods. It was concluded from this study that vacuum aspiration was superior with regard to time in hospital, duration of bleeding, and frequency of gastrointestinal side effects, but vaginal PG application was simpler (43). This would be particularly true if one, rather than repeated application(s), of PG was also effective.

The PGE analogs appear to have fewer side effects than the F analogs; they are still, however, somewhat unstable, and further work is needed to develop more stable analogs. Developmental work under way suggests that it should be possible within the next few years to have available a vaginal suppository containing a PG which can be self-administered during the first 56 days of amenorrhea, and which would be at least 90 per cent effective, and have a low incidence of side effects. Development of orally active analogs is also possible. Thus there appears great promise in the prostaglandins for a useful addition to our contraceptive armamentarium.

## MALE CONTRACEPTIVES

Although the balance is now being redressed, there has until recently been much less research on development of male contraceptives than on those intended for women. Furthermore, the need to maintain libido and potency in the male is paramount, and the close morphological and functional relationship of spermatogenic and androgenic functions makes many methods unacceptable. There are three major areas in which control of male fertility could be achieved: interference with (1) spermatogenesis, (2) sperm maturation, and (3) sperm transport.

Interference with spermatogenesis might be achieved by differential suppression of follicle-stimulating hormone (FSH) secretion, although there is some debate as to whether FSH alone controls spermatogenesis. There is considerable evidence that a water-soluble polypeptide in the testis (known as *inhibin*) may regulate gonadotropin secretion in vivo (15, 41). If this is true (and the question is somewhat controversial) (44), then this substance, or analogs of it, might be used for contraception in the male. Such a possibility is clearly far in the future.

Nearer to reality are the studies made in recent years using steroids, in various combinations, to suppress gonadotropin secretion and yet maintain testosterone concentrations. The most promising combinations have been comprised of a progestin (suppressing spermatogenesis, and production of FSH, LH, and testosterone) and an androgen to replace the endogenous testosterone production. One such combination is Danazol (17α-pregn-4-en-20-ynol [2,3-d] isoxazol-17-ol, 600 mg. per day by mouth) and testosterone oenanthate (200 mg. per month intramuscularly), which reduced sperm counts below 10 million in 12 weeks (40). After discontinuation of treatment, sperm counts returned to normal within 4 months. Other progestational agents, such as R2323, norethandrolone, megestrol acetate, medroxyprogesterone acetate, and norgestrienone, when combined with androgen either by injection or subcutaneous implant, have been shown to produce similar effects.

Thus the concept of combined androgen/progestin therapy is sound, and it seems only a matter of time before the most suitable combination is achieved. The major difficulty at the moment is the lack of an orally effective androgen without major side effects, such as the hepatotoxicity induced by methyl testosterone. It is still not clear what the contraceptive efficacy of such treatment will be in large-scale studies, or how acceptable it will prove in practice. The long delay before reduced sperm numbers are achieved, and the equally long delay before the return to fertility, seem likely to lead to reduced acceptability.

In addition to the progestin/androgen combinations, reversible suppression of sperm production in men can also be achieved by administration of an estrogen and an androgen (6), or a long-acting androgen alone (30). There is little information on the safety of long-term treatment of men with estrogens, and therefore the acceptability of this treatment is uncertain. With respect to the second approach, it remains to be demonstrated that sterility can be achieved without any elevation of average peripheral testosterone levels. The effects of chronically elevating peripheral testosterone levels remain unknown, but some concern exists as to the possible changes in prostatic growth and in the cardiovascular system.

All of the nonsteroidal compounds which are known to affect spermatogenesis directly are highly toxic and, generally, mutagenic, and thus hold no immediate promise for clinical use. Little work is being done with agents to interfere with sperm maturation or transport in the male because, with one exception, there are no promising leads. Some halogenated sugars related to α-chlorhydrin have shown promise as antifertility agents in rats and monkeys, but without the associated toxicity of this latter compound. They appear to affect metabolic activity of sperm in the epididymis within 4 to 5 days after oral treatment commences. Fertility returned 3 to 6 weeks after the end of treatment (44). It remains to be determined whether this early promise will be borne out.

## CONCLUSIONS

While the foregoing attests to the large amount of developmental work that is continuing world-wide in the search to develop new contraceptive methods, it is also clear that few of the new methods will be available in the immediate future. PG suppositories, medicated IUDs and vaginal rings, and perhaps androgen/progestin combinations may be available fairly soon. It will take a longer time to develop the promising contraceptive vaccine based on beta-hCG, the medicated devices (especially those containing spermicidal agents), and the long-term injectables. Forms of male contraception, other than the combination pills, are obviously very long-range projects. Thus the future holds promise, but it is unrealistic to expect any one new method to be available very soon or to provide a universal panacea. Various methods—both male and female—will be needed to suit different cultures, ethnic groups, and physiological conditions.

## REFERENCES

1. Bohn H: Nachweis und Charakterisierung von Schwangerschaftsproteinen in der Menschlichen Placenta, sowie ihre quantitative immunologische Bestimmung im Serum schwangerer Frauen. Arch Gynaekol 210:440, 1971

2. Bohn H: Isolierung and Charakterisierung des Schwangerschafts-spezifischen $\beta_1$-Glykoproteins. Blut 24:292, 1972

3. Bohn H: Nachweis und Charakterisierung von löslichen Antigenen in der menschlichen Placenta. Arch Gynaekol 212:165, 1972

4. Bohn H: Untersuchungen über das schwangerschaftsspezifische $\beta_1$-Glykoprotein (SP$_1$). Arch Gynaekol 216:347, 1974

5. Bohn H: The protein antigens of human placenta as a basis for the development of contraceptive vaccine. In Development of Vaccines for Fertility Regulation. Copenhagen, Scriptor, 1976, p 111

6. Briggs M, Briggs M: Oral contraceptive for men. Nature 252:585, 1974

7. Cinader B, de Weck A: Immunological Response of the Female Reproductive Tract. Copenhagen, Scriptor, 1976, 99 pp

8. Das C, Talwar GP, Ramakrishnan S, Salahuddin M, Kumar S, Hingorani V, Coutinho E, Croxatto H, Hemmingson E, Johansson E, Luukainen T, Shahani S, Sundaram K, Nash H, Segal SJ: Discriminatory effect of anti-Pr-$\beta$-hCG-TT antibodies on the neutralization of biological activity of placental and pituitary gonadotropins. Contraception 18:35, 1978

9. Fenwick L, Jones RL, Naylor B, Poyser NL, Wilson NH: Production of prostaglandins by the pseudopregnant rat uterus, *in vitro*, and the effect of tamoxifen with the identification of 6-keto-prostaglandin F$_{1\alpha}$ as a major product. Br J Pharmacol 59:191, 1977

10. Gabelnick HL (ed): Drug Delivery Systems. A workshop sponsored by Contraceptive Development Branch, Center for Population Research, National Institute of Child Health and Human Development. Washington DC, US Dept Health, Education and Welfare, DHEW Publ No. (NIH) 77-1238, 1976, 414 pp

11. Goldberg E: Effects of immunization with LDH-X on fertility. Acta Endocrinol (Kbh) [Suppl 194] 78:202, 1975

12. Henzl MR, Mishell DR Jr, Velazquez JG, Leitch WE: Basic studies for prolonged progestogen administration by vaginal devices. Am J Obstet Gynecol 117:101, 1973

13. Hodgen GD, Nixon WE, Vaitukaitis JL, Tullner WW, Ross GT: Neutralization of primate chorionic gonadotropin activities by antisera against the subunits of human chorionic gonadotropin in radioimmunoassay and bioassay. Endocrinology 92:705, 1973

14. Huber SC, Piotrow PT, Orlans B, Kommer G: IUDs reassessed—A decade of experience. In Conn FG (ed): Population Reports Series B, No 2, B21–B48, Dept Medical and Public Affairs, G Washington Med Center, Washington DC, 1975

15. Krueger PM, Hodgen GD, Sherins RJ: New evidence for the role of the Sertoli cell and spermatogonia in feedback control of FSH secretion in male rats. Endocrinology 95:955, 1974

16. Kulkarni BD, Avila TD, Phariss BB, Scommegna A: Release of $^3$H-progesterone from polymeric systems in the rhesus monkey. Contraception 8:299, 1973

17. Kumar S, Sharma NC, Bajaj JS, Talwar GP, Hingorani V: Clinical profile and toxicology studies on four women immunized with Pr-$\beta$-hCG-TT. Contraception 13:253, 1976

18. Menge AC, Fuller B: Testis antigens of man and some other primates. Fertil Steril 26:473, 1975

19. Mishell DR Jr: Intravaginal rings for contraceptive use: an editorial comment. Contraception 12:249, 1975

20. Mishell DR Jr, Talas M, Parlow AF, Moyer DL: Contraception by means of a Silastic vaginal ring impregnated with medroxyprogesterone acetate. Am J Obstet Gynecol 107:101, 1970

21. Pharris BB, Erickson R, Bashaw J, Hoff S, Place VA, Zaffaroni A: uterine therapeutic system for long term contraception II. Clinical correlates. Fertil Steril 25:922, 1974

22. Ramakrishnan S, Dubey SK, Das C, Salahuddin M, Talwar GP, Kumar S, Hingorani V: Influence of hCG and tetanus toxoid injections on the antibody titers in a subject immunized with Pr-$\beta$-hCG-TT. Contraception 13:245, 1976

23. Ramwell PW, Shaw JE (eds): Prostaglandins. Ann NY Acad Sci 180:568 pp, 1971

24. Sacco AG: Antigenic cross-reactivity between human and pig zona pellucida. Biol Reprod 16:164, 1977

25. Sacco AG: Immunological specificity of antizona binding to zona pellucida. J Exp Zool 204:181, 1978

26. Salahuddin M, Ramakrishnan S, Dubey SK, Talwar GP: Immunological reactivity of antibodies produced by Pr-$\beta$-hCG-TT with different hormones. Contraception 13:163, 1976

27. Saxena BB, Hasan SH, Haour F, Schmidt-Gollwitzer M: Radioreceptor assay of human chorionic gonadotropin: detection of early pregnancy. Science 184:793, 1974

28. Scommegna A: Progesterone-releasing intrauterine devices. In Moghissi KS, Evans TN (eds): Regulation of Human Fertility. Detroit, Wayne State University Press, 1976, p 222

29. Shivers CA: Immunological interference with fertilization. Acta Endocrinol (Kbh) [Suppl 194] 78:223, 1975

30. Steinberger E, Smith KD, Rodriguez-Rigau LJ: Suppression and recovery of sperm production in men treated with testosterone enanthate for one year. A study of a possible reversible male contraceptive. Int J Andrology [Suppl] 2:748, 1978

31. Stevens VC: Female contraception by immunization with hCG—Prospects and status. In Nieschlag E (ed): Immunization with Hormones in Reproduction Research. Amsterdam, North Holland, 1975, p 217

32. Stevens VC: Effects of antibodies to hCG on reproductive events in women and female baboons. In Laumas KR (ed): Recent Developments in Contraceptive Technology. Proc Int Symp New Delhi, New Delhi, Ankur, 1976, p 147

33. Stevens VC: Perspectives of development of a fertility control vaccine from hormonal antigens of the trophoblast. In Development of Vaccines for Fertility Regulation. Copenhagen, Scriptor, 1976, p 93

34. Stevens VC: Immunological approaches to fertility regulation. Bull WHO 56:179, 1978

35. Tatum HJ: The first year of clinical experience with the Copper T intrauterine contraceptive system in the United States and Canada. Contraception 6:179, 1972

36. Tatum HJ: Metallic copper as an intrauterine contraceptive agent. Am J Obstet Gynecol 117:602, 1973

37. Tatum HJ: Copper-bearing intrauterine devices. Clin Obstet Gynecol 17(1):93, 1974

38. Tatum HJ: Clinical experience with copper-bearing intrauterine devices and some thoughts on these mechanism(s) of action. In Moghissi KS, Evans TN (eds): Regulation of Human Fertility. Detroit, Wayne State University Press, 1976, p 194

39. Tung KSK: Considerations for the assessment of the safety of potential vaccines containing reproductive specific antigens. In Development of Vaccines for Fertility Regulation. Copenhagen, Scriptor, 1976, p 127

40. Ulstein M, Netto N, Leonard J, Paulsen CA: Changes in sperm morphology in normal men treated with Danazol and testosterone. Contraception 12:437, 1975

41. Van Thiel DH, Sherins RJ, Meyers GH, DeVita VT: Evidence for a specific seminiferous tubular factor affecting follicle stimulating hormone secretion in man. J Clin Invest 51:1009, 1972

42. Victor A, Johansson EDB: Plasma levels of d-Norgestrel and ovarian function in women using intravaginal rings impregnated with dl-Norgestrel for several cycles. Contraception 14:215, 1976

43. World Health Organization, Special Programme of Research, Development and Research Training in Human Reproduction, Sixth Annual Report, 1977, 141 pp

44. World Health Organization, Special Programme of Research, Development and Research Training in Human Reproduction, Seventh Annual Report, 1978, 167 pp

45. World Health Organzation Task Force on Immunological Methods for Fertility Regulation: Evaluating the safety and efficacy of placental antigen vaccines for fertility regulation. Clin Exp Immunol 33:360, 1978

46. World Health Organization Task Force on the Use of Prostaglandins for the Regulation of Fertility. Prostaglandins for Abortion II. Single extra-amniotic administration of 0.92 mg of 15-methyl-$PGF_{2\alpha}$ in Hyskon for termination of pregnancies in the 10th to 20th weeks of gestation: An international multicenter study. Am J Obstet Gynecol 129:597, 1977

47. World Health Organization Task Force on the Use of Prostaglandins for the Regulation of Fertility. Prostaglandins and Abortion III. Comparison of single intra-amniotic injections of 15-methyl-$PGF_{2\alpha}$ and $PGF_{2\alpha}$ for termination of second trimester pregnancy: an international multicenter study. Am J Obstet Gynecol 129:601, 1977

48. Zipper J, Medel M, Pastene L, Rivera M, Torres L, Osorio A, Toscanini C: Four years experience with the Cu 7 200 device—endouterine copper fertility control. Contraception 13:7, 1976

# 8

# Methods of Sterilization in Men and Women

## Marguerite K. Shepard

Since the mid-1960s there has been a marked increase in the number of individuals seeking sterilization to limit childbearing. Prior to that time, sterilization was usually performed only for medical or obstetric indications or in cases of very large family size.

Several factors have been responsible for the change. Social factors include emphasis on small family size; increased freedom for women to develop careers and interests outside the home; separation of recreational from procreational sex; and earlier completion of childbearing, leaving a substantial number of years during which a couple is both sexually active and fertile. Technical factors include improved surgical and anesthetic techniques and the refinement of endoscopic techniques, permitting safe, rapid procedures with minimal postoperative recovery requirements. Finally, professional factors include increased willingness of physicians to terminate fertility in individuals of relatively young age with limited reproductive experience. The following discussion of sterilization will consider indications, methods, immediate complications, choice of procedure, long-term sequelae (side effects or consequences), and possibility of reversal.

## INDICATIONS

Indications for sterilization may be classified as medical, obstetric, genetic, or social. The majority of procedures currently performed fall into the last category. Medical indications for sterilization usually relate to illness in one of the partners, specifically: *1*) disease states in the female which would be exacerbated by the process of pregnancy, such as rheumatic heart disease, severe diabetes, severe hypertension, and severe kidney disease; *2*) disease states in the male partner, whose life expectancy is, as a result, severely limited, and who consequently does not wish to leave his spouse the responsibility of rearing young children in case of early widowhood. A general rule of thumb followed in the case of medically indicated sterilization is to sterilize the affected partner, if possible. Such a practice permits the healthy partner to maintain fertility, in the event that the unhealthy spouse dies.

Obstetric indications for sterilization apply to the female alone and consist of conditions such as a history of several cesarean sections or numerous previous deliveries, which are a threat to the patient's health if pregnancy ensues. Women who have had three cesarean sections are at increased risk for rupture of the uterus, with possible hemorrhage and death during pregnancy, labor, or delivery. Women who have had five deliveries are at increased risk for uterine rupture, postpartum hemorrhage, and abnormal fetal presentations during labor. These complications are related to the loss of muscle tone and elasticity which occurs in the uterus that has been repeatedly gravid.

Genetic indications for sterilization apply equally to males and females. As in the case of medically indicated sterilizations, the partner carrying the abnormality is the one who should be sterilized. If both are carriers of the

**103**

abnormality, the choice becomes a social one, left to the couple.

Although the discipline of genetics is making great strides toward the identification of carrier states and the intrauterine diagnosis of a number of debilitating, if not fatal, diseases, there are still a large number of diseases for which no such identification is possible. One prominent example is Huntington's chorea, which does not manifest itself until the affected individual is well into fertile years. As the transmission rate is 50 per cent, individuals potentially affected may elect sterilization, rather than risk transmission. Potential carriers of the most common autosomal recessive disorder in Caucasians, the gene for cystic fibrosis, may elect sterilization after the birth of one or two normal children.

The three aforementioned classes of individuals who elect to control fertility through sterilization for medical reasons constitute a far smaller group than those who choose sterilization for social reasons. However, as a group, they have a far higher incidence of regret and dissatisfaction over the procedure. Several studies indicate that this undesired sequel is the result of a decision forced by external circumstance, rather than one prompted by free choice of the individual or couple involved (2, 24, 25).

The "social" indications that are responsible for the large majority of sterilizations performed over the last several years are many and varied. Financial considerations, the ideal of small family size, the "zero population" movement, emotional inability to become involved in childbearing, desire for increased personal freedom, and lack of confidence in long-term use of temporary contraceptive measures are some of the more commonly cited reasons for requesting surgical sterilization.

The shift from a predominance of medical, obstetric, and genetic indication to one of social indications has resulted from a combination of patient demands and a relaxation of medical regulations regarding sterilization. Until the late 1960s, socially indicated sterilization procedures were governed by "the rule of the 120": if the patient's age, multiplied by the number of children, was greater than or equal to 120, sterilization was considered permissible. This rule was almost certainly developed as a safeguard against subsequent regret and desire for reversal of sterilization. The rationale behind such a rule is the assumption that any woman who fits the stated criteria would be uninterested in future pregnancy by virtue of her age or number of previous pregnancies, even in the event of divorce and remarriage or a catastrophe resulting in the death of her children. This assumption has not been supported by the experience of most clinics dealing with requests for sterilization reversal. A by-product of the current trend toward greater participation by patients in their own medical care has been a relaxation of physicians' rules regarding sterilization. Many physicians still have unwritten age and parity criteria, and many still refuse to sterilize childless individuals. However, any individual who appears to be mentally sound should be able, without too much difficulty, to find a physician who will perform a sterilization, regardless of age, parity, or marital status.

## METHODS

Methods of sterilization currently in use involve occlusion of the ducts which transport germ cells (ova or spermatozoa) in either sex, and removal of the uterus in the female. Removal of the gonads (testes or ovaries) will also result in sterilization. However, the process of castration (withdrawal of sex-hormone production and stimulation) which results from the latter procedure is undesirable. Castration is now only performed in the treatment of individuals suffering from hormone-dependent malignancies. Prior to the availability of modern surgical and anesthetic techniques, castration by irradiation of the ovaries was used for medically indicated sterilizations in women who were considered poor operative risks.

Current methods of sterilization include vasectomy, occlusion of the fallopian tubes by a variety of means, and hysterectomy. Each will be discussed in terms of technique, ease of performance, complications, and failure rates. Undesired sequelae of sterilization of procedures will be discussed as a separate topic.

### STERILIZATION OF MEN

Vasectomy is the only technique of surgical sterilization commonly practiced in males. The procedure is generally performed by a urologist, general surgeon, or family practitioner. The procedure may be safely and effectively performed in the physician's office, under local anesthesia.

Vasectomy may be approached by either of

two types of scrotal incision (Fig. 8–1). One requires a separate incision for each vas, made on the anterolateral aspect of the scrotum near its attachment to the body. An alternate approach utilizes a single incision in the midline of the scrotum, just below the base of the penis. From this incision each vas can be isolated in turn. For either approach, the incision length is about 0.5 to 1.0 cm.

Once the vas has been isolated, a number of techniques have been described to produce occlusion. In all cases, the vas is severed, after being separated from its fibrous sheath. The cut ends may be ligated with silk, cotton, or cat gut, clipped with metal clips, or coagulated with an electrocautery. In some cases, a 0.5- to 3.0-cm. segment of vas is removed; in others, not. The occluded ends may be

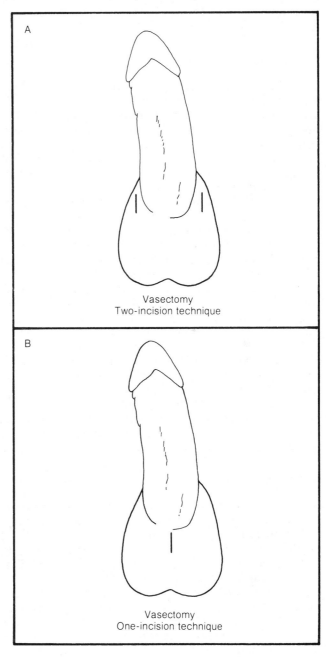

A

Vasectomy
Two-incision technique

B

Vasectomy
One-incision technique

**FIG. 8–1.** Vasectomy incisions.

dropped back into the sheath, turned back on themselves, or the sheath may also be severed and then clipped or sutured over the cut end of the vas (12, 23).

Attempts at reversible male sterilization, using plugs, clips, or stopcocks to occlude the vas, have not been successful. Leakage of sperm around the occluding device, or severe scarring may take place, causing permanent obstruction. These undesirable side effects have occurred too frequently to make the procedure practical (5).

## COMPLICATIONS

Immediate complications include wound infection (0.1–7.5%), hematoma (0.4–4.2%), symptomatic spermatic granuloma (0.4–4.2%), and epididymitis (1.8–5.6%). Spontaneous reanastomosis ranges from 0 to 3 per cent of reported cases, with a mean of 1 per cent (11, 23).

Spermatic granuloma is an inflammatory process which originates from the testicular side of the ligated vas. Pressure generated by continued spermatogenesis causes rupture at the point of occlusion, permitting sperm to extrude into the surrounding tissues, forming a granuloma, or mass. Forward progression of the sperm in the granuloma is considered responsible for successful recanalization between the two occluded segments of vas. Although a painful swelling is present in less than 5 per cent of cases, healed sperm granulomas at the vasectomy site have been found in 25 to 30 per cent of men requesting vasectomy reversal. Occasionally a spermatic granuloma will develop in the epididymis, causing epididymitis (inflammation). Subsequent scarring may cause occlusion of the sperm transport system at this point (29).

## SEQUELAE

Sequelae of vasectomy may be physical or psychological. Several careful studies of males before and after vasectomy indicate no significant change in the hormonal function of the testis. Spermatogenesis continues, although sometimes at a reduced rate. Silber, however, reports the possibility of a significant decrease in spermatogenesis at periods greater than 10 years after vasectomy. It appears that the sperm disintegrate and are resorbed in the epididymis (29).

Sperm autoantibodies that cause either agglutination or immobilization of sperm have been reported to occur in up to 60 per cent of men who have undergone vasectomy (1). The effect of these antibodies on the subsequent health of the individual appears to be negligible. However, the immobilizing antibodies may significantly affect future fertility, if reversal is requested.

Although there has been at least one report of an increased incidence of autoimmune connective tissue disorders in males, following vasectomy (21), it has not been confirmed by subsequent studies. At the moment, there appears to be no increased risk (6, 16).

Psychological sequelae that have been reported include impotence, anxiety, and exaggerated masculinity. The reported incidence of regret, in Western cultures, is about 3 per cent (14). Bloom and Houston (4) suggest that psychologic response to vasectomy requires further evaluation. Their review of the subject indicates that reports of increased sexual satisfaction may reflect a coping mechanism to allay concerns about the procedure. They suggest that there is a period of psychological adjustment to vasectomy that may extend for several years after the procedure before stabilization occurs. Rodgers and Ziegler (22) believe that many males initially look upon the vasectomy as a sacrifice, to save the female partner from surgery. This fact may then be used as a bargaining device to obtain her acquiescence in increased sexual activity.

## STERILIZATION OF WOMEN

### FALLOPIAN TUBE OCCLUSION

Fallopian-tube occlusion can be accomplished by removal, segmental resection, clipping, banding, burning (electrocoagulation), and chemical cauterization. All of the above techniques have been practiced utilizing an extrauterine approach. Burning and chemical cauterization have also been performed employing a transuterine approach.

The extrauterine techniques have been accomplished via infraumbilical, large and small abdominal, and vaginal incisions. The transuterine approaches involve insertion of an instrument through the cervix and uterine cavity to the tubal ostium (uterine opening of the fallopian tube).

Extrauterine procedures can be performed in conjunction with cesarean section or therapeutic abortion, shortly after delivery (puerperal), or as interval procedures (any time more than 6 weeks from the most recent delivery). The transuterine approaches have only been performed as interval procedures.

The transuterine approaches have been explored in an attempt to develop a sterilization procedure for females that is of the same order of risk, expense, and convenience as vasectomy is for males, and consequently can be performed in an office setting under local anesthesia. To date, none of these procedures has achieved a success rate that approximates those for vasectomy and conventional extrauterine tubal occlusion procedures. The transuterine techniques will be described, for the sake of completeness, but none are currently in use outside of a research protocol setting.

## METHODS OF APPROACH TO EXTRAUTERINE TUBAL STERILIZATION

The external surface of the fallopian tube can be reached through a variety of entry points into the abdominal cavity. The choice is generally dictated by the physician and depends on such factors as skill and familiarity with particular techniques, length of time since delivery, length of desired hospital stay and of desired postoperative recovery period, possible complications, and cosmesis. Success or failure of the sterilization is probably more dependent on the choice of occlusive procedure than on the method of approach.

Laparotomy. The conventional method of approach is by laparotomy (abdominal) incision. In the nonpuerperal patient, the incision is made in the lower abdomen. It may be longitudinal in direction, extending upward in the midline for a distance of about 4 in., starting at the pubic bone (Fig. 8–2A). As an alternative, a transverse incision of the same length can be made approximately 1 to 1½ in. above the pubic bone. This is usually just within the pubic hair line and is therefore more cosmetic (Fig. 8–2B). Both incisions provide easy access to the uterus and fallopian tubes for whichever procedure is desired. The required hospital stay is 2 to 4 days, and physical activity should be restricted for about a month after surgery to permit adequate wound healing.

Recently, the "mini-incision" has been developed in an attempt to reduce hospitalization and recovery periods. These incisions are about 1½ to 2 in. long, depending on the patient's weight (Fig. 8–2C). In order to have access to the tubes, some type of manipulating instrument must be placed transvaginally into the uterine cavity. The uterus is then rotated so that each tube in its turn is moved under the incision. The tube is pulled up through the incision and the desired occlusive procedure performed. The size of the incision necessarily limits visualization, which may be a great disadvantage in some difficult cases.

In the immediate puerperal period, the uterus extends almost to the umbilicus, necessitating a longitudinal incision beginning at the umbilicus and extending downward (Fig. 8–2E). A successful adaptation of the "mini-incision" which offers cosmesis is the subumbilical incision (Fig. 8–2F). The umbilicus of most women flattens and distends during pregnancy. A semilunar incision approximately 1 in. in length can be made in the crease at the lower margin of the umbilicus. The uterus is large enough to be manipulated without aid of an instrument, and the tube can easily be swung under the incision. As abdominal tone returns, the incision becomes inverted in the lower margin of the umbilicus and is barely visible. the postoperative recovery time is accomplished during the usual postpartum recovery period. If the procedure is performed within the first 24 hours of delivery, the patient is usually dismissed at the time she would have been for delivery alone.

Colpotomy. Another approach that is intended to be cosmetic is the colpotomy incision. In this technique the abdominal cavity is entered through an incision made in the posterior vaginal fornix (area behind the cervix), between the uterosacral ligaments. There are only a few thin layers of tissue between the upper posterior vagina and the pouch of Douglas, or cul de sac, the most dependent portion of the abdomen in the female. The ovaries and fallopian tubes may lie in the pouch of Douglas, and if not, they are generally within easy reach. The greatest problem with this approach is the risk of infection. The vagina can be cleansed, but not sterilized. The area cannot be cleansed as thoroughly as abdominal skin. Infection rates consequently run as high as 3 to 5 per cent whereas those for abdominal incisions are well under 1 per cent. The infections generally involve the tubes and

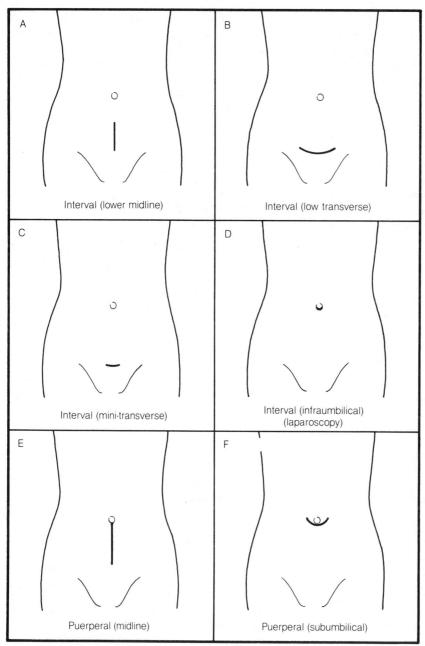

**FIG. 8–2.** Abdominal incisions used for tubal sterilization.

ovaries, and may be severe enough to require hysterectomy (27).

**Laparoscopy.** Currently the most popular and most reported approach is through the laparoscope, a fiberoptic telescope which permits excellent visualization of the pelvis through a half-inch-long incision made inside the lower margin of the umbilicus (Fig. 8–2D). The fallopian tubes may be grasped and manipulated through an accessory channel running in the same instrument as the telescope, or through a second incision about a quarter of an inch in diameter made in the lower midline, below the pubic hair line. The incisions are so small that superficial healing only is required, and the postoperative recovery period is no more than one or two days. Strenuous sports activities are generally avoided for about 4 or 5 days.

The infraumbilical entry is effected by first distending the abdominal cavity with gas, either carbon dioxide or nitrous oxide. A hollow tube with an inner spike is then forced through the abdominal wall, after the desired size of incision is made in the skin. Any bleeding that occurs usually stops promptly, since the area is devoid of large blood vessels. However, strenuous activity in the immediate postoperative period could cause recurrent bleeding from small vessels damaged in the initial entry process. This procedure has been performed without general anesthesia, utilizing intravenous sedation, and local anesthetics around the umbilicus. However, general anesthesia is more commonly utilized.

### TECHNIQUES OF TUBAL OCCLUSION

The existence of a variety of techniques for producing tubal occlusion reflects such disparate factors as desire for lowest possible failure rate, desire for potential reversibility, need for speed, and constraints on incision size.

Pregnancy has occurred after every type of sterilization procedure performed. Failures range from 0.1 to 3.0 per cent (27). The intricacy of the more exotic techniques does not appear to justify their use in spite of reported lower failure rates. These techniques tend to be more time-consuming and require more technical expertise than the commonly practiced methods.

Use in Laparotomy and Colpotomy. Tubal sterilization performed through the standard abdominal incision or the colpotomy incision generally utilizes either the Pomeroy technique or fimbriectomy. In the Pomeroy technique (Fig. 8–3A), the tube is grasped by its isthmus, or midsection. A plain catgut ligature is tied around the loop of tube, and the segment forming the loop is then cut away between the ligature points. The two cut ends of the tube fall away from each other over the next several days. The cut ends scar over, and a gap of about ½ to 1 in. is left between proximal and distal segments. This same technique can be used through any of the "mini-abdominal" incisions previously discussed.

Fimbriectomy (Fig. 8–3B) involves ligation and cutting away of the end of the tube possessing the fimbria. Only one ligature is required for each tube. Since the fimbriae are the essential part of the ovum pick-up mechanism, reconstruction of a tube occluded by fimbriectomy has little chance of success. This technique is not suited to mini-incisions, because the fimbriated end cannot be lifted through that incision. Other techniques less commonly performed are salpingectomy—total removal of the tube (Fig. 8–3C); cornual resection—ligation and cutting away of the tube where it joins the uterus (Fig. 8–3D); and the Irving procedure. The Irving technique (Fig. 8–3E) involves ligation and resection of the isthmus, as in the Pomeroy technique, but the proximal (nearest) segment of the tube is then looped back and buried in the uterine wall. Both salpingectomy and the Irving technique are more tedious and time-consuming than the Pomeroy procedure without substantially lower failure rates. Neither can be performed satisfactorily through a "mini-" incision. Cornual resection has an unacceptably high failure rate (27).

The Uchida technique (Fig. 8–3F) can be performed through conventional, as well as mini-incisions. However, it requires a considerable degree of manual dexterity. The isthmus of the tube is grasped, and the mesosalpinx, or fine membrane covering the tube, is injected with saline to create a bleb, or pocket. A slit is made in the bleb. The tube is pulled out, ligated in two places, and a 1½-in. segment excised. The proximal end of the tube is dropped into the pocket, and the edges of the slit are then purse-stringed around the distal end. Uchida reported from his personal experience a series of 5000 cases without a failure, but the technique requires more time to perform than most surgeons feel is justified (32).

Use in Laparoscopy. New techniques for occluding the tube had to be developed for laparoscopy because of the remote manipulative nature of this approach. The initial techniques involved coagulation (electric cautery), followed by cutting of the tube. Each tube is grasped in one or more places in the isthmic portion and coagulated, until a white burn scar develops for a distance of a 1-cm.-radius around the grasping forceps. Coagulation followed by cutting does not seem to improve the failure rate of coagulation alone. The greatest

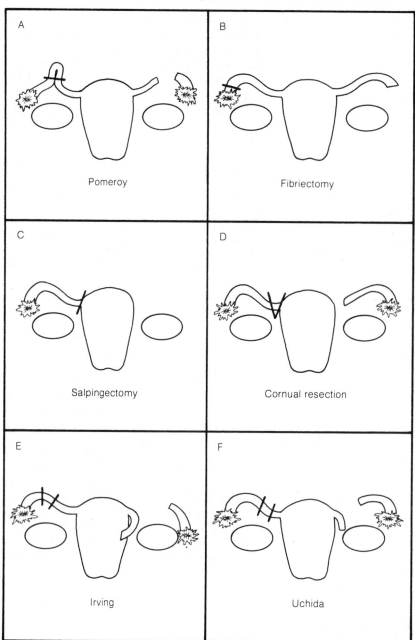

**FIG. 8–3.** Tubal ligation techniques.

risk of this technique involves inadvertent electrical or thermal burns from poor visualization or poorly insulated equipment. Although the incidence of such complications is generally less than 2 per cent, their elimination is desirable (27). To this end, several varieties of plastic clip (13) and inert silastic bands (37) have been developed that can be applied to, or slipped over, the tube. These techniques also produce less destruction of the tube than coagulation, which is desirable if reanastomosis (reversal of sterilization) should ever be contemplated.

**Use in the Transuterine Approach.** The transuterine approach to tubal occlusion can be performed blindly, or under direct vision using a hysteroscope (a fiberoptic telescope similar to the laparoscope). The blind techniques involve transcervical introduction of a curved metal or pliable plastic, hollow canula into the uterine cavity. The instrument is guided by touch along the lateral wall of the cavity until it drops into the cornual recess. A sclerosing agent, such as quinacrine or silver nitrate, is injected, with the purpose of scarring the tubal lining. Failure rates range from 3 per cent to 13 per cent. These are not acceptable by current standards (27).

The hysteroscope is used to direct a fine cautery probe into the tubal ostium. Electrocoagulation is then performed. Although the initial studies looked promising, subsequent efforts indicated unacceptably high complication and failure rates (7). Complications include development of fistulous tracts (openings) through the uterine wall, permitting transport of sperm into the abdominal cavity, and burns to loops of bowel lying adjacent to the uterus (7). Although Lindemann has reported no failures or complications, others have not been able to duplicate these results (15).

Research in the area of hysteroscopic sterilization continues; however, it appears doubtful that this method will enjoy the same popularity as laparoscopic sterilization.

## HYSTERECTOMY

Hysterectomy for the purpose of sterilization alone (rather than a treatment for uterine disease) has become an accepted procedure only since the mid-1960s; however, its use is still controversial. The various points of view concerning hysterectomy will be discussed in the section on choice of sterilization procedure.

As is the case with tubal sterilization, hysterectomy has been performed as both a puerperal and an interval procedure, and by both the abdominal and the vaginal routes. By far the largest number of reported sterilization hysterectomies have been performed vaginally as interval procedures, generally at least 3 or more months post partum.

The vaginal route is more popular than the abdominal route for cosmetic reasons, and because there is only one incision, instead of two, from which the patient must recover. It is difficult to compare the immediate outcomes

of the two techniques because the vaginal procedure is performed approximately ten to twelve times more frequently than the abdominal procedure for sterilization purposes (27).

The meager data available suggest that the complication and morbidity rate for abdominal sterilization hysterectomy is 12 per cent, or about half that for the vaginal approach. However, valid comparison is impossible, since no study comparing the two types of hysterectomy has ever been performed at one hospital, which would be essential to ensure that any difference in morbidity shown by the study could not be accounted for by differences in the training, aseptic technique, and expertise of the surgeons, or by the general health of the patient population. The available data suggest that by either route, the complication and morbidity rate is 2½ to 5 times higher than for tubal occlusion procedures (27). Postoperative recovery takes approximately 4 to 6 weeks. Following this, the patient may return to full activity.

Although sterilization hysterectomies performed in conjunction with cesarean section are in vogue in certain parts of the United States, they are generally frowned upon because they are associated with high incidence of serious complications, in the form of excessive blood loss and injury to the urinary tract. Occasionally, hysterectomy following cesarean section is necessary to adequately manage an obstetric emergency. However, desire for sterilization does not appear to constitute adequate justification for the increased risk of hysterectomy over that for tubal ligation performed in conjunction with the cesarean section (19, 20, 35).

Puerperal hysterectomy, that is hysterectomy performed within the first several days after delivery, has almost no advocates. If anything, this procedure is associated with higher complication and morbidity rates than cesarean section hysterectomy (3, 35). The possible savings in hospitalization and child-care arrangements cannot compensate for the increased risk.

Hysterectomy has been performed as a means of pregnancy termination in patients who also desire sterilization. The abdominal route is generally preferred over the vaginal because of increased uterine size and vascularity of the pelvic area related to pregnancy. The abdominal approach generally offers better control over bleeding than the vaginal approach. The complication and morbidity rate is of the same order as for interval vaginal hysterectomy. Thus, termination hysterectomy may logically be offered as a sterilization procedure in the patient who desires both end-results: nothing appears to be gained by utilizing separate procedures.

Sterilization by hysterectomy has almost a zero failure rate. However, between 20 and 25 cases of post-hysterectomy tubal and abdominal pregnancies have been reported in the medical literature (27). Less than half of these are the result of conceptions that took place during the same cycle as the operation. The remaining conceptions took place at a time remote from surgery and were presumably the result of tubo-vaginal fistulous tracts. Thus no sterilization procedure is 100 per cent sure, but hysterectomy best approximates this goal.

## SEQUELAE

The sequelae of sterilization fall into two categories—physical and psychological. The physical sequelae can be divided into two further categories—functional and organic. The two major physical sequelae that have been attributed to tubal sterilization are irregular vaginal bleeding and previously unexperienced pelvic pain. The combination of pain and/or irregular bleeding has been called the post-tubal-ligation syndrome. To date there has been no prospective adequately controlled study that proves incontrovertibly that such a syndrome exists. Both of these sequelae could be either functional or organic in nature (2, 4, 17, 18, 22, 25, 30, 31).

In functional disorders, it is presumed that the psychic stresses resulting from sterilization have been converted into physical symptoms such as pain or irregular bleeding. In organic disorders, it is assumed that the procedure itself has created a visible anatomic lesion which is responsible for either pain or bleeding. There has been at least one report of post-tubal-ligation pelvic pain that was presumably the result of adhesion formation between the ligation site and a loop of small intestine. The pain was relieved after lysis of the adhesions was performed (8).

An organic cause for irregular bleeding is more difficult to establish. Current theory suggests that tubal ligation may decrease the blood supply to the ovary, because one of the vessels supplying the ovary, a branch of the uterine artery that runs close to the tube, is cut during the procedure. The inference is that decreased blood supply interferes with normal secretion of ovarian hormones and the growth of the uterine lining, which may lead to irregular bleeding. Thus far, no convincing proof of this hypothesis has been offered (30).

When considering post-tubal-ligation pain and dysfunctional bleeding, it must be established that neither condition predated the operative procedure. If such were the case, it could not be said that the condition resulted from the tubal ligation. In actual practice, the existence of pain and dysfunctional uterine bleeding are considered indications for recommending hysterectomy, rather than tubal occlusion, for sterilization.

There are also strong correlations between post-tubal-ligation pain and bleeding and previous contraceptive practices. Many women who have used oral contraceptives are now electing sterilization as a means of contraception, because of the reported deleterious side effects of oral contraceptives, which increase in incidence with advancing age. It is well known that both menstrual bleeding and pain are decreased with oral contraceptive use. Therefore, if the patient experiences discomfort after sterilization, it is important to distinguish between pain and bleeding patterns that the patient has never experienced before, and those that differ from her experience on oral contraceptives but are similar to those experienced prior to use of that method. Many women may display an abnormal bleeding pattern after discontinuing oral contraceptives without undergoing tubal ligation. Since it is prudent to have an overlap, rather than a gap in contraceptive coverage, discontinuation of oral contraceptives usually occurs at the time of, or immediately following the tubal ligation procedure, making it difficult to identify the causative process with any certainty.

An additional factor that clouds the issue of post-tubal-ligation problems is that the incidence of irregular vaginal bleeding increases in women who are approaching the end of their reproductive life span (premenopausal), regardless of contraceptive practices. Extensive prospective controlled studies are needed before many of these questions can be answered.

Emotional sequelae of sterilization are generally related to loss of fertility, concerns over body image, and concerns over loss of sexual potency. The highest incidence of regret is reported in women who have sterilization procedures for medical or obstetric indications (2, 24, 25) and in those who have sterilization at the time of pregnancy termination (18). In the former group, the regret results from a decision forced by external circumstances, rather than made by free choice. In the latter group, the regret generally results from a double loss that of both the pregnancy and fertility.

Concerns over loss of sexual potency may follow loss of fertility in some patients. The most important reason for this attitude is the fact that many people make no separation between the procreational and recreational aspects of sexual intercourse. For these individuals, the chance of conception must be present for them to enjoy intercourse without guilt. The loss of menses following sterilization hysterectomy may have a two-fold effect. First of all, the absence of periods reminds the patient of her irrevocable loss of fertility and second, the lack of menses may be equated by some with the menopause. Menopausal women are erroneously considered by many to be lacking in sex drive, and so this association, too, is taken as evidence of a loss of sexual potency. Since ovarian function continues in women who have been sterilized by hysterectomy, there is no hormonal basis for these fears. Furthermore, sexual responsiveness may be related to established behavior patterns which will not be altered by gradual changes in hormonal levels that are experienced in a natural menopause.

Concerns over body image are more common in patients undergoing hysterectomy sterilization. Mathis (17) reports that women attributed four functions to the uterus: reproductive, menstrual, sexual, and a fourth function of serving as a source of general strength and effectiveness. Barglow (2) feels that women adjust to tubal sterilization better than hysterectomy because they are able to fantasize a failure of the sterilization, whereas the lack of menses in the hysterectomy patient confirms its permanence.

In general, one must be wary of the patient who fears a feeling of emptiness following hysterectomy, since she is highly likely to regret the procedure. However, it is worth probing farther, rather than taking her fears at face value. An occasional woman views her uterus as a plug or stopper that prevents infinite penile penetration during coitus. She simply needs reassurance that the vaginal vault is sewn over, after removal of the uterus.

## CHOICE OF PROCEDURE

The choice of sterilization procedure depends on a number of factors, including general health of the couple, stability of the relationship, economic and domestic situation, presence or absence of disease of the reproductive tract, acceptance of possible failure, desire of permanence, and attitude toward menses.

As previously noted, sterilization for medical or genetic reasons should be performed on the affected partner, if not contraindicated by the seriousness of the illness.

Patients electing sterilization should be informed that the procedure is intended to be permanent, and that if there is any uncertainty regarding future childbearing, a temporary method of contraception should be selected instead. Many patients who intend permanence at the time sterilization is requested later request reversal, for a variety of reasons. The most common are divorce and remarriage or catastrophic loss of life, as in house fires or traffic accidents.

## STERILIZATION: MALE VERSUS FEMALE

If a couple is choosing sterilization as a means of permanent contraception, they must decide which partner will undergo the procedure. Stability of the relationship and potential effect of the procedure on sexual function and body image are important considerations. If one is to consider the factor of risk, it must be approached from two points of view. The short-term risk of vasectomy is much lower than for tubal sterilization or hysterectomy, but the failure rate is higher. The mortality rate for all female sterilization procedures, including hysterectomy, is between 0.1 per cent and 0.3 per cent (27). Most deaths are related to the effects of general anesthesia. The mortality rate for vasectomy is essentially zero, because general anesthesia is not required. The complication and morbidity rate for female sterilization procedures ranges from 1 per cent to 2 per cent for laparoscopy procedures, to 35 per cent for hysterectomy (27). On the other hand, the complication and morbidity rate for vasectomy is 3 per cent to 5 per cent, and complications are minor. The failure rate for tubal sterilization procedures ranges from 0.1 per cent to 0.5 per cent, while that for vasectomy is 1 per cent (12). Deys and Potts (10) suggest that the choice of vasectomy over tubal ligation depends on whether or not the couple in question are "role dividers" as opposed to "role sharers". In the former relationship, males tend to dominate. They make all the economic decisions for the family, act as sole breadwinners, and generally assume the contraceptive responsibility. In the latter relationship, both partners share in wage earning and domestic chores, and the female partner tends to accept the responsibility for contraception. The inference is that in the former relationship the masculinity of the male partner is so well established that fertility is not required to affirm this, so that vasectomy may be the best choice. In the latter relationship the assumption by the male of traditionally feminine duties may erode these feelings of masculinity. The male partner must maintain fertility in order to affirm his masculinity, and in this situation, female sterilization may be preferable.

If the relationship is unstable, then sterilization should logically be chosen by the partner who is most desirous of avoiding further conceptions. From a personal point of view the female partner has a greater interest in being sterilized, as she is the one who has the physical responsibility of child-bearing. In many socioeconomic groups where the male partner obviously plays the dominant role, vasectomy is chosen as a means of deterring infidelity on the part of the female partner, since she will run the risk of pregnancy. The importance of individualization for each couple cannot be overemphasized.

## FEMALE PROCEDURES

If the female partner decides to be sterilized, she must then determine choice of method, timing, and approach.

### METHODS

Tubal sterilization, rather than hysterectomy, is suggested for women of young age and low parity, and for those who wish to maintain menstrual function and are without reproductive-tract pathology.

Hysterectomy is generally recommended for women who have demonstrable reproductive-tract pathology, such as dysfunctional uterine bleeding, chronic pelvic pain, repeated abnormal pap smears, and pelvic relaxation with urinary incontinence. All of these conditions are common indications for hysterectomy. Consequently, hysterectomy rather than tubal sterilization is suggested in these cases so as to avoid a second operative procedure. However, it must be emphasized that tubal sterilization should not be refused to the patient with any of these conditions who will not accept sterilization hysterectomy.

It does not appear justified to perform hysterectomy as prophylaxis against any of these conditions in a woman not symptomatic at the time of the sterilization request. A woman undergoing sterilization hysterectomy is not castrated. She is still advised to undergo an annual pelvic examination to evaluate ovarian size. An annual pap smear is sufficient to diagnose preinvasive cervical cancer. Therefore, prophylactic hysterectomy in the patient with normal pap smears is saving the patient nothing, as she still needs an annual examination. A review of the literature indicates that the maximum risk of a subsequent gynecologic procedure in women undergoing tubal sterilization regardless of pelvic pathology is 15 per cent (27). Therefore, a patient electing tubal sterilization has an 85 per cent chance of requiring no further operative procedure. (It is important to emphasize that the operative procedures reported are not all hysterectomies, but include minor procedures with no need for subsequent hysterectomy.)

On the other hand, if a woman has a negative feeling toward menstrual function and is aware of the increased short-term complication and morbidity rate and postoperative recovery time over that required for tubal sterilization, there appears to be no justification for refusing sterilization hysterectomy.

### TIMING

Timing may be dependent upon the patient's parity, desired family size, and chosen method of sterilization.

Tubal sterilization may be performed safely and effectively as puerperal or interval procedures or in conjunction with abortion. If sterilization following a pregnancy is dependent on fetal outcome, it is prudent to delay the procedure beyond the puerperium (first 6 weeks after delivery). Even with sophisticated pre-

and post-natal care, the first 28 days of life are the most precarious for the infant. If, on the other hand, the desire for sterilization is independent of fetal outcome, the immediate puerperium is the most convenient time for a tubal ligation.

If hysterectomy is elected for sterilization, the interval or termination procedure carries a much lower complication and morbidity rate than either the puerperal procedure or that performed in conjunction with a cesarean section.

### APPROACH

For tubal sterilization procedures, choice of approach and occlusion technique may be dictated by timing in relationship to delivery. For puerperal sterilization, the subumbilical incision utilizing the Pomeroy occlusive technique is the approach of choice. The procedure can be performed within 24 hours of delivery without requiring additional hospitalization or recovery period beyond that for a normal delivery. Laparoscopy must generally be deferred until 5 to 7 days after delivery because of uterine size. Thus hospitalization beyond the usual postpartum stay of 48 to 96 hours would be required.

If the interval sterilization or abortion-sterilization procedure is chosen, the laparoscopic approach appears to offer the following advantages: lowest morbidity, shortest hospital stay, lowest failure rate, and shortest recovery time. The choice of occlusivesprocedure may depend on the likelihood of request for reversal. In the patient in whom reversal is unlikely to be requested, cauterization is the procedure of choice. However, if reversal is more than a remote possibility, banding is preferable, since it causes less tubal destruction than cauterization. The advantage of cauterization over banding is that once the laparoscope is introduced for cauterization, both tubes may be occluded without removing the laparoscope. For the banding procedure, the laparoscope must be removed from the abdomen after the first tube has been banded in order to reload the instrument for occluding the second tube. Some time is lost, some gas is lost, and there is always the possibility that the sheath will slip out of the peritoneal cavity.

The interval laparotomy approach to tubal sterilization appears indicated if the surgeon is inexperienced in laparoscopy or if adhesions from previous abdominal procedures make adequate laparoscopic approach difficult or impossible.

If hysterectomy is chosen, the approach depends on individual anatomy and pregnancy status. Vaginal hysterectomy is generally utilized for interval procedures in women with several previous pregnancies. The abdominal approach is generally chosen either when abortion is requested or in nonpregnant patients with no pelvic relaxation. In the former case, the increased vascularity that accompanies pregnancy makes the abdominal approach preferable because greater control can be exerted over bleeding. In the latter case, lack of pelvic relaxation makes the vaginal approach technically difficult.

### REVERSIBILITY

Although currently offered sterilization procedures are intended to be permanent, it is clear that a certain proportion of the sterilized population eventually request reversal. Furthermore, a study by Shain (26) indicates that a significant segment of the population practicing mechanical or chemical contraception would accept a sterilization procedure if there were a fair guarantee of reversibility.

### FEMALE

Reversibility of female sterilization is not possible following hysterectomy. However, reversal may be possible following tubal sterilization. The success is related to the extent and location of tubal destruction caused by the original sterilization procedure. Success rates are highest if destruction is confined to a discrete area, such as occurs after laparoscopy banding or a Pomeroy tubal ligation. However, success rates are not at an acceptable level for people desiring temporary contraception. If conventional techniques for tubal repair are utilized, the chance of the patient's having an intrauterine pregnancy is generally no higher than 40 per cent (28). Gomel (11) has recently reported a 72% per cent intrauterine pregnancy rate following end-to-end reapproximation of tubal segments using microsurgical techniques. If the fimbriae have been removed, success rates with reversal generally are low, since the fimbriae appear to be necessary for ovum pickup.

Successful tubal repair after laparoscopic

coagulation is also difficult, because of the extensive tubal destruction caused by electrocoagulation. Wheeless (33) reports only one pregnancy in 11 patients utilizing conventional techniques. In contrast, Winston (36), using a microsurgical approach, has successfully restored fertility to 5 out of 8 patients sterilized by coagulation.

## MALE

Reanastomosis of the previously resected vas deferens is also being performed with considerable frequency. Techniques similar to those used for tubal reanastomosis, many utilizing microsurgical approaches originally developed for plastic, vascular, and neurosurgery, are employed. As with tubal reanastomosis, the incidence of successful pregnancy has been relatively low, generally from 5 per cent to 25 per cent, (29) despite the fact that approximately 30 per cent to 85 per cent of patients will have sperm in the ejaculate. Because of the disparity between patency and fertility, Silber (29) has conducted a detailed investigation of factors contributing to successful vasectomy reversal. Utilizing microsurgical techniques, he was able to achieve a 71 per cent pregnancy rate in an unselected population. Factors contributing to a favorable outcome were meticulous microsurgical technique, duration of less than 10 years from vasectomy to time of reversal, and presence of a sperm granuloma at the previous vasectomy site. The meticulous technique is important to ensure that the resulting space is large enough for adequate passage of a bolus of sperm and for appropriate union of the muscular layers, so that coordinated propulsion of sperm can take place. Those patients who had undergone vasectomy more than 10 years prior to reanastomosis had a higher incidence of spermatogenesis at infertile levels. Patients who had not formed a sperm granuloma tended to have marked dilatation of the vas on the testicular side and poor-quality semen, in terms of numbers and morphology of sperm. On the other hand, those who had formed a sperm granuloma tended to have a normal sized vas and good-quality semen. Silber has hypothesized that rupture of the ligation side, with release of pressure, exerts a protective effect on testicular function (29).

Since most vasectomy techniques emphasize steps to prevent sperm granuloma formation, in order to avoid failure, a decision regarding choice of occlusive method may have to be based on the likelihood that reversal may be requested.

At the moment it appears prudent to emphasize the intended permanence of all sterilization procedures and to be guarded about the probability of successful reversal.

## REFERENCES

1. Ansbacher R, Kwok KY, Wurster JC: Sperm antibodies in vasectomized men. Fertil Steril 23:640, 1972
2. Barglow P, Eisner M: An evaluation of tubal ligation in Switzerland. Am J Obstet Gynecol 95:1082, 1966
3. Bazley W, Crisp WE: Post-partum hysterectomy for sterilization. Am J Obstet Gynecol 119:139, 1974
4. Bloom LJ, Houston BK: The psychological effects of vasectomy for American men. J Genet Psychol 128:173, 1976
5. Bueschke EE, Zaneveld LJD: Development and evaluation of reversible vas occlusive devices. In Sciarra J, Markland C, Speidel JJ (eds): Control of Male Fertility. Hagerstown, Harper & Row, 1975, p 112
6. Crewe P, Dawson T, Tidmarsh E, Chanarin J, Barnes RD: Autoimmune implications of vasectomy in man. Clin Exp Immunol 24:368, 1976
7. Darabi KF, Roy K, Pichart RM: Collaboratored study on hysteroscopic sterilization procedures. In Sciarra JJ, Zatuchni DI, Speidel JJ (eds): Final Report in Risks, Benefits, and Controversies in Fertility Control. Hagerstown, Harper & Row, 1977, p 81
8. Daw E: (Letters to the editor): Post-sterilization mittelschmerz. Br Med J 3:701, 1972
9. Devi PR, Joshi AM, Moodbidri SB, Naik WK, Sushella PS, Stheth AR: Long term effects of vasectomy on pituitary-gonadal axis. Indian J Med Res 66:591, 1976
10. Deys CM, Potts M: Factors affecting patient motivation. In Sciarra J, Markland C, Speidel JJ (eds): Control of Male Fertility. Hagerstown, Harper & Row, 1975, p 210.
11. Gomel V: Tubal reanastomosis by microsurgery. Fertil Steril 28:415, 1978
12. Hackett RE, Waterhouse K: Vasectomy reviewed. Am J Obstet Gynecol 28:59, 1977
13. Hulka JF: Spring clip sterilization: one year follow-up of 1,000 cases. In Sciarra JJ, Droegemueller W, Speidel JJ (eds): Advances in Female Sterilization Techniques. Hagerstown, Harper & Row, 1976, p 51
14. Jones E: Vasectomy sequelae: empirical studies. J Reprod Med 19: 254, 1977
15. Lindemann HJ: Transuterine tubensterilisation per Hysteroskop. Geburtshilfe Frauenheilkd 33:709, 1973
16. Lucas PL, Rose NR: Immunologic consequences of vasectomy. A review. Ann Immunol (Paris) 129:301, 1978
17. Mathis JL: The emotional impact of surgical sterilization of the female. Okla State Med Assoc J 62:141, 1969

18. McCoy DR: The emotional reaction of women to therapeutic abortion and sterilization. J Obstet Gynaecol Br Commonw 75:1054, 1968
19. Mikal A, Begneaud WP, Hawen JP Jr: Pitfalls and complications of cesarean hysterectomy. Clin Obstet Gynecol 12:669, 1969
20. Patterson SP: Cesarean hysterectomy. Am J Obstet Gynecol 107:729, 1970
21. Roberts HJ: Thrombophlebitis after vasectomy. N Engl J Med 284:1330, 1971
22. Rodgers DA, Ziegler FJ: Effects of surgical contraception on sexual behavior. In Schima ME, Lubell I, Davis JE, Connell E (eds) Advances in Voluntary Sterilization. New York, American Elsevier, 1974, p 161
23. Schmidt SS: Technics and complications of elective vasectomy. Fertil Steril 17:467, 1966
24. Schneider H: Aussagen und ergebnisse nach tubensterilisation. Geburtshilfe Frauenheilkd 28:348, 1968
25. Schwyhart NR, Kutner SJ: A reanalysis of female reactions to contraceptive sterilization. J Nerv Ment Dis 156:354, 1973
26. Shain R: Acceptability of reversible versus permanent tubal ligation: an analysis of preliminary data. Fertil Steril 31:13, 1979
27. Shepard MK: Female contraceptive sterilization. Obstet Gynecol Surv 29:739, 1974
28. Siegler AM, Perez RJ: Reconstruction of fallopian tubes in previously sterilized patients. Fertil Steril 26:383, 1975
29. Silber SJ: Vasectomy and vasectomy reversal. Fertil Steril 29:125, 1978
30. Stock RJ: Evaluation of sequelae of tubal ligation. Fertil Steril 29:169, 1978
31. Thompson B, Baird D: Follow-up of 186 sterilized women. Lancet 1:1023, 1968
32. Uchida H: Uchida tubal sterilization. Am J Obstet Gynecol 121:153, 1975
33. Wheeless CR: Problems with laparoscopic sterilization using the electrocoagulation and resection technique. Fertil Steril 28:723, 1977
34. Wheeless CR Jr, Thompson BH: Laparoscopy sterilization. Review of 3600 cases. Obstet Gynecol 42:751, 1973
35. Wilson EA, Dilts PV Jr, Simpson TJ: Comparative morbidity of postpartum sterilization procedures. Am J. Obstet Gynecol 115:884, 1973
36. Winston RML: Microsurgical tubocornual anastomosis for reversal of sterilization. Lancet 1:284, 1977
37. Yoon IB, King TM: The laparoscopic Falope-Ring ™ procedure. In Sciarra JJ, Droegemueller W, Speidel JJ (eds): Advances in Female Sterilization Techniques. Hagerstown, Harper & Row, 1976, p 59

# 9

# Pregnancy Termination

## Paul Weinberg

## UNWANTED PREGNANCIES: ALTERNATIVE OPTIONS

The problem of unwanted pregnancy has been with us from ancient times to the present. Solutions to the problem differ from culture to culture. Infanticide and abortion are commonly practiced in many societies (see Chap. 18). In Western society, the major options available to the woman faced with an undesired pregnancy are marriage, single-parent rearing, offering the child for adoption, or pregnancy termination. Each of these has advantages and drawbacks for the mother in terms of physical and emotional health, and social acceptability.

### MARRIAGE

Marriage is commonly chosen: data from the United States indicate that in one of four marriages, the woman is already pregnant at the time of marriage (14). The major problem with opting for marriage as a solution to unplanned pregnancy is an increased incidence of separation and divorce in such marriages (10). Moreover, for most teenagers, this "solution" frequently means discontinuance of education, and frustration of life or career goals.

### SINGLE-PARENT REARING

The second option, single-parent rearing, is acceptable in some societies, particularly in Scandinavia, where maternity leave is common, day care centers are readily available, and no social stigma is attached to single par-

enting. In the United States these support services are usually nonexistent, and single-parent rearing is not widely accepted by society.

### ADOPTION

Carrying the child to term and then offering it for adoption is an option less frequently chosen since the legalization of abortion. Whereas some states still allow private placement, most have enacted laws that allow placement only by duly licensed agencies. This has significantly reduced the "gray-market baby" phenomena.

Homes for unwed mothers vary widely with respect to the services they furnish, many offering little in terms of continuing education and emotional support. Residence is usually required near term, thus imposing separation from the family. Many school systems still have no programs or structure that allow the pregnant teenager to continue her schooling. Consequently, adoption is usually not a positive growth experience for the mother.

### PREGNANCY TERMINATION

Pregnancy termination is the most utilized option. In the United States, there were 1.2 million abortions in 1976 and 1.3 million in 1977, with an estimated additional 0.5 million women who desired abortion but did not have available services (6). Prior to the legalization of abortion, in 1973, many women were forced to utilize extralegal practitioners, with maternal sepsis and mortality as frequent sequelae. Death rates from septic abortion have declined 19 per cent annually, following legalization (18). With present methodology, morbidity and mortality rates are quite low and are related to the length of gestation, rising as the length of gestation increases. For first-trimester procedures, total morbidity is only 5.5 per cent, with a mortality rate of 0.4:1,000 procedures. For second-trimester procedures, total morbidity is 35.8 per cent, with a mortality rate of 16:100,000 procedures (3). These mortality figures are lower than those for term delivery in the United States.

## METHODS OF PREGNANCY TERMINATION

The presently accepted methods of termination are dictated by, and thus are best understood in the context of, the length of gestation. In the clinical setting, the time elapsed in weeks from the first day of the last menses is utilized; gestational length is *approximately* 2 weeks less than this. Table 9–1 presents an overview of methods used in relation to weeks of amenorrhea.

## FIRST-TRIMESTER PROCEDURES

First-trimester procedures for termination of pregnancy are achieved with significantly less

morbidity than procedures undertaken in the second trimester. Thus a goal of termination services is to diagnose and terminate pregnancy as early as is feasible. Various diagnostic methods are available. The earliest objective findings on pelvic examination occur at 7 to 8 weeks. The cervix may be somewhat bluish (Chadwick's sign) and the uterine isthmus may show some softening (Helgar's sign). The uterus feels more globular, increasing in its anteroposterior diameter, prior to actual enlargement. Until recently, immunologic (agglutination) tests could not diagnose a pregnancy before 42 days, or 2 weeks past a missed menstrual episode. The newer radioreceptor assays can diagnose pregnancy at the time of the first missed menses. In addition, recent anthropologic data (11) demonstrate that a woman can determine that she is pregnant by subjective symptomatology, almost as early, and at almost as high a level of·confidence as the pregnancy test or physical examination.

### MENSTRUAL REGULATION

Menstrual regulation (extraction) (12) is a procedure which utilizes plastic intrauterine cannulas, up to 6 mm. in diameter, with a 50-cc. syringe as a source of suction to remove

**Table 9–1. Methods of Pregnancy Termination by Weeks**

| Weeks from last menses | | Comments | Applicable techniques |
|---|---|---|---|
| First trimester | 0 | First day of last menses | Menstrual extraction (regulation) [4–7 weeks] |
| | 2 | Fertilization | |
| | 4 | First missed menses; rapid receptor pregnancy test first valid | |
| | 6 | Agglutination pregnancy test first valid | |
| | 7 | Physical exam first valid for pregnancy diagnosis | Vacuum extraction (suction) [6–11 weeks] |
| | 12 | | Laminaria + suction (two-stage procedure) [11–15 weeks] |
| 2nd (mid-) trimester | 14 | | Research on prostaglandin, suppository or intramuscular [12–16 weeks] |
| | 16 | | |
| | 20 | Many centers limit procedures to under 20 weeks | Intraamniotic saline, urea, prostaglandin |
| | 24 | | Research techniques on prostaglandin suppositories |

the implanting morula. When performed at 2 weeks past a missed period, 80 per cent of women who are concerned that they might be pregnant are found to be so. Menstrual regulation requires no anesthesia, it requires less equipment than other termination procedures, and thus it is the least expensive method. Its disadvantages include a 2 to 4 per cent incidence of failure to remove the conceptus, a 20 per cent incidence of "unnecessary" procedures performed on the nonpregnant, and an occasional incomplete extraction, with subsequent infection. These disadvantages are largely avoidable.

With the newer radioreceptor pregnancy test, a positive test can be obtained prior to the procedure, providing assurance that it is necessary. If the procedure is performed at the optimum time, during the 5th and 6th week, the implantation site is less likely to be missed, and, because the uterine cavity is not large, incomplete evacuation is rare. At this time, "missing" of the pregnancy can still occur (2%). Thus it is necessary to either subject all of the removed tissue to microscopic analysis (to identify chorionic villi), or to repeat the pregnancy test in 2 weeks. This will still allow for a suction termination in those cases where extraction has failed. Menstrual extraction should not be utilized beyond 6 weeks, because the incidence of incomplete evacuation is unacceptably high at this time.

### SUCTION TERMINATION

At 7 weeks past a last menstrual period, pregnancy can be diagnosed by a routine agglutination pregnancy test. There are also objective breast changes and uterine enlargement on physical examination. From the 7th to the 12th week, the accepted method of termination is by suction abortion (3).

A suction apparatus generating 60 mm. of water vacuum is essential, as are plastic cannula, from 6 to 12 mm. in diameter. The procedure can be performed in an outpatient facility under local block anesthesia; however, some patients prefer general anesthesia. The technique is simple. After anesthesia, the cervix is grasped and is gradually dilated to admit a suction cannula 1 mm. smaller than the number of weeks of amenorrhea. The cannula is introduced into the uterine cavity, and suction is applied, aspirating the products of conception. The products must be identi-

fied grossly, and, ideally, should be studied microscopically. The practitioner may miss an unevacuated conceptus or more rarely an ectopic (tubal) pregnancy.

The results are excellent. There is a total morbidity of only 5.47 per cent (3). This morbidity generally is caused by incomplete evacuation with ensuing infection. On rare occasions, excessive hemorrhage or uterine perforation is encountered. Because of these rare complications, a free-standing facility must have immediate access to emergency hospital care. The following list summarizes the complications of first-trimester abortion.

*Complications of First-Trimester Abortion*

| | |
|---|---|
| Perforation | Hemorrhage |
| Failure to disrupt implantation | Incomplete evacuation |
| Excessive dilatation | Infection |

### THE "TWO-STAGE" PROCEDURE

Increasing experience has validated the "two-stage" procedure (5). It is applicable for the patient who presents for termination between the 12th to the 15th week of amenorrhea. A hydrophylic rod of seaweed, called *laminaria,* is inserted into the cervical canal 12 to 24 hours prior to the suction procedure. The laminaria dilates the cervix by imbibing body fluids and swelling to 2 to 3 times its original diameter. The following day, suction abortion is performed, as described above. However, cannulae of at least 12 mm. are employed. This "two-stage" procedure carries a risk of morbidity three times that of the suction procedure performed prior to the 12th week (3). This morbidity is still significantly less than that of mid-trimester procedures.

## SECOND-TRIMESTER PROCEDURES

Many clinics will not terminate pregnancies beyond 20 weeks gestation. Beyond 16 weeks, standard practice for termination consists of inserting a needle transabdominally (amniocentesis) and instilling an abortifacient solution (4). Some clinics utilize a hypertonic (20%) saline solution. Other clinics utilize hypertonic urea (53%) (20) or prostaglandin F2$\alpha$ (2). It is claimed that these agents are safer than saline solution. More recently, a combination of urea plus a small amount of prostaglandin has been advocated. This combina-

**Table 9-2. Complications of Mid-Trimester Abortion**

| | Saline | Urea | Prostaglandin |
|---|---|---|---|
| Infection | 6.3% | | 0.6% |
| Retained products | 27-35% | 13-24% | 32.0% |
| Transfusion | 0-3.6% | 0-3% | 1.2% |
| Failure to abort | 0-20% | 6.5-15% | 5.0% |
| Transplacental hemorrhage | 10-20% | Not reported | Not reported |
| Cervical perforation | Reported | Reported | 0.6% |
| Uterine rupture | Reported | Reported | 0.3% |
| Water intoxication | Associated with the use of oxytocin augmentation only | | |

tion provides a more rapid termination from time of injection, approximately 19 hours, as compared to approximately 30 hours with urea alone, and frequently avoids the use of oxytocin to induce or augment uterine contractility (13). This avoids the excessive water retention (water intoxication) sometimes caused by oxytocin. Mid-trimester procedures carry an eight- to nine-fold increase in morbidity over those utilized during the first trimester (3). Specifically, there is an increase in incidence of retained products, infection, bleeding, and cervical laceration. Table 9-2 summarizes these findings.

Because of the correlation between morbidity and length of gestation, medical care systems have a responsibility to provide early pregnancy diagnosis and easy access to services. They should also make the public aware of the importance of seeking termination early in pregnancy. Ideally, all terminations should be achieved in the first trimester. Nonetheless, in adolescent and lower socioeconomic populations, mid-trimester procedures are still quite common; the possibility of pregnancy is often denied, and access to services is limited.

In addition to the increase in morbidity, second-trimester procedures require 30 to 48 hours of hospitalization to ensure patient safety. These procedures are also more emotionally traumatic, due to the expulsion of the fetus and placenta: the patient experiences labor.

Recently it has been suggested (9) that evacuation by the vaginal route, by dilatation and evacuation, is as safe, or safer, than amniocentesis for mid-trimester termination. Many workers are dubious about this conclusion and fear that vaginal evacuation in such advanced pregnancies, especially in inexperienced hands, will lead to frequent major complications, such as hemorrhage and perforation.

## CURRENT RESEARCH

In the area of clinical research, the most promising development is the use of prostaglandin analogues in a vaginal suppository. Technical problems revolve around development of a vehicle for the suppository that will provide sustained release, and of an analogue of the drug that will provide acceptable success in terms of complete abortion, with few of the very annoying side effects of prostaglandin (i.e., nausea, vomiting, and diarrhea). Available data indicate that such self-administered abortion techniques may prove very acceptable (see Chap. 23), if there is assurance of safety.

## LEGAL AND ETHICAL CONSIDERATIONS

### LEGALIZATION OF ABORTION

In the United States, until relatively recent times, the majority of states had very restrictive abortion laws, dating back to the late 1800s. During the late 1950s and early 1960s, many states enacted laws similar to the American Law Institute's Model Penal Code. This model allowed legal abortion in certain situations—specifically, in the case of a threat to maternal life or health, rape or incest, or significant risk of congenital defect in the fetus.

In January, 1973, in a landmark decision, the Supreme Court of the United States (in a Texas case, called *"Wade* v. *Roe")* laid down certain guidelines for legal abortion (17). The decision states:

*1)* For the stage prior to approximately the end of the first trimester, the abortion decision and its effectuation must be left to the medical judgment of the pregnant woman's attending physician.

2) For the stage subsequent to approximately the end of the first trimester, the State, in promoting its interest in the health of the mother, may, if it chooses, regulate the abortion procedure in ways that are reasonably related to maternal health.

3) For the stage subsequent to viability the State, in promoting its interest in the potentiality of human life, may, if it chooses, regulate, and even proscribe, abortion except where it is necessary, in appropriate medical judgment, for the preservation of the life or health of the mother.

This Supreme Court ruling legalized abortion throughout the United States and invalidated all prior restrictive legislation. Since that time, most judicial activity has focused upon the areas of parental (in the case of minors), and spousal consent. In the case of *Central Missouri Planned Parenthood* v. *Danforth* (16), the Supreme Court held that a minor's consent to termination is valid and need not be accompanied by that of a parent. The general judicial consensus at the federal and district court level allows a woman abortion on her own consent, even if she is a minor or is married.

Despite its legalization, abortion is still opposed by certain religious and socioeconomic groups. The legalization decision has, in fact, led to a significant political polarization of "pro life" (antiabortion) and "pro choice" (pro abortion) forces. The result has been a potent single-issue political confrontation. Though some deny it, the polarization encompasses the allied issues of sterilization, contraception, and sex education; emotionally charged issues.

In effect, there has been a backlash in political, judicial, and legislative arenas against the legalization of abortion. Central to this polarization is the religious and ethical issue concerning the question of "when life begins"— that is, whether life begins at fertilization or at some point later in the gestational process. The related question of the definition of fetal viability is discussed later in this chapter. Voting patterns on the abortion issue have had real impact on some local and national elections. There are, and will be, an increasing number of cases testing various aspects of abortion, such as consent, medical practices, and even alleged criminality. There is a legis-

lative movement to invalidate the 1973 decision by constitutional amendment, obstensibly to give legal rights to the fetus (which it has never had, either in common or statutory law). An amendment, known as the Hyde Amendment, to the Department of Health, Education and Welfare appropriations bill, was passed in 1977. This amendment disallowed the use of any federal funds in furnishing termination services. A similar amendment was passed in 1978 to the Defense Department appropriations bill. These amendments deny the poor and military personnel on active duty and their dependents funds previously available for abortion unless the pregnancy to be terminated threatened the physical health of the mother, as attested to by two physicians, or resulted from rape or incest, promptly reported to law enforcement or public health authorities.

## VIABILITY OF THE FETUS

In any discussion of abortion, the ethical and moral implications of viability must be considered. A fetus is considered viable when it has attained the capability to survive in the extrauterine environment. Termination of pregnancy has been defined as "abortion," as opposed to homicide, when the fetus is still nonviable. There has never been a documented survival prior to the 21st week; therefore the age of the fetus may be regarded as a measure of viability. Various parameters have been used to determine fetal age. The prospective approach considers dating pregnancy from last menses. Retrospective parameters include fetal weight, crown rump and crown heel measurements of the fetus.

In Texas, abortion is defined as a pregnancy terminated through the 19th week, based on date of last menses. Other states commonly use a 500-g. fetal weight definition. The 1973 Supreme Court decision (17) refused to define viability. Most obstetrical texts define viability in terms of 1000 g. in fetal weight, or 28 weeks of gestational duration. Although with improved neonatal intensive care viability could doubtless be defined at lower fetal weight and gestational age, the outcome would be questionable, even with survival. Because of these considerations, most clinics will not perform elective termination beyond 20 weeks. This avoids any possibility of viability.

## DEMOGRAPHIC AND PSYCHOSOCIAL CONSIDERATIONS

### CHARACTERISTICS OF ABORTION PATIENTS

The Center for Disease Control, under its Joint Program for the Study of Abortion (JPSA/CDC) has published the most comprehensive study involving the demography and methodology of abortion (6). This research indicates that patients fall into the following three age groups, of relatively equal size: women under 19, 20 to 24, and over 25. Approximately 55 per cent are Caucasian, 30 per cent are black or of other minority racial or ethnic backgrounds, and 15 per cent are "unclassified." Approximately 75 per cent are unmarried, and 50 per cent have one or more living children. The JPSA data demonstrate that 25 per cent of pregnancies are terminated in the mid-trimester. This speaks poorly of education and of availability of early diagnostic, counseling, and termination services. It has also been shown that services are particularly inaccessible to the young, minority, poor, and rural population groups (3).

### THE ABORTION EXPERIENCE

Facilities offering services should provide adequate counseling, education, and emotional support before, during, and after the procedure. The provision of sexual information, particularly contraceptive advice, is essential. Although termination is not a pleasant experience, it should be a growth experience and thus, on balance, a positive, rather than a negative one.

Ideally, termination services should exhibit low repeat rates. Data from the Alan Guttmacher Institute (19), however, show an increase in the percentage of repeat abortion from 14.9 per cent, in 1974, to 23 per cent in 1976. This increase is misleading, in that it is based upon a preselected group of women, all of whom are sexually active and of proven fertility, as opposed to the female population at large. Nonetheless, every effort should be made to have the abortion patient become an acceptor and user of contraceptives. Such efforts have proven successful in several populations studied. Two studies demonstrate a 93 per cent contraceptive acceptance rate after abortion (7, 8).

Emotional sequelae are common. In one study (7), anxiety and depression were reported in as many as 86 per cent of patients, at the time of termination. However, in this same group of patients, only 15 per cent still reported these symptoms at the 4-month follow-up. In general, the rate of psychiatric illness after abortion is quite low (15). Women most likely to require psychotherapy after abortion are those with prior mental illness or deep-seated ambivalence that is not resolved (15). In one study (1), groups of patients who opted for early abortion, later abortion, or term birth were matched for parity, age, race, marital, social, and economic status. The findings indicated that self-esteem, alienation, and psychopathology were not significantly related to the option chosen.

The abortion issue is complex—biomedically, psychosocially, and philosophically. It has stirred, and will continue to stir, emotions that blur objectivity.

## REFERENCES

1. Athanasiou R, Oppel W, Michelson L, et al: Psychiatric sequelae to term birth and induced early and late abortion: a longitudinal study. Fam Plann Perspect 5:4, 1973
2. Brenner WE: Intra-amniotic administration of prostaglandin F2α to induce therapeutic abortion. Am J Obstet Gynecol 114(6):781, 1972
3. Cates W Jr, Schulz K F, Grimes DA et al: Effect of delay and method choice on the risk of abortion morbidity. Fam Plann Perspect 9(6):266, 1977
4. Chaudry SL, Hunt WB, Nortman J: Pregnancy termination in the mid trimester. Population Reports Series F:5, Sept 1976
5. Eaton CJ, Cohn F, Bollinger CC: Laminaria tent as a cervical dilator prior to aspiration-type therapeutic abortion. Obstet Gynecol 39:533, 1972
6. Forest JD, Tietze C, Sullivan E: Abortion in the United States 1976–1977. Fam Plann Perspect 10(5):271, 1978
7. Freeman EW: Abortion: subjective attitudes and feelings. Fam Plann Perspect 10(3):150, 1978
8. Gibbs CE, Weinberg PC: Legal abortion in Bexar County. Tex Med 75(2):92, 1975
9. Grimes DA, Schulz KF, Cates W et al: Mid trimester abortion by dilation and evacuation. N Engl J Med 296(20):1141, 1977
10. Hunt WB: Adolescent fertility-risks and consequences. Population Reports Series J:10, July 1976
11. Jordon B: The self-diagnosis of early pregnancy: an investigation of lay competence. Med Anthro 1(2):1, 1977
12. Kessel E, Brenner WE, Stathes G: Menstrual regulation in family planning services. Am J Public Health 65(7):731, 1975
13. King TM: The synergistic activity of intra-amni-

otic prostaglandin F2α and urea in the mid trimester election abortion. Am J Obstet Gynecol 120(5):704, 1974

14. Menken JA: The health and social consequences of teenage childbearing. Fam Plann Perspect 4(3):45, 1972
15. Pasnau RO: Psychiatric complications of therapeutic abortion. Obstet Gynecol 40(2):252, 1972
16. Planned Parenthood of Central Missouri v. Danforth, 428 US 52, 1976
17. Roe v. Wade, 410 US 113, 1973
18. Tietze C: Induced abortion. Reports on Population/Family Planning [Suppl] 14, 2nd ed, Dec 1977
19. Tietze C: Repeat abortions—Why more. Fam Plann Perspect 10(5):286, 1978
20. Weinberg PC, Linran JE, Linman SK: Intra-amniotic urea for induction mid trimester pregnancy termination. Obstet Gynecol 45(3):325, 1975

# 10

# Administration of Family Planning Programs

Richard A. Garcia
C. E. Gibbs
Mohammad M. Ahmad

Family planning is relatively new to the field of public health. As used in this chapter, *family planning* is defined as any action taken by individuals or couples to assure the desired number and spacing of children. Family planning programs are designed to provide the assistance or means with which to achieve these goals. In the United States such activity has also been referred to as *planned parenthood, birth control,* and *birth planning.* Planned Parenthood is also the corporate name of an international organization providing this type of service.

This chapter deals with administration of family planning programs. Administration consists of the following two major activities: *1)* organization of internal structure, and allocation of work force and resources, and *2)* direction and control of fiscal affairs, personnel, and other operational matters. The following definition of administration, introduced in 1936 by Gaus, White, and Dumock (4), is still valid:

[Administration is] the arrangement of personnel for facilitating the accomplishment of some agreed-upon purpose through the allocation of function and responsibilities. It is the relating of the efforts and capabilities of individuals and groups engaged upon a common task, in such a way as to secure the desired objective with the least friction and with the most satisfaction for those for whom the task is done and those engaged in the enterprise.

This definition indicates that although satisfaction of personnel is very important, the goals and integrity of the organization are of primary concern. In the event of conflict, personnel should adjust to a sound organizational structure, rather than modifying the structure to please individual whims.

## GENERAL ADMINISTRATIVE CHARACTERISTICS

### LINE VERSUS STAFF

Before discussing administrative principles, the distinctions between *line* and *staff* will be addressed. Misunderstandings created by confusion of these terms has led to considerable friction (7) and to the suggestion that the concepts of staff and line be discarded (2).

Much of this confusion is the result of conflicting definitions; each of the terms has two different meanings. One definition relates to functions performed, whereas the second relates to organizational authority. With respect to the first definition, *line* officers are those who are directly responsible for accomplishing organizational objectives. All others in the organization are considered *staff.* With respect to the second definition, *line* officers are those individuals who have relatively unlimited authority over those to whom direction is given. The authority of *staff* officers is restricted to specific functional areas.

Although there is significant confusion regarding the meaning of staff and line, these concepts are basic to management and play an important role in organizational structure.

## ADMINISTRATIVE PRINCIPLES

Established organizational principles apply equally well to private and public organizations. Pfiffner and Preshus (9) have identified certain basic organizational principles, including the following:

1. An organization should have a hierarchy, or "scalar process," with ascending and descending lines of authority and responsibility. There should be a broad functional base at the bottom and a single executive head at the top.
2. Every section and person must be answerable and accountable to the next higher level, and ultimately to the single head.
3. Principal sections should be created on the basis of functional or general purpose activities.
4. The number of sections should be sufficiently small to permit effective supervisory control. A rule of thumb is that an individual should supervise no more than seven to ten individuals.
5. Provisions should be made for staff services, such as planning or personnel management, to facilitate overall control and coordination of the organization.
6. The distinction between staff and line activities should be clearly identified and understood.

## POLICY-MAKING BODIES

Policy-making is primarily a function of governing bodies concerned with organizational goals and objectives. The formulation of policy and limits to agency activity is the responsibility of boards whose members are customarily appointed, rather than elected.

Ideally, governing boards should equitably represent the constituency the organization serves. However, conflict on the board is more likely to occur when its membership represents many diverse groups. When such conflict occurs, effective administrative action by the organization's chief executive officer may be weakened or curtailed. In such instances, joint action by impartial board members and the executive officer must occur to effect conciliation or effective compromise.

Conflict between governing-board members and the organization's chief executive officer may develop in various ways. First, the officer may consistently concur with the majority. In the event of a membership change, his or her impartiality would probably be questioned. Second, the chief officer may ignore the governing board or may fail to consult with it, or to provide the members with meaningful work to perform, or to abide by its recommendations. If the board lacks strong leadership, the chief officer's will may prevail. If the board has strong leadership, the board may attempt to assume the chief officer's functions and responsibilities. Third, the officer may refuse to accept responsibility, and may expect the board to accomplish his or her tasks.

The executive officer and the governing board have specific responsibilities and functions. The former must keep the board informed; provide access to all records; and, when board recommendations are not followed, provide an explanation. The governing board is responsible for hiring and dismissing the chief executive officer, determining general administrative and program policy, providing budget review and approval, and approving major personnel appointments.

### PRIVATE SECTOR

In the private sector, governing bodies are usually the constituent type, i.e., members are chosen for their personal qualifications and/or because they represent professional, social, religious, or other community interests. The greatest advantage of this type of board is that it facilitates communication between the organization and the community served. Examples are Planned Parenthood affiliates and neighborhood "free clinics."

### GOVERNMENTAL SECTOR

The government, or public, sector may use either a constituent and/or a technical board. For example, in addition to a constituent board, a public health agency may have a technical board to provide advice regarding problems in maternal care, engineering, law, and other professional or technical areas.

Within the governmental sector, general levels of administrative activities fall at the federal, state, and local levels.

**The Federal Level.** Federal boards are usually technical. Members advise appointed administrative officers and assist in formulation and interpretation of policy and legislation. Funding of programs and program initiatives on the international and national levels are influenced by these opinions.

**The State Level.** Members of state boards of health are usually appointed by the governor and approved by the senate. Ideally, board members are appointed for their professional, technical, or political competence and/or constituent representativeness. In practice, there is considerable variation. The number of members varies from three to fourteen. In some states candidates are nominated by the state medical association, and in at least one state are appointed directly by that association. In some cases all members must be physicians. In others, dentists, civil engineers, veterinarians, osteopaths, and attorneys are board members. However, in almost all cases, the population served—the lay public—is relatively unrepresented. Action to correct this situation is steadily increasing.

**The Local or Regional Level.** At the local or regional level, boards tend to be more representative of constituents than are those on the state or federal levels. This is partially the result of recent legislation, such as P.L. 93-641 (11), which mandated community involvement in federally funded health programs. In order to qualify for federal grant support, the following two conditions concerning constituent representation must now be met: *1)* local community initiative is required in determining needs and program content, and *2)* true consumers of the services must participate in the design and operation of the local program.

## PERSONNEL

Personnel management is a complex discipline; a general discussion is beyond the scope of this volume. For readers interested in this field, ample literature is available (3, 5, 13). This section addresses only those aspects of personnel management unique to family planning programs.

### THE ROLE OF THE PHYSICIAN

The physician's role in a family planning project varies among programs. In some, the physician is both medical director and chief executive officer. In others, she or he provides certain medical services, either under contract, or by referral from the program. Most commonly the physician is medical director, responsible for the quality of medical services provided, whereas the chief executive officer assumes administrative responsibilities. It is extremely important that cooperation and mutual assistance prevail between these individuals.

Regardless of the physician's specific role, she or he always retains responsibility for the following functions: identifying procedures to be performed, defining standards to be followed, offering leadership and direction to medical care, and assuring the quality of medical services. All medical care provided by the program should be supervised and/or directed by a physician who has received training in family planning and is accessible to patients and staff.

The physician should also assure that the program has written policy and procedure manuals which identify and describe in detail its basic services. These should include history, physical examination, laboratory tests, method selection, treatment procedures, and referral mechanisms. These services are delineated in greater detail later in this chapter.

### THE ROLE OF THE EDUCATOR

The family planning educator plays an important role in any family planning program. There are three main areas in which this individual can be effectively utilized: staff development, training of new personnel, and community education.

An important part of any family planning program is continuing education or staff development for its employees. This results in high employee morale, greater program effectiveness, and, eventually, in higher quality service for patients. The educator may function as a resource—making materials or personnel available to staff—or may actually provide the required training.

An equally important function is training of new personnel. Family planning programs require staff capabilities in the areas of sexuality, counseling, and medical knowlege. Most personnel seeking employment in such organizations have not had exposure to these skills. The family planning physician and educator must determine the minimum level of knowledge necessary to function effectively in a family planning setting. Minimum levels vary according to job function; for example, a registered nurse requires a much higher level of knowledge and skills than an appointment clerk. The functions, skills, and basic knowledge required for each position should be specified in written form.

The third function, providing community education, varies greatly among programs. Some emphasize this aspect of family planning and have created speakers' bureaus. Others deemphasize this activity and are very selective regarding speaking engagements or community exposure. Either way, the program educator must consider community education and expand or limit activities according to program policies.

### THE ROLE OF THE ADMINISTRATOR

Regardless of whether administrative duties are the responsibility of the program physician or of another individual, the required functions remain the same. The administrator is responsible, and accountable, to the governing body or board. However, in many respects the administrator's role in a health delivery program is different from that in other fields.

The operation of a health delivery program may be compared, conceptually, to the operation of a commercial enterprise, employing individuals of various skills and occupational levels, operating various types of equipment, and simultaneously performing dissimilar functions. A primary difference between the health administrator and the commercial manager lies in the managerial control function. The commercial manager controls all activity by issuing production orders, after first considering demand, and the capability and capacity of the organization. The health administrator does not determine production levels. This role is partially left to physicians, who determine the scope of services to be provided, within the parameters of available resources provided by the administrator, and for the rest, is uncontrolled. Limited control creates a difficult situation for the health admin-

istrator in his attempts to utilize scarce resources efficiently, in order to maximize production. Like the commercial manager, he is required to make decisions regarding questions of personnel scheduling and utilization, capital equipment purchases, and expansion or reduction of space or services. However, in addition to limited authority, the health care administrator faces several problems unique to his situation. For example, health, particularly contraceptive use, is an emotional issue, and fears or prejudices can impede the introduction of "rational," "logical," or "objective" methods. Moreover, the factors constituting "health" are very complex and signify different things to different groups. These difficulties, combined with the absence of strong economic or market forces, the absence of effective competition, the presence of a strong professional factor (the attitudes of physicians and nurses) in creating or determining demand for services, increasing public involvement, political intervention, and the need to coordinate different public, private, and voluntary agencies, impede the ready application of modern management methods in family planning.

Because of this difficulty, the health care administrator is dependent on good data information systems to facilitate decision-making processes. In order to be of use to an administrator, such systems must provide relevant, accurate data at timely intervals. The health administrator must constantly seek appropriate cost-reduction opportunities and make cost-avoidance decisions. To perform these critical functions, she or he must be trained in quantitative techniques and must be able to influence the formulation of organizational policy and decision-making.

It is through management processes that organizational objectives are achieved and resources appropriately acquired and allocated. Unfortunately, managerial perspectives and skills are often lacking in family planning programs. Consequently, established policies and procedures are often followed blindly, although they may hinder the attainment of program objectives.

### FACILITIES AND SUPPLIES

Family planning services should be provided in facilities that are readily accessible to patients, assure security and confidentiality, and are integrated with other community health agencies. The basic facility should be clean, uncrowded, comfortable, and characterized by a professional atmosphere.

All family planning facilities must meet all local and state building and safety codes. In the event that federal funds are utilized, federal codes regarding items such as facilities for the handicapped and designated areas for smoking and/or nonsmoking individuals must be met. Before any construction or renovation is instituted, it would be beneficial to review the "Minimum Requirements of Construction and Equipment for Hospital and Medical Facilities," a publication of the Department of Health, Education and Welfare (8).

Certain basic services may be found in any clinical facility. These should be housed in areas separated with respect to function, and include areas for: *1*) patient reception and waiting; *2*) restrooms; *3*) patient examination; *4*) consultation and education; *5*) laboratory; *6*) equipment and/or instrument cleaning and sterilization; *7*) maintenance; *8*) administration.

In some clinics, additional areas are provided for the following services: *1*) children's play; *2*) patient recovery; *3*) large group "rap" sessions; *4*) audio-visual information; *5*) conferences.

There should be sufficient supplies to conveniently satisfy the immediate needs of patients and clinic personnel. Depending on the range of services, items appropriate for IUD insertions or removal, diaphragm fitting, outpatient sterilizations or abortions, and laboratory samples should be available. A "crash" cart containing appropriate emergency supplies and resuscitation equipment should be immediately accessible and checked periodically. Contraceptive supplies providing a full range of hormonal substances and combinations should be included in the formulary. Nonprescription contraceptive items such as condoms, foams, creams, and jellies should be available in a variety of types. For programs providing "natural" family planning methods, basal body temperature thermometers and temperature charts should be stocked.

The medical director should periodically review the clinical formulary and make it available to all medical personnel. Only medi-cally justified and approved items should be listed.

## PATIENT RECRUITMENT

### STRATEGIES OF RECRUITMENT

As is true in most successful motivational efforts, the potential users must be reasonably certain that the suggested course of action is in their best interest and that future benefits will occur as a result of participation. In choosing the motivational strategies to be employed, it is necessary that the motivator understand the clientele, so that the strategy is compatible with the dominant characteristics of the target group. Equally important, the motivator must understand him- or her-self, and select a strategy congruent with his or her expertise and image. The strategy must "fit" the circumstances and person. The following three strategies have been traditionally employed within the context of family planning programs.

**The Goal of Personal and Family Socioeconomic Gain.** For many years, disadvantaged people have been encouraged to reduce their family size in order to make gains in their social or economic status. Improved housing, increased money for each family member, more time for each child, upward mobility, higher education, fewer family costs, increased personal development, and the like, have been cited as goals more readily achievable by smaller families. Although it is possible that these goals may lead to increased use of family planning, it is more likely that limitation of family size occurs as a result of upward mobility and an increased participation in middle-class life (see Chap. 19). In addition, utilization of this type of strategy is not really suitable for a worker in the health field, whose chief concern should be to improve the health of individuals.

**The Goal of Population Growth Limitation.** "A finite world equals a finite population"; "space-ship earth"; "consumption of resources"; "waste disposal"; "air, water, and land pollution"—and all the other phrases of the 1960s made a generation of Western man extremely conscious of the demographic aspects of family planning. Appealing to these concerns would appear to be a reasonable motivational strategy in planning national policy, international group relations, prevention of exploitation of limited resources, etc. However, individual decisions to enlist in a family planning program are usually not affected by demographic concerns. Like the strategy emphasizing socioeconomic gains, this strategy appears unbecoming for personal health workers, even though privately they may be very committed to zero population growth.

**The Goal of Health Improvement.** It should be apparent to the individual that his or her best interests are served by at least listening to, and perhaps following, unbiased suggestions given as preventative health measures. For example, it is fairly common knowledge that women over the age of 35 who bear children have a greater chance of having an abnormal child. It is also commonly understood that the degenerative diseases of age begin to make their appearance in adult women at about this same time. Therefore, perhaps a good place to begin discussing health matters related to family planning is with the subject of maternal age and health status. Another fact of considerable interest to women who expect to have more than one child is the increased safety for herself and her children if there is approximately 2 to 3 years spacing between the birth of one child and the conception of another. This information is often highly acceptable to people who otherwise think that the physician, in offering advice on family planning, is interfering in the right of a woman to have as many children as she wishes. The health worker might also point out that induced abortion is a health problem of great magnitude, and family planning is an appropriate method of reducing this hazard. Also, once the fifth baby has been born to a woman, there is good evidence that the likelihood of problems associated with maternal hemorrhage and other disorders increases. It behooves a helping person, then, to inform people of these possibilities.

The importance of good mental health must not be ignored. Some women do not want additional pregnancies, at least for the time being, and are threatened by the possibility of another pregnancy. It may be useful to initiate discussion demonstrating that enlistment into a scientifically oriented family planning program may significantly reduce fear of pregnancy and thus improve attitudes and ensure favorable family relationships.

Whether from a physical or mental health point of view, health-oriented suggestions from medical personnel are more palatable and more likely to be well received, understood, and given genuine consideration than advice derived from the two other strategies. For health personnel, it is probably best to resist the first two, and devote motivational efforts to elucidating the health benefits of modern family planning.

**TACTICS OF RECRUITMENT**

There are many opportunities to initiate the process of recruiting patients into family planning. Wherever health education efforts occur, family planning should have a role—in the internist's office, with the problems of chronic disease; in the premarital counselor's office; at the time of blood tests for premarital exams; in student health programs in colleges and universities; in health education classes in public school systems and churches; and in various types of mass media health education.

During pregnancy-related medical care, family planning is of obvious concern to both personnel and patient. Questions concerning desired family size and plans for contraceptive use should be asked at the first prenatal visit, the answers recorded, and indicated follow-up conducted. During a second pregnancy, it is advisable to inform the patient of the opportunities and advantages of permanent sterilization. Although it is likely that neither she nor her husband would be interested at this time, it facilitates consideration of this topic at a later date. Breast feeding, when discussed during the antepartum course, should be related to family planning with respect to method, timing, and risks. The proposed contraceptive program should be clearly outlined in the patient's medical chart. Following delivery, and prior to discharge, the patient should obtain appropriate education and information, and should enlist in follow-up activities. Prescriptions or supplies should be provided at this time. Tubal ligation is often performed a day or two after delivery and is eminently suited to many circumstances. However, many physicians and patients prefer to wait until after the 6 weeks' postpartum examination of mother and baby before committing themselves to a permanent procedure.

Abortion counseling and procedures should be accompanied by recruitment into family planning. No medical program committed to helping patients with abortion is complete without a thorough explanation and opportunity to begin family planning services.

During all other medical care of individuals of reproductive age, available family planning programs should be identified. This is especially true as the couple approaches the age when it is unlikely that they will want more children. During this period, it is appropriate to recommend changing from temporary contraception to some form of permanent sterilization. When it is necessary to recommend delay or cessation of childbearing, for health reasons, physicians must provide appropriate contraceptive supplies and information. Physical examinations in institutions such as prisons, and in long-term hospitalizations, should include comments about family planning services.

Less satisfactory than the above tactics are neighborhood recruitment efforts. Approaches range from store-front information and education sites to fully established medical clinics. These seem to have been important early in the family planning era, but appear less useful today. Nevertheless, in many areas they are the only kind of opportunity available. Least satisfactory is door-to-door, uninvited, and unsolicited, contact. Often this approach is unwelcome and liable to cost more in hostility to the program than is achieved in acceptance.

Patient referrals may also be useful. Asking a satisfied patient to tell her friends about the good care she is receiving enlists her even more strongly and simultaneously makes her realize her own usefulness. Such patient involvement should not be forced. Very often, a hint is all a patient requires to become an effective recruiter.

## EDUCATION AND INFORMATION

Patients must be well informed. They must understand all available methods and why it is in their best interest to use family planning. They should have a general idea regarding technique, effectiveness, risks, side effects, benefits to be expected, and the costs associated with each method. For example, IUD patients must be informed that their menstrual periods may be heavier, that occasional spotting may occur, and that there is a small risk of pregnancy associated with the method. They must also be told to be prepared to have an induced abortion if they conceive with the IUD in situ, or run serious risks if they elect not to do so.

Once informed, patients should select a method according to their individual needs and be carefully taught all necessary details. They should also understand how to obtain necessary services in the event of complications, side effects, or a move to another area. Follow-up visits must be arranged, and permission for outreach obtained, in the event that scheduled visits are not kept.

## FOLLOW-UP

Careful recording of all information in the patient's medical record is mandatory. An appropriate appointment log should be maintained, with a system of checking on missed appointments. A method of contacting "no show" patients should be part of each family planning program. A word of caution is needed here: many women utilizing family planning services do not want members of their families or neighbors to be aware of these activities. Under these circumstances, an obvious kind of follow-up would be injurious.

## PATIENT FLOW

A patient flowchart can easily be developed for any family planning delivery site. This is especially true in the outpatient or ambulatory clinic. The basic flowchart diagrammed in Figure 10-1 identifies typical key functions and decision-making areas involved in setting up a sterilization procedure. While the chart is not all-inclusive, the general flow can be quickly established.

Each program or clinic site should develop and evaluate a patient flowchart. In so doing, bottlenecks or confusion points frequently can be identified quickly. Specific items relating to uncoordinated activities, delays, and even losing of patients can be traced, and attempts to correct these problems can be initiated. In almost any problem where the solution depends upon logical sequencing of operations or proper positioning of required materials and personnel, a flowchart can be a valuable tool for analysis (see Chap. 11 for further discussion).

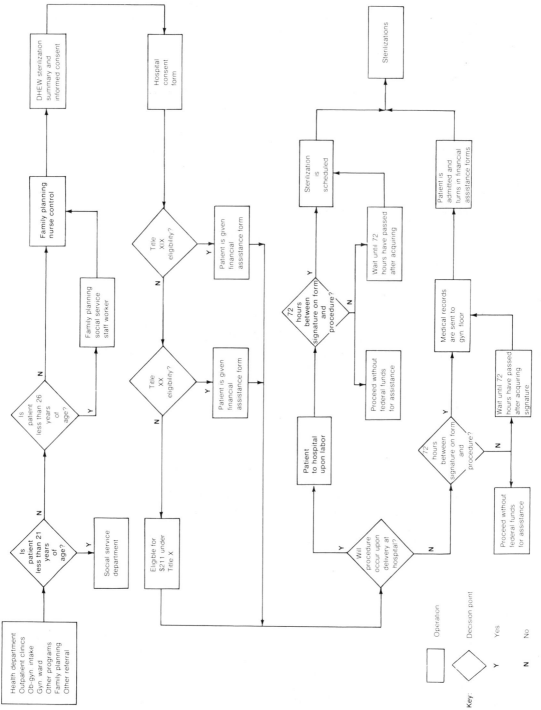

**FIG. 10-1.** Typical flow diagram of a specific family planning procedure (sterilization).

## SOURCES OF FUNDING

### FUNDING OF PROGRAMS IN THE UNITED STATES

Private family planning programs, primarily clinics operated by Planned Parenthood of America, have been in existence for over 50 years, with a history of impressive achievements in the face of formidable odds. Funds have been generated primarily through private fund-raising efforts, and (only within the last 10 to 15 years) from public sources. Public programs financed and administered by state and federal agencies are new in the United States, and for the most part, began with the passage of the Economic Opportunity Act of 1964.

This act established the Office of Economic Opportunity (OEO) as a federal agency given a mandate to deal with the problems of poverty affecting a fifth of the population of the United States. Some of the newly established poverty programs were delegated to OEO; others were placed under the responsibility of the Department of Health, Education and Welfare (DHEW), the Department of Labor (DOL), and the Small Business Administration (SBA).

The portion of the Economic Opportunity Act which relates directly to family planning activity is the Community Action Program, established under Title II, Part A. This act created a federally funded program which could award funds to either public or private nonprofit, local agencies to provide family planning services. The first direct OEO grant for family planning—an $8000 award—went to a private nonprofit organization in Corpus Christi, Texas, in 1965. This city had a large population of medically underserved, low-income Mexican-American families.

In order to qualify for federal grant money, three major conditions must be met. The first two, the need for local community initiative in determining needs and program content, and consumer participation in program design and operation, have already been mentioned. The third condition is that heavy emphasis must be placed upon breaking the poverty cycle by assuring the medically indigent access to low-cost family planning services. Published analyses (6) have documented the fact that among various approaches to comprehensive antipoverty action, family planning is one of the most effective in terms of cost-benefit analysis (see Chap. 13). It is highly cost-effective with respect to reducing the number of individuals living at, or below, the poverty level. The federal poverty level determines the definition of medical indigence and is derived from a schedule of income and family-size thresholds adjusted annually in accordance with changes in the Consumer Price Index. In 1979, this level was $6700 for a nonfarm family of four (1).

### GOALS AND PRIORITIES OF FEDERALLY FUNDED PROGRAMS

In family planning, even more than in other health programs, the need for specific and clear program policies and goals cannot be overemphasized. Over the years, certain policy guidelines have been established by federal legislation, and traditional medical ethics. These guidelines require that family planning services be accepted on a voluntary basis. Participation in any family planning program must not be used, or seen, as a prerequisite for any other form of public assistance. Any coercion of patients to use contraceptive methods is prohibited. Patients must be completely informed about all available methods of family planning; moreover, such information must be provided under the supervision of qualified medical personnel. Policy questions regarding controversial topics such as providing services to minors without requiring parental consent must be considered and resolved by individual programs within parameters set by the state. In this regard, formal adoption of written and publicized policy statements as soon as issues develop are of great value.

The basic goal of federally subsidized family planning programs is to make services equally accessible to all income groups. Recently, there has been an initiative by both the federal government and medical organizations to integrate services within comprehensive programs designed to meet the overall health and economic needs of the indigent.

Specifically, the following priorities led Congress to create funding mechanisms for family planning programs:

1. The need to improve maternal and child health and well-being.
2. The right of all individuals to freely determine the number and spacing of their children.

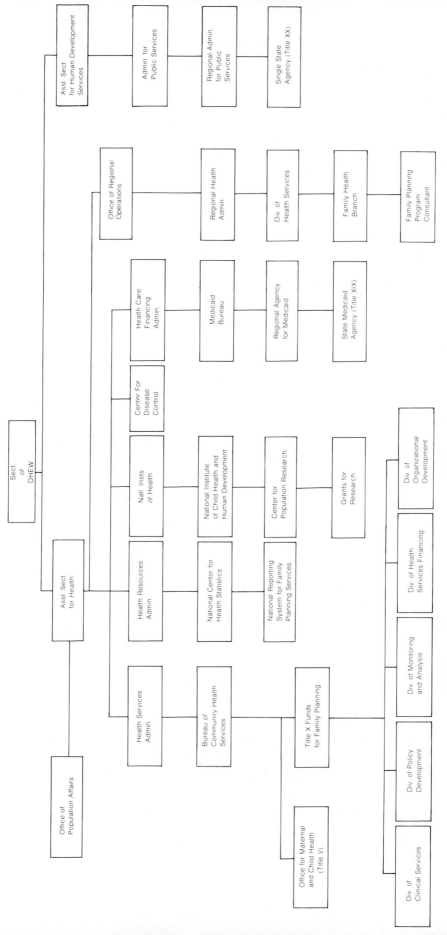

**FIG. 10–2.** Organizational structure of DHEW's family planning program activity.

3. The need to improve the economic well-being of our citizens.

These priorities shaped the congressional "intent" of laws authorizing federal programs, and administrative regulations or guidelines which influenced the manner in which appropriated funds were distributed. This "intent," whereby federal monies were to be distributed directly to local community agencies, was counter to President Nixon's "New Federalism" policy. The result was a shifting of the control of funds from federal to state or local officials, through various funding programs. The following section describes the various programs or "titles" by which these congressionally appropriated funds are distributed through the Health Services Administration (DHEW).

**TYPES OF FEDERAL FUNDING**

Title V, or the Maternal and Child Health Program. This title amended the Social Security Act in 1967 to upgrade maternal, infant, and child health services—and included family planning. The act is directed toward improving the overall health status of the medically high-risk population. Funds are allocated to states according to a "formula grant funding" system which considers total state population, income, and other health or social indices. The funds are distributed to the health departments of each state, which, in turn, allocate these monies to local maternal and child health activities. By federal regulation, at least 6 per cent of Title V funds must be used for family planning services. The federal funds make up 75 per cent of the total amount, with the local agencies providing, or "matching," the remaining 25 per cent. At the national level, responsibility is assigned to the Office for Maternal and Child Health, within the Bureau of Community Health Services (see Fig. 10-2).

Title X of the Public Health Service Act. This title is the major source of public family planning funds. The act defines the "right" of *all* individuals to have family planning services, and states that economic status cannot be used as a barrier to services; however, "priority in the provision of services will be given to persons from low-income families" (10). Because low-income individuals would have less access to family planning, programs funded through Title X must give priority to these consumers.

Title X funds are awarded on the basis of grant applications submitted by public organizations, (e.g., medical schools or public hospitals) or private, nonprofit organizations (e.g., Planned Parenthood of America, free-standing neighborhood clinics). Each applicant must present a detailed account of how the money will be utilized. Grant awards usually are for a one-year period, but may be renewed an unspecified number of times.

When a grant is approved and awarded, the grantee and the federal government enter into a direct relationship, through the grantee's particular DHEW Regional Office. For the sake of administrative effectiveness, DHEW has created ten regional offices. In some instances, for administrative or political reasons, project grants are awarded to an "umbrella" agency, such as a state family planning council or department of health, which, in turn, subcontracts with individual provider agencies. Under Title X, the federal government funds 90 per cent of the approved activity, with the local agency responsible for the remaining 10 per cent. At the national level, program responsibility is placed with the Office of Family Planning in the Bureau of Community Health Services (BCHS) which is part of the Health Services Administration (HSA) of DHEW (see Fig. 10-2).

Titles XIX (Medicaid) and XX (Social Services) of the Social Security Act. These titles were enacted to reimburse health care programs serving welfare recipients (Title XIX) and other needy or potentially needy persons (Title XX). The ultimate objective of these programs is to enable the poor to eventually become self-sufficient. The programs were initially created as a result of the 1967 Public Welfare Amendments (Title IV) to the Social Security Act. These amendments require states to offer family planning assistance to all families receiving public assistance, under the Aid to Families with Dependent Children (AFDC) program. The amendments were later modified and became the present Title XX program. Under both Titles XIX and XX, money is reimbursed to the states for specified services provided to certain categories of eligible recipients. The states, in turn, contract with approved providers of these services and reimburse the providers at an established rate per unit of service.

Title XIX (Medicaid) provides for reimbursement of costs incurred by the provision of approved family planning medical services to welfare recipients. Title XX provides for reimbursement costs incurred by the provision of educational services to welfare recipients and approved family planning medical and educational services to patients qualifying under the income and family-size threshold schedule previously discussed. The latter individuals are considered potential welfare recipients, in that one additional dependent would qualify them for such assistance.

Under Title XIX (Medicaid), overall state reimbursement is open-ended. These funds are administered by a Medicaid contractor within each state, and the program is generally supervised by the state's welfare agency. Some states, however, have created a Medicaid Division within the State Health Agency, and at least one state has a separate Medicaid Commission which administers the program. Family Planning services are funded at 90 per cent of the approved activity, with local agencies responsible for the remaining 10 per cent. At the national level, the agency responsible for Title XIX programs is the Medicaid Bureau of the Health Care Financing Administration (HCFA) or DHEW (see Fig. 10-2).

Title XX funds are administered by the state's welfare agencies, usually through the social service branch. Title XX also enjoys a 90 per cent/10 per cent match, and the responsible agency at the national level is the Administration for Public Services of the Office of Human Development (OHD) of DHEW (see Fig. 10-2).

## FUNDING OF INTERNATIONAL PROGRAMS

The legislation providing for international family planning program funding is the Foreign Assistance Act. Whereas domestic programs are administered through DHEW's Health Services Administration, international programs are administered through the Agency for International Development (AID) of the Bureau for Population and Humanitarian Assistance.

International programs are funded by the three following methods:

1. Support for international organizations
2. Funding of private agencies based in the United States which provide overseas services
3. Bilateral grants to foreign governments

The two international family planning organizations with the largest budgets obtain funding through methods *1* and *2*, respectively. They are the United Nations Fund for Population Activities (UNFPA) and the International Planned Parenthood Federation (IPPF). UNFPA is administered by representatives to the United Nations and is funded as an international organization. IPPF is administered by a coalition of private family planning associations, in nearly 100 countries. It is considered by AID as a private family planning agency based in the United States. The Family Planning International Assistance (FPIA) program is considered the international branch of the Planned Parenthood Federation of America.

There remains strong support in Congress for funding population programs through bilateral grants to foreign governments under existing foreign-assistance legislation. However, philosophical disagreement concerning both direction of, and prerequisites for assistance exists. One faction ties such aid to the preexistence of programs designed to reduce population growth. Other factions view the imposition of this condition on foreign governments as an insult.

## TYPES OF FAMILY PLANNING SERVICES

Two basic types of projects are found in family planning programs in the United States: hospital-based clinics and outpatient clinics. Some of the services not offered by the outpatient clinic and usually provided by the hospital-based clinic include: surgical services for complications resulting from family planning, inpatient sterilizations, and infertility diagnosis and/or treatment.

### HOSPITAL-BASED PROGRAMS

The hospital-based program usually offers a wide range of services to outpatients and inpatients. Because of relatively expensive inpatient costs, this type of project has a higher cost per individual served. Characteristically, high-risk patients compose a large portion of its population. High-risk factors include, but are not limited to, hypertension, age below 17 or over 35, previous cesarean section, high parity, diabetes, one or more previous abortions, or other medical problems (12). Referral agreements with surrounding outpatient clinics usually exist for surgical procedures or treatment of complications related to family planning services. The hospital-based program recruits most of its patients from the postpartum floor or from the gynecological service, and, in turn, refers many of these individuals to surrounding outpatient projects.

A hospital-based program has physiological, organizational, educational, and psychological advantages.

**Physiological Advantages.** The most effective period in which to provide birth control information is during, or immediately after, the first pregnancy and before the first postpartum ovulation (15). If contraception is not practiced post partum, approximately 50 per cent of all women will have conceived 90 days after the first postpartum menstrual period and 75 per cent within 1 year of this period (14).

**Organizational Advantages.** Maternity staff personnel and related facilities are easily adapted to providing family planning services for both postpartum and pregnant patients. In many cases, this simply involves the addition of contraceptive information to existing "mothers'" classes. Establishment of a parallel but separate organization would result in cost duplication of scarce resources.

**Educational Advantages.** During pregnancy and the early puerperium, the patient and partner are highly receptive to the ideas of child spacing and of maximizing maternal health. During the early postpartum period, the patient is under the medical and psychological care of personnel whom she trusts. Consequently, recommendations and advice of these individuals carry great weight in decision-making processes.

**Psychological Advantages.** When family planning is integrated within good maternal and infant care programs, it becomes politically more acceptable, since it is interpreted as part of an overall program to improve health, and not as a racist plot to curb births among minority populations. Hospital-based programs have, consequently, received unreserved approval from the general population.

## OUTPATIENT CLINICS

The outpatient clinic may be either a freestanding clinic or a part of a more comprehensive activity such as a primary care or maternal and child health clinic. Although the outpatient clinic does not offer the total range of services provided by the hospital-based clinic, it makes important contributions to the health of women of reproductive age and to that of infants and children.

As in the case of hospital-based projects, outpatient clinics contribute to cancer prevention through provision of annual pelvic examinations, breast examinations, and pap smears. Such examinations help to identify overall medical problems and often allow diagnosis of disease before it reaches an acute stage. Since many patients represent a combination of high reproductive risk and low socioeconomic status, they are in particular need of medical care. In most instances, the care they receive through family planning clinics is their only contact with modern medicine. Consequently, the outpatient clinic makes an important contribution toward improving overall health care and reducing high maternal and perinatal morbidity and mortality.

The characteristic aim of an outpatient clinic is to provide an acceptable level of medical care and protection for the majority, rather than highly specific protection for a few. This aim results in lower cost per patient with respect to both funds and time. While some degree of quality care may be sacrificed, the readily available services offered by these clinics is an important factor in the community's overall health delivery system.

## PROVISION OF MEDICAL SERVICES

All medical care in a family planning clinic should be provided under the direction, and/or supervision, of a licensed physician who has received training in family planning methods and services. This physician should be readily accessible to patients and staff members. Patient care provided by paraprofessionals should be based on an evaluation of the education, clinical skills, and experience of each individual. In areas where it is legally possible, these paraprofessionals should be supported by written standing orders issued by the medical director, which are effective when the physician is not physically present.

The Department of Health, Education and Welfare has published a manual identifying basic services which must be provided by any federally funded family planning program (10).

As a rule, the following items should be part of the standard medical history taken for a new patient:

1. Gynecologic and reproductive history: menstrual history; abortions; miscarriages; stillbirths; premature and/or live births; complications of pregnancy and deliveries; and vaginal and pelvic infections, including venereal disease.

2. Medical-surgical history: incidence of infectious diseases; cardiovascular, dermatologic, genitourinary, hematopoietic, metabolic, neoplastic, and neurologic conditions that demand special care in relation to either childbearing or birth control, and conditions that affect general health status.

The physical examination of new patient or a patient on an annual visit should consist of the following:

1. A concentration upon a thorough pelvic and breast examination, including a visualization of the cervix, and bimanual (including rectal) palpation. The examination should routinely include the thyroid, heart, lungs, and abdomen. This data should be updated during the annual visit.

2. If indicated—eyes (fundus), lymph nodes, skin, throat, and extremities should be checked.

3. Any contraindications to, or consequences of, contraceptives.

4. Any indications of sexually transmitted diseases.

The physical examination of male patients should focus on genital, rectal, and skin conditions and may include a throat examination.

The laboratory tests generally recommended for initial and annual visits are as follows: *1*) urinalysis for sugar and protein; *2*) hemoglobin or hematocrit; *3*) gonorrhea culture; *4*) papanicolaou smear.

Other laboratory tests which should be available, either on-site or by referral, include: urine pregnancy test; urine microscopic exam-ination; urine culture, and sensitivity tests for evaluation of pelvic or urinary tract infections; saline and KOH wet-mount of abnormal vaginal secretions; white cell count and differential; serologic tests for syphilis (mandatory, with positive gonorrhea cultures); antibody tests for herpes and rubella; blood type; sickle-cell screening; glucose tolerance test; semen analysis, for vasectomy follow-up; tuberculin tests (should be routine in areas of high risk); other cytologic studies and cultures, as needed.

More complex tests or other services which may be available only by referral are: chest x-rays; pelvic x-rays or sonography, for IUD location; mammography or thermography; colposcopy; biopsy of cervix, vagina, endometrium, or breast; amniocentesis; infertility diagnosis; sterilization procedures; abortion procedures; social services of some complexity.

In addition, complications resulting from family planning measures do occur, and there must be clearly defined referral procedures to immediately deal with these problems.

Treatment should be available, and provided to, patients with common clinical problems. It must be remembered that in many cases the only medical care available to these patients is that provided by family planning clinics. Updated protocols for the following conditions should be available: vaginitis; cystitis; cervicitis; condyloma acuminatum; pubic lice; nonspecific urethritis; herpes genitalis; anemia; gonorrhea; syphilis; immunizations.

All clinical material must be recorded in a standardized format developed by each particular program. The information must then be processed and stored in a confidential manner. Professional and clerical personnel with access to this information must be trained to respect and safeguard patient data, releasing such data only upon the patient's written consent.

A system of easy and rapid retrieval of medical records should be incorporated within every program. Two basic forms of indexing can be considered—alphabetical and numerical. Alphabetical indexing is functional in clinics with small populations. Clinics serving large numbers of patients should consider numerical indexing, particularly terminal digit filing systems, in cases of unusually large volume.

Recently, DHEW has indicated that family planning projects should also maintain a system of indexing patient records according to contraceptive method. This information must be readily accessible to the project and must not be dependent on individual record searches, or demand a prolonged turn-around time for computer processing. A prime example of the need for such a system occurred during the FDA Dalkon Shield recall. During this recall period, the FDA required family planning programs to contact all patients who had elected to use a Dalkon Shield. These patients were to be advised to return to a physician and have that particular IUD removed or replaced. Many projects were required to perform a manual search of all medical records, both active and inactive, in order to determine which patients to notify. This was both time-consuming and costly.

## COORDINATION OF ACTIVITIES

Public Law 93-641 was mentioned in the first section of this chapter with regard to constituency representation on governing bodies. This legislation not only affected the structure of boards but also influenced federally funded programs in other regards. P.L. 93-641 requires program review on a local level to ensure that ample and appropriate coordination between various health delivery programs and/or agencies exists. This legislation also requires program review, to prevent needless duplication or provision of unnecessary services within a certain geographic area. Only after local review and approval has been received will federal funding mechanisms be set into action to review the funding request. At this time, only those programs requesting federal financial assistance are required to enter this review process. However, it is expected that within the foreseeable future, all health-related programs, regardless of funding source, will be reviewed at the local level.

## REFERENCES

1. Community Services Administration: Community Services Administration Income Poverty Guidelines (Revised). 45CFR Part 1060.2-2. Washington, D.C., Dept. of Labor, May 7, 1979
2. Fisch GG: Line-staff is obsolete. Harvard Business Review 39:67, 1961
3. French WL: Personnel Management Process: Human Resources and Administration, 3rd ed. Boston, Houghton Mifflin, 1974
4. Gaus JM, White LD, Dimock ME: The Frontiers of Public Administration. Chicago, University of Chicago Press, 1936
5. George CS: Supervision in Action—The Art of Managing Others. Reston, VA, Reston Publishing, 1977
6. Jaffe FS: Short-term goals and benefits of United States family planning programs. Stud Fam Plann 5:105, 1974
7. Koontz H, O'Donnell C: Principles of Management, 4th ed. New York, McGraw-Hill, 1968, p 291
8. Minimum Requirements of Construction and Equipment for Hospital and Medical Facilities, Health Resources Administration (74–4000), Division of Facilities Utilization. Washington DC, Department of Health, Education and Welfare (DHEW), 1974
9. Pfiffner JMcD, Preshus R: Public Administration. New York, Donald Press 1967
10. Program Guidelines for Project Grants for Family Planning Services, Section 1001, Public Health Service Act (42USC300). Washington DC, DHEW, January 1976
11. Public Law 93–641, National Health Planning and Resources Development Act of 1974, 93rd Congress, January 4, 1975
12. Recommendations for the Regional Development of Maternal and Perinatal Health Services, Committee on Perinatal Health Toward Improving the Outcome of Pregnancy. White Plains, N.Y., National March of Dimes, 1976
13. Strauss G, Sayles LR: Managing Human Resources. Englewood Cliffs, Prentice-Hall, 1977
14. Taylor HC: A family planning program related to maternity services. Am J Obstet Gynecol 95:726, 1966
15. Zatuchni GI (ed): Post Partum Family Planning: A Report on the International Program. New York, McGraw-Hill, 1970

# 11

# Evaluation of Family Planning Programs

**Rochelle N. Shain**
**Mohammad M. Ahmad**

The previous chapter described services provided by family planning programs, from delivery of contraceptive methods and treatment of minor gynecologic disorders to education and follow-up. This chapter considers evaluation of overall program operations and of the quality of medical care. These topics, although interdependent, are discussed separately to facilitate exposition.

## PROGRAM EVALUATION

Evaluation of family planning programs answers two basic questions: *1)* How effective is a given project with respect to achieving its goals? and *2)* How efficiently are these tasks accomplished? The effectiveness of a program is evaluated in terms of the predetermined goals of the organization. Consequently, before evaluative measures can be developed and data collected, the program goals must be clearly defined, and priorities established.

The goals of family planning programs range from the very general, such as decreasing the economic dependency resulting from having too many children, to the very specific, such as reducing maternal mortality in a given hospital by a specific percentage. Typical goals include improving maternal and child health, reducing the discrepancy between the number of desired and actual births in a given area, providing services to a given percentage of a target group, increasing the contraceptive knowledge and practice of a specific population, decreasing the birth rate of the target group—and many others.

The successful delivery of contraceptive services is basic to all family planning programs and therefore will serve as a model to illustrate the development of evaluative procedures, the types of information which should be collected, and the ways in which these data are most appropriately analyzed. Many of the evaluative indices discussed, or the principles upon which they are based, can be modified to measure the attainment of other goals. During this discussion, reference will be made to the evaluation of certain more specific objectives as well.

Evaluative techniques are used to assess the effectiveness and efficiency of existing operations, and to test the utility of proposed innovations on a limited basis, before committing an entire program to them (1). The employment of such techniques fosters flexibility and a positive attitude toward innovation, and consequently encourages continuous improvement in services.

Evaluation is a valuable tool in the planning and administration of family planning projects, but it is not an end in itself. Unless the information it provides is used to improve services, it is an exercise in futility. In order to facilitate such feedback, the results of evaluative studies should be readily interpretable, and should be made available to program administrators in a systematic fashion (1).

## EVALUATING THE EFFECTIVENESS OF CONTRACEPTIVE PROGRAMS

### THE INCORPORATION OF EVALUATION INTO ROUTINE RECORD-KEEPING

The simplest and most efficient way of assessing the ongoing effectiveness of a family planning program is by integrating evaluation into the project's routine record-keeping procedures. Once this has been accomplished, reports can be generated automatically—monthly, quarterly, semiannually, and/or annually—as needed, to provide continuous, systematic feedback on the strengths and weaknesses of the program as a whole, or of any part of it. In this manner, minor problems are brought to light before they become major, and particular areas of strength are noticed, and, when feasible, emulated elsewhere in the program. Special periodic studies designed to answer particular needs serve as a supplement to this type of evaluation (8).

After the project's goals have been delineated, it is necessary to: *1)* determine criteria which can be used to judge whether or not a given goal has been attained; *2)* select appropriate measurements; *3)* determine the most effective way in which to analyze the measurements; and *4)* modify or develop the clinic record system to incorporate the items of information necessary for evaluation.

Three criteria are suggested as indicators of overall program effectiveness with respect to the successful delivery of contraceptive services. These include the demonstration of: concrete accomplishments in terms of services actually rendered, ability to satisfy clients, and ability to attract new clients from all strata of the target population.

### THE DEMONSTRATION OF CONCRETE ACCOMPLISHMENTS

The extent to which the first criterion has been successfully met is most simply estimated by what is commonly referred to as "measurements of effort" (9). "Effort," in this context, is the quantity of services provided, and the total number of unduplicated patients served during a specified time interval, such as 6 months or a year. Nonmedical services, such as outreach programs and community education, should also be measured. Measurements of

effort are the bases with which to compare the performance of a program at different periods of time, or of the program's various clinics, or of one project with others offering similar services. Thus, they serve as useful, although crude, indicators of program effectiveness and of general system failures. For example, a significant drop in the total patient load during a program's last 6 months of operation signals unspecified problems which should be further investigated. Measurements of effort are most meaningful when compared to the quantity of services the program or individual clinics expected to provide, and/or to the number of unduplicated patients they expected to serve (program goals). Moreover, if the particular family planning program serves a well-defined target population, such as all women in a given postpartum ward (19), measurement of effort is a meaningful and simply computed index of effectiveness, which involves dividing the number of acceptors by the number of women on the ward during a given period of time (9).

Measurements of effort alone are inadequate as evaluative indices. They do not provide sufficient information, and can be misleading. For example, a family planning program may, for several years, succeed in attracting large numbers of new clients, who subsequently drop out because of dissatisfaction with their care. Eventually, because of decreasing numbers of potential clients and unfavorable comments spread by word of mouth, the unduplicated patient count decreases. Measurements of effort would not detect shortcomings in the program until this point; in the interim, large numbers of patients would be lost. Consequently, what is also needed is a more refined index of program effectiveness measured in terms of patient satisfaction.

### THE DEMONSTRATED ABILITY TO SATISFY CLIENTS

Patient satisfaction is important for reasons other than its use as a criterion of program effectiveness: satisfied clients may prove to be the project's best, and least expensive, means of attracting new acceptors (8).

Patient satisfaction is measured by many methods. Two of the more important of these are the clinic continuation rate (CCR) and objective patient interviews. The CCR, or the extent to which clients seeking nonpermanent methods of contraception continue to return for services and supplies, indicates patient satisfaction, provided the given clientele is not unusually mobile, and the providers remain accessible (8). A rough approximation of this index can be derived by dividing the number of previously served clients who visited the clinic at least once during the year $x + 1$ by the total patient load in year $x$, exclusive of individuals who came for sterilization (9).

After careful exploration of average continuation rates in other clinics within the same community, administrative personnel should determine realistic goals for their own program. These goals may be modified (usually annually) as the program matures. The actual CCRs attained by the project as a whole and by its individual clinics should be calculated according to the various methods of contraception prescribed, and should be presented in tabular form. In this manner, comparisons between different clinics and between actual and expected rates can be readily made and problem areas easily discovered (8). As illustrated in Table 11-1, if Clinics 1 and 3 are expected to retain 75 per cent of their clients, and Clinic 2 is expected to retain 80 per cent, CCRs indicate that Clinic 3 is doing an inadequate job of retaining all types of clients, and Clinic 1 of retaining patients for whom oral contraceptives have been prescribed. The low CCR of Clinic 3 may suggest an overall lack of quality care and courteous service, and/or a disregard of particular cultural needs in that geographic location. The low CCR for oral-contraceptive patients in Clinic 1 merits further investigation, and a possible follow-up study of the clients in question. The CCR can also be computed for patients according to various demographic characteristics, such as age, level of education, etc. However, before doing so, program administrators should determine that such additional information can be utilized to improve existing services. The clinic continuation rate should be distinguished from the contraceptive continuation rate. The latter is discussed in Chapter 12.

Another indicator of patient satisfaction is the degree to which patients refer friends and family for services. This index is called the "patient-to-patient referral rate" and is calculated by dividing the number of clients referred by previously served patients during a given time interval (usually 1 year) by the total number of new patients during that same time period (9). This index should be computed for the program as a whole and for its individual clinics, and presented tabularly, so that trends can be observed over the course of time.

## THE DEMONSTRATED ABILITY TO ATTRACT NEW CLIENTS FROM ALL STRATA OF THE TARGET POPULATION

Ideally, a family planning program identifies its target population and then strives to recruit a realistic proportion of those individuals as clients. One criterion by which to judge a program's success is its ability to attract acceptors from all sectors of the target population in question. It is possible that a program and/or several of its clinics are drawing a majority of new clients from one element of the target group, such as the best-educated, or from a given age category, and are failing to attract other elements which are as numerous, and equally in need. In such a case, although quotas may be achieved, the unduplicated patient count as well as the quantity of services provided will be significantly lower than a program's potential. It is therefore important for administrative personnel to recognize the types of clients they are not reaching and then to institute appropriate changes in recruitment strategy, educational approaches, or overall patient care (8).

To measure differential acceptance, program directors should define their target population in terms of its most salient characteristics, such as age, ethnicity, level of education,

**Table 11-1. Clinic Continuation Rates by Method of Contraception**

|  | Total | Oral | IUD | Diaphragm | Foam/ Condoms | Rhythm |
|---|---|---|---|---|---|---|
| Clinic 1 | .65 | .39 | .87 | .92 | .63 | .78 |
| Clinic 2 | .82 | .80 | .95 | .60 | .78 | .81 |
| Clinic 3 | .32 | .32 | .26 | .35 | .25 | .12 |
| Total | .60 | .50 | .69 | .62 | .55 | .57 |

**Table 11–2. Frequency Distribution of New Clients by Clinic and Age of Woman**

|          | Total | Under 18 years | 18–25 years | 26–34 years | 35 & over |
|----------|-------|----------------|-------------|-------------|-----------|
| Clinic 1 | 1500  | 90             | 500         | 710         | 200       |
| Clinic 2 | 2000  | 60             | 700         | 940         | 300       |
| Clinic 3 | 2500  | 150            | 900         | 1000        | 450       |
| Total    | 6000  | 300            | 2100        | 2650        | 950       |

(Adapted from Pedersen H, Elkins H, Sinquefield JC: A Simplified Client Record System for Family Planning Programs. Chicago, Community and Family Center, University of Chicago, 1972, p 34)

**Table 11–3. Percentage Distribution of New Clients by Clinic and Age of Woman**

|          | Total | Under 18 years | 18–25 years | 26–34 years | 35 & over |
|----------|-------|----------------|-------------|-------------|-----------|
| Clinic 1 | 100   | 6.0            | 33.0        | 48.0        | 13.0      |
| Clinic 2 | 100   | 3.0            | 35.0        | 47.0        | 15.0      |
| Clinic 3 | 100   | 6.0            | 36.0        | 40.0        | 18.0      |
| Total    | 100   | 5.0            | 35.0        | 44.0        | 16.0      |

(Adapted from Pedersen H, Elkins H, Sinquefield JC: A Simplified Client Record System for Family Planning Programs. Chicago, Community and Family Center, University of Chicago, 1972, p 34)

and number of living children. This procedure is most readily accomplished for a population confined to a well-demarcated area. Administrative personnel can sample all new clients during a specified time period, usually a year, with respect to the distribution of selected characteristics. Differential acceptance rates, according to the characteristics in question, should be computed, and presented in the form of a frequency table and/or a percentage distribution table, as illustrated by Tables 11–2 and 11–3. In this manner, comparisons between clinics, and between actual and expected distributions, are readily made. For example, a contraceptive program serving all postpartum women in a given county hospital may find that 25 per cent of all patients who deliver here are 17 years of age or younger. Administrative personnel would consequently expect women of this age to constitute approximately 25 per cent of their program's annual enrollees. Table 11–3, however, reveals that only 5 per cent of the program's new clients are seventeen or younger. Further investigation is required to determine the reason. The problem could lie in discriminatory attitudes toward young, sexually active single women on the part of recruitment or clinic personnel, or in other areas.

Differential acceptance and continuation rates can also be used to measure program success in attracting a specific segment of the population. For example, a project's goal may be to devote at least half of its resources to women who are in high risk of experiencing complicated pregnancies, due to diabetes, high parity, advanced age, hypertension, etc. The program can determine the extent to which it has attained this goal by measuring the percentage of high-risk women that it has served during a given period of time. The goal of another program may be reduction of birth rates. Such a project would be especially interested in recruiting clients early in their childbearing careers, in order to have the greatest impact upon future reproductive behavior. Administrative personnel, in this instance, may use differential acceptance and continuation rates in order to measure the program's success in attracting women in the younger age groups, or those of low parity and in maintaining them as active clients (8).

**ITEMS TO BE INCLUDED IN THE CLINIC RECORDS**

In order to effectively integrate evaluation into routine record-keeping procedures, the following information should be collected: the client's name, identification number, full address, date of birth, years of education completed, socioeconomic status (this can be measured by wife's, husband's, or parent's occupation, as applicable), number of currently living children, number of children desired or expected, previous use of contraception, contraceptive method prescribed, date of prescription (when applicable), source of referral to project, date of enrollment into project, kept and missed appointments, type of visit (initial, annual, medical problem, resupply, etc.), services received during each visit (physical examination, patient education, pre- or post-counseling, outreach, laboratory procedures, etc.), and recontact information (the name, address, and telephone number of a person who should always know the client's whereabouts) (8). This last item is needed in the event that follow-up studies are undertaken. Such persons should not be contacted for research purposes without the client's prior permission. Some clients are particularly hesitant to disclose such information because they are seeking contraceptive services without the knowledge of family or friends. The collected data must also include any specific characteristics of the target population, such as whether or not they are considered to be in the high-risk category.

Other items of information should be collected as dictated by the needs of the particular family planning program. Only those items which will actually be used to help administrators make current decisions, judge current progress, or formulate future programs should be included in clinic records. Unless evaluation remains simple and inexpensive, in terms of actual financial outlays and in manpower demands on staff and patient time, it grows cumbersome, and loses its value. Moreover, if evaluation consumes a disproportionate amount of clinic resources, the provision of services is likely to suffer. Information requested of patients should take the form of a printed questionnaire, to minimize the interviewer's influence and thus ensure uniformity in data collection (1, 8, 9).

Processing of data can be performed manually. However, inexpensive packaged programs which can be adapted for use in small computers are now available. Computerized data processing is often more reliable and more efficient, and, particularly in the cases of large family planning programs, may prove to be less expensive than manual retrieval and analyses (1, 2, 8).

### SPECIAL EVALUATIVE STUDIES

Special follow-up studies can be conducted periodically to supplement the information obtained through the family planning program's system of continuous evaluation. Such studies serve many purposes, perhaps the most valuable of which is the isolation of factors responsible for program ineffectiveness, as indicated by the CCR, differential acceptance rates, measurements of effort, and/or other indices. For example, a given clinic may have an unusually low CCR, which demands im-

mediate investigation. The first step in such a follow-up study is designing a detailed interview schedule requesting information about patient attitudes toward all aspects of clinic operations, and reasons for nonattendance at the clinic. All patients, or a random sampling of them, who did not return for services during a given period of time, are contacted and interviewed in their homes. Interviewers should be well-trained, sensitive individuals, fluent in the clients' mother tongue. Moreover, they should convey the impression of objectivity, that is, of having no stake in the program's success. Under these conditions, clients are less likely to fear that their uncomplimentary remarks will be offensive, and are thus apt to express their feelings more candidly than they would otherwise do. If possible, interviewers should be hired for this purpose alone, and should not be affiliated with clinic operations (1).

It is rarely possible to locate all of the individuals who previously were clients; nor is it usually possible to elicit cooperation from all concerned. However, sufficient information can be collected from the individuals who participate in the study to help isolate the factors responsible for the clinic's low CCR.

Clients may drop out of a family planning program for many reasons. Administrative personnel are particularly interested in ascertaining whether these factors are avoidable or nonavoidable. Despite a given clinic's provision of quality care, it is powerless to maintain a high CCR if its clients are unusually mobile. Nor can clinic personnel be held responsible for a woman's desire to have a child, her cessation of sexual activity, or the onset of menopause or of a serious illness. On the other hand, program directors must be made aware of, and correct, the following conditions, should they prove to be sources of program ineffectiveness: curt and discourteous treatment by personnel, long waiting periods, inconvenient clinic hours, inadequate explanations concerning the use of a particular contraceptive method, and lack of privacy during counseling sessions (9). Other conditions, such as problems with babysitters or with transportation, and even disapproving husbands, may be eliminated, depending upon the objectives and resources of a given program.

The attainment of certain program goals cannot be adequately measured without recourse to sources of data outside the project itself, such as hospital records. Follow-up studies can be effectively used to tap this data base. For example, the goal of a particular project may be to improve the maternal and child health of the medically indigent (see Chap. 10). One way of ascertaining how well this goal has been met is to obtain infant and maternal morbidity and mortality statistics from the area's hospital(s) and observe changes in these statistics with time. Changes should begin to be noticeable approximately 1 year following the opening of clinic facilities. It must be understood, however, that significant drops in mortality and morbidity rates cannot be attributed to family planning alone. A host of factors, such as improved nutrition and expansion of obstetrical staff and facilities, whose influence cannot be measured, still cannot be ignored.

Special evaluative studies are also usefully employed as experimental tools. It is important that family planning programs maintain a flexible and open attitude toward new ideas, so as to continuously improve program organization and service delivery. However, as we have already mentioned, not all "promising" new ideas prove beneficial, and they should be tested, on a limited scale, before committing an entire project to their use (1, 8). For example, a director may want to develop a certain type of outreach program, believing it will increase acceptance rates, and, thus, the use of clinic facilities. Another may want to remind patients of their upcoming appointments by phone, mail, a home visit, and/or any combination of these, in an attempt to decrease the number of "no-shows." Yet a third may be considering supplying patients with oral contraceptives every 6, as opposed to every 3 months, in order to improve his program CCRs. In each of these situations, an experiment can be devised to evaluate the extent to which the proposed innovation actually improves program effectiveness. For example, the "show" rates of clients who are reminded of their upcoming appointments (by whichever method) should be compared with those of a control group (1, 8). If the program's show rate is increased by reminding patients of their appointments, administrative personnel must decide whether the improvement is significant enough to warrant the additional expenses involved in its implementation—that is, whether or not the proposed innovation is cost-effective.

## EVALUATING THE EFFICIENCY OF CONTRACEPTIVE PROGRAMS

If a project is to be successful, particularly in times of dwindling resources, it must not only attain its goals, but must accomplish them at the lowest possible cost. Although program effectiveness and efficiency are usually interdependent, it is possible for a given project to meet its goals at the price of considerable inefficiency. In this instance, costs would be needlessly high. On the other hand, family planning programs should not try to cut costs to the point where patient care suffers, or where clients have to wait an inordinately long time to be served. The cost to the patient, in this case, could ultimately prove excessively high, and clinic continuation rates would probably fall. A family planning project should strive to provide quality care at the lowest possible cost to itself, in terms of expenditures, and to its patients, in terms of waiting time. To satisfy both of these ends, costs must be carefully monitored (2). Clinic design, particularly the series of steps patients are required to follow during their visits (patient flow) should also be carefully planned to make optimal use of available resources. Evaluation of program efficiency is needed, with respect to both costs and general clinic operations.

### COST-EFFICIENCY ANALYSIS

Family planning projects should integrate measures of cost-efficiency, in addition to measures of program effectiveness, into their routine record-keeping procedures. Clinics should maintain an accurate daily account of all supplies dispensed and the number of hours worked by each type of personnel. An equally accurate record of daily accomplishments— that is, the number of visits to the facility, the number of unduplicated patients served, and the number and type of services rendered— should also be kept. At the end of each month, or at least of each quarter, the total costs of operating the program and its individual clinics should be estimated. All expenditures, such as salaries, supplies, overhead, transportation, communication, etc., should be included. These data should then be compared to the clinic's respective accomplishments, so that measures of cost-efficiency, expressed primarily in terms of cost per clinic visit and per unduplicated patient, may be determined. To calculate the cost per clinic visit, total costs are divided by total number of visits; likewise, to calculate the cost per unduplicated patient, total costs are divided by the number of unduplicated clients. The expenditures used in the numerator must have been incurred during the same period of time in which the services in the denominator were performed. Both of these measures may be used as bases by which to compare the efficiency of one's own program at various times, of the program's various clinics, and of one's own program with that of other projects (2, 11).

If these indices are significantly higher than the national or regional average for similar clinics, or than what experienced cost accountants believe they should be, it is likely that the program or clinic is operating inefficiently (2). Inefficiency can be caused by many factors, such as poor staffing patterns, an inaccessible location or one which is unsuitable for other reasons, overly expensive facilities, excessive loss of supplies through theft, the inability to attract and/or maintain an adequate patient load, and other factors. Some factors can only be investigated through follow-up studies. Others can be checked through scrutiny of clinic records. For example, if a disproportionate amount of total clinic expenditures is spent on physical accommodations and overhead, the clinic may be housed in too expensive a facility. If a significant proportion of supplies cannot be accounted for, either in inventory or as having been dispensed to patients, theft should be suspected. If records reveal that a disproportionate amount of total salaries is being spent on administrators, counselors, or on personnel from any given category, the family planning program is probably overstaffed with that type of employee. This possibility is easily checked by observing clinic operations; such an investigation will reveal which employees are working at full productivity, and which jobs can be consolidated (2).

## COMPARING THE COSTS OF DISSIMILAR PROGRAMS

When comparing different family planning programs, with respect to costs per unduplicated patient or per visit, caution must be exercised not to attribute differentials in such costs solely to differences in efficiency. Differentials in per-capita costs may be due, at least

partially, to other factors (15). For example, programs may differ with respect to the range of services provided, years of operation, patient volume, budget size, institutional setting, and cultural characteristics of clientele. These factors influence costs interdependently. Programs offering a comprehensive range of services, including community education, can be expected to have higher per-capita costs than projects offering only the basic minimum (11). More equitable comparisons between dissimilar programs can be made if each project determines its costs with respect to serving a given type of patient, such as women given oral contraceptives, or providing a given type of service, such as patient education.

It is particularly difficult to compare cost data from new programs with those of well-established projects. During the initial stages of development, family planning programs invest significant sums of money into furnishing and, when necessary, remodeling clinic facilities; training staff; and purchasing an adequate inventory of supplies. The program's fixed operating costs are very high compared to the actual number of patients served. Consequently, new projects usually have much higher per-capita costs than other programs. In time, as the new project attracts increasing numbers of clients, its costs should become more in line with the services it provides (2).

Costs of serving clients also tend to vary inversely with patient volume and budget size—at least up to a certain point (11, 15). Large programs can take advantage of economies of scale and thereby decrease their per-capita expenditures. Costs also tend to be considerably lower in urban than in rural areas, because rural clients are more widely dispersed. Rural clinics would therefore tend to have fewer clients than their urban counterparts, and spend a disproportionate share of their resources on transportation (15). Because overhead expenses are generally lower, hospital-based clinics are often less costly to operate than free-standing facilities (15). Certain client characteristics, such as particular cultural backgrounds, have also been known to influence program costs. For example, a family planning project may be forced to spend a disproportionate amount of its resources on patient education and counseling, in order to overcome its clients' failure to keep appointments. Consequently, whereas it is possible to use cost data to compare the efficiency of dissimilar programs, such data are more effectively and validly used to compare programs similar in setting and scope.

## THE USE OF COST-EFFICIENCY MEASURES AS EXPERIMENTAL TOOLS

Cost-efficiency measures are also very effectively employed as experimental tools by which to evaluate the efficiency of alternative operating procedures. For example, administrative personnel can compare the costs involved in sterilizing linens with those incurred by purchasing disposable supplies, to determine which procedure is more cost-effective. The costs of hiring additional clerks can also be compared to those of instituting computer-based data processing.

## EVALUATING THE EFFICIENCY OF OVERALL CLINIC OPERATIONS

Studies of staffing patterns and patient flow should be conducted periodically, to evaluate the efficiency of clinic operations. Various managerial techniques can be utilized in this regard, perhaps the most basic of which is flowcharting. The evaluator must first become thoroughly familiar with clinic operations, and then must diagram the actual steps patients are required to take during different types of visits, such as an annual examination, or a "resupply" visit. The average lengths of time required to proceed from one step to another—for example, from initial intake to education—should be documented through sampling techniques (9).

Different symbols, most commonly a rectangle, diamond, and ellipse, are used in a flowchart to denote the various steps. A rectangle symbolizes any defined operation, such as a physical examination. A diamond indicates that a decision must be made; such a decision is a switching operation, determining which, of a number of alternative paths, is to be followed. A letter *Y* and *N* following the diamond respectively signify the answers "yes" and "no" in response to the question posed. An ellipse is a terminal point, serving both as entry to, and exit from, the flow. Arrows indicate the direction of the flow, which normally proceeds, on the chart, downward, and to the right.

Figure 11–1 illustrates a simplified flowchart for patients served at a typical family planning clinic (see Chap. 10 for a detailed presentation of a specific procedure—sterilization). Patients are greeted at the front desk, where they sign in. New patients, and those making an annual visit, are directed to a special room where, as a group, they receive instruction in the biological basis of reproduction and are introduced to the various contraceptive methods. Such instruction is usually scheduled once or twice a day. Consequently, new and annual clients are often told to arrive at the same time. While they are being instructed, others are being screened by the clerk. She or he collects all the information necessary for administrative and evaluative purposes and initiates all the paperwork associated with laboratory procedures. New and annual clients proceed to the screening step following patient education. The paperwork involved in processing these clients is considerably more extensive than that required by patients who have come for other types of visits.

After being screened, those individuals who only require a resupply of contraceptive materials are directed to a nurse or an aide, who checks their blood pressure and perhaps their weight, and questions them with regard to any problems they may be experiencing. If there are no problems requiring the physician's attention, these patients receive their supplies and a new appointment, and then leave. Patients who do require a physical examination proceed to a different nurse or aide who determines their weight and blood pressure, performs the necessary laboratory procedures, and precounsels them with regard to their choice of contraceptive method. The nurse also takes a full medical history, in the case of new patients, and notes any changes or new information, in the case of previously served clients. The patient is then prepared for a physical examination, following which she is again counseled by the nurse or aide, who reviews the instructions associated with the prescribed contraceptive method. The client receives her supplies and a new appointment, and leaves.

Flowcharting is very useful, because it forces administrative personnel to become intimately aware of the actual workings of the system, particularly its bottlenecks and other shortcomings. For example, after constructing the flowchart depicted in Figure 11–1 and timing the intervals between steps, the evalua-

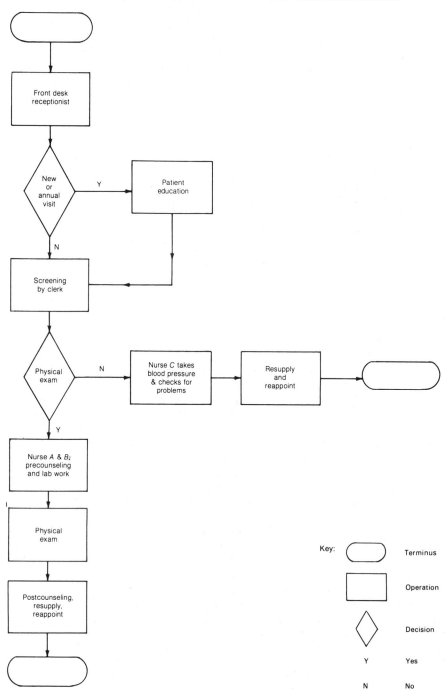

**FIG. 11–1.** Flowchart of a family planning clinic.

tor or program director may learn that patients must wait for a prolonged period of time to be screened. Although the clerk may be overburdened with waiting clients, Nurses *A* and *B* may be relatively idle because patients are not being processed rapidly enough. Moreover, Nurse *C* may be periodically idle because of the uneven and unpredictable flow of clients who seek her services. After further study, the program director may decide to hire an additional clerk. However, in order to improve the efficiency of clinic operations, she or he should first consider reorganizing staffing patterns for greater flexibility. Nurses *A, B,* and/or *C* could be directed to assist the clerk with patient screening to alleviate the bottleneck at this point in the flow. Consideration should also be given to redesigning the flow so that resupply patients bypass the screening clerk entirely and proceed directly to Nurse *C.* In order to accomplish this, the receptionist must separate patients requiring a physical examination from those who only require contraceptive supplies. This change should equalize the burden presently placed entirely on the clerk, and thereby increase operational efficiency. Further study could also be made of the patient-educator's role. Perhaps she or he could also help screen clients.

In addition to periodic assessment of program efficiency, flowcharting may be effectively used to follow up patients' complaints. Clients may, for example, complain of discourteous service on the part of certain clinic personnel, or of long waiting periods. After studying clinic operations through flowcharting, administrative personnel may discover that a given employee's irritability and curt treatment of clients is due to poor staffing patterns. This clerk may be overburdened by work. Administrators may also learn that unusually long waiting periods are due to understaffing, inefficient staffing patterns, poor scheduling of patients, and/or to other factors.

Flowcharting is also an indispensable aid during the planning stages of clinic design. Whether establishing a new clinic or instituting innovations within an already established facility, flowcharting is an effective way of pretesting alternative operational procedures before deciding to implement any of them.

## EVALUATION OF MEDICAL CARE

Providing medical care is the most important service of family planning programs, particu-larly for the indigent, who often do not have access to other medical facilities. Consequently, the quality of such care must be subjected to routine scrutiny, preferably as an integral part of health care delivery.

Evaluation of medical care in family planning programs is accomplished by the "medical audit." Medical audit, or quality care assessment, is usually defined as a measurement of health care quality through systematic investigation of patient data (3, 14).

## ROLE OF THE MEDICAL AUDIT IN FAMILY PLANNING

The purpose of the medical audit in family planning is to assure that patients using specific contraceptive methods are receiving the full benefit of medical care, with the fewest complications. The need and demand for quality care assessment and assurance is particularly important for family planning service grantors, providers, and consumers. This area is characterized by a lack of readily measurable criteria of success, differences in stated goals among various grantors, and marked differences in skills and knowledge among program administrators. Moreover, the patient selects his or her preferred method of contraception and decides whether to continue using it. Freedom of choice is essential in family planning to assure that contraceptive use remains free of external pressure and that full confidentiality is maintained. However, this very freedom makes quality care assessment particularly imperative.

Despite these factors, there has been little effort to design a uniform system of medical care evaluation for family planning programs. Consequently, existing systems of quality care assessment are fragmented, and are utilized in piecemeal fashion. Although many medical programs have made considerable progress in evaluating medical care, family planning has not kept pace with other health services in this respect.

## APPROACHES TO MEDICAL CARE EVALUATION

The evaluation of medical care involves measurement or comparison of an instance of care against a given standard (4). A standard is the minimally acceptable level of performance. Medical audits usually detect and emphasize underutilization of services or errors of omission, rather than overutilization or errors of commission (5).

The extent of overutilization can be determined by tallying the number of procedures or services performed on a sample of patients who do not normally require these procedures (5). Extent of underutilization is more difficult to assess. Methods of approaching this problem are still in incipient stages of development and can be broadly classified as: *1*) the process approach, and *2*) the outcome approach.

## THE PROCESS APPROACH

This approach focuses upon the providers' performance. It involves an assessment of how resources are used, including actual patient management, as evidenced in patient records, record abstracts, encounter forms, and direct observation (4, 12, 13). Proponents of this approach believe that if the proper services are performed, the outcome will automatically be satisfactory. This type of review is most appropriately utilized when explicit standards of care are defined prior to the audit by a medical staff group or a body of external experts, followed by random sampling, and checking of records to determine whether or not the program is meeting these criteria (12).

An example of this approach in a hospital setting is offered by Huntley and his coworkers. Charts of all patients seen in a hospital clinic were reviewed weekly to determine if clinic criteria for history, physical and laboratory tests, and plans for continuous patient care had been met. The results indicated that 13 per cent of the charts contained abnormal findings which were not being pursued (7).

The process approach is commonly used in family planning to determine if clients are being prescribed contraceptive methods for which there are major contraindications. When rapid feedback is possible, as with computerized medical record systems, process criteria can also be used as guidelines for actual delivery of care. For example, the computer can be programmed to detect and "flag" records belonging to patients with thrombophlebitis for whom an oral contraceptive has been prescribed.

## OUTCOME APPROACH

Outcome studies are concerned with the impact of care, that is, with what actually happens to the patient. Outcome as regarded by a growing number of scientists as the most accurate or important index of the quality of health care (18). Its use in family planning, however, has not yet been established. Whereas inpatient review lends itself to outcome evaluation, most ambulatory or outpatient evaluation projects, particularly those in family planning, are difficult to assess in this manner. In inpatient care, the desired outcome is successful amelioration, or cure, of a given disease state. In family planning most patients are not ill; for those who are, there is no easily definable episode of illness. Therefore, it is difficult to assign a beginning and end-point for the outpatient problem. Secondly, family planning patients are less likely to receive a specific diagnosis. Most audit and data systems rely heavily on the diagnostic codes used in clinic settings. Family planning patients present with problems, but do not go through a discharge diagnosis. Therefore a diagnostic coding system usable in the family planning outpatient setting is lacking. Third, family planning outpatient medical records are not uniform and are seldom complete. Consistent, comprehensive records ideally follow the patient from history-taking and physical examination through laboratory tests, to definitive diagnosis, appropriate management, and subsequent course. Family planning records rarely reach this ideal, and the inconsistency and frequent inadequacy of individual record-keeping systems make outcome review difficult. Fourth, the physician has less control over the family planning patients' adherence to instructions or prescribed measures, as discussed earlier. Lastly, in family planning clinics, patients are often seen by a number of different physicians. The information recorded by these practitioners is often not comparable, in definition or in terminology. Because of these factors, and because the desired outcome of family planning—avoidance of pregnancy, either permanently, or for a given period of time—is difficult to measure, the outcome approach to medical evaluation in family planning is rarely used.

When it is employed, its most common use involves measurement of side effects or complications of a given contraceptive method, within a specified time frame. Charts are randomly sampled to determine incidence of problems within a given population, such as women who use the pill.

## IMPORTANCE OF MEDICAL RECORDS

In order to complete a medical audit, adequate medical records for every patient must be maintained. They must be completely and accurately documented, readily accessible, and systematically organized, to facilitate the retrieval and compilation of information. Each entry must be signed. A record must be maintained of every patient encounter with the staff, the reason for the encounter, and any action taken. The medical record must contain sufficient information to identify the patient, justify diagnosis or clinical impression, and warrant treatment or end results (6).

In addition to the items listed in the discussion of clinic records in the first part of this chapter, all medical records must contain detailed clinical data, including medical history data, management instructions, and a listing of all procedures which were performed and their results. Chapter 10 delineates the minimal procedures which must be performed.

Every physician must sign his or her entries into the medical record for the purpose of documentation. A physician should also initial the entries of a nurse midwife, nurse practitioner, or other appropriately trained person for whom the physician is responsible. Records should be retained and preserved, either in the original or on microfilm, for a period of time not less than that determined by the state's statute regarding medical record retention. In the absence of specific state requirements, federal guidelines suggest 3 years (10).

## AN EXAMPLE OF MEDICAL CARE EVALUATION: THE ORAL-CONTRACEPTIVE PATIENT

Patients using hormonal contraceptives have been selected as an example because they constitute the largest portion of contraceptive users in the United States who are not already sterilized (16, 17). Moreover, there are particularly controversial arguments regarding side effects, contraindications, and complications. The following discussion addresses only the specific medical requirements which must be documented for oral-contraceptive users. This example could, however, be readily modified to fit the needs of patients using other methods, such as the intrauterine device (IUD).

Medical records are randomly selected from among pill users during a given time frame, usually the preceding 12-month period. Documentation must be found for the following items: *1*) the performance of all required procedures (for example, physical examination and various types of laboratory tests) described in the previous chapter; *2*) the absence of *absolute* contraindications to the oral contraceptive. For example, the absence of thrombophlebitis, estrogen-dependent neoplasia, severe liver disease, and undiagnosed uterine bleeding, should be appropriately checked; *3*) the presence or absence of *relative* contraindications, such as diabetes, heart disease, renal disease, and hypertension. Evidence must also be provided that all such contraindications were being adequately managed. For example, hypertensive patients must be frequently monitored, so that their blood pressure levels do not exceed a critical level. Patients with cardiac or renal disease should also be closely supervised. Moreover, in federally funded clinics, diabetic patients must be referred to appropriate medical clinics for monitoring; *4*) the absence and presence of side effects or complications with appropriate management. In the case of *no* side effects, a written statement to this effect should be included; *5*) adequate recording of history, including age and social habits such as smoking and alcohol or drug abuse; *6*) verbal and written consent, preceded by appropriate education and instruction, especially regarding potential side effects, types of complications, and their severity; *7*) an appointment for a return visit, and information necessary for follow-up, *8*) if the audit occurs at a time when the client is scheduled for a return visit, evidence that the patient either returned for a visit or was followed up. Waiting period from time of nonappearance to follow-up varies according to program.

As a result of this audit, the medical director can assess quality and consistency of the care received by oral contraceptive patients, and initiate changes where they are needed.

## REFERENCES

1. Bogue DJ (ed): Family Planning Improvement through Evaluation. A Manual of Basic Principles. Chicago, Community and Family Study Center, University of Chicago, 1970
2. Bogue DJ: Cost Effectiveness Analyses of Family Planning Programs. Chicago, Community and

Family Study Center, University of Chicago, 1973

3. Christoffel T: Medical care evaluation: an old new idea. J Med Educ 51:83, 1976

4. Christoffel T, Loewental M: Evaluating the quality of ambulatory health care: a review of emerging methods. Med Care 15:877, 1977

5. Eisenberg JM, Williams SV, Garner L et al: Computer-based audit to detect and correct overutilization of laboratory tests. Med Care 15:915, 1977

6. Hopkins CE, Hetherington RW, Parsons EM: Quality of medical care: a factor analysis approach using medical records. Health Serv Res 10:199, 1975

7. Huntley RR, Steinhauser R, White KE et al: The quality of medical care: techniques and investigation in the outpatient clinic. J Chron Dis 14:530, 1961

8. Pedersen H, Elkins H, Sinquefield JC: A Simplified Client Record System for Family Planning Programs. Chicago, Community and Family Study Center, University of Chicago, 1972

9. Polgar S, Jaffe F: Evaluation and recordkeeping for US family planning services. Public Health Rep 83:639, 1968

10. Program Guidelines for Project Grants for Family Planning Services, Section 1001, Public Health Service Act (42USC300), DHEW, January, 1976

11. Reardon MJ, Deeds SG, Dresner NA, Diksa JH, Robinson WC: Real costs of delivering family planning services. Implications for management. Am J Public Health 64:860, 1974

12. Reichman S: Quality assessment and ambulatory care. Bull NY Acad Med 52:75, 1976

13. Rosenberg C, Donabedian A, Greenberg SM, Guck JK, Sillman FH, Knutson R, Reichman S, Morehead MA: The professional responsibility for the quality of health care. A discussion of methods. Panel discussion. Bull NY Acad Med 52:86, 1976

14. Sanazaro PJ: Medical audit, continuing medical education and quality assurance. West J Med 125:241, 1976

15. Sparer G, Okada L, Tillinhast S: How much do family planning programs cost? Fam Plann Perspect 5:100, 1973

16. Westoff CF: Trends in contraceptive practice: 1965–1973. Fam Plann Perspect 8:54, 1976

17. Westoff CF, Jones EF: Contraception and sterilization in the United States, 1965–1975. Fam Plann Perspect 9:153, 1977

18. Williamson JW: Evaluating the quality of patient care: a strategy relating outcome and process assessment. JAMA 218:564, 1971

19. Zatuchni GI: Overview of program: two-year experience. In Zatuchni GI (ed): Postpartum Family Planning: A Report on the International Program. New York, McGraw-Hill, 1970, p 30

# 12

# Costs and Benefits of Family Planning Programs

## Harold D. Dickson

Most organized family planning programs are designed to provide services to persons who are either unable to pay for them or who, regardless of ability to pay, would face high risk of social or medical problems in the event of pregnancy, due to such conditions as hypertension, diabetes, or age (under 18 or over 35). In either case, such programs usually rely on funding from government at various geopolitical levels. Simultaneously, other programs intended to produce better systems of education, justice, overall health care, and transportation are seeking limited tax funds. Consequently, family planning programs must consider how they can effectively convince those who allocate government funds that a share should be allotted to them. Arguments in favor of family planning programs may stress either the long-term (30–100 years) or short-term (1–5 years) benefit to society. The *potential* long-term benefits of an active and successful family planning program may include reduced demand for schools, transportation, legal, and health systems, thus cutting costs to the government and releasing resources for capital investment, which (if income were distributed properly) could improve the standard of living for all. I emphasize the word *potential,* because the nature of the long-term impact is controversial. The economy is flexible and can respond to increased population readily; population pressures create increased demand for consumer goods and, perhaps, an environment which stimulates the creation of new products.

Therefore, as noted by Simon (18), there may not be substantial long-term benefits. The methods for assessing long-term benefits will be discussed in a later section.

Long-term benefit is not a powerful argument for funding specific family planning services, since governmental decision-makers would prefer to see *short-term* (1–5 years) benefits and savings. The major emphasis in this chapter will therefore be upon short-term benefits.

## SHORT-TERM COST-BENEFIT ANALYSIS

In presenting the short-term benefits of family planning to a government, one of two major strategies may be stressed. The first involves the concept of *reducing unwanted births;* the second emphasizes the *lowering of desired family size.* For reasons which will be made clear in the course of the discussion, the strategy of unwanted births is probably the more effective one; it provides the focus for this chapter.

The lowering of desired family size, by altering families' perceptions of, or the actual, *personal* benefits and costs of having an additional child, is an unstated objective of many family planning programs, especially in less-developed countries. For example, a government might attempt to increase families' perceptions of (or perhaps actual) costs of an additional child by reducing allocations to subsidized child care, schooling, and housing, and by providing widespread information

**153**

**Table 12-1. Percentage Distribution of Exposed[a] Women, According to Current Use of Specific Contraceptive Method Among Women Who Do Not Desire Future Birth (World Fertility Survey)**

| | No method used | Any method | Ineffective only | Effective | Sterilization Female | Sterilization Male | Pill | IUD | Injection | Condom | Female local | Douche | Withdrawal | Rhythm | Abstinence | Other |
|---|---|---|---|---|---|---|---|---|---|---|---|---|---|---|---|---|
| **Asia & Pacific** | | | | | | | | | | | | | | | | |
| Bangladesh | 86 | 14 | 5 | 9 | 1 | 1 | 5 | 1 | NA | 1 | 0 | 0 | 1 | 2 | 2 | 0 |
| Fiji[b] | 26 | 74 | 7 | 67 | — 43 — | | 9 | 7 | NA | 7 | NA | NA | 3 | 3 | NA | 2 |
| Indonesia | 47 | 53 | 7 | 46 | 1 | 0 | 27 | 14 | [c] | 4 | 1[c] | 0 | — 4 — | | | 3 |
| Korea, Rep. of | 44 | 56 | 12 | 44 | 3 | 6 | 13 | 13 | 0 | 8 | 0 | 0 | 4 | 7 | 1 | 0 |
| Malaysia | 48 | 53 | 15 | 38 | — 11 — | | 20[d] | 1 | [d] | 5 | — 0 — | | 4 | 5 | 4 | 3 |
| Nepal | 91 | 9 | 0 | 9 | 0 | 7 | 1 | 0 | 0 | 0 | 0 | 0 | 0 | 0 | 0 | 0 |
| Pakistan | 85 | 15 | 4 | 11 | 3 | 0 | 3 | 2 | NA | 2 | 1 | NA | 0 | 0 | 3 | 0 |
| Sri Lanka | 47 | 54 | 20 | 34 | 20 | 1 | 2 | 8 | 1 | 3 | 0 | 0 | 2 | 12 | 6 | 0 |
| Thailand | 44 | 56 | 4 | 52 | 14 | 5 | 20 | 10 | 3 | 1 | 0 | 0 | — 4 — | | | 1 |
| **Latin America** | | | | | | | | | | | | | | | | |
| Colombia | 44 | 56 | 16 | 40 | 8 | 0 | 16 | 11 | 1 | 2 | 3 | 1 | 7 | 6 | 1 | 1 |
| Costa Rica | 16 | 84 | 13 | 71 | 29 | 2 | 20 | 5 | 4 | 10 | 2 | 0 | 5 | 6 | 1 | 1 |
| Dominican Republic | 43 | 57 | 14 | 43 | 30 | 0 | 9[e] | 4 | [e] | 2 | — 3 — | | 6 | 2 | NA | 0 |
| Mexico | 52 | 48 | 11 | 37 | 7 | 1 | 15 | 9 | 2 | 1 | 2 | 0 | 6 | 5 | NA | 0 |
| Panama | 26 | 74 | 10 | 64 | 41 | 1 | 16 | 4 | 1 | 1 | 2 | 1 | 4 | 3 | 2 | 0 |
| Peru[f] | 54 | 46 | 29 | 17 | 6 | 0 | 5 | 2 | 1 | 2 | 1 | 5 | 5 | 15 | 4 | 1 |

NA = not available

[a] All currently married, nonpregnant, and fecund women, including those sterilized for contraceptive purposes

[b] Fiji—Definition of exposed excludes those in postpartum abstinence

[c] Indonesia—Injection included with female local methods

[d] Malaysia—Injection included with pill

[e] Dominican Republic—Injection included with pill

[f] Weighted sample

(Kendall M: The World Fertility Survey: current status and findings. Popul Rep [M], No.3:73, 1979)

about the costs of childbearing. Policies to reduce family benefits of childbearing could involve greater encouragement of female employment, so that a woman's satisfaction might come more from work than from children; increased social security for the elderly, so that large numbers of children are not needed to provide income for the nonworking elderly; and improved maternal and infant care, so that the probability of children living past the age of ten is improved, and therefore a continuing source of child-parent relationships can be obtained with fewer children. Haveman (8) presents an excellent discussion of why such policies encouraging broad-based social change may be more effective than family planning service delivery programs in changing desired family size. Nonetheless, because a span of 5 to 10 years would be necessary to effect such changes, this approach is not as direct as the "unwanted birth" strategy.

Furthermore, data from the National Fertility Survey (7) and the World Fertility Surveys (12) provide a great deal of support for the "unwanted births" strategy, and suggest that, in fact, desired family size is already low in many countries. Based on the findings of the 1955 and 1960 Growth of American Families Studies, and the 1965 National Fertility Survey, Cutright and Jaffe (3:121) report that "low-income and marginal-income wives *desired* about the same number of children as higher-income wives and . . . most had used or expected to use some form of fertility control, . . . but had more unwanted or untimed births than higher-income wives . . . due to use of less effective birth control methods." If this is the case, short-term (3–5 years) governmental cost savings can be made solely through family planning educational and clinic efforts, and it is unnecessary to change perceptions of desired family size. The 1979 report by Sir Maurice Kendall, Project Director for the World Fertility Survey (12), provides evidence that even in less developed countries, approximately 20 to 30 per cent of the women surveyed want no more children, but are not using *effective* family planning methods to prevent pregnancy. In Peru, 61 per cent of the currently married, fecund women in the survey wanted no more children, and 46.1 per cent had not wanted their last child or current pregnancy. Two important tables from the World Fertility Survey are repeated here as Tables 12–1 and 12–2. The first illustrates the

**Table 12–2. Percentage of Exposed\* Women Who Want No More Children and Are Not Currently Using Contraception, in 15 Developing Countries**

| Country | Sample Size | *Of all currently married women, % who are exposed and want no more and are not using:* | |
|---|---|---|---|
| | | *Any method* | *Modern method* |
| **Asia & Pacific** | | | |
| Bangladesh† | (N = 5767) | 45 | 47 |
| Fiji‡ | (N = 4650) | 10 | 12 |
| Indonesia | (N = 7868) | 13 | 15 |
| Korea, Rep. of | (N = 5051) | 25 | 32 |
| Malaysia | (N = 5802) | 17 | 22 |
| Nepal | (N = 5501) | 21 | 21 |
| Pakistan | (N = 4663) | 26 | 27 |
| Sri Lanka | (N = 6163) | 22 | 31 |
| Thailand | (N = 3482) | 20 | 22 |
| **Latin America** | | | |
| Colombia | (N = 2827) | 22 | 30 |
| Costa Rica | (N = 2684) | 7 | 12 |
| Dominican Republic | (N = 1808) | 17 | 23 |
| Mexico | (N = 5640) | 21 | 26 |
| Panama | (N = 2723) | 14 | 19 |
| Peru | (N = 5061) | 25 | 38 |

\* All currently married, nonpregnant, and fecund women, including those sterilized for contraceptive purposes
†Bangladesh only—Some women were asked: "Do you want another child soon?"
‡Fiji only—excludes women in postpartum abstinence

(Kendall M: The World Fertility Survey: current status and findings. Popul Rep [M], No. 3:73, 1979)

contraceptive methods used, and the second the percentage *of all currently married women* who are exposed, *and* want no more children, *and* are not using either a modern method or any method. The percentage of such women ranges from 12 per cent, in Costa Rica, to 47 per cent, in Bangladesh. In these countries, the figures are conservative estimates of need because they do not include the unmarried group, who, although somewhat less exposed, may still have contraceptive needs. Therefore, short-term costs and benefits can become important and politically acceptable, particularly considering the government officials' need for short-term payoff. Any social program that can demonstrate true, direct dollar savings to the government, equivalent at least to the program's cost, probably will receive priority for the allocation of limited tax funds.

To make a case for this approach, it is necessary to specify a goal for a target group of persons for whom the government is spending substantial funds for childbirth and child care and compute the 1 to 5 (preferably 1) year potential savings of direct government expenditures, due to a reduction of unwanted births through more effective contraception.

## ASSESSING SHORT-TERM BENEFITS THROUGH THE "UNWANTED BIRTHS" STRATEGY

The suggested procedure for assessing short-term benefits is summarized as follows:

1. Determine the size of the *target population in need* of family planning services.
2. Determine government *expenditures* per child for unwanted children born to the focus group.
3. Estimate the *additional couple years of protection* provided by the family planning program to this group, by examining contraceptive continuation rates.
4. Estimate the number of *unwanted births averted.*
5. Compute the government *cost savings* for the averted births.
6. Compute the direct *government expenditures* for the family planning program that were required to avert the births mentioned.
7. Compare the savings to the expenditure incurred to derive the estimated *net benefit* to the treasury.

Each of these steps will be discussed in greater detail along with the desired method of data collection. A rule-of-thumb method of estimation is provided for those decision-makers who require only a general notion of the short-term benefits of a given program.

### DETERMINING THE SIZE OF THE FOCUS GROUP IN NEED

It is first necessary to define the focus group in need. The women in the target group will have the following characteristics:

1. Of child-bearing age (typically 15–44)
2. Fecund, and not currently pregnant
3. Sexually active
4. *Not wanting* to become pregnant during the next year, for either social, economic or medical reasons

5. Presently using a relatively ineffective contraceptive method, and likely to continue employing it, or not likely to use an effective method without assistance in the form of education and low-cost services, and *not* likely to have an abortion in the event of an unwanted pregnancy

If a program is already in operation, the planner should determine the number of women being served who fit these criteria upon their initial contact with the program. A questionnaire should be administered, either at the initial contact with a clinic or at the time of the most recent pregnancy termination (delivery or abortion).

When results are required for a program which has not yet begun, and the planner is trying to gather evidence of need, a community (door-to-door) sample survey should be conducted. If this is not possible, women in medical care clinics should be interviewed. If no survey is possible, the method used by Dryfoos (4) is suggested as a way to derive a quick estimate of the size of the target population.

Dryfoos (4) has demonstrated that in the United States, the size of the group in need can easily be estimated by first determining, from census data, the number of females in the age groups 15–19, 20–29, and 30–44, who are in the low-income category (a minor from a high-income family is considered to be in this group), and therefore are unlikely to be able to afford effective contraception. The marital status of the females in such age groups is determined, and the *percentage* of persons in each of the age/marital status groups who, due to fecundity, sexual activity, desired family size, and current and estimated future pregnancy status are in need of subsidized family planning services is determined from Table 12–3. Then need is computed by multiplying the number of females in the group by the percentage of women in need, shown as the bottom row of Table 12–3. This table, from the 1975 Dryfoos article (5), demonstrates the factors used to derive these percentages.

To illustrate the usefulness of the table, the first column will be explained. It contains the factors for low-income females, 15 to 19 years old, who are married, with husband present. To estimate the number in need of a program, using the 1975 results, the family planning program planner could multiply the size of

**Table 12–3. Estimated Percentage of Low-Income Women in Need of Family Planning Services, 1970 and 1975, by Age and Marital Status, Showing Component Factors Used by Dryfoos**

| Need and component factor, 1970 and 1975 | Percent, by age and marital status | | | | | | | | |
|---|---|---|---|---|---|---|---|---|---|
| | *15–19* | | | *20–29* | | | *30–44* | | |
| | MHP | PM | NM | MHP | PM | NM | MHP | PM | NM |
| Fecund | | | | | | | | | |
| 1970 | 100 | 100 | 100 | 91 | 89 | 97 | 67 | 71 | 86 |
| 1975 | 100 | 100 | 100 | 90 | 88 | 97 | 66 | 70 | 86 |
| Sexually active | | | | | | | | | |
| 1970 | 100 | 31 | 31 | 100 | 65 | 65 | 100 | 65 | 65 |
| 1975 | 100 | 40 | 40 | 100 | 75 | 75 | 100 | 75 | 75 |
| Not pregnant or trying | | | | | | | | | |
| 1970 | 46 | 100 | 100 | 82 | 100 | 100 | 97 | 100 | 100 |
| 1975 | 44 | 100 | 100 | 82 | 100 | 100 | 97 | 100 | 100 |
| Need: point-in-time | | | | | | | | | |
| 1970 | 46 | 31 | 31 | 75 | 58 | 63 | 65 | 46 | 56 |
| 1975 | 44 | 40 | 40 | 74 | 66 | 73 | 64 | 53 | 65 |
| Ratio not pregnant or trying: 12 months/point-in-time | | | | | | | | | |
| 1970 | 1.67 | | | 1.18 | | | 1.02 | | |
| 1975 | 1.71 | | | 1.18 | | | 1.02 | | |
| Need: 12-month period | | | | | | | | | |
| 1970 | 77 | 31 | 31 | 88 | 58 | 63 | 66 | 46 | 56 |
| 1975 | 75 | 40 | 40 | 87 | 66 | 73 | 65 | 53 | 65 |

Key:
MHP = married, husband, parent
PM = previously married
NM = never married

(Dryfoos J, Fam Plann Perspectives 7:175, July/Aug 1975)

this target group by 0.75, as shown in the bottom row.

The 0.75 is derived as follows:

1. According to the second row of the table, 100 per cent of the 15–19 year-old females who are married with husband present are estimated to be fecund.

2. Of the fecund group, 100 per cent are sexually active, as shown in the 4th row of the table.

3. Of the sexually active, 44 per cent are not pregnant or trying to become pregnant, according to the data in row 6 of the table.

4. At a given point in time, the need is then 44 per cent of the 15–19 year-old married females with husband present. This figure is obtained by multiplying the figures in items 1–3 above: (100% fecund × 100% sexually active × 44% not pregnant or trying and dividing by 10,000.

5. Then, to account for changing pregnancy status over the period of a year (some who were formerly pregnant deliver, pass the stage of postpartum amenorrhea, and be-

come at risk for pregnancy), the point-in-time need is multiplied by a factor of 1.71 (row 10) to obtain the final results (44% × 1.71) = 75% of the 15–19 year-old, low-income females who are married, with husband present.

Of the 20–29 year-old, low-income married females with husband present, 87 per cent are in need of family planning services. This figure was derived by multiplying the factors in the 4th column as follows: (91% fecund × 100% sexually active × 82% not pregnant or trying × 1.18 ratio of point-in-time need to annual need divided by 10,000) = 87 per cent in need.

Calculation factors are provided for two different years (1970 and 1975) to illustrate the extent of change that can occur within a 5-year period. Some changes are substantial and thus indicate the need to conduct sample surveys on a routine basis at least every other year. However, the Dryfoos factors were presented here only as a temporary measure to use until a data base from a given program and service area can be accumulated. The Dryfoos method does not provide the exact number of women in "need," as defined in the "focus group," and it does not provide an estimate of the number likely to use an effective method and likely to have an abortion in case of an unwanted pregnancy. However, an assumption about the proportion of women in the target group in need (as Dryfoos defined it) who are likely to use an ineffective method and/or to have an abortion in case of an unwanted pregnancy could be made from a small sample of persons, and the result should be close enough to appropriately adjust the size of the focus group for planning purposes. If a program has not yet started, the number of acceptors of various contraceptive methods should be estimated from the total group in need, to determine the number who would participate in the family planning program.

### DETERMINING GOVERNMENT EXPENDITURES FOR UNWANTED CHILDREN BORN TO THE FOCUS GROUP

The questionnaire used to determine the size of the focus group in a specific program should include questions on the estimated *use* of various services for the last child (future child, if they have no children, are pregnant, or plan to have children), such as prenatal care, hospital or other delivery, postpartum and pediatric care for the first year of life, public financial assistance, public housing, and (if they are working), day care services. Once the group's use rate is known, it can be multiplied by the *average dollar* cost of providing the care, to obtain the total costs.

In order to identify the services covered by government, the mother should be asked about the financial arrangements covering each instance of care. In an excellent article on short-term costs and benefits of family planning programs in the United States, Jaffe (10) computed 1970 governmental costs *per birth* averted as shown in Table 12–4.

These are low estimates, because they exclude subsidized day-care and taxes lost from lost income for those low-income mothers who work. In addition, costs would be incurred for future day-care and schooling. A short-term cost-benefit determination *should* include some estimate of subsidized day-care that could be reduced by a substantial reduction in births.

The government expenditures saved for each birth averted become the "benefits" side of a short-term cost-benefit analysis. Next it is necessary to determine the extent of protec-

**Table 12–4. Government Costs per Birth Averted (1970)**

| Item of Care | U.S. government expenses per unwanted birth |
|---|---|
| a. Cost of maternity and pediatric care for the infant year 1970–71 was $971 | |
|   (1) Hospital component of $701 × government share of 0.25 | $437.00 |
|   (2) Ambulatory care of $270 × government share of 0.25 | 67.00 |
| b. Public assistance cost of $798.77 per recipient for financial assistance, social services, administration, and food stamps × 16% (percentage of low-income individuals receiving public assistance) | 128.00 |
| Total *minimum* government costs per birth averted = | $632.00 |

tion (and therefore births averted) provided by the family planning program.

### ESTIMATING COUPLE YEARS OF PROTECTION

A "couple year of protection" results from a contraceptive acceptor continuing to use a method effectively for 1 year. This concept involves determining the number of acceptors of a particular method and the corresponding contraceptive continuation rate. "The proportion of women practicing contraception at a given time interval after acceptance" is defined as the continuation rate (14). Continuation rates traditionally refer to time spans of up to 3 years, varying according to the method being used at the time of acceptance. Consequently, it is necessary to relate family planning program activity in a given year to the births averted in the following years due to the couple years of protection provided to the focus group. One way to accomplish this, for all but sterilization cases, is to classify the focus population served during a year by method, and then divide the groups into initial, and previous, acceptors who are still continuing with the given method. The average number of months of contraceptive protection provided during the year under question to each group is then determined, and no attempt to determine the length of time contraception continued past that year would be needed.

The following case will serve as an example: a *sample* of 400 persons (the total focus-group population = 4000) is followed to determine the average months of effective contraceptive use during the year in question. Assume that the sample is distributed as shown in Table 12–5. In this case, the couple months of protection for the initial acceptor *pill* users would be computed as 4000 total in the focus group × 0.375 proportion of initial acceptors using the pill × 6 months' average use = 9000 months. Dividing by 12 provides 750 couple years of protection. Similar calculations are made for each group, and the total couple years of protection for each group is added, to determine the overall total.

Another method for determining the couple years of protection for all methods except sterilization is shown by Laing's (13) description of the effect of family planning programs in the Philippines. He considered the couple years of protection obtained by *initial acceptors* throughout the 3-year period following the year during which they were seen in the family program. The total couple years of protection derived during that year and the two following years were *attributed* to the activity in the initial year. The use of this technique would work well if the ratio of initial acceptors to continuing patients remained relatively constant each year. Laing (13) illustrated the continuation rate for selected months after acceptance, as shown in Figure 12–1 for each method. The curves distinguish between the "first method" and "all-method" results. The "first method" rate measures the extent of continuation of the first method chosen at the time of initial acceptance. The "all-method" rate refers to the continuation of *any* method, regardless of the initial choice of methods.

The percentage of acceptors still using a contraceptive method during ensuing months after initial acceptance will eventually decline, as shown in Fig. 12–1. As noted by Laing

(13), this exponential decay curve can be represented by a formula

$$C_t = ae^{bt}$$

where: $C_t$ = the cumulative continuation rate for ordinal month $t$ following acceptance.

$a$ and $b$ are obtained by the regression equation (see Chap. 27 for discussion of regression and curvilinear regression analysis), when the natural logarithm of $C_t$ ($LnC_t$) is the dependent variable and $t$ is the independent variable, to obtain the formula:

$$Ln\ C_t = (Ln\ a) + b(t)$$

Where the regression coefficients are ($Lna$) and ($b$), the coefficient $b$ will be a negative value. Most of the rest of the discussion refers to the absolute value of $b$, notated as $|b|$. The antilog of the first regression coefficient ($Lna$) will be taken to determine $a$. Then ($a/|b|$) will give the mean period of contraceptive continuation. The months of effective contraception (MEP) provided by a program is calculated as:

$$MEP = CE(a/|b|)e^{-|b|(OPA)}$$

where     ($a|b|$)   is computed as described in the previous paragraph

    OPA = months of overlap of contraceptive practice with postpartum amenorrhea, during which the method is not needed and therefore provides no protection from pregnancy

    CE = index of contraceptive effectiveness

$$CE = 1 - \left[ \frac{PL(PR_n)\ (12/EFGR - GPA)}{(a/|b|)\ (e^{-|b|(OPA)}e^{-|b|(n-0.5)})} \right]$$

**Table 12–5. Data Used to Compute Average Months of Protection**

|  | No. in sample | % of total | Mean months of use of couples in the sample |
|---|---|---|---|
| **Initial acceptors** | | | |
| Pill | 150 | 37.50 | 6 months |
| IUD | 25 | 6.25 | 8 months |
| Foam & condom | 25 | 6.25 | 5 months |
| **Previous acceptors** | | | |
| Pill | 175 | 43.75 | 4 months |
| IUD | 15 | 3.75 | 9 months |
| Foam & condom | 10 | 2.50 | 3 months |

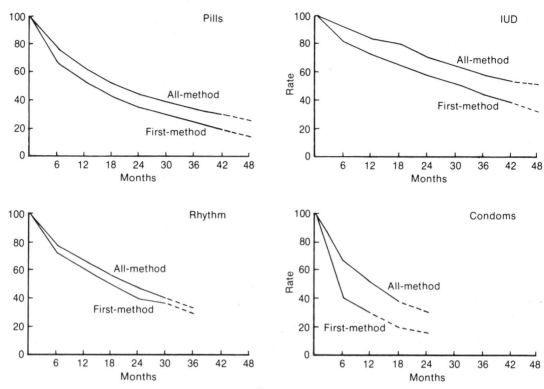

NOTE: Dotted lines denote that the number of cases entering the indicated month is less than 50 but greater than 19.

**FIG. 12–1.** Continuation rates by month after initial acceptance, according to contraceptive method. The Philippines, 1970–1974. The "first-method" rate measures the extent of continuation of the first method chosen at the time of initial acceptance. The "all-method" rate refers to the continuation of any method, regardless of the initial choice of methods. (Adapted from Laing JE: Stud Fam Plann 9(6):150, June 1968)

where    PL = proportion of post-acceptance pregnancies that result in live birth

$PR_n$ = probability that any woman who has accepted will become pregnant by the $n$th month following acceptance

$n$ = number of months following acceptance that are considered for the analysis

GPA = average number of months of gestation and postpartum amenorrhea per birth interval

EFGR = expected annual general fertility rate

In Table 12–6, Laing illustrated the assumptions used in computing each of the above values for the Philippines. The rate that best measures total couple years of protection is the all-method one. Table 12–7 illustrates the re-

sultant values that Laing calculated to show the months of *effective* protection (MEP). The MEP would have to be divided by 12 to obtain the necessary figure of couple years of protection.

One other technique used to calculate couple years of protection is shown by Osteria (14). He suggests a relatively simple formula for computing the couple months of protection for a given method, which is:

$$CMP = A\ (m^1 + m^2 + m^3 + \ldots + m^{n\ \text{months}})$$

$A$ = total acceptors of a given method

$m = \sqrt[24]{C}$

where $C$ = 2-year continuation rate

$\sqrt[24]{C}$ = the 24th root of $C$

= $C$ to the power of $(\frac{1}{24})$

$n$ months = 42.5 − average age of acceptors where 42.5 was assumed to be the upper limit of fecundity

**Table 12–6. Assumptions Utilized by Laing in Computing the Months of Effective Protection (MEP) for the Philippines (1970–74)**

| Input | Pills | IUD | Rhythm | Condoms |
|---|---|---|---|---|
| | | Methods first accepted | | |
| | | *First-method Inputs* | | |
| $a$ = $a$ in the formula $C_t = a \times e^{-|b|t}$ | 0.8360 | 0.9420 | 0.8850 | 0.7210 |
| $|b|$ = absolute value of $b$ in the formula $C_t = a \times e^{-|b|t}$ | 0.0360 | 0.0210 | 0.0310 | 0.0830 |
| PR = probability of a female acceptor becoming pregnant $n$ months following acceptance | 0.0772 | 0.0755 | 0.3281 | 0.1385 |
| $n$ = number of months considered after acceptance | 42.0000 | 42.0000 | 30.0000 | 14.0000 |
| OPA = months overlap of postpartum amenorrhea with contraceptive use | 0.7600 | 1.8700 | 1.4100 | 1.3800 |
| EGFR = expected annual general fertility rate | 0.4030 | 0.4030 | 0.4360 | 0.3500 |
| GPA = average months of gestation and postpartum amenorrhea | 16.200 | 15.4000 | 15.9000 | 17.7000 |
| PL = proportion of postacceptance pregnancies that result in a live birth | 0.8400 | 0.8400 | 0.8400 | 0.8400 |
| | | *All-method Inputs* | | |
| $a$ = $a$ in the formula $C_t = a \times e^{-|b|t}$ | 0.8770 | 1.0090 | 0.9370 | 0.8760 |
| $|b|$ = absolute value of $b$ in the formula $C_t = a \times e^{-|b|t}$ | 0.0266 | 0.0150 | 0.0278 | 0.0475 |
| PR = probability of a female acceptor becoming pregnant $n$ months following acceptance | 0.1988 | 0.1341 | 0.3569 | 0.2750 |
| $n$ = number of months considered after acceptance | 46.0000 | 44.0000 | 32.0000 | 21.0000 |
| OPA = months overlap of postpartum amenorrhea with contraceptive use | 0.7600 | 1.8700 | 1.4100 | 1.3800 |
| EGFR = expected annual general fertility rate | 0.4030 | 0.4030 | 0.4360 | 0.3540 |
| GPA = average months of gestation and postpartum amenorrhea | 16.2000 | 15.4000 | 15.9000 | 17.7000 |
| PL = proportion of postacceptance pregnancies that result in a live birth | 0.8400 | 0.8400 | 0.8400 | 0.8400 |

(Adapted from Laing JE: Stud Fam Plann 9 (6): 150, June 1968)

In the same article (13:195), the 2-year "all-method" continuation rates for 1968 are presented; these rates are shown in Table 12–8.

As previously stated, the CMP is divided by 12 to derive couple years of protection.

Taylor (20) suggests first-, second-, and third-year continuation rates of 0.85, 0.72, and 0.60 for the IUD and 0.72, 0.45, and 0.27 for the pill. The rate of 0.72 for the IUD and 0.45 for the pill would be used as $C$ in the Osteria method. These rates seem to be in a range consistent with the Osteria findings and also with the Laing approach of dividing $a$ by $|b|$ to derive, for the IUD, a mean of 3.66 years of protection, using the "first-method" continuation rates, and 5.6 years of protec-

**Table 12–7. Laing's Computed Results for Months of Effective Protection\***

| Rate | Pills | IUD | Rhythm | Condoms |
|---|---|---|---|---|
| | | First method | | |
| First-method | | | | |
| CE | 0.949 | 0.963 | 0.796 | 0.616 |
| CMP | 23.200 | 44.100 | 28.500 | 8.700 |
| MEP | 21.400 | 41.500 | 21.800 | 4.800 |
| All-method | | | | |
| CE | 0.902 | 0.947 | 0.810 | 0.637 |
| CMP | 33.000 | 67.300 | 33.700 | 18.400 |
| MEP | 29.100 | 61.900 | 26.300 | 11.000 |

\* Computed results for months of effective protection (MEP), contraceptive effectiveness (CE), and couple months of protection (CMP), given the assumptions shown in Table 12–6.
(Laing, JE: Stud Fam Plann 9 (6): 150, June 1968)

**Table 12–8. Two-year Continuation Rates, by Age Group, for Different Methods; Philippines, 1968**

| Method and age (years) | Two-year continuation rate |
|---|---|
| Pill | |
| 15–29 | 0.384 |
| 30 and older | 0.607 |
| IUD | |
| 15–29 | 0.652 |
| 30 and older | 0.757 |
| Rhythm | |
| All ages | 0.282 |

(Osteria TS: Stud Fam Plann 4 (7): 191, July 1973)

tion using the "all-methods" continuation rate.

In the case of a person who has been sterilized, the method of computing couple years of protection is to subtract the current age of the individual from a selected upper-limit age for female childbearing. Osteria (14) chose 42.5 years as the average maximum age. The definition of the focus group given at the beginning of this chapter would have 44 years as the upper limit, but the demographic data of the locality or nation under study will dictate the appropriate age to use.

**ESTIMATING BIRTHS AVERTED**

If the focus group has been identified, as indicated in Step 1, the couple years of protection should lead directly to an estimation of *births averted*, as will be shown in this section. Before presenting the method, it should be mentioned that deriving births averted from couple years of protection is not the ideal way to derive this estimate. The ideal method of computing births averted would be to introduce a program in certain randomly selected target populations whose birth rates are high and equivalent to those in a control group and then compare the differential birth rates in each area. Unfortunately, this is rarely possible in a program which is already in progress; moreover, it is difficult to justify deliberately restricting services. Cutwright and Jaffe (3) used cross-sectional multiple regression analysis to determine the relationship between the change in birth rates and the degree of program activity in various regions of a country. This kind of analysis cannot always be accomplished by an individual program because each program has only one site to work with; consequently, the couple years of protection

method is most practicable for most *individual* programs.

Calculation of births averted from couple years of protection requires an estimate of the probability of pregnancy if women in the target group are without effective contraceptive protection. Since the focus group was defined, in the earlier part of this chapter, as persons not wanting to become pregnant and not likely to use, on their own, effective birth control methods or abortions, the probability of pregnancy is difficult to estimate with existing data. General population data will tend to underestimate the probability of pregnancy during an unprotected year. The general rule of thumb that has been used for less developed countries is that 3 couple years of protection lead to one birth averted. This implies that given less effective contraceptive methods (rhythm, withdrawal), it would require 3 years of average coital frequency for conception to occur. This figure is derived from observing birth intervals of the general fecund, exposed population.

Jaffe (10) uses a figure of 7 years for the United States population, which would give a 0.14 probability that an unprotected person-year would result in a pregnancy. Based on the 1975 National Fertility Study, in which women originally interviewed in 1970 were resurveyed, Westoff and McCarthy (21) calculated the number of unwanted births between the time of the last wanted child and the time of the interview. The results were given for 1, 2, 3, 4, 5, 10, and 15 years of exposure since the last wanted child, as shown in Table 12–9. The table indicates, for example, that for every 1000 black females ex-

**Table 12–9. Estimated Births per Unprotected Year (U.S.)**

| Years exposure since last unwanted pregnancy | Births per 1000 persons for once-married females | |
|---|---|---|
| | All persons | Blacks |
| 1 | 11 | 68 |
| 2 | 77 | 211 |
| 3 | 139 | 345 |
| 4 | 174 | 431 |
| 5 | 208 | 526 |
| 10 | 342 | 832 |
| 15 | 397 | 1034 |

(Data from: Westoff C, McCarthy J: Fam Plann Perspectives 11(3), 147, May/June 1979)

posed for 5 years after the last wanted birth, there were 526 births. This would mean that for each person coming to the clinic, the probability of an unwanted birth would be 0.105 $\left(\frac{526 \text{ births}}{1000 \text{ persons}} \div 5 \text{ years}\right)$. The probability per year for persons that are protected for 3 years since the last wanted birth is 0.115, but for 10 years of protection the yearly probability is 0.0832, and for 15 years the probability falls to 0.06. The probability estimate used would depend upon the length of time that passed after the last wanted birth before the family planning program began to provide services. If clients are asked about this length of time on the survey given when persons first arrive at the clinic, a distribution of years since the last wanted birth can be produced and multiplied by the appropriate probabilities of an unwanted birth. In the absence of such a distribution, a figure of 0.1 births per unprotected year could be used. The Jaffe figure of 7 couple years per birth averted would give 0.14 (1 ÷ 7) probability per couple year of protection. The Westoff results probably understate the probability of pregnancy when unprotected because the data applies to all persons, not just to those using relatively ineffective methods. Therefore the Jaffe figure of 7 couple years of protection = 1 birth averted would provide a reasonable lower bound for the United States, and the figure of 3 couple years of protection = 1 birth averted would provide an upper bound.

### SAVINGS FROM BIRTHS AVERTED

The total savings from births averted is computed by multiplying the number of births averted, from Step 4, by the 1-year governmental expenditures per birth averted, as computed in Step 2. The minimum funds that a government should be willing to spend for an effective family planning effort are thus derived.

### GOVERNMENT PROGRAM EXPENDITURES

The focus group, by definition, is not able to pay for modern contraception. Consequently, the budget or fees for service granted by the *government* to family planning programs becomes the relevant expenditure figure. Even if other members of society (such as physicians, health centers, etc.) subsidize the services,

these nongovernment subsidizers do not necessarily realize the short-term dollar benefits. The three major problems in cost determination are selection of the appropriate time period, identification of the source of funds and costs by method, and deciding whether or not the services were being delivered in a minimum-cost fashion.

Time Period. There is a minimum delay of 9 to 24 months between provision of a couple year of protection and a resultant averted birth. Consequently, the computation of the expenditures for preventing a given number of unwanted births should be *based* on the year in which the protection was provided, but *compared* to savings from births averted that occur during a future period, or sets of periods. Let us assume that the rate of inflation is similar to the interest rate the government has to pay to borrow money. For an adequate comparison, the money that is saved in future periods can be estimated in terms of the prices during the year in which the family planning funds were expended. The benefits from a sterilization that is performed in year *1* may extend for several years into the future, but it is suggested that all births averted be attached to year *2* after the family planning program funds were expended. As long as the rate of inflation and the interest rate which the government must pay for 3–5 year notes are similar, savings can be calculated in this way. However, if the inflation rate differs substantially from the interest rate, then the savings from each year in the future should be computed (to include the inflation in medical care prices and intensity of service use) and then discounted to the present, using a discount rate which is estimated by the interest rates on 3–5 year government securities. The formula is as follows:

$$\text{Present discounted value} = \sum_{i=1}^{k} \frac{(\text{dollar expenses saved in year } i)}{(1 + r)^i}$$

when $r$ = the rate of interest

Sources of Funds and Costs per Method. A family planning program may obtain funds from various sources, including national, regional, and local governments, private agencies, individual fees for service, government-funded fees for service, and private donations.

The funding received from each source should be specified in total and preferably in detail, by type of *method,* so that the government's cost per birth averted may be computed and compared to total government savings from program activity. For example, it may be desirable to indicate that the government subsidized the total costs of sterilizations and thereby achieved a certain number of births averted, but subsidized only half the costs of pill users and therefore achieved a lesser degree of births averted. Some government officials may argue that if they contributed even a small portion of the total costs, they should be able to count *all* births averted as resulting from government monies, because the funds were used as "seed money" to encourage generation of other funds, but family planners do not have to agree.

The costs for each method should be determined by, first, identifying the *direct* costs that can easily be associated with a given method, such as hospitalization (for sterilization procedures), equipment, supplies, some personnel, pill supplies, etc. The remaining costs should be divided according to the number of clinic visits required per year for persons using each type of *method.* Correa, Parrish, and Beasley (2) provide a very detailed example of how costs are allocated to *methods* (although not by source of funding) and arrive at the following costs per patient:

|        | *1967* |
| *Method* | *Cost per patient in U.S.* |
| --- | --- |
| Pill | $ 69.42 |
| IUD | 51.84 |
| Foam | 65.69 |
| Other | 114.25 |

Then the couple years of protection for each method and the corresponding births averted should be related to these costs to derive a *cost per birth averted* for each method.

It would also be helpful to determine the proportion of the cost per birth averted contributed by each funding source. Osteria (14) demonstrates that the source of funds for the family program in the Philippines includes the International Planned Parenthood Federation (19% of the total), the Pathfinder Fund (12% of the total), USAID (62.2%), the Population Council (5.9%), the Ford Foundation (0.2%), and all others (0.7%). Although Osteria did not report the births averted by each funding source, the latter could be identified. When a funding source provides general funds that are not tied directly to a certain method, then the costs and births averted can be distributed to that source in the same proportion as the funds which they contribute to the total program. However, if a funding source restricts its contribution to a specific method, that funding source could be told what percentage of the costs of providing that method they had contributed. Correspondingly, they should be told the percentage of the couple years of protection provided by that method, and the resulting percentage of births averted.

**Minimizing Costs.** If an individual program is to argue that it has short-term benefits, it must ensure that costs per birth averted are at a minimum when compared to other projects with a similar client mix. Most programs which allocate a high percentage (about 60%) of their budget to personnel (as do family planning programs) can be made more cost efficient. Reardon and his coworkers (15), in an excellent study of the cost components of family planning programs, showed the average costs per patient for various *methods* in 1974, and the associated maximum and minimum costs among projects studied throughout the United States (see Table 12–10).

The high variability revealed in the range of unit costs could be due to differences in number of visits, patient cooperativeness, low- or high-risk status, effectiveness in maintaining patients on a contraceptive device, mix of new and continuing patients, or in cost efficiency (see Chap. 11). To ensure cost efficiency, two things are required: *1)* monitoring systems with which to evaluate staff productivity and

**Table 12–10. Average Cost per Patient for Various Methods (U.S., 1974)**

| Item | Average | Min. | Max. |
| --- | --- | --- | --- |
| Annual cost per oral contraceptive patient | $ 72.70 | $18.10 | $187.50 |
| Annual cost per IUD patient | 97.40 | 27.30 | 293.40 |
| Annual cost per diaphragm patient | 71.00 | 26.30 | 141.90 |
| Cost per male sterilization | 48.40 | 1.30 | 106.80 |
| Cost per female sterilization | 224.70 | 25.80 | 550.00 |

*2)* ability to compare costs with those of similar clinics. The latter requires participation in a common reporting system. If the costs per patient are not at least close to the average, it may not be possible to demonstrate a sizeable difference between program costs and benefits.

### FIGURING NET BENEFIT TO THE GOVERNMENT

Compare the cost saving per unwanted birth averted to the program operating cost per birth averted to determine if at least most program costs can be recovered by the government. Jaffe (10) showed a benefit-cost ratio of between 1.8:1.0 and 2.5:1.0 in the United States program. Osteria (14) showed a savings per birth averted in the Philippines which were equivalent to ten United States dollars, but he did not indicate government costs. In Singapore, Kee and Tee (11) showed an average cost per birth averted of $91 ($114 for oral contraceptive users, $45 for condom users, $54 for IUD users, and $70 for users of other methods) but did not report the dollar benefits of averting these births. Both the costs for averting the births and the dollar saving benefits are needed to determine the value of a family planning program.

### Example of Computing the Short-term Benefit/Cost Ratio in a Local Program.

As an example of how a local program could compute the short-term cost and benefits for a single age group, assume that a clinic is serving a group of 500 females who are 25 years of age. The survey given at the initial visit showed that all were fecund, not currently pregnant, and sexually active. None wanted to become pregnant. Of the total, 80 per cent were using an ineffective method prior to the program and would continue to do so without the program. Of this group, 90 per cent were unwilling to have an abortion, in case of an unwanted pregnancy. Therefore, the focus group is 500 persons × 0.8 (used ineffective methods) × 0.9 (unwilling to have abortion) = 360 persons.

A short questionnaire was given to all 360, and among them, 200 had previously had a child. For the most recent birth, the use of health and financial services were estimated (by interviewers who talked with the clients) as shown in Table 12–11.

For the 200 persons surveyed, the cost to state and local government, per birth, was $268,000, and $309,000 was paid by the federal government, resulting in a total of $577,000, or $2885 per birth. A total of 100 persons out of the 360 in the focus group had an unplanned child; the average time period between the last planned and the unplanned child was 5 years.

Based on data on the persons using the clinic, the data shown (in decades) in Table 12–12 reflects the methods being used by initial and previous acceptors and the average months of protection provided *during the year* by that method (except for sterilization, where the months of protection for future years up to age 44 are assigned to the current year).

The 3425 months of protection, divided by 12 months per year, results in 285 couple years of protection. The 285 years of protection divided by the 5 years of exposure required for birth results in 57 births averted due to the program activity for the year. In the survey of infant and birth costs to the government, the total government savings would be $2885 per birth averted, providing a total dollar savings of $2885 × 57 births = $164,445, of which $66,173 (computed as follows: [268,000/-

**Table 12–11. Costs for Births Not Averted in Sample Focus Group**

| | Total costs in the 200 families | Amount of the expenses paid by | |
| --- | --- | --- | --- |
| | | State and local government | Federal government |
| Prenatal care | $ 20,000 | $ 4,000 | $ 12,000 |
| Hospitalization of mother and child in 1st year | 200,000 | 120,000 | 40,000 |
| Postpartum care | 20,000 | 6,000 | 3,000 |
| One year pediatric outpatient care | 40,000 | 12,000 | 12,000 |
| Public assistance | 300,000 | 120,000 | 180,000 |
| Day-care nursery | 60,000 | 6,000 | 36,000 |
| Income taxes lost from lost work | 26,000 | | 26,000 |
| | $666,000 | $268,000 | $309,000 |

**Table 12–12.  Average Months of Protection Provided to Members of Focus Group During One Year**

| | Number of persons in the focus group | Total months of use after end of postpartum amenorrhea |
|---|---|---|
| Initial acceptors by method | | |
| Pill | 190 | 1140 |
| IUD | 20 | 160 |
| Other | 10 | 70 |
| Sterilization | 5 | (44 yrs. − 25 yrs.) × 12 mos. × 5 persons = 1140 |
| Previous acceptors, by method | | |
| Pill | 100 | 600 |
| IUD | 25 | 225 |
| Other | 10 | 90 |
| | 360 | 3425 months of protection |

666,000] × 164,445) would be a reduced cost to state and local government.

As long as the federal, state, and local expenditures in the program are less than $164,445 per budget year, a short-term positive ratio between benefit and cost exists. If the program's unit expenditures are similar to the average costs of the programs studied by Reardon and his coworkers (15), the approximate total costs (in 1974 dollars) could be computed as shown in Table 12–13.

Even if the $39,020 is multiplied by 1.77 to account for 10 per cent inflation per year in medical care prices since 1974, the total would only be $69,065, providing for *this* example project only a ratio between benefit and cost of 2.38 to 1.

## LONG-TERM COST BENEFIT ANALYSIS

The discussion in this chapter has assumed that if family planning programs are operated in a cost-conscious fashion and with a well-defined target population, the prevention of unwanted births will have sufficient short-term economic benefits to cover a high proportion of operating costs. If there are no short-term benefits, because government ex-

penditures for health and financial services to children do not exist (e.g., in developing countries), the long-term benefit approach may have to be considered.

Reliance on family planning as a major tool for economic development over the long term is a controversial matter. There is considerable disagreement as to whether decreasing the birth rate will, in fact, benefit the economy in developing countries. The models for assessing the impact of various strategies of development are constantly being revised and refined. The assumptions used in the models must be based on rather tenuous data, and the results, therefore, could be equally tenuous. However, in a society where the masses are living on the verge of starvation, family planning, when combined with an aggressive capital investment program and an adaptable population, could possibly assist sufficiently in the growth process to be beneficial in ways shown below by the macroeconomic models.

Two of the macroeconomic models are presented by Enke (6) and Isbister (9). In the Enke model the flow of development proceeds in the following stages:

1. The country, through family planning or other policies, achieves a low birth rate.

**Table 12–13.  Total Program Costs Per Year (by Method)**

| Method | Total number using method* | Cost per patient year | Total |
|---|---|---|---|
| Pill | 402 | $ 73 | $29,346 |
| IUD | 63 | 97 | 6,111 |
| Other | 28 | 71 | 1,988 |
| Sterilization | 7 | 225 | 1,575 |
| | 500 | | $39,020 |

* Applied the same proportions as used with the 360 patients to the *total* of 500 patients being served

2. Due to the sudden drop in the birth rate, there are fewer people, but the same labor force, so per capita income increases.

3. More income per capita leads to increased savings, because families do not have to spend every penny on food or shelter.

4. Increased savings, if held in a financial institution or retained by the government, can facilitate more investment, particularly in the purchase of capital equipment (tools that can assist in the production process).

5. More capital equipment means greater production, with the same or fewer workers. Also, with the widespread use of equipment, ideas are generated for further technological change. This results in even greater productivity.

6. Greater productivity will mean higher income per capita, and, *if* income is distributed according to productivity, higher standards of living for many.

7. Higher income per capita, in a less developed country, may mean better nutrition, better health care for infants, and, as a result, more population. However, by the time the population has increased, the productivity of the average worker will have risen; thus, the per-capita income will remain high.

Enke made the following assumptions for a country with a 1970 population of 10 million, a per-capita income of $150, and a crude birth rate of 44 per 1000: fertility could be halved within 30 years, and by 1985, 22 per cent of the population between the ages of 15 and 49 would be practicing effective birth control. He notes:

A large birth-control program might directly cost about $5 a year per acceptor. About 25 per cent of the population aged 15 through 49 would have to practice contraception on an average to halve the gross reproduction rate in 30 years. During this period the total cost might be roughly $200 million for a less-developed country that started with a population of 10 million. Accumulated benefits could be $16 billion. The benefits to cost ratio is roughly 80 to 1 (6).

Isbister (9) modeled the Mexican economy through a somewhat different approach. He divided the economy into sectors—manufacturing, services, and agriculture—and considered both demand and supply elements of the economy. The flow of activity proceeds as follows:

1. Birth control programs lead to lower population growth, which, in turn, may eventually mean lower total population.

2. Lower population leads to less demand for food; as a result, to a lower *price* for food (or for all agricultural output).

3. Low agricultural prices generate very little increased consumption, because food is a basic necessity of life; thus, its demand is not very dependent upon price. Therefore, lower prices mean lower wages for agricultural sector employees.

4. Lower agricultural wages will drive many persons from agriculture into manufacturing. The increased supply of labor in the manufacturing sector will cause wages to decrease.

5. Lower wages in this sector mean increased profits for manufacturers. The manufacturer *can* lower prices and *gain* substantially increased sales because consumption of manufactured goods is more dependent upon price than consumption of foodstuffs (the demand for manufactured goods is elastic).

6. Increased profits mean increased availability of funds for capital investment, either directly or indirectly, through businessmen's savings.

7. More investment means greater overall production productivity per worker.

8. Greater productivity per worker *can* mean increased wages and more income per capita.

Isbister believes that the effects of declining fertility on savings may be either positive or negative, depending on the responsiveness of consumers to prices and workers to wage rates. In Mexico, given the assumptions shown in the data, birth control is likely to raise the savings rate long enough to free the country from poverty. Further, he notes that the more responsive food purchases are to lower prices, the less impact fertility control will have upon profits and saving (9).

As may be expected, models such as these have come under wide criticism. An erroneous determination of the degree of responsiveness of the dependent variable to the independent variables of any equation of the model, low initial starting values, or faulty behavioral assumptions could give a falsely positive prediction of future economic benefits. For example, savings behavior is important to each model, yet very little hard evidence exists regarding such behavior in less developed countries, especially in light of high rates of inflation in these countries, and expectations of higher future income. In both models presented, the major positive impact is derived from the money released for investment. It could be argued that an economic developer should spend the funds directly in investment, rather than wait 5 to 15 years for the influence of family planning programs to be felt. For example, Conroy (1, p. 29), in a review of the literature, notes Bogue's optimism regarding the family planning movement and his assumption that the masses of people are ready to curtail their fertility, and states that "confidence in this assumption is rapidly dissipating." Conroy (1) further discusses problems with cost analyses of prevented births (most of which have been overcome in the methodology proposed in this chapter), analytical models, and macroeconomic simulation models, and concludes that due to the absence of good empirical data, the results of analytical models are indeterminate; that macroeconomic models based on Western notions of economic modeling may be incorrect when applied to less developed countries; and that economic growth probably has more impact on fertility than family planning recruitment efforts. He suggests more specific regional studies which could synthesize data with analytical models.

Suits and Mason (19) have begun such work in a simulation model and have so far indicated that family planning programs generate economic development, which in turn produced an estimated *economic* benefit of $850 (in U.S. dollars) per birth averted, in a wide variety of less developed countries, with the benefits equally divided between participating families and society at large. Moreover, Enke (6) notes that even family planning programs that spend a relatively large portion of their budget on patient recruitment in less developed countries would require less than 5 per cent of the total funds allocated to economic development. Therefore Enke believes that it should not be necessary to choose between *only* family planning and *only* direct capital investment.

An important book by Simon entitled *The Economics of Population Growth* (18) is suggested as useful reading for administrators or researchers in the field of family planning because it serves as a point of departure for further research. Simon distinguished between the more and the less developed countries and considers time frames beyond the 30 to 50 years generally considered in economic development models. Although he agrees that very high fertility has a negative effect within the 30 to 50 year time frame, he convincingly argues that a moderate, but not necessarily low, rate of growth is highly desirable in the long run: *moderate growth* can create greater economic mobility, new jobs, a more productive work force, less risk for investment, and, therefore, improved productivity and capital formation. Simon also suggests that population growth provides developing countries with an incentive to invent new technology, in order to avoid impending doom (18).

Serow (17), however, has noted that Simon does not adequately include the economic law of diminishing returns (which states that with fixed resources, increased workers will add less and less to additional production of goods and services) in his model and ignores the possibility that a less developed country can obtain technology from more developed nations without having to produce new inventions themselves.

Regardless of criticism, Simon remains skeptical of the validity of the generally accepted theory that low population growth is beneficial. In the preface to his book he says, "I began to work in the field of population economics for the same reason that many others do: I thought population growth, along with all-out war, to be one of the two fearsome threats to mankind and civilization. So I respect the motivations and intentions of many of those people with whose conclusions and recommendations I no longer agree" (18:*xxiii*).

Obviously, population economics is a highly controversial field, with many conflicting theories and models, and little hard evidence to give them firm support. There is a great need for more well-funded, long-term, country-specific research which will permit us to make more accurate statements about possible long-term benefits of family planning. Consequently, the focus of this chapter has been on short-term cost benefit analyses, particularly the *unwanted births* strategy, which offers the most direct and practicable approach to demonstrating the economic benefits of family planning—especially for individual local programs.

# REFERENCES

1. Conroy ME, Folbre HR: Population growth as a deterrent to economic growth: a reappraisal of the evidence. Paper prepared for the Project on Cultural Values and Population Policy of the Institute of Society, Ethics, and Life Sciences, February 1976. Institute of Society, Ethics, and the Life Sciences, The Hastings Center, Hastings-on-Hudson, New York
2. Correa H, Parrish VW, and Beasley JD: A three year longitudinal evaluation of the costs of a family planning program. Am J Public Health 62:1647, Dec, 1972
3. Cutright P, Jaffe F: Impact of Family Planning Programs on Fertility: The U.S. Experience. Praeger, Washington, D.C., 1977
4. Dryfoos J: A formula for the 1970's: estimating need for subsidized family planning services in the United States. Fam Plann Perspectives 5(3):145, Summer 1973
5. Dryfoos J: Women who need and receive family planning services: estimates at mid-decade. Fam Plann Perspectives 7(4):172, July/Aug 1975
6. Enke S: Birth control for economic development. Science, 164:798–802, May 1969
7. Freedman R, Whelpton PK, Campbell AA: Family Planning, Sterility and Population Growth. New York, McGraw-Hill, 1959
8. Haveman RH: Benefit-cost analysis and family planning programs. Population and Development Review 2,1:37, 1976
9. Isbister J: Birth control, income distribution, and the rate of saving: the case of Mexico. Demography 10:1, Feb 1973
10. Jaffe F: Short term costs and benefits of United States family planning programs. Fam Plann Perspectives 9(2):77, Mar/Apr 1977
11. Kee WF, Tee QS: Singapore: a cost effect analysis of family planning program. Stud Fam Plann 3(1):8, Jan 1972
12. Kendall M: The world fertility survey: current status and findings. Popul Rep Spec Top Monogr 7:4, 1979
13. Laing JE: Estimating the effects of contraceptive use on fertility: techniques and findings from the 1974 Philippine National Acceptor Survey. Stud Fam Plann 9(6):150, June 1968
14. Osteria TS: A cost-effectiveness analysis of family planning programs in the Philippines. Stud Fam Plann 4(7):191, July 1973
15. Reardon MJ, Deeds SG, Dreshner NA, Diksa JM, Robinson WC: Real costs of delivering family planning services—implications for management. Am J Public Health 64:860, Sept 1974
16. Ryder NB, Westoff CF: Reproduction in the United States. Princeton, Princeton University Press, 1971
17. Serow W: Book review of *The Economics of Population Growth,* by Julian Simon. Southern Economic J 46:2, Oct 1979
18. Simon J: The Economics of Population Growth. Princeton, Princeton University Press, 1977
19. Suits D, Mason A: Measuring gains to population control results from an econometric model. Presented at the annual meeting of the Population Association of America, Atlanta, Georgia, April 13–15, 1978
20. Taylor H: Human Reproduction. Cambridge, Mass., MIT Press, 1976
21. Westoff C, McCarthy J: Sterilization in the United States. Fam Plann Perspectives 11(3):147, May/June 1979

# Demographic

# Aspects

# of Population

# Change

Demography is the study of the size, composition, and distribution of human populations. Changes in these three factors are a direct result of the processes of fertility (births), mortality (deaths), and migration (residential movement). Chapter 13 explores the nature of demography and introduces the materials and perspectives fundamental to its study. Chapter 14 first discusses basic features of populations, and second presents demographic data and particular methods used in demographic analysis.

The demographic transition, a perspective which attempts to explain how, and to some extent why, populations change their sizes over time, is given attention in Chapter 15. Chapter 16 addresses population change, with emphasis on fertility reduction, including such facilitating factors as economic development and organized family planning programs. Finally, in Chapter 17, case studies of Mexico, India, China, and the United States, focusing on their demographic past, present, and future, are presented. The purpose of the final chapter of Part Three is to increase understanding of the extent to which social and economic factors, population policies, birth control programs, and technology interact to influence the birth rate.

# 13

# Nature and Implications of Population Growth

### Dudley L. Poston, Jr.

The objective of this chapter is to introduce demographic concepts of population change. The demographer brings a somewhat different set of concepts, methods, and data to the study of population change from those of the biologist, medical scientist, and anthropologist. Without delving directly into the fundamentals of demography, the demographic approach will be illustrated by examining current trends in population, and then suggesting what these portend for the future.

## WHAT IS DEMOGRAPHY?

In the most general sense, demography may be defined as the scientific study of human populations—their size, composition, and distribution—and the changes that occur in these phenomena through the processes of fertility, mortality, and migration. Demographers are concerned with how large (or small) populations are—their size; how the populations are composed according to age, sex, race, and other attributes—their composition; and how the populations are distributed in space, e.g., how rural or how urban they are—their distribution. Of equal or greater importance, demographers are concerned with changes, in the course of time, in the size, composition, and distribution of populations, particularly as these result from the processes of fertility, mortality, and migration (births, deaths, and migrations).

Not only do demographers observe and describe the size, composition, and distribution of human populations, and the changes resulting from fertility, mortality, and migration; they are also drawn to the question of why these phenomena operate and change in the way they do. That is, why do populations increase (or decrease) in numbers; why do they become older or younger; why do they become more urban or more rural? Some demographers employ strictly demographic variables to answer these questions, while others use nondemographic variables (frequently those from sociology, economics, psychology, etc.). The former group is following a *formal* demographic approach in developing explanations (as exemplified by Chap. 14), while the latter group is using a *social* demographic approach (as exemplified by Chaps. 15 through 17).

Let us draw on current demographic data to illustrate the differences between these two approaches. Take the demographic question of why populations are distributed the way they are in space. Countries differ with respect to the proportion of their residents who live in large cities. For example, in 1970, 38 per cent of the population of the United States lived in cities with more than one million inhabitants; the corresponding percentages for China (People's Republic) and Thailand were 10 per cent and 6 per cent, respectively. Why do these differences exist? In an attempt to answer this question, the *social* demographer would go beyond purely demographic concerns and would probably focus on the processes of industrialization and modernization, where the *formal* demographer would rely solely on demographic kinds of explanations.

Let us take another example, that of population growth rates. It is estimated that the rate of population growth in 1978 for the United States is 0.6 per cent; the rates for the People's Republic of China and for Thailand are 1.4 per cent and 2.3 per cent, respectively (see the data chart in Appendix 1). Why are these countries growing at such different rates? The formal demographer might develop an answer to this question by looking at the birth rates of these countries. The United States has a birth rate of 15:1000 people in the population; that is, in 1978, the United States added 15 persons to its population each year through fertility, for every 1000 persons in the population, whereas China and Thailand have birth rates in 1978 of 22:1000 and 33:1000, respectively. The formal demographer might thus observe that Thailand is growing at a more rapid rate than the United States because it has a higher birth rate.

In answering the same question, the social demographer would perhaps look first at birth rates, but then would go beyond this demographic consideration to nondemographic factors which may be affecting the birth rates. The social demographer would ask what leads the country to such high (or low) birth rates. Perhaps the economy has something to do with it (poorer countries have higher birth rates). Prehaps the level of industrialization in the country has an impact (the more industrialized countries generally have lower birth rates than less industrialized countries). Whatever the reasons, the social demographer goes beyond demography (i.e., beyond a consideration involving only demographic variables such as birth or death rates) in formulating answers.

## DEMOGRAPHIC COMPONENTS OF POPULATION GROWTH

Before examining contemporary demographic data for the populations of the world and then asking what these empirical patterns suggest about the future, it is appropriate to focus first on the basic demographic components of population growth. It has been implied in preceding paragraphs that change in the size of a human population during a given time-interval occurs in a very limited way; change may only result from the influences of three components: births, deaths, and migrations. That is, a population may change its size over a given interval by adding the number of persons born

during the period, subtracting those dying during the interval, and by adding the number of persons moving to the area, and subtracting those moving away. There are no other ways for a population to change its size. Regarding change in the population of the world, obviously, only the first two components are operable.

The dynamics of population change may be represented in a form known as the population equation:

$$P_2 = P_1 + B - D \pm M$$

where $P_2$ is the size of the population at the end of the time interval;

$P_1$ is the size of the population at the beginning of the interval;

$B$ is the number of births occurring in the population during the interval;

$D$ is the number of deaths occurring in the population during the interval; and

$M$ is the net number of migrants moving to, or away from, the population during the interval.

Using data (expressed in thousands) for the United States between 1970 and 1977, the equation becomes the following:

|  1977<br>population =<br>(216,333) |  1970<br>population +<br>(203,305) | |
| --- | --- | --- |
| 1970–1977<br>births<br>(23,870) | 1970–1977<br>– deaths<br>(13,982) | 1970–1977<br>+ net migrants<br>(3,140) |

Demographers have developed a broad description and explanation of population change by focusing generally on the first two components of the above equation: births and deaths. This explanation, known as the demographic transition, is an attempt to answer the question of why most populations have tended to change their size in the course of time. The theory of the demographic transition is discussed in detail in Chapters 15, 18, and 19.

## CURRENT TRENDS IN FERTILITY AND MORTALITY

A knowledge of contemporary birth and death rates, and of their variability from country to country, is necessary if one wishes to understand the implications that the demographic components provide for the future of world population. Since migration contributes only slightly to population change among the countries of the world, this component of the demographic equation is not covered in the following discussion.

Before beginning this section, a linguistic inconsistency must be clarified. English-speaking demographers and medical scientists use the term *fertility* differently. Demographers generally distinguish between the ability to produce children and the actual production of children. Among demographers, the former is known as *fecundity,* the latter as *fertility.* Medical scientists, however, do not make such a distinction, using the term *fertility* to refer to reproductive ability.

French-speaking and Spanish-speaking demographers (like their English counterparts) also distinguish between potential and actual reproduction but they reverse the English usage of the two terms. Thus, French-speaking demographers use the term *fertilité,* and Spanish-speaking demographers the term *fertilidad,* to refer to reproductive ability, and they use *fécondité* and *fecundidad,* respectively, to refer to actual reproductive performance. In using the terms in this and subsequent chapters, we follow the usage of English-speaking demographers (1).

## FERTILITY

The basic way of quantifying fertility is by examining the number of births produced in a population in a given time period (usually 1 year) per 1000 members of the population. This is a very crude procedure for measuring fertility, but it will suffice for this introductory discussion. (More refined measures will be discussed in the next chapter.) It is known as the crude birth rate (CBR), and is expressed as follows:

$$CBR = \frac{\text{births in the year}}{\text{population at mid-year}} \times 1000$$

Using data for Mexico, in 1978, the equation becomes:

$$CBR = \frac{2,809,800}{66,900,000} \times 1000 = 42$$

The answer, 42, means that there were 42 babies born in Mexico in 1978 for every 1000 persons in the Mexican population. Referring to Appendix 1, we observe that crude birth rates range, in 1978, from a low of 10, in the Federal Republic of Germany, to a high of 52, in Niger. The world's rate is 31.5.

If we rank the major areas and countries of the world in terms of their fertility, they may be placed generally into one of three groups, on the basis of their crude birth rates: low fertility (CBRs under 20), medium fertility (CBRs from 20 to 39), and high fertility (CBRs above 40). According to the data in Appendix 1, all of North America, virtually all of Europe, and the USSR are in the low-fertility group (CBRs under 20), and nearly all of Africa (important exceptions are Egypt and Mauritius) are characterized by high fertility (CBRs above 40). Most of the Asian countries, except for East Asia, also report crude birth rates above 40, while the East Asian countries, including Japan, both Chinas, and South Korea, have rates in the high teens and low to mid-twenties.

The Latin American countries are found at all three levels of fertility. Middle and Tropical South America (except for Colombia, Costa Rica, Guyana, Panama, and Venezuela) are generally areas of high, and near-high, fertility, while most of the Caribbean and Temperate South American countries are in the medium-fertility group. Uruguay, Argentina, Cuba, and the Bahamas, however, have rates in the very low 20s, and Barbados has a rate of 19.

Another way of portraying the fertility data in Appendix 1 involves grouping the countries according to their stages of economic development. For the sake of discussion, countries with per-capita gross national products (GNP) in 1978 of $2000 or more (in U.S. dollars) will be referred to as *developed,* while countries with per-capita GNPs below $2000 will be classified as *developing* (see the last column of Appendix 1). Although there are important exceptions, the developed countries are characterized by low crude birth rates, the developing countries by medium to high rates. Southwest-Asian countries, such as Kuwait, Qatar, and the United Arab Emirates, along with Venezuela and Libya (all members of the Organization of Petroleum-Exporting Countries), are the major exceptions, with high birth rates (all in the mid- to high 40s, except for Venezuela), and high levels of GNP. The extent to which modernization and development provide reasonable explanations of fertility variation among the countries of the world will be discussed in more detail in later chapters.

## MORTALITY

As with fertility, an easily understood and easily interpreted method for quantifying mortality is the crude death rate (CDR), or the number of deaths in a population in any given year, per one thousand members of the population. It may be expressed as follows:

$$CDR = \frac{\text{deaths in the year}}{\text{population at mid-year}} \times 1000$$

Again using data for Mexico, in 1978, the equation is the following:

$$CDR = \frac{535,200}{66,900,000} \times 1000 = 8$$

This means that in Mexico, in 1978, there were 8 deaths for every 1000 persons in the population. Looking again at Appendix 1, crude death rates in the countries of the world range, in 1978, from lows of 5 in Kuwait, Singapore, Hong Kong, Taiwan, Costa Rica, the Bahamas, and Cuba, to highs of 26 in Malawi, and 25 in Mali, Upper Volta, and Ethiopia. The range of crude death rates is narrower than the range for crude birth rates, for the countries of the world in 1978.

Except for Northern Africa, with CDRs generally in the mid- to high teens, African countries south of the Sahara have the highest death rates in the world, almost always above 20. The Asian countries, for the most part, report death rates in the mid- to upper teens, except for East Asia, with death rates of 10 or below. The North and Latin American countries, the USSR, and countries in Oceania and in Southern Europe have the lowest crude death rates in the world, rates almost always below 10. The remaining European countries (those in the northern, western and eastern parts) have death rates generally in the low to mid-teens. Most countries of the world have crude death rates below 20.

If the countries of the world are categorized as "developed" or "developing," and their crude death rates examined, the kinds of clear distinctions which emerged when studying fertility do not appear. Low-death-rate countries are found in both groups. This does not mean that both the developed and developing countries of the world have the same general mortality experiences, however. For although the crude death rates are low in most countries of the world, members of the populations in the developed countries have greater longevity (i.e., they live longer) than those in the developing countries (see, for example, column 10 of Appendix 1).

One now begins to see why crude death rates are crude, a topic that will be investigated in greater detail in the next chapter. Here it is sufficient to note that most developing countries have low crude death rates because they have large numbers of young persons in their populations, and young people have low death rates. Hence a measure such as the CDR, which gauges the number of deaths per 1000 persons in the population (without regard to their ages) is not capable of distinguishing between countries with high longevity, e.g., the developed countries, and countries with very young populations, but without high longevity, e.g., most of the developing countries. Crude death rates do provide a rough notion of the distribution of deaths in the countries of the world, but they do not elucidate the underlying reasons for this pattern.

## POPULATION GROWTH

With a knowlege of crude birth and death rates, one can proceed directly to the rate of natural increase, by subtracting the CDR from the CBR. Continuing with the example of Mexico in 1978, with its CBR of 42 and CDR of 8, it is clear that this country had a net gain of 34 persons for every 1000 members of its population. The rate of natural increase is usually represented in percentage terms, that is, per 100 persons. Thus, Mexico's rate of natural increase in 1978 was 3.4 per cent. Appendix 1 indicates that rates of natural increase range from a high of 3.9 per cent in Libya and Kuwait to a low of −0.2 per cent in the Federal Republic of Germany, the German Democratic Republic, and Luxemburg.

Further, the population growth rate may be determined by adding the rates of natural increase and net migration. For most countries the growth rate is due almost entirely to the difference between births and deaths. Kuwait, Israel, Australia, the Federal Republic of Germany, and Switzerland are exceptions in that portions of their population increase are due to net gains through migration. Similarly,

Puerto Rico, Jamaica, Martinque, Trinidad and Tobago, and Surinam are exceptions in the other direction: some of their population increase is offset by net losses through migration. But for most countries, migration is insignificant in accounting for population change from one year to the next. Therefore, the rates of natural increase and of population growth are usually equivalent.

## THE POPULATION OF THE FUTURE, AND ITS IMPLICATIONS

What may be deduced about our demographic future from a knowledge of current demographic trends? An interesting, indeed intriguing, set of projections about the future may be entertained by setting forth a series of assumptions about the future course of fertility and mortality in each country of the world. If a number of dates in the future are set as alternative times when the countries will reach replacement-level fertility, while making additional assumptions about mortality, it is possible to predict when each country will stop growing in size, and how large each of them will be when this occurs.

## MEASURES OF REPRODUCTION AND LIFE EXPECTANCY

To carry out the above exercise, fertility and mortality measures somewhat more complex than the crude rates developed earlier are required. Rates are needed which provide information on the levels of fertility and mortality in populations without regard to their age structures. Measures particularly appropriate are, for fertility, the net reproduction rate, and, for mortality, the expectation of life at birth. For purposes of this discussion, these measures will be discussed only in a general way. These and other measures will be developed and examined more systematically in the next chapter.

The net reproduction rate (NRR) is a fertility measure which tells how many daughters born to the average woman in the population will reach, or survive to, childbearing age. This rate is independent of the population's age structure and illustrates the extent to which the population is reproducing itself. If the rate is about 1, the country's current generation of childbearers is having children at levels necessary to replace themselves with a

generation of about the same size, provided that the fertility and mortality conditions remain the same. If the rate is above 1, they are producing a generation larger than their own; if less than 1, a generation smaller. For instance, the net reproduction rate of the United States, in 1975, was 0.9, in Mexico, 2.8, and in the Federal Republic of Germany, 0.7 (6).

The mortality measure to be used in this exercise, years of life expected at birth, refers to the average number of years of life a newborn baby may expect to live. This measure is derived from the life table, and, like the net reproduction rate, is independent of the population's age structure. Column 10 of Appendix 1 provides life expectancy data for the various countries of the world. The values range from a high of 75 years, in Iceland, Norway, and Sweden, to a low of 38 years in a number of African countries.

Many countries today have net reproduction rates at replacement levels or lower, among them the United States, Canada, both Germanies, Denmark, Sweden, Finland, Japan, and others. However, most of these countries continue to grow, even though their childbearing women are not replacing themselves. Because of their previous demographic histories, acting through their current age structures, these countries have an excess number of potential parents. This means that even with below-replacement levels of fertility (i.e., NRRs of less than 1), more babies are born into the population in a year than members leave it through death. For example, the United States had 1.2 million more births than deaths in 1974, despite a net reproduction rate lower than the replacement level of 1. It is important to remember that populations with net reproduction rates at or below replacement levels are not automatically no-growth populations. Put in another way, countries with replacement, or below-replacement, levels of fertility are not necessarily stationary (i.e., zero population growth) countries. This also means that once a country reaches replacement-level fertility, it will not stop growing immediately. Since it often has one or more large generations of childbearers already built in, its numbers will continue to increase until its age structure becomes less conducive to growth, that is, until the proportion of its members in the older ages becomes larger, and the proportion of women in the childbearing ages becomes smaller (3).

## POPULATIONS PROJECTIONS

Given the above information, a set of four different projections about the future of the population of the world and its countries may be made, each one starting from demographic conditions as of 1970 (3). Each projection differs from the others with respect to when it is assumed that replacement-level fertility (an NRR of 1) is attained, and then maintained. Specifically, the first projection assumes that every country of the world reaches replacement-level fertility by 1980 to 1985, the second by 2000 to 2005, the third by 2020 to 2025, and the fourth by 2040 to 2045. Regarding mortality, expectation of life at birth is assumed to increase in each country between now and the first half of the next century. By 2045 to 2050, it is assumed to have stabilized at an average of 74 and 75 years, for females in the developing countries and in the world at large, respectively.

Assuming that replacement-level fertility will be attained by 1980 to 1985 (projection 1) (perhaps an unrealistic assumption, given current fertility levels), the population of the world would continue to increase until about the year 2100, when its size would peak at 6.4 billion (the population of the world in 1975 was estimated to be almost 4 billion—see Appendix 1). Projection 2 assumes that replacement-level fertility will be reached by the turn of the century, and, if countries follow this course, the world's population will continue to increase for another 100 years, reaching a maximum size, in the year 2100, of 8.4 billion. If replacement-level fertility is achieved by 2020 to 2025 (projection 3), the world will continue to grow until about the year 2120, and its total population then will be 11.2 billion. Finally, if the world does not arrive at an NRR of 1 until 2040 to 2045 (projection 4), it will not stop growing until about 2150, with a maximum population, then, of about 15.1 billion.

These projections show that the future size of the world's population, when it finally stops growing, could be anywhere from 6.4 billion to 15.1 billion. Of course, if the major assumption behind the fourth projection, that the world will reach replacement-level fertility by the years 2040 to 2045, is not met, then the world's population will continue growing beyond the year 2150 and will attain a size larger than 15.1 billion.

Although the above projections do not suggest the theoretically maximum size of the world's population, they do indicate the minimum attainable. If replacement-level fertility around the world is achieved by 1980, the world population will finally stop growing, more than 100 years later, with a population of about 6.4 billion, an increase of almost 2.5 billion over its present size. But this is hardly a realistic projection. Many countries of the world today show net reproduction rates of between 2 and 3: Algeria, Ghana, Southern Rhodesia, Honduras, Jamaica, Ecuador, Paraguay, Iraq, Lebanon, Pakistan, Thailand, and Turkey are only selected examples (see 6:518–527). With so many showing these rates, it is unreasonable to assume that all of the countries will be characterized by an average NRR of 1 in the few years between now and 1980 to 1985.

The second projection allows somewhat more time, until the turn of the century, for the countries to achieve replacement-level fertility. Given this situation, the world would grow in size until it reached a population of 8.4 billion. How reasonable is it to expect that this assumption will be met? Thomas Frejka, the architect of these model projections, provides an insightful response: this projection illustrates "developments that would take place if the demographic transition (mainly the fertility decline in the developing countries) were relatively fast and the change in fertility behavior from traditional to modern were attained within about one generation" (3:22).

Projections 3 and 4 may be more realistic expectations, in that they give more time in which the developing countries might reduce their fertility. But since they provide more lead time, there will be more than a corresponding increase in the numbers of children born in the interim periods. Hence, if replacement-level fertility is not reached until about the year 2020, the world will finally stop growing about 100 years later, with a total population of 11.2 billion (projection 3). If an additional 20 years is allowed before replacement-level fertility is attained, the world's total population will be 15.1 billion by the middle of the twenty-second century (projection 4). Frejka notes that this last projection signifies the kinds of developments "that might occur if the demographic transition in the developing countries were to take as much time as it did in Western Europe" (3:22).

Whatever the set of projections one chooses for focus, the preceding analysis, at the very least, helps to clarify the future, and the population growth potential, of the world. It illustrates well, within broad limits, what "can and cannot be expected to occur at least within the next 50 years or so" (2:201). Each country of the world, by virtue of its current age structure, has a certain potential for future population change in the years ahead, a potential for future growth which remains, even if replacement-level fertility were to occur immediately. Consideration of the above sets of population projections and their attendant assumptions helps to clarify this built-in momentum.

## TWO ALTERNATIVE SCENARIOS

Before leaving this discussion of the future of the world's population, let us compare the present world demographic situation with two scenarios for the future incorporating materials from the projections just described. These scenarios concern the distribution of populations in the future, and the relative size of populations in the developed and developing countries. It is already known that many countries are currently at, or near, replacement-level fertility. These constitute the majority of the countries of the developed world. A fairly reasonable assumption is that all of the developed world will reach replacement levels of fertility by 1985, as is assumed in the first set of projections. In this context, the developed world includes the countries of Europe, North America, Oceania, and the USSR.

Regarding the developing countries, the assumption of replacement fertility by 1985 is not at all a realistic one, as we have noted above. Perhaps the most optimistic scenario

finds the developing countries reaching replacement-level fertility by the period 2000 to 2005. A less optimistic alternative, but, some would argue, a more realistic one, gives the developing countries an additional 40 years to reach replacement-level fertility, as in Projection 4.

Given these alternatives, Table 13–1 compares the distributions of the populations of the major areas of the world in 1975 with two possibilities for the year 2150: the first alternative assumes that the countries of the developed world will have reached replacement-level fertility by the period 1980 to 1985, and that the countries of the developing world (the areas of East Asia, South Asia, Africa, and Latin America) will have reached replacement-level fertility by the period 2000 to 2005. The second alternative for the year 2150 assigns the same patterns for the developed countries as in the preceding, but assumes that the developing countries will have reached replacement-level fertility by the period 2040 to 2045. The data here are drawn from Frejka (4) and Peck (5).

Examining first the distributions of population in the world's areas by size, for the developing countries there is a substantial difference between the first and second alternatives for the year 2150. Moreover, the sizes, under both alternatives, are considerably greater than those in 1975. South Asia, with 1.2 billion in population in 1975, would increase to 3.2 billion by 2150, under alternative 1, or 7.2 billion under alternative 2. Latin America has a population of 324 million, in 1975, and it would increase to 824 million by 2150, under alternative 1, or 1.7 billion under alternative 2.

**Table 13–1. Distributions of Populations by Size and Percentage for Eight Major Areas of the World in 1975, and Two Alternatives for 2150**

| Area of world | 1975 | | 2150 (#1) | | 2150 (#2) | |
|---|---|---|---|---|---|---|
| | Size (millions) | Percentage | Size (millions) | Percentage | Size (millions) | Percentage |
| Total world | 3,967 | 100.0 | 8,267 | 100.0 | 15,644 | 100.0 |
| East Asia | 1,006 | 25.4 | 2,060 | 24.9 | 3,456 | 22.1 |
| South Asia | 1,249 | 31.5 | 3,163 | 38.3 | 7,197 | 46.0 |
| Europe | 473 | 11.9 | 591 | 7.1 | 591 | 3.8 |
| USSR | 255 | 6.4 | 336 | 4.1 | 336 | 2.2 |
| Africa | 401 | 10.1 | 933 | 11.3 | 2,008 | 12.8 |
| North America | 237 | 6.0 | 330 | 4.0 | 330 | 2.1 |
| Latin America | 324 | 8.2 | 824 | 10.0 | 1,696 | 10.8 |
| Oceania | 21 | 0.5 | 30 | 0.3 | 30 | 0.2 |

(Source of data: Frejka T: Reference Tables to the Future of Population Growth. New York, Population Council, 1973; Peck JM: Population Bulletin 29: October, 1974)

The populations of the developing countries under these two alternatives differ by a factor of about two. Allowing these countries an additional 40 years in which to reduce their fertility to replacement levels means that their populations will be twice as large then as they would have been if replacement-level fertility had been achieved by the turn of the century.

In 1975, one-fourth of the world's population resided in East Asia (principally in the People's Republic of China, and in Japan); nearly one-third in South Asia (mostly in India, Indonesia, Pakistan, and Bangladesh); and about one-tenth in Africa. The developed world (Europe, USSR, North America, and Oceania) contained about one-quarter of the world's population. Under the most optimistic demographic conditions (alternative 1), by the year 2150 the South Asian countries will have increased their representation to more than 38 per cent of the world's total, the Latin American countries to 10 per cent, and the African countries to more than 11 per cent. The other areas, including East Asia, will have decreased their respective proportions of the world's population—the European countries by more than four percentage points.

If the world's demographic future proves to be better approximated by the second alternative, in the year 2150 the patterns of change just described will be even more dramatic. The South Asian countries, with a population of more than 7 billion, will contain nearly one-half of the world's people. As already noted, the African and Latin American countries will more than double their populations over those which would have been obtained under the first alternative, but their proportions of the world's population will remain approximately the same. The other areas of the world will lose even greater shares of the world's population than would have been the case under the first alternative.

## MILITARY AND POLITICAL IMPLICATIONS

These differences in relative population size between the major areas of the world could have important military and political implications. Indeed, the balance of world power could well be changed by the year 2150, particularly if the second scenario is the operable one. Whichever alternative results, substantial alterations in the distribution of the world's population will occur, and these changes will surely have profound social, economic, and political implications. Of course, there is another possibility, and that is that major areas of the world, such as South Asia, will have neither the land base nor the potential for productivity and distribution to accommodate populations as large as those projected, especially under the second alternative. If this proves true, the populations will not increase quite as rapidly as assumed, but the cause will probably be increased mortality, rather than decreased fertility.

It would appear that the future course of the world's population depends, for the most part, upon the actions taken by the developing countries, assuming that currently low fertility levels in the developed world are maintained. Consequently, as Frejka has observed, in the demographically less developed countries, "the point in time when fertility levels approximating replacement are reached are crucial moments for the nature of their future long-term population growth. . . . 'The sooner the better' counts here more than in other fields. . . . The population growth potential of most less-developed countries is very high. . . . [Consequently], the eventual size of the population in the developing countries is closely related to the nature of their demographic transition: Will it be a matter of one generation or of two or more generations?" (2:201–202).

The preceding pages have attempted to introduce demographic aspects of population change. They were meant to illustrate the strategies followed, and the questions asked, by demographers in their quest for more knowledge regarding patterns of change in human populations.

## REFERENCES

1. Federation Internationale de Gynecologie et d'Obstetrique and The Population Council, Human Reproduction, Vol 2, Population. Cambridge, MIT Press, 1976
2. Frejka T: The Future of Population Growth: Alternative Paths to Equilibrium. New York, John Wiley & Sons, 1973
3. Frejka T: The prospects for a stationary world population. Sci Am 228:15, 1973
4. Frejka T: Reference Tables to the Future of Population Growth. New York, Population Council, 1973
5. Peck JM: World population projections: alternative paths to zero growth. Population Bulletin 29 (October), 1974
6. United Nations, Demographic Yearbook: 1975. New York, United Nations, 1976

# 14

# The Basic Population Model and the Data and Methods of Demography

**Dudley L. Poston, Jr.**
**Harley L. Browning**

The last chapter briefly considered the nature of demography. Although this book is primarily concerned with reproduction, it is necessary to address the broader areas of demography, because an understanding of what is truly distinctive about the discipline is needed. In the view of many people, including some demographers, the field of population is almost entirely descriptive in nature, consisting of little more than arrays of data taken from censuses and vital registers. Consequently, many social and biological scientists believe demography to be theoretically and analytically barren. Unfortunately, this misconception is fostered by the rather mundane, "bookkeeping" type of work that preoccupies some demographers. Our goal is to demonstrate that demography can, if properly conceived, be an analytically rigorous enterprise.

All disciplines have certain core features or central concerns by which they can be identified. In the case of demography, this core feature is the "basic population model." By model, we mean a specification of the key components of a system, how they are interrelated, and how they change through time. In other words, models should provide insight into the functioning of a given phenomenon. As we shall try to demonstrate, the basic population model is a general model of the features of a population, one that can be fruitfully applied to a wide range of subject matter. Its basic

logic is applicable to many problems in fields other than demography, and its potential has not been sufficiently exploited.

The specification of the population model relies heavily upon a seminal article by Norman Ryder, "Notes on the Concept of a Population" (2), where he follows the leads established decades ago by Alfred J. Lotka, who, as Ryder notes, is "the man most responsible for modern demography." Ryder's article succinctly describes the characteristics of the basic population model and then relates it to some of the central concerns of the social sciences: the nature of structure as opposed to process, the interrelation of micro (individual) and macro (aggregate) levels of analysis, and the study of social changes. He identifies the theme of his work as "the way in which the concept of a population forces the sociologist to give time a central place in his theory and research" (2:448).

The core of population study is formal demography. For Ryder (2:448), "[f]ormal demography is the deductive study of the necessary relationships between the quantities serving to describe the state of a population and those serving to describe changes in that state, in abstraction from their association with other phenomena." The key terms in this definition which identify the basic population model as fundamentally mathematical in nature are *deduction,* and *abstraction.* Both the strengths and the limitations of the model derive from these characteristics.

## ELEMENTS OF THE BASIC POPULATION MODEL

### DEFINITION OF A POPULATION

*A population is an aggregate of individuals defined in spatial and temporal terms* (2). An aggregate is not necessarily a group, which (in sociological terms) requires some forms of interpersonal interaction and the development of a sense of communality. Thus, all that is required to identify the population of the United States is to specify its territorial boundaries for some specific date or span of time. Subpopulations of the United States, such as Mexican Americans or women who are in the childbearing age range, are similarly identifiable.

### DYNAMIC QUALITY OF POPULATION ANALYSIS

*Population analysis inherently is dynamic, because attention automatically is focused on changes in the population in the course of time* (2). Because it is extremely rare for any particular population to be exactly constant in the course of time, change is taken for granted in population analysis, more so than in many areas of social science which rely on static analytical models.

Change in the size of a given population can be expressed by the "population equation" (already stated in the preceding chapter, in slightly different form):

$$\text{Population}_{\text{Time 2}} = \text{Population}_{\text{Time 1}} + (\text{Births-Deaths}) + (\text{Inmigration-Outmigration})$$

The population equation depicts a closed and determinate model, provided the area remains the same, since population change can take place *only* through the operation of the three basic demographic processes: fertility, mortality, and migration. Put differently, a population changes in terms of two forms of entry (births and inmigration) and two forms of exit (deaths and outmigration); therefore, no other variables need be considered. Of course, if one wishes to determine *why* fertility or mortality is at a certain level, or *why* in- and out-migration rates vary, many other variables must be introduced. But, as discussed later in this chapter, these are not the concerns of formal demography, but those of social demography.

### MICRO- AND MACRO-DYNAMIC QUALITIES

*The basic population model is both microdynamic and macrodynamic in nature* (2). This means that processes of change can be identified at both the individual and the aggregate level. Indeed, this distinction lies at the very heart of the population model, for it introduces Lotka's distinction between the persistence of the individual and the persistence of the aggregate. All human beings are born, live for some period of time, and then die. But an aggregate is not temporally limited, provided enough individuals continue to enter the population to replace those exiting: the aggregate is immortal. But aggregates, both in terms of the changes in numbers and characteristics of those entering and exiting, can experience changes not reducible to the individuals who constitute the population. To illustrate, individuals, upon entering a population (either by birth or immigration) can only "age" by becoming older, but the aggregate not only can become older —it can become "younger," provided that births exceed deaths, and inmigrants are younger than outmigrants. The racial composition of a neighborhood will change if more members of one race enter than of another race. Indeed, all human institutions and organizations (e.g., churches, schools, armies, clubs) can be conceived in these terms, and one way social change can be studied is by monitoring the compositional change caused by entrances and exits.

### THE LIFE CYCLE AND COHORT ANALYSIS

*Age is the key variable in demographic analysis, for it reflects the passage of time* (2). Age is subject to metric measurement; it thus provides a precise statement of the time spent by individuals within the population, as well as identifying changes in the aggregate. Demographers have developed two key concepts to deal with these age-related changes: the life cycle and the cohort. The former allows charting the life course of individuals in terms of key events, i.e., age of entry into and exit from formal education, entry into full-time employment and subsequent retirement, first marriage, births of first and last children. The cohort is a less commonly known concept and is defined as an aggregate of individuals who experience important events in their life cycles at the same time. The defining event generally is year of birth, but it could also be year of entry into college, year of birth of first child, or year of retirement, etc. Within this context, we can better appreciate Ryder's words (2:449): "Age as the passage of personal time is, in short, the link between the history of the individual and the history of the population."

Cohorts are valuable analytically because they are subpopulations intermediate between the behavior of individuals and that of the total population. Thus, in terms of birth cohorts, "the population at any moment in time is a cross-section of cohorts . . . stacked in uniformly staggered fashion, each atop its predecessor in time" (2:450). In the United States we customarily identify a Depression cohort, a World War II cohort, a baby-boom cohort, each representing groups of people born during different time periods, and each suggesting a different socioeconomic context for reproduction.

The central place of time in the demographic model is linked to the notion of an "at-risk" population (that is, the group or subgroup actually exposed to the risk of experiencing the event). By taking into account sex, one can calculate the number of births and the number of deaths within each age interval and time interval per person-year of exposure. Much of formal demography is occupied with working through the logico-mathematical relationships among these variables.

But where is migration in this formulation? It is excluded, because until now, formal demography has not yet been able to satisfactorily incorporate migration into a "complete deterministic model." The difficulty is not with outmigration, for conceptually it is similar to mortality, and the "risk" of outmigration can be determined for either the total population or various subpopulations. Inmigration, by contrast, cannot be subjected to such calculations. The risk of inmigration is not known, because the at-risk population itself is often unknown. Because of this limitation, formal demographic techniques are, strictly speaking, suitable only for "closed" populations, where migration is absent or plays a very minor role. Since most populations are not closed, this restricts the usefulness of formal demography in many situations.

Even given the limitations of this approach,

it is fair to say that in the last three decades some of the most impressive and enduring accomplishments in the field of population have been made in formal demography. Many features of the basic population model have been developed, and the fruitfulness of the demographic approach and its core concerns have been demonstrated.

## DATA AND METHODS OF DEMOGRAPHY

Having examined the basic population model, the focus of this chapter now is directed to a consideration of the data and methods of demography. What is the nature of the data used by demographers, and what kinds of procedures and methods are employed in the reduction, manipulation, and analysis of these data?

## SOURCES OF DEMOGRAPHIC DATA

There are three basic sources of demographic data: censuses, registers, and surveys. Censuses and registers may be distinguished from one another in that the former are conducted decennially (or quinquennially, in some countries) while the latter, theoretically at least, are compiled continuously. In fact, registration data are compiled and published annually or monthly.

### CENSUSES

A census may be defined as "the total process of collecting, compiling, and publishing demographic, economic, and social data pertaining, at a specified time . . . , to all persons in a country or delimited territory" (4:3). Its overall objective is to develop data and information on the size, composition, and distribution of the population in question. Thus a typical census will include data on the size of the population and subpopulations under study, as well as data on their sex and age composition and their educational composition (levels of illiteracy, levels of educational attainment, and extent of school attendance). Many censuses will also contain information on the economically active and inactive population (industrial and occupational composition of the active population). Other data often included pertain to country of birth and

| | | **1. WHAT IS THE NAME OF EACH PERSON** who was living here on Wednesday, April 1, 1970 or who was staying or visiting here and had no other home? | **2. HOW IS EACH PERSON RELATED TO THE HEAD OF THIS HOUSEHOLD?** |
|---|---|---|---|

**DO NOT MARK THIS COL-UMN**

*Print names in this order* — *Head of the household / Wife of head / Unmarried children, oldest first / Married children and their families / Other relatives of the head / Persons not related to the head*

**2.** *Fill one circle.*

*If "Other relative of head," also give exact relationship, for example, mother-in-law, brother, niece, grandson, etc.*

*If "Other not related to head," also give exact relationship, for example, partner, maid, etc.*

**(1)** Last name _____
First name _____ Middle initial
- ○ Head of household
- ○ Wife of head
- ○ Son or daughter of head
- ○ Other relative of head— *Print exact relationship* →
- ○ Roomer, boarder, lodger
- ○ Patient or inmate
- ○ Other not related to head— *Print exact relationship* ↗

**(2)** Last name _____
First name _____ Middle initial
- ○ Head of household
- ○ Wife of head
- ○ Son or daughter of head
- ○ Other relative of head— *Print exact relationship* →
- ○ Roomer, boarder, lodger
- ○ Patient or inmate
- ○ Other not related to head— *Print exact relationship* ↗

**(3)** Last name _____
First name _____ Middle initial
- ○ Head of household
- ○ Wife of head
- ○ Son or daughter of head
- ○ Other relative of head— *Print exact relationship* →
- ○ Roomer, boarder, lodger
- ○ Patient or inmate
- ○ Other not related to head— *Print exact relationship* ↗

**(4)** Last name _____
First name _____ Middle initial
- ○ Head of household
- ○ Wife of head
- ○ Son or daughter of head
- ○ Other relative of head— *Print exact relationship* →
- ○ Roomer, boarder, lodger
- ○ Patient or inmate
- ○ Other not related to head— *Print exact relationship* ↗

**(5)** Last name _____
First name _____ Middle initial
- ○ Head of household
- ○ Wife of head
- ○ Son or daughter of head
- ○ Other relative of head— *Print exact relationship* →
- ○ Roomer, boarder, lodger
- ○ Patient or inmate
- ○ Other not related to head— *Print exact relationship* ↗

**(6)** Last name _____
First name _____ Middle initial
- ○ Head of household
- ○ Wife of head
- ○ Son or daughter of head
- ○ Other relative of head— *Print exact relationship* →
- ○ Roomer, boarder, lodger
- ○ Patient or inmate
- ○ Other not related to head— *Print exact relationship* ↗

**(7)** Last name _____
First name _____ Middle initial
- ○ Head of household
- ○ Wife of head
- ○ Son or daughter of head
- ○ Other relative of head— *Print exact relationship* →
- ○ Roomer, boarder, lodger
- ○ Patient or inmate
- ○ Other not related to head— *Print exact relationship* ↗

**(8)** Last name _____
First name _____ Middle initial
- ○ Head of household
- ○ Wife of head
- ○ Son or daughter of head
- ○ Other relative of head— *Print exact relationship* →
- ○ Roomer, boarder, lodger
- ○ Patient or inmate
- ○ Other not related to head— *Print exact relationship* ↗

**9.** *If you used all 8 lines* —Are there any other persons in this household?     Yes     No
*Do not list the others; we will call to get the information.*

**10.** Did you leave anyone out of Question 1 because you were not sure if he should be listed—for example, a new baby still in the hospital, or a lodger who also has another home?     Yes     No
*On back page, give name(s) and reason left out.*

**FIG. 14–1.** U.S. Census of Population, 100% questionnaire.

| 3. SEX | 4. COLOR OR RACE | DATE OF BIRTH | | | 8. WHAT IS EACH PERSON'S MARITAL STATUS? |
|---|---|---|---|---|---|
| | | 5. Month and year of birth and age last birthday | 6. Month of birth | 7. Year of birth | |

Header details:

- **3. SEX** — Fill one circle
- **4. COLOR OR RACE** — Fill one circle. If "Indian (American)," *also give tribe.* If "Other," *also give race.*
- **5. Month and year of birth and age last birthday** — *Print*
- **6. Month of birth** — *Fill one circle*
- **7. Year of birth** — *Fill one circle for first three numbers* / *Fill one circle for last number*
- **8. WHAT IS EACH PERSON'S MARITAL STATUS?** — *Fill one circle*

*Make no mark in this margin*

Repeating person entry (×8):

| 3. SEX | 4. COLOR OR RACE | 5. Month / Year / Age | 6. Month of birth | 7. Year (first three) | 7. Year (last) | 8. Marital status |
|---|---|---|---|---|---|---|
| ○ Male ○ Female | ○ White ○ Negro or Black ○ Indian (Amer.) *Print tribe →* ○ Japanese ○ Chinese ○ Filipino ○ Hawaiian ○ Korean ○ Other– *Print race* | Month ___ Year ___ Age ___ | ○ Jan.-Mar. ○ Apr.-June ○ July-Sept. ○ Oct.-Dec. | ○ 186· ○ 187· ○ 188· ○ 189· ○ 190· ○ 191· ○ 192· ○ 193· ○ 194· ○ 195· ○ 196· ○ 197· | ○ 0 ○ 1 ○ 2 ○ 3 ○ 4 ○ 5 ○ 6 ○ 7 ○ 8 ○ 9 | ○ Now married ○ Widowed ○ Divorced ○ Separated ○ Never married |

*Make no mark in this margin*

---

**11.** Did you list anyone in Question 1 who is away from home now— for example, on a vacation or in a hospital?　Yes　No
*On back page, give name(s) and reason person is away.*

**12.** Did anyone stay here on Tuesday, March 31, who is not already listed?　Yes　No
*On back page, give name of each visitor for whom there is no one at his home address to report him to a census taker.*

26:1

citizenship of the population, their ethnic heritage, language, and religion (3, Vol. I).

In the actual enumeration of the population, censuses are conducted on either a de jure or de facto basis. In the case of a de jure enumeration, the census covers the entire territory of the country and all persons, according to their normal place of residence within the country. A *de facto* enumeration also covers the entire territory of the country, but categorizes each person in the population according to his geographical location on the day of the census undertaking.

Presented in Figure 14–1 is one of the questionnaires used in the 1970 United States Census of Population. This questionnaire was administered to all households in the country, and is hence known as the 100 per cent questionnaire. Other questionnaires used in the 1970 U.S. Census included questions on education, occupation, income, mobility, and other topics, but were administered only to samples of the population.

Census-taking had its origins in ancient Egypt, China, and Rome, among other places, although only a few of these enumerations have survived. Coverage was highly suspect, because women and children were seldom included; moreover, the objective of the censuses often was the determination of fiscal and military obligations (3, Vol. I). Today, censuses are important to the functioning of most governmental bodies. Indeed it has been estimated that during the decade between 1965 and 1974, about 55 per cent of the world's population had been enumerated (6). This estimate does not include the People's Republic of China, with nearly a quarter of the world's population; China last conducted a census in 1953.

### REGISTERS

Whereas censuses provide a cross-sectional portrayal of the size, composition, and distribution of the population, registration systems involve the identification of demographic events (typically, births and deaths) as they occur. While censuses are static in their administration, registers are dynamic and continuous.

Aside from a few known registrations in very early times, perhaps the most famous landmark in the history of registration systems is the 1532 English ordinance requiring that weekly Bills of Mortality be collected and published by the parishes of London. Shortly thereafter, weddings and baptisms were also recorded, and in 1563, the Council of Trent required that all parishes in Europe and in the New World maintain registers. Registration systems were required in Protestant parishes by the early 1600s (3, Vol I).

Registration systems today are usually confined to the events associated with the demographic processes of fertility and mortality: live births, deaths, marriages, and divorces. Registration systems involving geographic mobility (migration within countries) are largely restricted to the Scandinavian countries, some Eastern European countries, and the Far East. As an example of an actual registration certificate, Figure 14–2 is a copy of a death certificate currently in use in Texas. Similar certificates are used for the registration of the other events.

### SAMPLE SURVEYS

Demographers frequently employ a third type of data source, sample surveys, often because censuses and registration systems do not always contain the extensive kinds of information needed to address some of the more critical demographic questions. This is particularly true regarding the analysis of fertility. Therefore, surveys are often conducted in order to collect more detailed information. By administering these surveys to a carefully selected sample of the larger population, demographers are better able to uncover underlying patterns in demographic behavior than would be possible with materials from censuses and registration systems.

An important research program currently under way in many countries of the world involves the organization, development, and analysis of sample surveys focusing on fertility. The World Fertility Survey is a massive collective effort to gather high-quality data on fertility levels and fertility regulation in 35 developing, and 17 developed countries. Moreover, 14 additional developing countries are expected to participate in the World Fertility Survey at a later point in time. The questionnaires contain, minimally, items regarding individual women's pregnancies, births, marital history, and use and knowledge of contraceptive procedures and methods. Information on the backgrounds of both husband and wife is

CERTIFICATE OF DEATH

STATE OF TEXAS   STATE FILE NO.

1. PLACE OF DEATH
   a. COUNTY

2. USUAL RESIDENCE (Where deceased lived. If institution: residence before admission)
   a. STATE   b. COUNTY

b. CITY OR TOWN (If outside city limits, give precinct no.)   c. LENGTH OF STAY in 1 b.   c. CITY OR TOWN (If outside city limits, give precinct no.)

d. NAME OF (If not in hospital, give street address) HOSPITAL OR INSTITUTION   d. STREET ADDRESS (If rural, give location)

e. IS PLACE OF DEATH INSIDE CITY LIMITS?   YES ☐   NO ☐   e. IS RESIDENCE INSIDE CITY LIMITS?   YES ☐   NO ☐   f. IS RESIDENCE ON A FARM?   YES ☐   NO ☐

3. NAME OF DECEASED (Type or print)   (a) First   (b) Middle   (c) Last   4. DATE OF DEATH

5. SEX   6. COLOR OR RACE   7. Married ☐   Never Married ☐   Widowed ☐   Divorced ☐   8. DATE OF BIRTH   9. AGE (In years last birthday)   IF UNDER 1 YEAR Months | Days   IF UNDER 24 HRS. Hours | Minutes

10a. USUAL OCCUPATION (Give kind of work done during most of working life, even if retired)   10b. KIND OF BUSINESS OR INDUSTRY   11. BIRTHPLACE (State or foreign country)   12. CITIZEN OF WHAT COUNTRY?

13. FATHER'S NAME   14. MOTHER'S MAIDEN NAME

15. WAS DECEASED EVER IN U.S. ARMED FORCES? (Yes, no, or unknown) (If yes, give war or dates of service)   16. SOCIAL SECURITY NO.   17. INFORMANT

18. CAUSE OF DEATH [Enter only one cause per line for (a), (b), and (c).]   INTERVAL BETWEEN ONSET AND DEATH
   PART I. DEATH WAS CAUSED BY:
   IMMEDIATE CAUSE (a)_____
   Conditions, if any, which gave rise to above cause (a), stating the underlying cause last.   DUE TO (b)_____
   DUE TO (c)_____
   PART II. OTHER SIGNIFICANT CONDITIONS CONTRIBUTING TO DEATH BUT NOT RELATED TO THE TERMINAL DISEASE CONDITION GIVEN IN PART I(a)   19. WAS AUTOPSY PERFORMED?   YES ☐   NO ☐

20a. ACCIDENT ☐   SUICIDE ☐   HOMICIDE ☐   20b. DESCRIBE HOW INJURY OCCURRED. (Enter nature of injury in Part I or Part II of Item 18.)

20c. TIME OF INJURY   Hour   Month   Day   Year   a.m.   p.m.

20d. INJURY OCCURRED   WHILE AT WORK ☐   NOT WHILE AT WORK ☐   20e. PLACE OF INJURY (e.g., in or about home, farm, factory, street, office building, etc.)   20f. CITY, TOWN, OR LOCATION   COUNTY   STATE

21. I hereby certify that I attended the deceased from_____ 19_____ to_____ 19_____ and last saw the deceased alive on_____ 19_____ Death occurred at_____ m. on the date stated above, and to the best of my knowledge, from the causes stated.

22a. SIGNATURE   (Degree or title)   22b. ADDRESS   22c. DATE SIGNED

23a. BURIAL, CREMATION, REMOVAL (Specify)   23b. DATE   23c. NAME OF CEMETERY OR CREMATORY

23d. LOCATION   (City, town, or county)   (State)   24. FUNERAL DIRECTOR'S SIGNATURE

25a. REGISTRAR'S FILE NO.   25b. DATE REC'D BY LOCAL REGISTRAR   25c. REGISTRAR'S SIGNATURE

— BUREAU OF VITAL STATISTICS   TEXAS DEPARTMENT OF HEALTH   MEDICAL CERTIFICATION   VS-112, REV. 1/58

**FIG. 14–2.** Texas certificate of death.

also collected. Beyond these core items, most countries include additional questions on such topics as fertility regulation, family planning, abortion, and factors other than contraception which are known to affect fertility. To date (late 1978) ten developing nations have published the preliminary results of their surveys (5).

Having considered the basic sources of demographic data, attention is now directed to the methods of demography. Mortality methods will be examined first, and then fertility methods.

## BASIC DEMOGRAPHIC METHODS

Numerous procedures exist for quantifying the various concepts used by demographers (3). In this section, only the most basic methods are covered, principally those which receive the greatest attention from demographers and lay persons alike. The reader is directed to Shryock and Siegel (3), where approaches for measuring the various and assorted components of composition and distribution, as well as migration, are comprehensively discussed.

**MORTALITY METHODS**

In this section, the crude death rate (CDR), the age-specific death rate (ADR), the standardized death rate (SDR), and the life table will be covered. Calculations for rates of any kind are based on the following formula:

$$\text{Rate} = (\frac{E}{PR})k, \qquad (1)$$

where $E$  is the number of events occurring over a particular time period (usually 1 year);

$PR$ is the number of persons exposed to the risk of the event occurring to them during the time period;

$k$  is a constant, usually 1000.

When $E$ is divided by $PR$, and the resulting fraction multiplied by $k$, the result indicates the rate at which the event occurs to every $k$ persons (for example, 1000 persons) over the course of the time period studied. Greater accuracy is achieved as the denominator is increasingly restricted to those persons in the population who are actually exposed to the particular event, (the population "at risk")— for example, individuals within a particular age group. The following discussion describing differences between the crude and the age-specific death rates illustrates this point.

**The Crude Death Rate.** Numerator data for the study of mortality are often obtained from death-certificate tabulations, a product of population registration systems. Those data on mortality events (the $E$ in equation 1) may be related to population data taken from censuses (the $PR$ in equation 1 or 2). The resulting rate, known as the *crude death rate* (CDR), may be represented as follows:

$$CDR = (\frac{D}{PR})k, \qquad (2)$$

where $D$  is the number of deaths occurring in a population over a given period (usually 1 year);

$PR$ is the size of the population at the mid-point of the time interval;

$k$  is a constant of 1000.

The crude death rate represents the number of deaths occurring over a given period per 1000 members of the entire population. It must be interpreted with extreme caution, especially when comparisons are made between countries, because it is greatly affected by the age composition of the population. It is thus a very rough measure of the population's mortality level. It is commonly expected, for example, that the death rate will be lower in developed countries, such as the United States, than in underdeveloped countries, because of differences in health and general living conditions. However, a comparison of crude death rates among certain countries may not follow this pattern: e.g., a country with a higher percentage of young people might have a lower death rate than a country with a high percentage of old people, regardless of level of development.

Look, for example, at Appendix 1. Crude death rates are listed for most countries in the world as of approximately 1978. Mexico is a very young country: 46 per cent of its population is under 15 years of age. Its crude death rate of 8 is very low, yet its per capita gross national product is much less than that of the United States. (See the last column of the Appendix.) The United States has a crude death rate of 9.4, a rate of more than one death per 1000 *greater* than that of Mexico. This apparent anomaly is explained by differences in age structure: the median age in the United States is about 29 years, and only 24 per cent of its population is under 15 years of age. In other words, the United States has a higher crude death rate than Mexico because there are, proportionately, more older persons in its population.

**Age-specific Death Rates.** In order to account for age distribution, demographers frequently compute death rates for each of the population's age groups. The age-specific death rate for age group $a$ ($ASDR_a$) may be represented as follows:

$$ASDR_a = \frac{D_a}{PR_a} \times k, \qquad (3)$$

where $D_a$  is the number of deaths occurring to persons of age $a$ over a given time period (usually 1 year);

$PR_a$ is the mid-year number of persons in the population of age $a$;

$k$  is a constant of 1000.

The age-specific death rate represents the number of deaths of persons of a particular age over a given period, per 1000 members in the population of that age. ASDRs computed for each age, or age group, in the population may be referred to as a schedule of age-specific death rates.

Schedules of age-specific death rates for Taiwan and for the United States, circa 1960, are found in Table 14-1. In Taiwan, there were approximately 7.9 deaths for every 1000 persons in the 1 to 4 year age group, compared to 1.1:1000 in that age group in the United States. The reader should inspect the age-specific death rates for the remaining age groups, and compare Taiwan with the United States. The data in this table indicate that, at every age, the age-specific death rates were lower in the United States than they were in Taiwan.

Observe now the crude death rates as of 1960, listed at the base of the table, which indicate that the United States had a higher (not a lower) crude death rate than Taiwan. Why is this so? Taiwan is much like Mexico with respect to age composition. Taiwan had a lower crude death rate than the United States because its population was younger.

The crude death rate is merely a weighted average of a schedule of age-specific death rates; the weights are the proportions of the population at each age. For this reason, the magnitude of the crude death rate is greatly influenced by age distribution.

**Standardized Death Rates.** Crude death rates would not be an appropriate measure of mortality differences in two populations, particularly if their respective age structures are known, or thought to be, dissimilar. Schedules of age-specific death rates could be used, but these could prove to be cumbersome, because so many figures must be handled and compared. A summary measure, without the methodological constraints of the crude death rate, is the standardized death rate (SDR). This approach computes a weighted average of the age-specific rates in a given population, using as weights the age distribution of a standard population. The formula is:

$$SDR = \Sigma \ ASDR_a \left( \frac{P_a}{P} \right), \qquad (4)$$

where $P_a$ is the proportion of persons of age $a$ in a standard population; and

$$P = \Sigma P_a$$

To illustrate, death rates in India will be compared with those in Sweden. The appropriate measure of mortality in this situation is one which employs age-specific death rates, but not the actual populations of the given countries, because they are so dissimilar with respect to age. A standard, such as the age distribution in the population of the world, is substituted for both populations, and is used as the base from which to calculate age-specific death rates. The rates of these two countries may now be compared, with the assurance that age differences do *not* account for any part of the difference in these rates. (Sex is another basis for standardization; age-sex-standardized death rates could also be computed.) Table 14-2 illustrates the age-standardized death rate procedure.

**The Life Table.** The final topic to be discussed in this section is a statistical model of mortality known as the life table. It is used generally in studies of longevity and population growth, "as well as in making projections of population size and characteristics and in studies of widowhood [and] orphanhood. . . . In the simplest form of the life table, the entire table is generated from age-specific mortality rates. . . ." (3, Vol. II:429).

Table 14-3 illustrates a life table for white

**Table 14-1. Age-Specific Death Rates: Taiwan and the United States, 1960**

| Age | Taiwan 1960 ASDR | U.S. 1960 ASDR |
|---|---|---|
| Under 1 | 32.4 | 27.0 |
| 1-4 | 7.9 | 1.1 |
| 5-9 | 1.1 | 0.5 |
| 10-14 | 0.8 | 0.4 |
| 15-19 | 1.4 | 0.9 |
| 20-24 | 2.3 | 1.2 |
| 25-29 | 2.2 | 1.3 |
| 30-34 | 2.8 | 1.6 |
| 35-39 | 3.6 | 2.3 |
| 40-44 | 5.0 | 3.7 |
| 45-49 | 6.6 | 5.9 |
| 50-54 | 10.8 | 9.4 |
| 55-59 | 17.1 | 13.8 |
| 60-64 | 25.5 | 21.4 |
| 65-69 | 41.1 | 31.4 |
| 70-74 | 63.9 | 46.9 |
| 75-79 | 99.6 | 71.3 |
| 80-84 | 199.5 | 115.7 |
| 85+ | | 196.3 |
| Crude death rate | 6.9 | 9.5 |

(Source of data: Shryock HS, Siegel JS: The Methods and Materials of Demography, Vol. 2. Washington, D.C., U.S. Government Printing Office, 1975, p 401)

**Table 14–2. Illustration of Procedure for Standardizing Death Rates for India and Sweden, Using Composition of the World as Standard**

| | Standard population (world in mid-1960, in proportions) | Age-specific death rates (ASDRs) | | Expected deaths in standard population | |
|---|---|---|---|---|---|
| | | India | Sweden | India | Sweden |
| | A | B | C | A × B = D | A × C = E |
| Under 1 year | .030 | 164.9 | 15.3 | 4.947 | .459 |
| 1–4 years | .111 | 23.1 | 1.0 | 2.564 | .111 |
| 5–14 years | .226 | 4.4 | 0.4 | .994 | .090 |
| 15–24 years | .181 | 6.2 | 0.7 | 1.122 | .127 |
| 25–44 years | .261 | 9.8 | 1.3 | 2.558 | .339 |
| 45–64 years | .146 | 23.3 | 7.7 | 3.402 | 1.124 |
| 65–74 years | .032 | 64.8 | 32.7 | 2.074 | 1.046 |
| 75 years and over | .013 | 159.6 | 119.9 | 2.075 | 1.559 |
| Total | 1.000 | — | — | 19.736 | 4.835 |

Standardized rate (SDR): India = Σ D = 19.7.    Sweden = Σ E = 4.8.
(Source of data: Bogue D: Principles of Demography. New York, Wiley & Sons, 1969, p 552)

**Table 14–3. Part 1: Life Table for White Males: United States, 1969–1971**

| Age Interval | Proportion dying | Of 100,000 born alive | | Stationary population | | Average remaining lifetime |
|---|---|---|---|---|---|---|
| Period of life between two ages (1) | Proportion of persons alive at beginning of age interval dying during interval (2) | Number living at beginning of age interval (3) | Number dying during age interval (4) | In the age interval (5) | In this and all subsequent age intervals (6) | Average number of years of life remaining at beginning of age interval (7) |
| $x$ to $x + t$ | $_tq_x$ | $l_x$ | $_td_x$ | $_tL_x$ | $T_x$ | $\overset{\circ}{e}_x$ |
| Days | | | | | | |
| 0–1 | 0.00892 | 100,000 | 892 | 273 | 6,793,828 | 67.94 |
| 1–7 | .00527 | 99,108 | 522 | 1,625 | 6,793,555 | 68.55 |
| 7–28 | .00139 | 98,586 | 138 | 5,668 | 6,791,930 | 68.89 |
| 28–365 | .00462 | 98,448 | 454 | 90,686 | 6,786,262 | 68.93 |
| Years | | | | | | |
| 0–1 | .02006 | 100,000 | 2,006 | 98,252 | 6,793,828 | 67.94 |
| →1–2 | .00116 | 97,994 | 114 | 97,937 | 6,695,576 | 68.33 |
| 2–3 | .00083 | 97,880 | 81 | 97,840 | 6,597,639 | 67.41 |
| 3–4 | .00072 | 97,799 | 71 | 97,763 | 6,499,799 | 66.46 |
| 4–5 | .00059 | 97,728 | 57 | 97,700 | 6,402,036 | 65.51 |
| 5–6 | .00054 | 97,671 | 52 | 97,645 | 6,304,336 | 64.55 |
| 6–7 | .00051 | 97,619 | 50 | 97,594 | 6,206,691 | 63.58 |
| 7–8 | .00048 | 97,569 | 47 | 97,546 | 6,109,097 | 62.61 |
| 8–9 | .00044 | 97,522 | 43 | 97,500 | 6,011,551 | 61.64 |
| 9–10 | .00039 | 97,479 | 38 | 97,460 | 5,914,051 | 60.67 |
| 10–11 | .00034 | 97,441 | 32 | 97,425 | 5,816,591 | 59.69 |
| 11–12 | .00032 | 97,409 | 32 | 97,393 | 5,719,166 | 58.71 |
| 12–13 | .00039 | 97,377 | 38 | 97,358 | 5,621,773 | 57.73 |
| 13–14 | .00055 | 97,339 | 54 | 97,313 | 5,524,415 | 56.75 |
| 14–15 | .00080 | 97,285 | 77 | 97,246 | 5,427,102 | 55.79 |
| 15–16 | .00107 | 97,208 | 104 | 97,156 | 5,329,856 | 54.83 |
| 16–17 | .00134 | 97,104 | 130 | 97,039 | 5,232,700 | 53.89 |
| 17–18 | .00156 | 96,974 | 152 | 96,897 | 5,135,661 | 52.96 |

**Table 14–3. (Continued)**

| Age Interval | Proportion dying | Of 100,000 born alive | | Stationary population | | Average remaining lifetime |
|---|---|---|---|---|---|---|
| Period of life between two ages (1) | Proportion of persons alive at beginning of age interval dying during interval (2) | Number living at beginning of age interval (3) | Number dying during age interval (4) | In the age interval (5) | In this and all subsequent age intervals (6) | Average number of years of life remaining at beginning of age interval (7) |
| $x$ to $x + t$ | $_tq_x$ | $l_x$ | $_td_x$ | $_tL_x$ | $T_x$ | $\overset{o}{e}_x$ |
| 18–19 | .00172 | 96,822 | 167 | 96,739 | 5,038,764 | 52.04 |
| 19–20 | .00181 | 96,655 | 175 | 96,568 | 4,942,025 | 51.13 |
| 20–21 | .00190 | 96,480 | 183 | 96,388 | 4,845,457 | 50.22 |
| 21–22 | .00201 | 96,297 | 193 | 96,200 | 4,749,069 | 49.32 |
| 22–23 | .00205 | 96,104 | 198 | 96,005 | 4,652,869 | 48.42 |
| 23–24 | .00203 | 95,906 | 195 | 95,809 | 4,556,864 | 47.51 |
| 24–25 | .00195 | 95,711 | 187 | 95,618 | 4,461,055 | 46.61 |
| 25–26 | .00184 | 95,524 | 175 | 95,436 | 4,365,437 | 45.70 |
| 26–27 | .00173 | 95,349 | 165 | 95,267 | 4,270,001 | 44.78 |
| 27–28 | .00165 | 95,184 | 157 | 95,105 | 4,174,734 | 43.86 |
| 28–29 | .00162 | 95,027 | 154 | 94,950 | 4,079,629 | 42.93 |
| 29–30 | .00165 | 94,873 | 157 | 94,795 | 3,984,679 | 42.00 |
| 30–31 | .00170 | 94,716 | 161 | 94,635 | 3,889,884 | 41.07 |
| 31–32 | .00176 | 94,555 | 167 | 94,471 | 3,795,249 | 40.14 |
| 32–33 | .00183 | 94,388 | 173 | 94,302 | 3,700,778 | 39.21 |
| 33–34 | .00192 | 94,215 | 181 | 94,125 | 3,606,476 | 38.28 |
| 34–35 | .00203 | 94,034 | 191 | 93,939 | 3,512,351 | 37.35 |
| 35–36 | .00217 | 93,843 | 204 | 93,741 | 3,418,412 | 36.43 |
| 36–37 | .00235 | 93,639 | 219 | 93,529 | 3,324,671 | 35.51 |
| 37–38 | .00256 | 93,420 | 239 | 93,300 | 3,231,142 | 34.59 |
| 38–39 | .00281 | 93,181 | 262 | 93,050 | 3,137,842 | 33.67 |
| 39–40 | .00310 | 92,919 | 288 | 92,775 | 3,044,792 | 32.77 |
| 40–41 | .00340 | 92,631 | 315 | 92,474 | 2,952,017 | 31.87 |
| 41–42 | .00372 | 92,316 | 343 | 92,144 | 2,859,543 | 30.98 |
| 42–43 | .00409 | 91,973 | 377 | 91,785 | 2,767,399 | 30.09 |
| 43–44 | .00452 | 91,596 | 414 | 91,389 | 2,675,614 | 29.21 |
| 44–45 | .00501 | 91,182 | 457 | 90,953 | 2,584,225 | 28.34 |
| 45–46 | 00555 | 90,725 | 504 | 90,473 | 2,493,272 | 27.48 |
| 46–47 | .00612 | 90,221 | 552 | 89,945 | 2,402,799 | 26.63 |
| 47–48 | .00673 | 89,669 | 603 | 89,368 | 2,312,854 | 25.79 |
| 48–49 | .00739 | 89,066 | 658 | 88,737 | 2,223,486 | 24.96 |
| 49–50 | .00812 | 88,408 | 718 | 88,049 | 2,134,749 | 24.15 |
| 50–51 | .00892 | 87,690 | 782 | 87,300 | 2,046,700 | 23.34 |
| 51–52 | .00980 | 86,908 | 852 | 86,482 | 1,959,400 | 22.55 |
| 52–53 | .01081 | 86,056 | 930 | 85,591 | 1,872,918 | 21.76 |
| 53–54 | .01194 | 85,126 | 1,016 | 84,618 | 1,787,327 | 21.00 |
| 54–55 | .01318 | 84,110 | 1,109 | 83,556 | 1,702,709 | 20.24 |
| 55–56 | .01452 | 83,001 | 1,205 | 82,399 | 1,619,153 | 19.51 |
| 56–57 | .01594 | 81,796 | 1,304 | 81,144 | 1,536,754 | 18.79 |
| 57–58 | .01745 | 80,492 | 1,404 | 79,790 | 1,455,610 | 18.08 |
| 58–59 | .01906 | 79,088 | 1,508 | 78,334 | 1,375,820 | 17.40 |
| 59–60 | .02077 | 77,580 | 1,611 | 76,775 | 1,297,486 | 16.72 |
| 60–61 | .02258 | 75,969 | 1,716 | 75,111 | 1,220,711 | 16.07 |
| 61–62 | .02451 | 74,253 | 1,820 | 73,344 | 1,145,600 | 15.43 |
| 62–63 | .02657 | 72,433 | 1,924 | 71,471 | 1,072,256 | 14.80 |
| 63–64 | .02879 | 70,509 | 2,030 | 69,494 | 1,000,785 | 14.19 |
| 64–65 | .03120 | 68,479 | 2,136 | 67,411 | 931,291 | 13.60 |

**Table 14-3. (Continued)**

| Age Interval | Proportion dying | Of 100,000 born alive | | Stationary population | | Average remaining lifetime |
|---|---|---|---|---|---|---|
| Period of life between two ages (1) | Proportion of persons alive at beginning of age interval dying during interval (2) | Number living at beginning of age interval (3) | Number dying during age interval (4) | In the age interval (5) | In this and all subsequent age intervals (6) | Average number of years of life remaining at beginning of age interval (7) |
| $x$ to $x + t$ | $_tq_x$ | $l_x$ | $_td_x$ | $_tL_x$ | $T_x$ | $\overset{o}{e}_x$ |
| 65–66 | .03386 | 66,343 | 2,246 | 65,220 | 863,880 | 13.02 |
| 66–67 | .03674 | 64,097 | 2,355 | 62,919 | 798,660 | 12.46 |
| 67–68 | .03977 | 61,742 | 2,456 | 60,514 | 735,741 | 11.92 |
| 68–69 | .04284 | 59,286 | 2,540 | 58,016 | 675,227 | 11.39 |
| 69–70 | .04597 | 56,746 | 2,608 | 55,442 | 617,211 | 10.88 |
| 70–71 | .04916 | 54,138 | 2,662 | 52,807 | 561,769 | 10.38 |
| 71–72 | .05262 | 51,476 | 2,708 | 50,122 | 508,962 | 9.89 |
| 72–73 | .05655 | 48,768 | 2,758 | 47,389 | 458,840 | 9.41 |
| 73–74 | .06118 | 46,010 | 2,815 | 44,603 | 411,451 | 8.94 |
| 74–75 | .06647 | 43,195 | 2,871 | 41,759 | 366,848 | 8.49 |
| 75–76 | .07231 | 40,324 | 2,916 | 38,866 | 325,089 | 8.06 |
| 76–77 | .07843 | 37,408 | 2,934 | 35,941 | 286,223 | 7.65 |
| 77–78 | .08472 | 34,474 | 2,921 | 33,014 | 250,282 | 7.26 |
| 78–79 | .09103 | 31,553 | 2,872 | 30,117 | 217,268 | 6.89 |
| 79–80 | .09749 | 28,681 | 2,796 | 27,283 | 187,151 | 6.53 |
| 80–81 | .10466 | 25,885 | 2,709 | 24,530 | 159,868 | 6.18 |
| 81–82 | .11273 | 23,176 | 2,613 | 21,870 | 135,338 | 5.84 |
| 82–83 | .12127 | 20,563 | 2,494 | 19,316 | 113,468 | 5.52 |
| 83–84 | .13012 | 18,069 | 2,351 | 16,894 | 94,152 | 5.21 |
| 84–85 | .13942 | 15,718 | 2,191 | 14,623 | 77,258 | 4.92 |
| 85–86 | .15033 | 13,527 | 2.034 | 12,510 | 62,635 | 4.63 |
| 86–87 | .16321 | 11,493 | 1,875 | 10,555 | 50,125 | 4.36 |
| 87–88 | .17666 | 9,618 | 1,699 | 8,768 | 39,570 | 4.11 |
| 88–89 | .18947 | 7,919 | 1,501 | 7,169 | 30,802 | 3.89 |
| 89–90 | .20145 | 6,418 | 1,293 | 5,771 | 23,633 | 3.68 |
| 90–91 | .21344 | 5,125 | 1,094 | 4,579 | 17,862 | 3.49 |
| 91–92 | .22684 | 4,031 | 914 | 3,574 | 13,283 | 3.30 |
| 92–93 | .24152 | 3,117 | 753 | 2,740 | 9,709 | 3.12 |
| 93–94 | .25767 | 2,364 | 609 | 2,060 | 6,969 | 2.95 |
| 94–95 | .27426 | 1,755 | 481 | 1,514 | 4,909 | 2.80 |
| 95–96 | .29014 | 1,274 | 370 | 1,089 | 3,395 | 2.67 |
| 96–97 | .30431 | 904 | 275 | 766 | 2,306 | 2.55 |
| 97–98 | .31784 | 629 | 200 | 529 | 1,540 | 2.45 |
| 98–99 | .33085 | 429 | 142 | 358 | 1,011 | 2.36 |
| 99–100 | .34324 | 287 | 98 | 238 | 653 | 2.27 |
| 100–101 | .35479 | 189 | 67 | 155 | 415 | 2.20 |
| 101–102 | .36553 | 122 | 45 | 100 | 260 | 2.13 |
| 102–103 | .37550 | 77 | 29 | 62 | 160 | 2.08 |
| 103–104 | .38471 | 48 | 18 | 39 | 98 | 2.02 |
| 104–105 | .39320 | 30 | 12 | 24 | 59 | 1.98 |
| 105–106 | .40101 | 18 | 7 | 15 | 35 | 1.94 |
| 106–107 | .40818 | 11 | 5 | 8 | 20 | 1.90 |
| 107–108 | .41475 | 6 | 2 | 5 | 12 | 1.86 |
| 108–109 | .42075 | 4 | 2 | 3 | 7 | 1.82 |
| 109–110 | .42624 | 2 | 1 | 2 | 4 | 1.79 |

(National Center for Health Statistics: United States Life Tables: 1969–1971. DHEW Publication No. (HRA) 75-1150. Washington, D.C.: U.S. Government Printing Office, 1975)

males in the population of the United States for the period from 1969 to 1971. Observe that there are seven columns for the life table. Using this life table as an example, each of the columns may be defined as follows:

*Column 1: Age interval x to x + t.* This column refers to the interval in years between two birthdays. The sixth row of the life table in column one is 1–2, and refers to that period of life between the first and second birthdays. Entries on the life table for the 1–2 group refer to that portion of the population who are between their first and second birthdays. (The *x* used in the life table refers to the age on the birthday at the beginning of the interval.)

*Column 2: Proportion dying($_t q_x$).* This is the proportion of the population alive at the beginning of the age interval who will die before reaching the end of the age interval. Again referring to age interval 1–2, column 2 for this age group informs us that .00116 of the persons alive at the beginning of this interval will die before reaching their second birthday. The data in this column are determined from age-specific death rates. For most of the age groups in the population, except for the very oldest and the very youngest (where special considerations and calculations are needed (see 3, Vol. II:433–443), the probability of dying (the $_t q_x$ function) may be determined with the following formula:

$$_t q_x = \frac{ASDR_x}{1 + \frac{1}{2} ASDR_x} \tag{5}$$

*Column 3: Number living at the beginning of the age interval ($l_x$).* This column refers to the number alive at the beginning of the age interval. It represents the difference between column 3 and column 4 of the *preceding age interval.* Turning to age interval 1–2, 97,994 is the difference between column 3 and column 4 in the age interval 0–1, or 97,994 = 100,000 minus 2,006. The table thus indicates that for each 100,000 white males born in the United States, 97,994 were living at the beginning of age interval 1–2.

*Column 4: Number dying during the age interval ($_t d_x$).* This column refers to the number of persons who will die during the age interval. Column 4 equals column 2 multiplied by column 3 of the *same age interval.* Turning to age interval 1–2, 114 equals .00116 multiplied by 97,994. The table thus indicates that 114 persons will die after their first birthday, but before they reach their second birthday.

*Column 5: Stationary population in the age interval ($_t L_x$).* This column refers to the number of years lived by the life-table cohort (which begins with 100,000 members at birth) during the age interval. Once again referring to age interval 1–2, 97,937 years were lived by the life-table cohort during this interval. This figure is less than the number in the life-table cohort at the beginning of the age interval ($l_1 = 97,994$) because some members of the cohort died during the interval. Values of $_t L_x$ are not calculated directly, but follow a series of formulas depending upon the age of the group (see 3:433–443, for further information).

*Column 6: Stationary population in this and all subsequent age intervals ($T_x$).* This is the sum of the number of years lived by the life-table cohort at this and all subsequent ages. In general terms,

$$T_x = \sum_{i\ =\ x}^{\infty} {}_t L_x \tag{6}$$

One can also obtain the $T_x$ value by using both columns 5 and 6 with the following formula:

$$T_x = T_{x+1} + {}_t L_x \tag{7}$$

Referring to age interval 1–2, and using formula 7, we note that $T_1$ is 6,695,576. This number equals $T_2$ (6,597,639) + $_t L_1$ (97,937).

*Column 7: Average remaining lifetime ($e_x$).* This column refers to the average number of years that persons in the age interval may expect to live. This column is also known as life expectancy. Column 7 equals column 6 divided by column 3 of the same age interval. Referring again to age interval 1–2, 68.33 (column 7) is obtained by dividing 6,695,576 (column 6) by 97,994 (column 3). The table thus suggests that persons in this age group can expect to live on the average an additional 68.33 years beyond their first (or *x*th) birthday.

**FERTILITY METHODS**

There are numerous procedures for quantifying the fertility of a population. In this section, the crude birth rate (CBR), the general fertility rate (GFR), the age-specific fertility rate (ASFR), the total fertility rate (TFR), the gross reproduction rate (GRR), and the net reproduction rate (NRR) will be examined.

**The Crude Birth Rate.** As with the crude death rate, the numerator data for the CBR are derived from birth-certificate tabulations, and the denominator data are usually taken from census enumerations. The formula for the crude birth rate is as follows:

$$CBR = \left(\frac{B}{PR}\right) k, \qquad (8)$$

where $B$ is the number of births occurring in the population over a given period of time (usually 1 year);

$PR$ is the size of the population at the mid-point of the time interval;

$k$ is a constant of 1000.

The crude birth rate represents the number of births occurring in the population over a given time interval, usually 1 year, per 1000 members of the population. Lay persons employ the CBR more often than any other fertility measure, but it is one of the most inaccurate. The denominator is not really indicative of the population exposed to the risk of the event: all males, prepuberty females, women past the childbearing age, and other women who cannot have children are included. Because of this inadequacy, the CBR, like the CDR, should be interpreted with caution.

**The General Fertility Rate.** Demographers frequently refer to rates more refined than the crude birth rate. A rate which employs a denominator better approximating the population exposed to the risk of childbearing (that is, the event of birth) is the general fertility rate (GFR). It is obtained by dividing the number of births recorded in the population during a specified time interval, usually 1 year, by the total number of females between the ages of 15 and 49 in that population at the mid-point of the given time interval, and then multiplying the result by a constant of 1000. The formula for the general fertility rate is:

$$GFR = \frac{B}{P_{f\,(15-49)}} k \qquad (9)$$

where $B$ is the number of births occurring in the population over a given period of time (usually 1 year);

$P_{f(15-49)}$ is the number of females between the ages of 15 and 49 in the population at the mid-point of the time interval;

$k$ is a constant of 1000.

The GFR may be interpreted as the number of births in the population during a certain year per 1000 women of childbearing age. The GFR thus is more representative of the true fertility situation than the CBR. The principal limitation of the GFR is that it does not consider differences in the age distribution of women 15 to 49 among different populations. For example, if two populations (A and B) were compared, and population A proportionately had more women in ages 20 to 29 (the prime childbearing ages) than population B, and the fertility rates in corresponding age groups were generally equivalent, population A would nonetheless have a higher general fertility rate (GFR) than population B. Since fertility varies by age, a fertility rate which accounts for differences in age distribution is required.

**Age-specific Fertility Rates.** One satisfactory approach is to compute fertility rates for the specific age groups of the population of women exposed to the risk of childbearing. Fertility rates of this type are known as age-specific fertility rates. They may be computed for each individual age group of women in the 15 to 49 year category—for example, a fertility rate specific for women aged 23 years. More commonly, age-specific fertility rates are computed for each of the seven five-year age groups of women in the following childbearing years: 15–19, 20–24, 25–29, 30–34, 35–39, 40–44, 45–49.

The general formula for the age-specific fertility rate for age group $a$ (any one of the specific age groups) is:

$$ASFR_a = \frac{B_a}{P_{f(a)}} \times k \qquad (10)$$

where $B_a$ is the number of births in the population over a given period of time to women in age group $a$ (where $a$ is one of seven five-year age groups, 15–19, 20–24, . . . 45–49);

$P_{f(a)}$ is the number of women in age group $a$ in the population at the mid-point of the time interval;

$k$ is a constant of 1000.

Table 14–4 contains data on the number of births in the population of Texas in 1970 by age of mother. Column 4 of this table repre-

#### Table 14-4. Age-specific Fertility Rates: Texas, 1970

| Age group (1) | Number of births to women of specified age (2) | Number of women of specified age (3) | ASFR (4) |
|---|---|---|---|
| 15–19 | 46,526 | 538,518 | 86.4 |
| 20–24 | 90,106 | 484,457 | 186.0 |
| 25–29 | 56,337 | 386,051 | 145.9 |
| 30–34 | 23,697 | 330,031 | 71.8 |
| 35–39 | 10,616 | 322,428 | 32.9 |
| 40–44 | 3,104 | 334,311 | 9.3 |
| 45–49 | 224 | 324,786 | 1.0 |

(Source of data: Texas State Department of Health: Texas Vital Statistics, 1970, Austin, Texas; United States Bureau of the Census: 1970 Census of Population. PC(1)-B45. Texas, Washington, D.C., U.S. Government Printing Office, 1971)

sents the age-specific fertility rates for each of the seven age groups; it shows clearly that fertility varies with age. For every 1000 women in the 20–24 year age group, there were 186 births. For the age group 40–44, there were slightly more than 9 births.

The ASFRs are particularly useful in the two following respects: (*1*) they reveal the pattern and extent of the age differential in childbearing; (*2*) they are the raw material for many of the remaining fertility measures, including the total fertility rate (TFR).

The data in the first three columns of Table 14–4 also allow the computation of the general fertility rate. Following the formula for the GFR previously presented, $B$ is obtained by summing the seven figures in column 2 ($B = 230,610$); $P_{f(15-49)}$ is obtained by summing the seven figures in column 3 (2,720,-582). $B$ is divided by $P$, and the result is multiplied by 1000, yielding a figure of 84.8. This number means that for every 1000 women between the ages of 15 and 49 living in Texas in 1970, there were 84.8 births.

**The Total Fertility Rate.** Rather than using a schedule of age-specific fertility rates to reflect the fertility performance of a population, demographers frequently employ a summary rate. One of the more frequently used is the total fertility rate (TFR).

The TFR is an estimate of the number of children a cohort of 1000 women would bear if they all went through their reproductive years (ages 15–49) exposed to the age-specific fertility rates in effect in a population at a specified time. The formula for the total fertility rate is the following:

$$TFR = \Sigma(ASFR)\,t \qquad (11)$$

where $ASFR$ is the age-specific fertility rate for

each group of women in the childbearing years;

$t$ is the width of the age interval; if the age groups are 15–19, 20–24, ... 45–49, then the width of these age groups, or $t$, would be 5.

To compute this rate for a particular population at a particular time, the age-specific fertility rates for the age groups are added; the result is then multiplied by the interval into which the age groups are divided. For example, if the population is divided into age groups by five-year intervals, one adds the ASFRs for these (ASFR for 15–19 + ASFR for 20–24 + ASFR for 25–29 ... + ASFR for 45–49), and then multiplies the result by 5, the age-group interval.

Returning to the data and rates in Table 14–4, the sum of the seven age-specific fertility rates is 533.3; it is multiplied by 5, yielding a TRF of 2666.5. This number means that if 1000 women passed through their childbearing years exposed to the age-specific fertility rates characteristic of Texas women in 1970, they would bear 2666.5 babies, or 2.67 children per woman. The TFR is generally regarded as the best single cross-sectional measure of fertility, because it is rather closely restricted to the childbearing population and is not influenced by differences in age structures. Thus TFRs of different countries may be validly compared.

**The Gross Reproduction Rate.** The gross reproduction rate (GRR) is a refinement of the total fertility rate in that it is concerned only with female births, that is, the births of future childbearers. The gross reproduction rate may be determined by multiplying the total fertility rate by the proportion of births

**Table 14–5. Net Reproduction Rate Computation: Texas, 1970**

| Age group (1) | ASFR × 5 (2) | $B_f/B$ (3) | $1_x/1_0$ (4) | Columns (2) × (3) × (4) (5) |
|---|---|---|---|---|
| 15–19 | 0.432 | 0.4878 | 0.97636 | 0.205 |
| 20–24 | 0.930 | 0.4878 | 0.97331 | 0.442 |
| 25–29 | 0.730 | 0.4878 | 0.96996 | 0.345 |
| 30–34 | 0.359 | 0.4878 | 0.96554 | 0.169 |
| 35–39 | 0.165 | 0.4878 | 0.95996 | 0.077 |
| 40–44 | 0.046 | 0.4878 | 0.95097 | 0.021 |
| 45–49 | 0.003 | 0.4878 | 0.93793 | 0.001 |
| | | | Net Reproduction Rate (NRR) = | 1.260 |

that are female. The formula for the gross reproduction rate is:

$$GRR = TFR \times \frac{B_f}{B} \qquad (12)$$

where *TFR* is the total fertility rate;

$B_f$ is the number of female births; and

$B$ is the number of total births.

Since about 105 males are born for every 100 females, $B_f/B$ is usually 0.4878 (1).

**The Net Reproduction Rate.** A further refinement of the total fertility rate is the net reproduction rate, a measure of generational replacement. It may be defined as "the number of daughters that would be born to a cohort of newborn girls during their lifetimes assuming the continuation of the age-specific fertility and mortality rates of a given year. Unlike the total fertility rate, it also takes into account the fact that some women will die before or during the reproductive age span (1:11). As an index of generational replacement, an NRR of 1 indicates that on the average each female produces one female who herself survives to the age of parenthood.

The net reproduction rate may be determined by multiplying each age-specific fertility rate by the proportion of female births to all births; this number is then multiplied by the proportion of daughters surviving to the age indicated for each of the age-specific fertility rates. The NRR is calculated by summing these results. The formula for the net reproduction rate is:

$$NRR = \Sigma \left( ASFR \times \frac{B_f}{B} \times \frac{l_x}{l_0} \right) \qquad (13)$$

where *ASFR* is the age-specific fertility rate;

$B_f/B$ is the proportion of female births to all births; and

$l_x/l_0$ is the probability of surviving to age *x* for females.

Table 14–5 provides the information needed for computing, and thus illustrating, the net reproduction rate. The age-specific fertility rates are taken from Table 14–4 before multiplying them by the constant of 1000. They are multiplied here by the width of the interval, 5. Since data are not directly available for sex of babies by age of mother, the constant 0.4878, which indicates the proportion of all births that were female, has been used. The probability of surviving to each age $(l_x/l_0)$ has been computed for each age category with life-table data for females in the United States, 1969 to 1971, published by the National Center for Health Statistics. (These life-table data are also the basis for the female portion of the life tables presented in Table 14–3). According to Table 14–5, the net reproduction rate in Texas in 1970 was 1.260, a figure slightly above the level (1.0) needed for replacement.

**REFERENCES**

1. Bouvier LF: U.S. population in 2000—zero growth or not? Population Bulletin 30, December, 1975
2. Ryder NB: Notes on the concept of a population. Am J Soc 69:447, 1964
3. Shryock HS, Siegel JS: The Methods and Materials of Demography. Washington DC, US Government Printing Office, 1971
4. United Nations: Principles and Recommendations for National Population Censuses. New York, United Nations, 1958
5. Vaessen M: World fertility survey: The current situation. Int Fam Plann Perspect Dig 4:73, 1978
6. Weeks J: Population: An introduction to Concepts and Issues. Belmont, Cal, Wadsworth, 1978

# 15

# The Demographic Transition

**Harley L. Browning**
**Dudley L. Poston, Jr.**

*In traditional societies, fertility and mortality are high. In modern societies, fertility and mortality are low. In between, there is the demographic transition (3).*

Behind this innocuous statement lie some of the central problems of our time, involving the nature, significance, and timing of development. The demographic transition involves a profound change in the nature of societies and their organization. No known society has ever entered the third stage of low fertility and low mortality without also becoming industrialized and "modern." As will be demonstrated, the most problematic feature of the demographic transition is fertility change. At times, fertility analysis appears to be ahistorical and limited to the micro levels involving only individuals and couples, i.e., studying the effects of education and female participation in the labor force on family size. This is a legitimate mode of analysis, but a sense of the broad sweep of history, of the various levels of development, and of their effects on demographic processes, is also necessary.

## WHAT IS THE DEMOGRAPHIC TRANSITION?

Instead of describing the temporal sequence of the demographic transition in the customary way, by presenting a generalized depiction of the demographic transition model, reference is made to two concrete cases, Denmark and Korea. The former is an example of a European country that has completed the transition, whereas Korea is an Asian Third World

country very much in the middle, transitional stage.

### DENMARK

In Figure 15–1, the crude birth and death rates from Denmark are plotted for more than one and one-half centuries, from 1800 to 1970. At the beginning of the period, the birth rate was a bit over 30, and it fluctuated narrowly in the lower 30s until about 1885, after which it dropped, with occasional interruptions, to about 15:1000 in 1970. The death rate also was near 30:1000 in 1800, but showed great swings (reflecting the effects of contagious disease) until about 1870, although the trend line was declining. In the last 100 years, it has rather smoothly dropped to 10:1000, or less, showing less variation than the birth rate.

### KOREA

Korea is shown in Figure 15–2 as an example of a developing country for the period 1910 to 1975 (the data are for all of Korea through 1945; thereafter, only for South Korea). As is usual with developing countries, the time interval is much shorter than for Western European countries. Despite lack of data, it is known that prior to 1910, births and deaths were in a state of near equilibrium, appropriate to the first stage of the demographic tran-

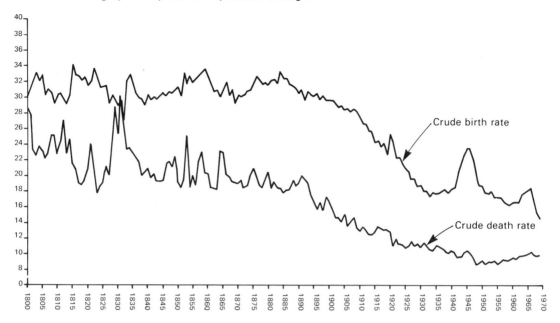

**FIG. 15-1.** Annual crude birth rates and crude death rates (per 1000 population) Denmark, 1800–1970. (Source of data: Mitchell, BR: European Historical Statistics, 1750–1970. New York, Columbia Univ. Press, 1976, pp. 105–121)

sition. When Korea was annexed by Japan, in 1910, two things happened: the birth rate rose from 38:1000 to about 45:1000 in 1930, and the death rate declined from 37:1000 to about 25:1000. Both trends were a response to Japanese colonial practices. The political stability introduced was an important factor in the rise of the birth rate; the death rate declined primarily in response to programs in hygienic and medical services initiated by the Japanese. The birth rate fell somewhat during the 1940s, and then rose sharply after the end of the Korean war, probably due to delayed unions and the reunion of couples separated during the war. From a high of 45:1000 in 1960, the birth rate dropped more than a third to 29 in 1975, one of the sharpest declines within the Third World. The birth rate nonetheless remained high relative to the death rate (9:1000). The resultant rapid rates of population growth places South Korea in the transitional stage.

## HOW DOES THE TRANSITION OCCUR?

All countries have their own particular historical development which affects the form of their demographic transition. However, the cases of Denmark and Korea are helpful in making generalizations that fit relatively well-developed countries, on the one hand, and developing countries, on the other.

The Danish patterns clearly show that the death rate in earlier periods demonstrated extreme fluctuations, for brief intervals even rising above the birth rate, due to the effects of disease and famine. Since 1900, the curve has smoothed out, displaying only small fluctuations. The birth rate showed much less fluctuation in the early period, but then demonstrated a very striking "blip" representing the post-World War II baby boom. Unfortunately, the Korean case begins very late (1910), so the first stage of the demographic transition cannot be plotted. Almost no developing countries have adequate statistics for this stage.

Fertility levels in the developing countries generally are appreciably higher than those in the European countries were before the decline. In Denmark, the birth rate fluctuated within the lower thirties for many years. Korea, with a reported birth rate of 38:1000, in 1910, was on the low side, but it reached a high of 45:1000 in 1930 and 1960. A number of countries—Rwanda and Zambia, to cite two African examples—have birth rates today of 50:1000 or above (see Appendix 1).

The reductions in mortality are occurring much more rapidly in the developing coun-

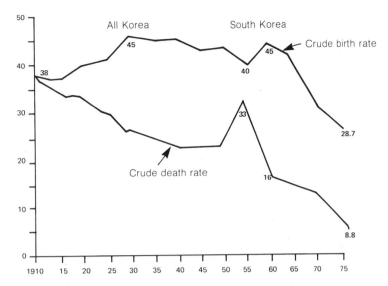

**FIG. 15–2.** Crude birth rates and death rates (per 1000 population) Korea, 1910–1975. (Source of data: Kwon TH, et al.: The Population of Korea. Seoul, Seoul National University, 1975. Rates for 1975 taken from Population Reference Bureau: World Population Data Sheet, 1975)

tries than they did in the European countries. There is nothing remotely comparable in European history to the decline in the death rate in South Korea from about 25:1000, in 1950, to 9:1000, in 1975. Again, put in rough terms, the amount of decline currently occurring in developing countries took three to four times as long in Europe.

A number of Western European countries had a safety valve during the period of their most rapid rate of growth which is not available to developing nations. They sent out tens of millions of their citizens as emigrants to other parts of the world, primarily to the New World.

As a consequence of the above generalizations, we conclude that developing countries in the transitional stage are experiencing considerably faster rates of population growth than the now developed countries did when they passed through the comparable period. In general terms, developing countries have per-annum rates of growth of 3 per cent or more, whereas European countries had rates of only about one-half this figure (8).

## WHY DOES THE TRANSITION OCCUR?

Until now, aspects of the "how" of the demographic transition, particularly questions relating to the magnitude and tempo of mortal-

ity and fertility decline, have been addressed. These are very important considerations, but are limited to the descriptive level of analysis. For an adequate understanding of the demographic transition, it is necessary to go beyond the demographic variables into the realm of social structure.

### DENMARK

The period from the mid-1700s to the mid-1900s was a time when Denmark changed from an agricultural to an industrial country. In 1801, only 20 per cent of the population lived in towns and cities, whereas by 1965, 63 per cent of the population was urban. In 1801, 76 per cent of the labor force was engaged in agriculture; by 1965, this figure had dropped to 14 per cent. Income per capita (in fixed prices) quadrupled between 1870 and 1960. Compulsory education was institutionalized in the early 1800s (8). These structural changes are generally characteristic of Northwestern Europe during this period.

### KOREA

Korean demographic change was influenced by a different set of factors. Japanese colonial rule, as already noted, had a major impact, particularly with regard to preventing infectious diseases. Quarantines were enforced at the seaports to prevent epidemic diseases from entering the country. Preventive programs were also initiated for tuberculosis and small-pox; vaccination was enforced at the local level in 1915; and public hospitals were established in each province. The development of transportation networks, mainly railways, facilitated the distribution of goods and services throughout the country and thus, indirectly, was an important factor in the mortality decline (5).

After World War II, the South Korean economy deteriorated and the colonial-built health systems collapsed, but it was the Korean war which dramatically increased the death rate. The large reduction in deaths after the war was in many ways a response to the dissemination of antibiotics and programs introduced by United Nations agencies. Unlike the mortality declines in Europe, which were brought about jointly by medical and public health innovations and a rise in level of living, in South Korea the major part of the decline was due to externally introduced improvements in medicine and public health. This pattern is characteristic of Third World countries.

The drop in the birth rate was unusually great between 1960 and 1975 and is attributable to various factors. Infant mortality decreased significantly, and couples gradually realized that they no longer needed to give birth to many children in order to have a reasonable number survive to adulthood. Moreover, with increasing urbanization, children become more of a liability than the asset they had been in rural settings. Family planning programs, eventually to include abortion, were instituted in 1962. Their services and target groups have expanded, and they have become more widely accepted by the population as a whole (5).

**A GENERALIZED TREATMENT**

Denmark and Korea may serve as the basis for a more general discussion of the "why" of the demographic transition. It is doubtful that one can properly speak of a theory of the demographic transition which satisfies scientific canons, but in the last 30 years or so, a fairly large literature on the subject has developed (4, 8). Basically, the argument for the first stage of the demographic transition hinges on population survival: high fertility is necessary

because mortality is high. Consequently, societies have to develop a variety of beliefs and practices that are supportive of high reproductive levels. These are primarily centered on family and kinship organization.

The forces of modernization have altered the conditions of this state of near-equilibrium. (We use the term *equilibrium* in a qualified sense; population growth at the societal and global levels did take place, but so slowly that it required thousands of years for the earth's population to double, prior to the beginning of the Industrial Revolution in 1650.) The effect first was experienced as a decline in mortality. (See Chaps. 18 and 19 for a different perspective.) There is agreement that the beginnings of mortality decline in Europe were stimulated not so much by medical or public health innovations as by a general improvement in levels of living. In the last century, of course, control of contagious disease achieved remarkable success. Moreover, control programs could be introduced to countries by outside international agencies with very little structural change required internally.

The intermediate stage of the demographic transition generated very rapid rates of population growth, because the level of fertility remained high for some time after mortality had declined substantially. The "gap" appears to have lasted longer, but was narrower for the European countries than for now developing countries. Because the latter have not completed the process to the third stage, where both fertility and mortality are low, it is uncertain how long their gap will last.

The reasons for both the decline of mortality and the consequent drop in fertility are often stated in general terms; that is, modernization, industrialization, and urbanization are evoked. Although it is true that fully industrialized and urbanized societies do have relatively low mortality and fertility, these concepts are too broad and inclusive to illuminate the specific ways by which the declines were brought about.

Although the factors inducing the decline in mortality had, until recently, seemed evident—industrialization improved the overall standard of living, and this was accompanied by significant improvements in medicine, personal hygiene, and public health—there is now a continuing debate as to what were the key factors, even concerning a country with some of the best historical data—England. McKeown (7) argues that for nineteenth-century England, improvements in nutrition were instrumental in reducing the death rate. His contention that medical services, personal hygiene, and public health efforts had virtually no effect in the early phase of the decline has not been widely accepted. There simply is insufficient evidence at this time, even for England, to resolve the issue, and for other countries the situation is even more obscure.

The causal linkages for fertility are perhaps even more complex. Underlying the global concepts of industrialization and urbanization are such specific determinants of fertility as women's participation in the labor force, and the role of the family. Most commentators stress the manner by which the normative, institutional, and economic supports for the large family were eroded, and the small family became predominant. The increasing importance of urbanization affects the family by altering its role in production: compared to rural families, the urban family is less often the unit of production, and the value of children is considerably lessened. At the same time, urban families must meet considerably higher demands for consumption by their children, especially for education and recreation. In brief, those changes reduce the economic value of children and increase their cost (4) (see Chaps. 19 and 22).

Unfortunately, it is difficult, if not impossible, to obtain adequate data on the value and cost of children over long periods of time, as is possible with trends in urbanization. Family reconstruction studies have undeniably furthered our understanding of European communities, but they can provide explanation only to a certain point, beyond which the only recourse is inference. The European Fertility Study, under the direction of Ansley Coale, at Princeton, has for years conducted careful studies for a number of countries, utilizing subnational provincial units. Results indicate that the generalized interpretation of the demographic transition is not always appropriate—the fact that in France fertility began to decline *before* much urbanization or industrialization occurred is a particularly striking exception—and the whole matter is much more complex than had been anticipated (4).

### CHANGE AND RESPONSE

Davis (2) interprets the demographic transition within a framework of "change and response," that is, "not only continuous but also reflexive and behavioral." By *reflexive*, he means that a decline in mortality will have an impact on fertility. He specifies *behavioral* because individuals and couples must continually make decisions in terms of certain goals and then act to achieve them. Davis believes that couples seek "to avoid relative loss of status," especially in economic dimensions, and that when past successes in controlling mortality are perceived as threatening family status, couples resort to a variety of means to control their fertility. In his analysis of fertility trends in post-World War II Japan, he argues that the Japanese "quickly postponed marriage, embraced contraception, began sterilization, utilized abortions and migrated outward" (2:349). This "multiphasic" response facilitated a fertility decline in 40 years that took at least 60 years in the United States. In Ireland the pattern of responses was different, with large-scale out-migration, delayed marriage, and celibacy assuming great importance. Davis emphasizes the complexity of responses followed, but the motivating force which he stresses is the "fear of invidious deprivation."

## APPLICATION OF DEMOGRAPHIC-TRANSITION THEORY TO DEVELOPING COUNTRIES

Knowledge of demographic-transition experiences may only have limited, if not ambiguous, application for developing countries (8). There are certain differences between the developed and developing countries which appear to represent obstacles to the timely and "natural" decline of fertility in the latter. Other differences appear to favor or encourage rapid and prompt fertility decline in developing countries. A review of these two types of differences will explain Teitelbaum's (8) conclusion that the application of demographic-transition theory to developing countries may not be appropriate, and that predictions based upon it will vary with the factors considered.

### DIFFERENCES NOT FAVORING RAPID FERTILITY DECLINE

Differences between developed and developing countries which militate *against* a rapid decline in the developing countries include the following (some of which have already been discussed): *1*) the rapid mortality declines in the developing countries "have often resulted largely from imported technologies which can be transferred with relative ease and are only marginally related to the pace and level of general development" (8:422). *2)* Fertility levels in the developing countries today are higher than they were in European countries prior to the transitions. *3)* The higher-than-average rates of population growth occasioned by death rates lower than birth rates were often mitigated in the European countries by international migration, an outlet not available today at the same levels to the developing countries. *4)* Owing to the above differences, rates of population increase are significantly higher in the developing countries than they were at similar periods in the European world. *5)* The developing countries have much younger populations, because of their higher birth rates, than did the developed countries at similar periods. Hence they are characterized by far greater momentum for additional growth. As Teitelbaum notes, "even in the unlikely event that fertility in developing countries declined *within the next decade* to the 'replacement level' now characteristic of developed countries, the population of the developing world would nonetheless continue to grow for 60 to 70 years, and by the year 2050 would have reached a size nearly 90 per cent greater than its 1970 level" (8:423). *6)* There are fewer opportunities in developing countries for occupational and rural-to-urban mobility than there were in the European countries when they experienced their transitions. These opportunities provided alternative life styles and are believed to have had an influence on family and reproductive values. In developing countries today, however, the higher natural increase has produced a much greater demand for nonagricultural employment than can be met. *7)* Opportunities for female participation in the labor force in the developing countries are more limited than they were in the European countries. *8)* Owing to their high birth rates, the developing countries are experiencing difficulties in expanding their educational facilities so that all those who are eligible may be served. "This means deferment of the goals of universal education, along with its hypothesized effects upon fertility behavior in transition" (8:423). In theory, these factors appear to argue against an orderly and "natural" decline of fertility in the developing countries.

## DIFFERENCES FAVORING RAPID FERTILITY DECLINE

The differences between Europe's and the developing countries' transition experiences which may facilitate a more rapid fertility decline in the latter include the following: *1)* social and economic development has been more rapid in some developing countries than was the case in Europe. To the extent that these advances accelerate fertility decline, some developing countries should anticipate a swift completion of their demographic transition. *2)* The developing countries have significantly more advanced and effective contraceptive and abortion technologies available to them than did the European countries during their transition years. *3)* In nineteenth-century Europe, the "large" family was the norm throughout the world. "In contrast, the 'demonstration effect' of the European transition has provided modern legitimacy for the small family norm and evidence that its achievement is feasible. . . ." (8:423). *4)* Government leaders today are more aware than their nineteenth-century predecessors of the effects which large populations have on national development. Indeed, many developing countries are engaging in economic and demographic planning and forecasting, endeavors that received little attention in nineteenth-century Europe. *5)* International assistance programs (through the United Nations and related types of agencies) are available today to provide outside resources and expertise to developing countries. These facilities were not available during the European transitions. *6)* There is some demographic evidence in developing countries that where fertility decline has been experienced, the pace has been more rapid than was the case in Europe. This more rapid decline may be due to factors such as those just addressed.

There is little doubt that there are important differences between pretransition Europe and developing countries today. Depending upon which differences the analyst wishes to accentuate, future fertility decline in the developing countries may be predicted as more, or less, rapid and orderly than it was in Europe. Its pace, and rate, of change will vary if one set of differences plays a greater role than another. Hence Teitelbaum's suggestion that the European transition experiences provide ambiguous, or, at best, limited guidance about the course of fertility in the developing world.

## CALDWELL'S RESTATEMENT OF TRANSITION THEORY

Recently, Caldwell has called for a "restatement" of demographic-transition theory (1). His research experience is not in Europe, but in sub-Saharan Africa in general, and in Ghana in particular. He believes that the "conventional wisdom" of the theory has led to "an inadequate understanding of the way in which birth levels first begin to fall," and this, in turn, has produced "unnecessary hysteria about the likely long-term size of the human race. . . ." (1:321).

Although Caldwell is not entirely clear on this point, he maintains that "emotional" nucleation of the family is crucial for lower fertility. Emotional nucleation occurs when parents become "less concerned with ancestors and extended family relatives than they are with their children, their children's future, and even the future of their children's children" (1:352). In many Third World countries, he feels that this will be brought about by "westernization," specifically, by importing the western conception of the family.

Caldwell maintains that to say that people in developing countries are "irrational" because they continue to have large families is to profoundly misunderstand these societies; fertility behavior is rational in virtually all societies, regardless of their level of development. He argues that there are fundamentally two types of societies: "the first where the economically rational response is an indefinitely large number of children and the second where it is to be childless" (1:322). But why, from an economic point of view, should couples want either an unlimited number of children or none at all? Caldwell explains that it depends upon the direction of intergenerational flows of wealth and services. If the flows run from children to their parents or other

adults, it is entirely rational for parents to want to have large families. In "modern" societies, where the flow is from parents to children, small families are to be expected (see Chaps. 19 and 22).

Caldwell believes that the importation into the Third World of this "concept of the predominance of the nuclear family with its strong conjugal tie [as well as the] concept of concentrating concern and expenditures on one's children, . . . ." is absolutely necessary. The penetration of family nucleation and "the reversal of the intergenerational wealth flow . . . into the Third World in the next half century, almost inevitably . . . will *guarantee* slower global population growth" (1:356, [italics added]).

In setting forth Caldwell's basic ideas, we have not attempted to demonstrate that his view is the correct one, but rather to suggest that although the demographic transition is a basic feature of social change, more investigation is needed before demographers fully understand why it occurs.

## REFERENCES

1. Caldwell JC: Toward a restatement of demographic transition theory. Pop Dev Rev 2:321, 1976
2. Davis K: The theory of change and response in modern demographic history. Pop Index 29:345, 1963
3. Demeny P: Early fertility decline in Austria-Hungary: a lesson in demographic transition. Daedalus 97:502, 1968
4. Knodel J, van de Walle E: Lessons from the past: policy implications of historical fertility studies. Pop Dev Rev 5:217, 1979
5. Kwon H, Lee H, Chang Y, Yu E: The Population of Korea. Seoul, South Korea, Population and Development Studies Center, Seoul National University, 1975
6. Matthiessen PC: Some Aspects of the Demographic Transition in Denmark. Copenhagen, Denmark, Kobenhavns Universitets Rond Til Tilvejebringelse Af Laeremidler, 1970
7. McKeown T: The Modern Rise of Population. New York, Academic Press, 1976
8. Teitelbaum MS: Relevance of demographic transition theory for developing countries. Science 188:420, 1975

# 16

# Planned Intervention in Population Change

**Harley L. Browning**
**Dudley L. Poston, Jr.**

Since the origins of nation states, governments and their leaders in one way or another have had to evaluate the human resources of their countries, including their distribution and the changes brought about by varying death and birth rates. However, only recently have large-scale efforts been introduced through which governments intervene directly in the operation of population processes.

## FACTORS ACCOUNTING FOR INTERVENTION OR NONINTERVENTION

There are several reasons why governments have been slow in attempting to deal directly with population factors. For one thing, information has been lacking; censuses have not been common until relatively recently, and they often are taken only at long time intervals, thus reducing their effectiveness as instruments for planning policy. Moreover, governments often have not had the kind of comprehensive organization and skilled personnel that facilitate the manipulation of population factors. Leaders have been ignorant of the role of population variables, partly because of the lack of information, but also because demography has not emerged as a distinct specialty until recently; indeed, demographers still do not occupy high positions in the hierarchy of governmental advisors.

There is also considerable variation in terms of the willingness and ability of governments to deal with the three main population variables: fertility, mortality, and migration. Of

the three, governments have put their greatest efforts into the control of mortality. Saving lives is unambiguously positive, and no government has ever avowed other than a policy of mortality reduction. There is, however, great variation in governmental commitment of funds and personnel toward this end.

Migration has been the object of governmental intervention, but most frequently under crisis conditions. War is one prominent occasion where there have been massive transfers of populations across national borders and sometimes within countries. Religious and political persecutions have also led to significant population redistribution. In none of these cases, however, is migration, whether international or internal, part of a long- or intermediate-term plan for population change. The impetus, in other words, comes from other sources. Increasingly, population redistribution is viewed as integral to national policies for economic growth and development, but the actual administrative mechanisms available to affect redistribution in any precise manner are limited. Totalitarian countries, by their very nature, should be able to monitor and affect population distribution, but even where citizens are subject to close control and surveillance by means of identity and food-ration cards, it has not been easy to regulate migration. Truly effective population policies must always have something of a coercive feature about them if they are to be completely successful. But governments, whatever their political natures, have been reluctant to put their coercive powers to use for population ends, except in such clear-cut instances as the effort to control contagious disease.

Nowhere is this more evident than with respect to fertility. Unlike mortality, where there is near unanimity in fostering programs that will reduce the risk of death, there is no consensus regarding fertility control. There are many reasons why fertility control is such a sensiti e issue, often a source of such contentiousness and bitterness that government officials avoid it as a "no-win" situation; however, the primary factor appears to be that reproduction lies at the core of the values, practices, and norms that affect one of society's most central and important institutions, the family.

Until recently, the partial and inconsistent efforts by the state to intervene in the reproductive practices of their populations have largely been pronatalist—that is, the concern has been to increase, rather than retard, the rate of population growth through various material and nonmaterial incentives. Only in the last three decades has the "population problem," with its Cassandra-like prophesies of impending doom, particularly for the developing countries of the world, led governments to reluctantly acknowledge the effect of population change on the developmental process.

## SOURCES OF OPPOSITION TO FAMILY PLANNING PROGRAMS

As noted, programs to reduce mortality rarely, if ever, are opposed, whereas few governments have attempted to develop and implement long-term and comprehensive plans for the redistribution of the population through migration. Consequently, population specialists and government officials alike regard the reduction of the birth rate as the most direct way to reduce the overall rate of growth. But it is precisely this component of population change that has aroused the most opposition. The organized provision of birth control services has been a controversial issue for approximately a century, since it was first fostered by private organizations in Great Britain, and later in the United States, until the present time when it has become a worldwide phenomenon.

## THE IDEOLOGICAL COMPONENT

Unease about "tampering" with the process of reproduction may have been felt by many, but has not often been articulated; however, on another level, particularly in the media, a strong ideological component has developed in the opposition to birth control programs. This is especially true in Third World countries, where population policies easily become intertwined with other issues, thus becoming highly politicized. In most Third World countries, programs to reduce birth rates do not initially originate in indigenous groups or organizations, but are imported from developed countries. Given the wariness and generalized distrust with which Third World countries regard the actions of developed countries, the imported birth control programs are not warmly wlecomed, particularly when they are often tied in one degree or another to foreign aid. Stycos (11) has classified the different sources of opposition to population control programs in Latin America, but his analysis is equally applicable to many other parts of the Third World. The following paragraphs summarize his analysis.

**Nationalists.** A strong force cutting across the entire political spectrum is nationalism. Of whatever political persuasion, nationalists are united in their belief that the destiny of their country requires a large and growing population. To hold one's own in the international political arena, it is argued, bigger is better. Large populations mean more economic and military power to discourage incursions of the aggressive developed countries or of other, hostile Third World countries. Where the population density is low and large areas are not populated, as in Brazil and some African countries, a fast-growing population is needed to colonize and develop lagging regions. For many nationalists, birth control programs are defeatist and even cowardly, for they imply the inability of a people to meet the challenge of growth. The theme of national virility is never completely absent in these arguments.

**Conservatives.** Conservatism is often, but not invariably, associated with religious groups—i.e., Catholics, Muslims, Fundamentalist sects. The conservative position considers birth control programs to be contrary to natural law (however defined), and yet another step in the weakening of the foundation of society—the family, and kinship structure. Inevitably, this position leads to a consideration of woman's proper role; the conservative position is that a woman's place is in the home, as wife and mother.

Conservatives also value patriotism and the "integrity" of the nation; consequently, they generally align with the nationalists in opposition to "foreign" birth control programs. At times they share the leftist concern with "imperialist" intervention.

**Leftists.** The ideological basis for this position is mainly Marxist. Marxist doctrine on population reverts to the strong attacks that Marx mounted on Malthus, generating an ideological dispute which, to this day, has colored the discussion of the relation of population to resources. In its most simplistic form, the Marxist argument is that each form or mode of economic organization—e.g., feudalism, capitalism, socialism—has its own law of population growth; hence, there are no universal laws applicable to all societies. More than this, the roots of the population problem are found in certain types of economic organization. Thus, the advanced capitalist system is indeed overpopulated, because of its need to generate a reserve army of the unemployed. In a socialist society, with its different economic organization, the problem of overpopulation simply does not exist. This position is still advanced, even though all socialist countries from Cuba to China have extensive programs offering a wide range of birth control services.

In the Third World countries, the leftist opposition to birth control is often linked to opposing the United States as an "imperialist" power seeking to impose its will on "dependent" countries. They believe that the "imperialists" want to curb population growth in Third world countries in order to take a larger share of the world's resources.

Marxists also oppose birth control programs, because they believe that uncontrolled growth will aggravate economic problems (although this is inconsistent with their position that population growth has nothing to do with development), and increase social tensions and class conflict, thus eventually bringing about the expected revolution. To the extent that birth control programs ameliorate social conditions, they delay the revolution, and therefore should be opposed.

## THE 1974 WORLD POPULATION CONFERENCE AT BUCHAREST

Nearly all of the ideological positions that impinge on population control programs were represented in the landmark meeting held in Bucharest in 1974. There had been world population conferences before, but they were professional gatherings of population specialists, debating primarily technical matters. In Bucharest, 136 member states of the United Nations were in attendance and were represented primarily by governmental and political personnel, rather than population specialists.

Because large international conferences can be in session for only a limited time, generally a couple of weeks at most, participants must rely upon their secretariats to prepare background documents and a draft of a plan of action. During the conference these documents are debated and then approved by the conference participants, customarily with only minor modifications. The 1974 World Population Conference was organized around a similar format.

The U.N. Secretariat had spent more than 2 years in preparation for the conference, consulting with population experts and member governments, conducting four symposia in Cairo, Honolulu, Stockholm, and Amsterdam on various themes, as well as formulating the Draft World Population Plan of Action. As Finkle and Crane (2) have noted in their analysis of the "Politics of Bucharest," the inspiration for the conference came principally from the United States, and to a lesser degree from a small number of Western European and Asian nations which had, for some time, been promoting fertility reduction. The Bucharest meeting was designed as the culmination of the World Population Year, during which a great deal of publicity had been given to population issues. The conference organizers wanted to convince governments to devote greater resources and effort to dealing with population problems, including specifying target numbers and dates for reducing rates of population growth.

The hopes of the organizers of the conference were shattered once the meeting began. There was much conflict—more than 300 amendments to the draft plan were introduced and debated—and for a time it appeared that the conference would adjourn without any plan at all. Unexpectedly, several Third World countries, particularly Algeria and Argentina, led a well-organized attack on the draft plan. What went wrong? It is clear that the planners of the conference (most of whom were either from the developed countries, or strongly influenced by them) underestimated the political nature of the meeting and the fact that most Third World countries saw the international conference not so much as a forum for a discussion of population targets and the appropriate policies necessary to achieve them as an opportunity to advance the broader objectives of economic and social development. This theme has reappeared in all recent international conferences, regardless of the topic under consideration, whether it was food, or the status of women. Bucharest was the first international conference scheduled after the U.N. General Assembly adopted, in May, 1974, a Declaration and Programme of Action on the Establishment of a New International Economic Order. Fundamentally, this document called for a redress of the economic and political imbalances between the developed and the developing countries. As a consequence, population questions, as such, receded into the background, while the representatives debated the merits of the New International Economic Order.

To maintain, as some participants did, that the sole theme of Bucharest was "development is the best contraceptive" is to ignore the diversity of positions represented. Mauldin and his coworkers (6:359) were able to assign nearly all attending countries to the following five major positions: *1) Population growth is desirable.* China argued that rapid growth would enable Third World countries to defend their interests against the superpowers. Other countries, such as Brazil, encouraged growth in order to people their lightly populated countries. Among developed countries, France saw rapid expansion as a stimulus for economic growth. *2) Population growth is not an important variable.* Many African and Latin American countries believed that genuine economic and social development and the elimination of inequities are the most critical problems, and that their successful resolution, as opposed to the "artificial" way of birth control programs, will bring about an eventual reduction in fertility. *3) Rapid population growth intensifies problems in socioeconomic development.* Many developing Asian countries, Western European countries, and the United States adopted this position. While rapid population growth, in and of itself, is not seen as the cause of economic and social problems, it is believed to intensify the effects. The best strategy,

therefore, is to have both strong development programs *and* vigorous population control, for they are basically complementary. *4) Population is a key variable in socioeconomic development.* Only a few countries, notably Bangladesh, gave this much emphasis to population factors. *5) There is no need for population policy.* Most Eastern European countries argued that population problems are strictly a consequence of developments in capitalist countries. In socialist countries, population trends automatically adjust to economic and social forces; consequently, programs affecting population are unnecessary.

The political representatives of countries at Bucharest acknowledged the high levels of population growth in Third World countries, but they did not view them with alarm. They emphasized that each country is a sovereign entity and has to formulate its own position. Concern was expressed about the depletion of resources, the need for international assistance programs, and the status of women in development.

The revised Plan of Action reflected these changes in emphasis from the earlier version. It represented a conciliatory position which developed in the last days of the conference, allowing the 136 national delegations to approve the plan. This agreement was something of a surprise, considering the vehemence with which the different positions had been maintained. Probably a number of countries signed the plan, not because they agreed with all its provisions, but because, as Finkle and Crane (2:107) remark, "almost all countries saw it as politically advantageous to perpetuate the process by which complex economic and social problems of global importance are dealt with in the United Nations."

The Plan of Action has received various interpretations. Berelson (1:143–144) holds that "the Plan downgraded the current programmatic emphasis without putting another correctly in its place. At the same time, it legitimated so wide a range of population-related activities that countries and international organizations could continue present activities without violating any provisions of the Plan. Thus the basic paradox: the Plan has a 'new look' while it justifies the old one." Miro (7:421) reviewed reactions to the plan in the 3 years following the conference, calling it "an inherently political document." The plan received more attention than might have been anticipated, and Miro believes it is a "potentially strong political instrument." Yet she notes that the plan has not as yet served as a guide for dealing with population matters for international bodies, particularly the United Nations.

## THE SPREAD AND EFFECT OF FAMILY PLANNING PROGRAMS

The previous discussion may have led the reader to conclude that the conditions for developing population programs, and specifically birth control programs, in countries throughout the world, and especially in the Third World, are not at all propitious—that existing programs are under ideological attack from many sides, threatening their very existence. Yet this is not the case. Family planning is increasing as never before. It encounters less and less opposition, even within countries which were strongly opposed only a few years ago. China, for example, was one of the loudest voices opposing population policies at Bucharest, but domestically it apparently continues to develop one of the most comprehensive and effective control programs in the world (see Chap. 17).

The major question addressed in this section is, To what extent have family planning programs in the developing world become more (or less) prevalent since the 1960s, and what are their effects on contraceptive use?

## ACCEPTANCE OF FAMILY PLANNING

One of the more useful family planning program statistics is that which measures the number of new acceptors. There are problems, of course, with this type of statistic; two principal ones are misreporting, and the fact that the statistics do not report the discontinuation of contraceptive use after acceptance. Nevertheless, an examination of materials of this kind for selected points in time provides an indication of changes in the acceptance of family planning services.

Program data on the number of new acceptors are available for most developing countries for selected years since 1965. However, official family planning program acceptance data are not available for the People's Republic of China, or for Vietnam. This is particularly unfortunate, since the combined population of these two developing countries is close to one billion. Moreover, there is evidence that China is characterized by an extensive family planning program, and that the similarly impressive family planning network in Vietnam, begun in 1962 in the North, was extended to the South in 1975, following unification (8, 9, 10, 12). The numbers to be analyzed would be significantly larger if these countries were included.

Table 16–1 presents data on the number of new acceptors of family planning for the developing countries of the world, by region, for four points in time during the period from 1965 to 1975. These data reflect an impressive expansion of family planning services in the developing world. The number of new acceptors has grown from nearly 2.5 million, in 1965, to more than 17 million in 1975, an increase of 600 per cent. The number in the Latin America/Caribbean region, with its largely Catholic population, has grown from a mere 36,000 new acceptors, in 1965, to more than 2 million, 10 years later. The growth in Africa has been slower, but this region is expected to increase its momentum in the coming decade (12:27). The South Asian region had the greatest number of new acceptors in 1965—nearly 2 million. By 1975, the region increased its number of new acceptors by over

**Table 16–1. New Acceptors of Family Planning Programs: Countries of the Developing World (Excluding China and Vietnam) by Region, Selected Years between 1965 and 1975**

| Region | Number of new acceptors (in thousands) | | | |
|---|---|---|---|---|
| | 1965 | 1970 | 1974 | 1975 |
| All regions | 2,484 | 9,118 | 12,646 | 17,385 |
| South Asia | 1,823 | 6,068 | 5,708 | 9,668 |
| East/Southeast Asia | 602 | 1,623 | 4,089 | 4,537 |
| Latin America/Caribbean | 36 | 705 | 1,816 | 2,020 |
| W. Asia/North Africa | 20 | 639 | 839 | 962 |
| Sub-Saharan Africa | 3 | 83 | 194 | — |

(Watson WB (ed): Family Planning in the Developing World: A Review of Programs. New York, Population Council, 1977, Table 5; Tsui AO, Bogue DJ: Population Bulletin 33:1978, Table 10)

**Table 16–2. Percentage Distribution of Contraceptive Methods Chosen by New Acceptors in 1975: Countries of the Developing World (Excluding China and Vietnam), by Region**

| Region | Total | Method of Contraception | | | | |
| | | Steriliza-tion | IUD | Pill | Abortion | Condom/other |
|---|---|---|---|---|---|---|
| All | 100 | 18.0 | 15 | 28 | 2.0 | 37 |
| South Asia | 100 | 28.0 | 9 | 7 | 2.0 | 54 |
| East/Southeast Asia | 100 | 5.0 | 20 | 54 | 0.4 | 21 |
| Latin America/ Caribbean | 100 | 3.0 | 34 | 47 | 7.0 | 10 |
| W. Asia/North Africa | 100 | 1.0 | 17 | 73 | 2.0 | 7 |
| Sub-Saharan Africa | 100 | 0.1* | 12* | 71* | 0.1* | 17* |

* Percentage distribution based on data from only six countries: Botswana, Ghana, Kenya, Lesotho, Mauritius, and Uganda.
(Watson WB (ed): Family Planning in the Developing World: A Review of Programs. New York, Population Council, 1977, Table 5; Tsui AO, Bogue DJ: Population Bulletin, 33:1978, Table 10)

400 per cent, to nearly 10 million. These numbers clearly reflect the influence of India, with its large population and long-term family planning program efforts.

## TYPES OF CONTRACEPTIVE METHODS CHOSEN

Another type of family planning program statistic is presented in Table 16–2: methods of contraception selected by new acceptors in 1975. For countries of the developing world, nearly one-fifth of the new acceptors chose sterilization, about one-third the pill, and 15 per cent the intrauterine device. Combined, over 60 per cent of the new acceptors in 1975 chose one of the three most effective contraceptive procedures. In South Asia, the most popular choice was sterilization, but the oral contraceptive was preferred in the remaining regions of the developing world. The less effective contraceptive methods, such as the condom and foam, were selected by slightly more than one-third of all new acceptors. Given the greater popularity of the more effective methods among new acceptors, the impact of the programs on fertility decline should be more dramatic and influential than if the more traditional, and less effective contraceptives had been chosen (12).

## PREVALENCE OF CONTRACEPTIVE USE

Another consideration is the degree of coverage of the "at-risk" population. Specifically, how prevalent is contraceptive use among married women of reproductive age (MWRA)? This is a crucial statistic for determining how extensive a particular program is in a country.

Data are available on contraceptive use among married women of reproductive age for an assortment of developing and developed countries; for some, information is available for more than one point in time. These materials are presented in Table 16–3.

Before examining this table, note that the denominator used in computing these percentages is the number of married women between the ages of 15 and 44. It is important to remember that many of these women have no current need to contracept, because they are pregnant, trying to become pregnant, postpartum, or sterile. Still others may be separated from their husbands on a temporary basis and have no current need for contraception. Country-by-country comparisons such as we will make with the data in Table 16–3 thus may not be entirely valid, since the proportions of women in the above categories vary significantly in the different regions and countries of the world (8).

Table 16–3 has two important features. First, there is a major difference in the percentage of married women of reproductive age using contraception in the developed countries compared to the percentage in the developing countries. Whereas in most of the developed countries approximately two-thirds of the MWRA utilize some method of contraception, this is the case in only a few of the developing countries. With the exception of nine countries (Costa Rica, Trinidad and Tobago,

**Table 16–3. Percentage of Married Women of Reproductive Age (MWRA) Currently Using Contraception: Selected Countries and Years**

| Country | Year | Percentage of MWRA using | Country | Year | Percentage of MWRA using |
|---|---|---|---|---|---|
| *Developing countries* | | | Costa Rica | 1976 | 34 |
| | | | Dominican Republic | 1976 | 24 |
| **Africa** | | | Ecuador | 1975 | 6 |
| Egypt | 1975 | 21 | | 1974 | 3 |
| Ghana | 1976 | 2 | El Salvador | 1976 | 10 |
| Kenya | 1971 | 2 | Guatemala | 1974 | 4 |
| Mauritius | 1976 | 37 | Haiti | 1976 | 5 |
| | 1971 | 25 | Mexico | 1976 | 20 |
| Morocco | 1974 | 7 | | 1973 | 13 |
| | 1969 | 1 | Paraguay | 1975 | 10 |
| Tunisia | 1977 | 18 | Trinidad & Tobago | 1971 | 44 |
| | 1971 | 12 | | | |
| **Asia** | | | *Developed countries* | | |
| Bangladesh | 1976 | 5 | **Asia** | | |
| Hong Kong | 1976 | 61 | Australia | 1971 | 66 |
| | 1969 | 42 | Melbourne | 1950–1954 | 66 |
| India | 1976 | 18–20 | Japan | 1975 | 61 |
| | 1969 | 7–8 | | 1965 | 56 |
| Indonesia | 1977 | 19 | | 1950 | 20 |
| | 1971 | 0.5 | **North America** | | |
| Iran | 1975 | 17 | Canada, Toronto | 1968 | 63 |
| | 1969 | 3 | United States | 1973 | 70 |
| Korea, South | 1976 | 34 | | 1970 | 65 |
| | 1972 | 30 | | 1965 | 64 |
| Malaysia, West | 1975 | 43 | **Europe** | | |
| | 1969 | 6 | Belgium | 1975–1976 | 87 |
| Nepal | 1976 | 17 | | 1966 | 76 |
| | 1971 | 3 | Czechoslo- | | |
| Philippines | 1976 | 22 | vakia | 1970 | 66 |
| | 1972 | 8 | Denmark | 1970 | 67 |
| Singapore | 1976 | 77 | England & Wales | 1967 | 69 |
| | 1970 | 45 | Finland | 1971 | 77 |
| Taiwan | 1977 | 61 | France | 1972 | 64 |
| | 1971 | 44 | Hungary | 1974 | 75 |
| Thailand | 1976 | 32 | | 1966 | 64 |
| | 1971 | 10 | Netherlands | 1975 | 71 |
| Turkey | 1968 | 35 | | 1969 | 59 |
| **Latin America** | | | Poland | 1972 | 57 |
| Colombia | 1974 | 31 | Yugoslavia | 1970 | 59 |
| Bogota | 1974 | 51 | | | |
| | 1969 | 37 | | | |
| | 1964 | 27 | | | |

(Nortman D: Population Bulletin 32:1977, Table 2)

Mauritius, Hong Kong, South Korea, West Malaysia, Singapore, Taiwan, and Turkey), less than one-third of the MWRA use contraception in the developing world. Most reports from China suggest that it should also be listed with the exceptions, but since actual data are not available, it cannot be included (8:10).

The second major aspect of Table 16–3 is that for at least a few of the developing countries for which information is available for more than one period of time, a marked rise in contraceptive use has occurred in a short time. For example, in India, the number of MWRA using contraception increased from about 8 per cent, in 1969, to nearly 20 per cent by 1976. Contraceptive use in Indonesia rose from less than 1 per cent of MWRA in 1971, to 19 per cent in 1977, and, in Thailand, from 10 per cent to 32 per cent in only 5 years.

Among Latin American countries for which data are available, similar dramatic increases are found. In Bogota, Colombia, the number of MWRA using contraception increased from 27 to 51 per cent between 1964 and 1974. Mexico, too, has seen an increase, although somewhat more modest than those already cited: in 1973, 13 per cent of its MWRA were using contraception; 3 years later, the percentage had increased to 20 (8:14). Thus, for those few developing countries with data, Table

16–3 suggests a very rapid diffusion of family planning programs.

## THE ROLES OF ECONOMIC DEVELOPMENT AND FAMILY PLANNING PROGRAMS IN FERTILITY DECLINE

A major debate within contemporary demographic circles concerns the extent to which two major classes of factors influence, or determine, the course of fertility within a country. Are factors representing developmental efforts the principal determinants of fertility decline, or are factors dealing directly with the supply of family planning services, that is, program efforts, the major determinants? We will address this question from an empirical point of view, drawing upon current demographic research. Several recent methodologically sound and sophisticated studies permit a far superior and more definitive response than has been possible previously.

One aspect of the debate reverts to the demographic-transition experiences of the European countries during the eighteenth and nineteenth centuries. Until recently it was believed that modernization and industrialization were principally, if not solely, responsible for the onset and continuation of fertility decline in the European countries. Developmental factors such as increased literacy, improvements in social and economic status, urbanization, heightened participation of women in the labor force, and decreased infant and maternal mortality motivated couples to limit the size of their families; hence the eventual transition in the European countries from high to low fertility.

Historical demographers have recently suggested that the causes of fertility decline in Europe were not so direct and clear-cut. Indeed, fertility decline appears to have occurred under a host of conditions and determinants. In many countries the declines were closely associated with development and modernization, but developmental factors were not the prime determinants in all countries. Knodel and van de Walle (3) have noted that fertility decline began at approximately the same time in England and in Hungary. But whereas the former had already experienced considerable urbanization and industrialization, the latter "was at a substantially lower level of development as measured by any conventional socioeconomic indices" (3:6). Further, in the rural areas of a number of European countries, including Germany, fertility declines appeared "long before the conventional signs of socioeconomic development were evident" (3:6).

Despite this less than definitive appraisal of the influences of modernization factors on fertility decline, there are government leaders and policy practitioners who cling strongly to the belief that the only path to fertility decline is modernization. As noted earlier in this chapter, a major slogan at the recent World Population Conference in Bucharest was "development is the best contraceptive." Although representatives from many developing countries recognized the role that family planning services should play in their countries' fertility control policies, the actual empirical relationships have never been clarified. In the remaining section of this chapter it will be shown that both developmental and programmatic (family planning) determinants are important, and that fertility reductions are most dramatic when both sets of factors are operable.

## RECENT DEMOGRAPHIC STUDIES

Recently (in 1978), two pairs of demographers examined the conditions accompanying fertility decline in the developing world during the late 1960s and first half of the 1970s. Mauldin and Berelson (5), of the Population Council, investigated the influences of developmental and programmatic factors on crude birth rate changes in 94 developing countries between 1965 and 1975. Tsui and Bogue (12), of the Community and Family Study Center of the University of Chicago, examined the varying impacts of the same two sets of variables on changes in the total fertility rates between 1968 and 1975 for 89 developing countries. Both studies report impressive fertility declines for most countries during the given time intervals, and conclude that both developmental and programmatic factors have influenced this development. Importantly, both studies identify organized family planning programs as having a very real and independent effect, over and above the effects of developmental factors.

### THE TSUI AND BOGUE APPROACH

The statistical analysis by Tsui and Bogue primarily involved a multivariate regression, in which the countries' total fertility rates in

1975 were in the "estimated" or "predicted" position of the equation. The "independent," or "predictor," variables were those dealing with development and family planning effort. Also included as an independent variable were the countries' 1968 total fertility rates (TFR). As the authors observed, this form was preferred because it yielded a lagged regression. Moreover, "it reduces the amount of prediction error and locates the 1975 TFR relative to its 1968 value. If the predicted 1975 TFR is 4000, the amount of TFR change depends on the 1968 value, whether it be 2500 or 3800. Change in fertility can then be obtained after the fitted regression line is estimated by substituting values for [the independent variables] and the 1968 TFR" (12:30).

The authors then selected five independent variables to represent modernization and development: per capita gross national product, percentage of urban residence, infant mortality rate, percentage of employed females in agriculture, and the female school enrollment ratio. Other variables reflecting modernization were excluded because they were highly correlated with one or more of the five. Since the impact of modernization and development on fertility is not presumed to be instantaneous, data were used for the five variables as of 1968.

To gauge the degree of family planning services, Tsui and Bogue used the measure of "family planning effort," constructed earlier by Lapham and Mauldin (4). It applies 15 family planning programmatic criteria (e.g., whether fertility reduction is included in the official planning policy of the country; whether contraception is readily and easily available throughout the country; whether there is an adequate family planning administrative structure), to each country. A scale ranging from 0 to 30 is developed which is based on the answers to the 15 criteria questions for each country. A "yes" receives two points, a "qualified yes" one point, and a "no" zero points. The scoring was done on the basis of the countries' family planning situations in 1972.

These five modernization variables, the one family planning programmatic variable, and, as noted earlier, the 1968 total fertility rate, were entered as independent variables into a regression equation, with the 1975 total fertility rate as the dependent variable. The major findings of the analysis are reported in Table

**Table 16–4. Standardized Regression Coefficients for 1975 TFR Regressed on 1968 TFR, Five 1968 Socioeconomic Indicators, and the 1972 Family Planning Effort Score: 89 Developing Countries**

| Variable | Standardized regression coefficient |
|---|---|
| TFR, 1968 | 0.626 |
| Per capita GNP, 1968 | 0.067 |
| Percentage urban, 1968 | −0.017 |
| Infant mortality rate, 1968 | 0.070 |
| Percentage of employed females in agriculture, 1968 | −0.003 |
| Female school enrollment ratio, 1968 | −0.089 |
| Family planning effort score, 1972 | −0.308 |
| Multiple coefficient of determination ($R^2$) | = 0.860 |

(Tsui AO, Bogue DJ: Population Bulletin 33:1978, Table 12)

16–4 in the form of standardized partial regression coefficients for each of the independent variables. In the regression equation computed for all 89 developing countries, the influence of the family planning variable is second only to that of the 1968 total fertility rate. Its impact on the 1975 fertility rate is greater than any of the five modernization variables. And the direction of the family planning coefficient is negative, as expected. That is, increases in the family planning services variable lead to decreases in the 1975 fertility variable, holding constant the influences of the five modernization variables and the 1968 fertility rate. This analysis suggests that family planning effort has both a significant, as well as an independent, influence on fertility.

**THE MAULDIN AND BERELSON APPROACH**

The Mauldin and Berelson analysis examines the decline of fertility among developing countries of the world during the period from 1965 to 1975. The authors were especially interested in discovering the degree to which developmental factors and family planning program factors contribute to changes in the fertility rate, both collectively and separately. A description of this study is included here because, unlike the Tsui and Bogue analysis, it examines approaches to declining fertility rates in various ways. But regardless of the approach taken, the same basic conclusion emerges: developmental factors and family planning factors work together most effectively and have a joint impact on declining fertility rates.

Mauldin and Berelson used the crude birth rate (CBR) as their measure of fertility and analyzed its decline between 1965 and 1975 in 94 developing countries. The authors recognized the methodological and conceptual liabilities involved in the employment of the crude birth rate (see Chap. 14). Nevertheless, they chose it, because "of its greater familiarity to the general reader and because of its availability" (5:94).

A comparison was made, however, early in their analysis, between declines in the crude birth rate and the total fertility rate between 1965 and 1975. The ten-year changes in the two rates are so highly related ($r = 0.97$) as to be identical, for all practical purposes.

The authors conducted an extensive search of the social science literature in an attempt to identify the major modernization variables, or "social setting variables," as they refer to them. In their examination of over 100 variables, they considered theoretical relevance to the problem and availability of data. They selected seven variables as basic indicators of social setting: adult literacy, primary and secondary school enrollment, life expectancy, infant mortality rate, number of males aged 15–64 in the nonagricultural labor force, gross national product per capita, and population in cities of 100,000+. These seven variables were used singularly in some analyses, and combined into a social-setting index in others. (See Chap. 19 for a discussion of yet another variable, equity in resource distribution.)

The family planning services variable used by Mauldin and Berelson was the index of program effort developed by Lapham and Mauldin (4) and is identical to the index used by Tsui and Bogue in their analysis.

Mauldin and Berelson's first approach involved regressing the 1965–1975 crude birth rate changes on the seven social-setting variables and the program effort variable, both for the year 1970. The multiple coefficient of determination ($R^2$) between the seven social-setting variables and CBR decline among 94 countries was 0.66, but it increased to 0.83 when the program effort variable was added. The authors concluded that "program effort adds substantially to the multiple $R^2$ of such factors, and in effect breaks through the plateau of small increments among these factors,

presumably as another kind of influence. Another demand factor that similarly extended the correlation would surely be considered a major influence on CBR decline" (5:105).

The authors also compared the standardized regression coefficients (the betas) for the program effort index with a single index assembled from the seven social-setting variables. The impact of program effort on CBR decline was substantially stronger than that of the social-setting index; the betas were 0.75 and 0.22, respectively.

Mauldin and Berelson (5:106) next turned to an investigation of the same question through the application of path analytic procedures. They wanted to determine the extent to which both "social setting and program effort exert a direct impact on fertility decline" and to what degree social-setting factors influence program effort. Their results suggest that program effort has a significantly stronger direct effect on fertility decline than social setting. However, social setting has a sizable indirect influence on fertility decline by operating through program effort. They concluded that "again both factors are important, but in this (path) analysis two-thirds of the total effect of social setting is filtered through program effort, and the total effect of program effort is more than that of social setting in a ratio of 89:67, or 4:3" (5:106).

In another approach, the authors attempted to disentangle the interaction effects of the social-setting and program effort variables on fertility decline. They found that the social-setting variables were less highly related to the fertility decline before family planning programs were instituted than after they were organized. This test also suggests the importance of the two sets of factors operating jointly on fertility decline.

The authors engaged in still additional analyses. They conducted an analysis of changes in the rate of fertility decline, assuming that "it is the change in the socioeconomic variables over time that makes for fertility reduction rather than their state at a given time" (5:107). Their results indicated that changes in the social-setting variables accounted for about as much of the fertility decline as social-setting data at 1970 levels; moreover, the influence of the program variable, along with the social-setting change data, on fertility decline was not altered significantly from the earlier test.

Another procedure involved lagging the social-setting variables, since "it is often put forward that whereas socioeconomic factors are prime determinants of the level of fertility, there is a lag of some years between achievement of a given level of socioeconomic status and the reduction of fertility to a corresponding level" (5:108). The results were not very different from the earlier tests, before or after the program effort variable was introduced into the equation. Lastly, the authors altered their fertility measure to reflect absolute CBR decline rather than percentage CBR decline, suggesting that perhaps percentage reductions are less significant for policy-makers and social scientists than the absolute declines. The patterns of the general relationships remained virtually the same when absolute declines were used.

## CONCLUSIONS

The various approaches and procedures used by Mauldin and Berelson, along with the important analysis of Tsui and Bogue, permit the following generalizations. First, factors associated with social setting have a close relationship with fertility declines. The most developed countries do much better than those that are not as highly developed. (See Chap. 19 for an anthropological approach to this question.) Second, family planning program factors, the program effort, exert an independent and significant impact on fertility, over and above that of the social-setting factors. Third, the greater the period the program has been in existence, the more substantial its impact on fertility, although there are some deviant countries. Fourth, and most important, results of all the analyses conducted indicate that both sets of factors are influential, and that they work most effectively together (5:124).

Mauldin and Berelson reach the following conclusion:

Countries that rank well on socioeconomic variables and also make substantial program effort have on average much more fertility decline than do countries that have one *or* the other, and far more than those with neither. The policy implications are that, if a country wants to reduce its fertility, it should seek a high degree of modernization . . . and it should adopt a substantial family planning program. . . . In short . . . one could conclude that the Bucharest judgment that family planning effort is of little consequence is itself of little consequence (5:124).

## REFERENCES

1. Berelson B: The world population plan of action: where now? Pop Dev Rev 1:115, 1975
2. Finkle JL, Crane BB: The politics of Bucharest: population, development and the new international economic order. Pop Dev Rev 1:87, 1975
3. Knodel J, van de Walle E: Lessons from the past: Policy implications of historical fertility studies. Paper presented at annual meetings of the American Public Health Association, Washington DC, 1977
4. Lapham RJ, Mauldin WP: National family planning programs: review and evaluation. Stud Fam Plann 3:31, 1972
5. Mauldin WP, Berelson B: Conditions of fertility decline in developing countries, 1965–1975. Stud Fam Plann 9:89–147, 1978
6. Mauldin WP, Choucri N, Notestein FW, Teitelbaum M: A report on Bucharest. Stud Fam Plann 5:357–395, 1974
7. Miro C: The world population plan of action: a political instrument whose potential has not been realized. Pop Dev Rev 3:421, 1977
8. Nortman D: Changing contraceptive patterns: a global perspective. Population Bulletin 32 (entire volume), 1977
9. Nortman D, Hofstatter E: Population and family planning programs: A factbook, 8th ed. Reports on Population/Family Planning, 1976
10. Nortman D, Hofstatter E: Population and Family Planning Programs, 9th ed: A Population Council Factbook. New York, The Population Council, 1978
11. Stycos JM: Ideology, Faith and Family Planning in Latin America. New York, Mcgraw-Hill, 1971
12. Tsui AO, Bogue DJ: Declining world fertility: trends, causes and implications. Population Bulletin 33, 1978

# 17

# Four Case Studies: Mexico, India, China, United States

**Dudley L. Poston, Jr.**
**Harley L. Browning**

This chapter discusses the demographic past, present, and future of Mexico, India, China, and the United States. A primary concern is the extent to which social and economic development factors, population policies, and actual birth control campaigns and technology have interactively influenced the birth rate. The importance of the different factors varied from country to country. A factor which seemed quite influential in the country might not be influential at all in another.

The selection of Mexico, China, India, and the United States as the subject of case studies is based on a number of considerations. These countries are the largest (China), second largest (India), fourth largest (United States), and eleventh largest (Mexico) in the world. Moreover, their combined 1978 population size of 1.85 billion inhabitants represents nearly 45 per cent of the world's population of 4.2 billion.

In terms of population policy, socioeconomic development, and birth control programs, the four countries are not identical, thus providing additional rationale for their selection. Only one (the United States) may be classified as developed, according to most social and economic criteria. The remaining three are at various stages within the "developing" category. Further, fertility change has interacted with population policy differently in the various countries. The United States has experienced substantial fertility decline (considerably more than the other three countries)

in the absence of organized family planning and a federally sponsored population policy. India has established significant family planning programs (as early as 1952), but these have had little impact on fertility. China may be characterized as representing an "on again, off again" approach to family planning and birth control, but has apparently made remarkable advances toward the reduction of its birth rate. Mexico still has a high birth rate, but only recently has its government endorsed family planning as a major policy ingredient. Simultaneously, it has made marked advances in certain areas of social and economic development.

Fertility reduction is exceedingly complex, in terms of both concept and process. The countries profiled in this chapter will provide reasonably complete illustrations of this complexity.

## MEXICO

### TWO DISTINCTIVE FEATURES

Mexico is a large and rapidly growing country in the Third World. With a population of 66.9 million, it ranks second in population to Brazil, within Latin America, and eleventh in the world as a whole (see Appendix 1). It is not Mexico's size that makes it attractive as a case study; rather, there are two features of Mexican development that warrant attention. Despite considerable structural change since the

1910 revolution and a strong economy since World War II, its birth rate did not decline, as would have been predicted by demographic-transition theory. In other words, fertility in Mexico remained high for decades after the changing socioeconomic structure presumably had established the appropriate conditions for a decline.

The second distinctive feature of the Mexican experience is the suddenness with which government policy toward birth control programs has shifted. Until recently, virtually all government officials believed that rapid population growth was positive, or at least not detrimental, for the country's development. Family planning programs were not banned, but they received no public encouragement or support. Yet within several years a complete turnabout occurred, with population planning not only sanctioned, but encouraged. The current president of Mexico, Lopez Portillo, has proclaimed reduction of the birth rate from 42 to 25:1000 as a target to be attained before he leaves office in 1982.

## SOCIAL AND DEMOGRAPHIC TRENDS

At the beginning of the twentieth century, the Mexican census recorded a population of 13.6 million, not a large population for a country with an extensive land area. At the time of the 1910 revolution, Mexico had the classic characteristics of a developing country: only one-fifth of its population lived in urban areas; four-fifths of the employed males worked in agriculture; and four-fifths of the male population was illiterate. The male life expectancy was only an estimated 37 years. (For a good review of Mexico's demographic development, see 13).

The 1910 revolution caused many dislocations, and it was not until the 1930s that the country began to recover. In 1940, the population of 20.2 million had grown less than 50 per cent above the 1900 figure. World War II stimulated the Mexican economy and ushered in a period of sustained economic growth which lasted approximately three decades, until the early 1970s (32). Structurally, this was a period of intense change. Mexico shifted from one-quarter to one-half urban. Sustained growth was particularly intense in metropolitan centers, such as Mexico City, Guadalajara, and Monterrey—the consequences of heavy migration from rural to urban areas. This was

paralleled by the sectoral shift in employment from agriculture into manufacturing and service industries. Education also improved, with the percentage of males who were literate doubling from 40 per cent to 80 per cent over the 30 years.

Life expectancy also showed marked improvement, with the male figure rising from 40 years at birth, in 1940, to 61 years in 1970 (that of females is approximately 3 years greater). According to Hernandez (15), the crude death rate, which had been in the range of 33 to 35 (per thousand) in 1900, and 23 in the period 1935–1939, declined to 10 during 1969–1971. A substantial part of the decline was caused by a sharp drop in infant mortality: from 289 (per thousand live births), in the period 1899–1901, to 124 in 1939–1941, to 66 in 1969–1971. The decline is primarily attributable to public health measures and somewhat better living conditions for the population as a whole.

While mortality decreased markedly, the birth rate showed only small declines, from as high as 46 (per thousand) in the period 1900–1909, to 45 in the 1940s, to 44 in the 1960s (see Fig. 17–1 for trends since 1955). The plunging death rate, when coupled with a high and slowly declining birth rate, raised the rate of natural increase in the period from 1940 to 1970 from about 2.2 per cent per annum to almost 3.5 per cent, at which level Mexico became one of the fastest-growing countries in the world (15).

Probably the best way to understand Mexico's demographic transition is to examine data provided by Berelson (4) and reported in Table 17–1, on "threshold values" for seven development variables: life expectancy, infant mortality rate, adult literacy, school enrollment, nonagricultural labor force, per-capita gross national product, and percentage of never-married females, aged 15 to 19. Berelson notes that the choice of variables is arbitrary—others could have been selected, but would not have materially affected the results—and the threshold values themselves are arbitrary, to an extent, because there are not enough data to allow for more than a mid-range choice of specific values. In any event, it is the overall pattern, rather than any particular variable, that is important (see Chap. 16).

With these caveats in mind, Table 17–1 demonstrates that Mexico currently meets the threshold values for fertility decline for all seven variables. The country is comparable to

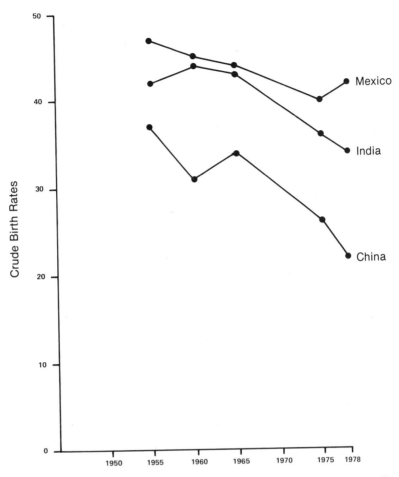

**FIG. 17–1.** Trends in crude birth rates through 1978: Mexico, India, and China. (Sources of data: [Crude birth rates through 1975]: Maudlin WP: Studies in Family Planning (Apr., 1978), Table 1; [Crude birth rates for 1978]:, Population Reference Bureau, World Population Data Sheet, 1978)

**Table 17–1. Approximation to Seven Threshold Values for Selected Countries (Circa 1970)**

| Category and country | Life expectancy | Infant mortality rate | Adult literacy | School enroll-ment | Nonagri-cultural labor force | Per capita GNP | Females, 15–19, never married | Number of thresholds met |
|---|---|---|---|---|---|---|---|---|
| *Threshold values* | 60 yrs. | 65 | 70% | 55% | 55% | $344 | 80% | est. 1975 |
| Mexico | 62 | 68 | 74 | 69 | 54* | 996 | 79 | 7 |
| Chile | 62 | 79 | 88 | 83 | 57 | 811 | 91 | 6 |
| Colombia | 60 | 76 | 76 | 63 | 44 | 432 | 86 | 5 |
| Venezuela | 57 | 49 | 82 | 75 | 57 | 1837 | 84 | 7 |
| India | 48 | 130 | 33 | 40 | 32 | 140 | 43 | 0 |
| China | 60 | — | — | — | 34 | 170 | — | ? |

\* The figure in the original table is given as 42, an error.
(Adapted from Bernard Berelson: Population and Development Review 4, Dec., 1978, Table 4)

Chile, which Berelson is "certain" will achieve a birth rate of 20:1000 by the year 2000. The contrast with India, the next case study to be examined, is especially marked, for the latter does not meet one of the threshold values, although its current birth rate is lower than Mexico's. Berelson's assignment of India to the "possible," rather than the "unlikely," category (e.g., Pakistan, Nigeria), for achieving a birth rate of 20:1000 by the year 2000 represents a hope that the family planning experience and government commitment will be sufficient to overcome structural conditions.

## POLICY REVERSAL ON FAMILY PLANNING

In the 1930s, Gilberto Loyo, the dean of Mexican demographers, argued that Mexico was underpopulated in terms of its area and resources; consequently, he advocated a higher growth rate (20). In the 1960s, Loyo altered his position: "I believe that Mexico's population growth has until now not hindered its economic development, but that it could diminish the rhythm of economic development in the coming years if it continues at the growth rate of the early 1960s. Furthermore, I believe that the accelerated growth of the population of Mexico is a fundamental fact which must be taken in account in the planning and execution of economic and social policies" (20:186).

As a demographer, Loyo was aware that the situation of the 1930s differed from that of the 1960s: a population of 17 million in 1930, and a per-annum rate of growth of 1 per cent, as compared to a population of 36 million in 1960, and a 3 per cent rate of growth. He was perhaps the first person with important government affiliations to publicly counter official pronatalist policy. It should be noted, however, that even at this time the Mexican government permitted pharmaceutical industries (mainly foreign controlled) to manufacture and distribute contraceptives, allowed private family planning organizations (e.g., Associacion Pro-Salud Maternal) to operate, though on a very small scale, and supported El Colegio de Mexico, a graduate-level educational institution whose Center for Demographic Studies had as its spokesman the noted economist, Victor Urquidi. Urquidi used public, as well as academic, forums to expound the disadvantages of unprecedentedly high rates of population growth (34).

Throughout the 1960s, the Mexican government and its spokesmen continued to maintain its traditional pronatalist position in national and international forums. Indeed, during the presidential campaign tours in 1970, the eventual victor, Luis Echeverria Alvarez, continually assumed a hard stance on family planning, saying, "I do know that we need to populate our country" (22). Pictures of him with his family (including eight children) were widely distributed. In office, Echeverria maintained this position for slightly less than 2 years.

Suddenly, in April of 1972, the government announced a national family planning program under the slogan of "responsible parenthood." The extensive clinical facilities of the social security system (Seguro Social) were empowered to provide counseling and contraceptive devices to the population. Although this system is based almost exclusively in urban areas, it can reach far more women than the private organizations. A new Law of Population was debated, and then passed, by the Mexican legislature in 1974. It provided legitimate status for population planning and policies within a government context. A National Population Council was established within the government to address population matters. By allocating a considerable proportion of its funds to television cartoons and radio jingles that advocate small families, the council is publicizing the new orientation toward family planning.

Urquidi has observed that the government is proceeding rather cautiously, with its spokesmen stressing that family planning is only a means, and not an end in itself (34). The goal is development and better living standards—hence family planning can in no way be considered a substitute for other development programs. This approach was followed by Mexico at the 1974 World Population Conference at Bucharest, where it took a middle position in the ideological confrontation. Nonetheless, the government permitted one of its top officials, Antonio Carrillo Flores, to accept appointment as the Secretary General of the World Population Conference, and he played a conciliatory role through his tenure.

Lopez Portillo has strengthened the policy established by his predecessor, Echeverria. Opening the 18th congress of the International Union for the Scientific Study of Population in Mexico City, in August, 1977, Lopez Portillo stated that "man is the principal problem of man: of man and of his planet earth. The real frontier of this problem is population. . . ." (26). He demonstrated the relevance of population factors for a number of pressing national problems, though never once did he mention family planning as a solution.

Why did the Mexican government make such a radical change regarding population policy? Such a move was clearly at variance with the position advocated for many years, and it unquestionably involved certain political risks. The Catholic church and the active leftist groups opposed population control. However, pressure to change emerged from a number of sources. The private family planning associations, particuarly Associacion ProSalud Maternal (APROSAM) and the Foundation for Population Studies (FEPAC) helped pave the way for the policy reversal. Further, Mexico's medical profession facilitated the change "through research findings and expressed concern over . . . high rates of infant and maternal mortality and illegal abortion" (22:15). It is likely that there was pressure from the Mexican drug industry in the 1960s, as well. Also, the various Mexican demographic research organizations (for example, El Colegio, and the Mexican institute of Social Studies) "helped fuel public discussion and understanding of population issues during the 1960s" (22:15).

It is also of interest to note that in December, 1972, a mere 2 weeks before the Mexican government was to initiate its new program (although some months after Echeverria's pronouncement) "a collective pastoral of the 80 Mexican bishops announced their support of the new government family planning policy" (22:17). This provided excellent publicity for the new program at a very strategic point in time. On a broader scale, economic factors must have been important. From the 1940s through the 1960s, the Mexican economic "miracle" had been able to sustain the growth of the economy at high levels, around 6 per cent per annum. Consequently, even though annual population growth was very high, at 3 per cent to 3.5 per cent, there still could be a per-capita increase of roughly 3 per cent— quite respectable, within a world context. But by the 1970s, Mexico's economy began to experience serious difficulties, and the margin of economic growth above population increase evaporated, creating a situation where negative growth occurred for several years. Perhaps

Echeverria, once in office, became aware of the grim realities that are often obscured by political rhetoric. The task of providing decent jobs for the ever-larger cohorts entering the labor force is truly a staggering one. It is no coincidence that the volume of undocumented workers from Mexico entering the United States has increased substantially over the last decade, creating a major problem in the relationship between the two countries.

There was virtually no opposition to the government's change in policy. As noted, the Catholic church certainly did not stand in the way. Indeed, the bishops reinterpreted *Humanae Vitae* by focusing on "the very real and excruciating emergency for most Mexican families: the population explosion" (27:17). Nor did other important Mexican groups create serious difficulties. Perhaps this reflected a growing appreciation of Mexico's difficult position, or the fact that strong, direct opposition to the Mexican government is not readily undertaken by any group.

## THE FUTURE OF MEXICAN FERTILITY

The course of Mexican fertility over the next several decades is difficult to predict, but it is possible that a relatively rapid decline may take place. In Latin America, Potter, Ordonez, and Measham have documented a striking decrease in Colombian fertility in only a few years (28). But even if Mexican fertility does decline rapidly, the demographic momentum built up over the past decades of rapid growth has formed an age-structure which will ensure much larger population (see Chap. 13). Indeed, if Mexico were to attain a net reproduction rate of 1 by the years 2000–2005 (a possible, but by no means certain, event), its population would reach a stationary state in approximately 2075, when it would number about 170 million, that is, 100 million more than at present. Even with massive direct intervention in population matters, this figure will represent a great challenge for the Mexican government and people.

## INDIA

### SOCIAL AND DEMOGRAPHIC TRENDS

The two most populous countries of the world, China and India, share a common border, have long illustrious histories, and are predominantly agrarian societies. But they are very different with respect to ethnicity, religion, government, and the nature of their population programs. India, among larger developing countries, was the first to explicitly recognize the need for governmental intervention in population issues. In the First Five-Year Plan draft of 1951, the Indian Planning Commission recognized family planning as a way to improve health; among contraceptive practices, sterilization was endorsed. Yet in the quarter-century since the plan was approved, India has had indifferent success in lowering its population growth rate. In fact, Berelson (4) classifies India only among the "possible" category of countries likely to reach a crude birth rate of 20:1000 by the year 2000. Why is it so difficult for India to reach population goals, and what are its current prospects?

In his classic study entitled *The Population of India and Pakistan,* Kingsley Davis (10) used censuses from 1871 to 1941 to analyze population processes as they were embedded within the country's complex and long-developing social structure. Since then, a number of capable Indian demographers, such as Visaria and Jain (37), have assumed the task of interpreting demographic changes.

Present-day India, after the separation of Pakistan and Bangladesh, ranks seventh in the world in land area. Its existence is conditioned by a monsoon climate characterized by marked annual and regional variations in rainfall; periodic droughts and floods often endanger the sustenance of millions of people. About two-thirds of the economically active population, in 1971, were primarily engaged in agriculture. India remains largely a village society, with only 20 per cent of the total population living in areas designated as urban (37).

Large as its population is, its growth rate in the twentieth century has not been as rapid as that in many developing countries. The Indian population grew from 238 million in 1901, to 319 million in 1941, an increase of 34 per cent. In the next 40 years, by 1981, the population probably will have more than doubled, to approximately 700 million. The growth rate in the 1961–1971 censal period was about 2.5 per cent per annum, below the 3.0–3.5 per cent rates in many Third World countries, because of lower birth rates (38–40:1000) and higher death rates (15–17:1000) (see Fig. 17–1 for birth rate trends since the 1950s).

Economically, India's fortunes have fluctuated during the past decades. The increase in rate of population growth, starting in 1921, was accompanied by economic gains, partly deriving from British stimulation during World War I. The world depression adversely affected India, but World War II again served as an even stronger stimulus to the economy, leading to peaks in urbanization and labor transfers into the nonagricultural sector. Mitra notes that industrialization has declined in recent decades, while the population growth rate has accelerated (21).

## POPULATION POLICIES AND PROGRAMS

Though India was an early advocate of governmental intervention in population change, financial support for its first two five-year plans during the period between 1951 and 1961 was modest. No precedents were available for developing an effective program to serve the needs "of a largely illiterate agricultural population dispersed among over half a million villages" (37). The first decade was devoted largely to research, and there was a growing realization that clinics were not well suited to reach the mass of population. In the 1960s, emphasis shifted to a community extension approach which utilized "auxiliary nurse-midwives, family planning health assistants" (37). Primary emphasis was given to sterilization, as intrauterine devices (IUDs) were not as acceptable as initially anticipated. Mass vasectomy camps were established in many states during the early 1970s, but were discontinued after several years. The stringent laws governing abortion were also relaxed during this time.

Programs in population control thus moved by fits and starts, subject to variations in funding and the adoption and discontinuation of various approaches. Yet the government steadily became convinced that the growth rate had to be cut substantially. During Indira Gandhi's tenure, this belief was forcefully expressed in the April, 1976, National Population Policy, which stated that the rate of population growth had to be treated as a top national priority and commitment and that population control was crucial in effecting desired social transformation and economic independence. Specifically, the government established the target of reducing the birth rate from 35:1000, in 1974, to 25:1000 in 1984.

This, in conjunction with the expected mortality decline, would reduce the rate of natural increase to 1.4 per cent per annum (21, 24).

To effect this decline, a variety of policies and programs were advocated, including raising the legal age at marriage, tying the amount of financial assistance allocated by the federal government to the states to the performance of family planning units in each state, and establishing stronger directives for sterilization, paving the way for legalizing compulsory sterilization. "It was a package of directives, disqualifications, and entitlements addressed to the state and the individual. It was a document of persuasion with unmistakable overtones of compulsion" (21:290).

Compulsion there was, especially the harsh measures introduced in certain states which sought to vigorously pursue compulsory sterilization programs. "It represented the conversion of the government's administrative resources into an engine of oppression, corruption, and fraud" (21). Sterilization quickly became a political issue that swelled to major proportions during the national elections of 1977. While it is impossible to determine the exact contribution of this issue, it doubtless played a decisive role in defeating the Congress Party, after 30 years of power.

## WHY HAS IT BEEN DIFFICULT TO REDUCE THE BIRTH RATE?

It is advisable to pause and explore the reasons why India has found it so difficult to reduce its birth rate, so much so that the government finally engaged in heavy-handed coercion in an attempt to achieve this goal.

The country's diversity plays a role. Although 83 per cent of the population reports Hinduism as their religion, there are many Hindu sects, creating more diversity than would superficially appear. Hindi, designated the official administrative language, is the native tongue of only 30 per cent of the population. Included in the national constitution as meriting "state encouragement" are 14 other major languages. In addition to diversity of languages, Indian caste groups are based on religion, region, and occupational clustering; whereas the system is less rigid than formerly, it is still basic to the country's social organization (37).

India's administrative structure is complex and often cumbersome. Since 1947 the country has been a parliamentary democracy based on the British model. There are 22 states, which vary greatly in population, with some (e.g., Uttar Pradesh, with nearly 100 million people) more heavily populated than many of the larger countries of the world. States are divided into district levels (387, in 1976), the primary administrative units (37). At all levels Indian bureaucratic practices are notoriously inefficient and corrupt.

The educational system has saturated the country with university graduates who are underemployed. Simultaneously, most of the population remains illiterate. In 1971, only 29 per cent of the population (39.5 per cent of the males and 18.7 per cent of the females) was literate. Thus, a key variable in effective contraceptive use, female literacy, still remains very low, even relative to other Third World countries (4, 37).

To understand what is happening in India, it is necessary to study the village, where the great majority of the population live. Cassen's review of the living conditions of the rural poor in India provides little grounds for optimism (7).

The fabric of India's rural society resists or absorbs most attempts at change. Governmental actions have made India's villages more tolerable places for many people to remain; but a large share of the benefits of these actions has accrued to the better off. For the mass of the poor, there is little sign of improvement in terms of their ability to acquire the basic necessities of food, clothing, fuel and decent housing (7:65).

Recently, the reasons why the Indian peasant resists family limitation have been more widely appreciated in the West as rational responses (18). The male head of the poor Indian household believes that many children, or rather many male children, are desirable because they make significant contributions, generally as day laborers, to family income and resources. This reasoning is consistent with Caldwell's theory regarding the direction of intergenerational wealth and service flows, as reviewed earlier in Chapter 15. Mamdani's *The Myth of Population Control* (18) effectively sets forth this position. He fails, however, to mention that what may be rational and economically rewarding for the heads of household may not produce the same benefits for the wives (Mamdani evidently did not talk to them), the children (in terms of their entire work careers), and the society at large, where short-term solutions may be disastrous from a long-term perspective (see Chaps. 18 and 19 for further discussion of individual versus societal needs).

## WHAT IS INDIA'S DEMOGRAPHIC FUTURE?

It is hard to disagree with Cassen's judgment that rapid fertility decline will not occur in India without substantial improvement in living conditions—income, education, and health—for the rural poor (7). Currently there is little indication of such changes. As demonstrated in the next section, the Chinese example suggests that it is possible to introduce substantial changes in village environments, including provision of birth control services, over a relatively short period. This has been possible because of Chinese political organization, which is quite different from that of India.

Nortman (24) has carefully analyzed the likelihood that the Indian government will achieve its revised target of fertility reduction. Indira Gandhi's Five-Year Plan for the years 1979 to 1984 was to lower the birth rate to 25:1000. The present government hopes to achieve a birth rate of 30:1000 by 1983. Nortman presents several alternative models that could lead to this goal, but the task confronting India is a formidable one. In March, 1977, when the government changed hands, approximately 25 million of an estimated 108 million couples were practicing contraception under the government program. Twenty-two million of the 25 million had been sterilized (24). But to meet the revised target of 30 births per 1000 by 1983, Nortman's model would require an increase from the present 24 per cent of couples using contraception to 67 per cent, during a 5-year period. This would require adoption of sterilization among a populace still resentful of the coercive measures attempted only a few years ago. Nortman counsels Indian policymakers to set more realistic targets, so as to minimize the likelihood of continued program failures (24).

Meanwhile the Indian population continues to grow. Cassen and Dyson (8) have produced a series of population projections based on new data and revisions of old data. Combining six sets of fertility assumptions with three sets of mortality assumptions, they provide 18 separate projections. The projections for total population in the year 2000 range from a low of 798.5 to a high of 1119.8 million. By 2011, 13 of the 18 projections exceed the billion mark. For India, then, the question of reaching a billion in population is not a matter of *if,* but rather of *when* (8).

Cassen and Dyson have also projected the number of years if will take India to attain a stationary population, and its size at that time. Their nine projections suggest that the Indian population would stabilize within 150 years, with a resulting size of 1249 to 1796 million, roughly either a doubling or a tripling of its current population. Another intriguing projection incorporates periodic catastrophes which would minimally double the death rate for several years. This "medieval mortality" pattern does not greatly impact on the population, for the population would still increase to well over a billion. Finally, Cassen and Dyson make two projections based on radical political and social change, such that the present slow fertility and mortality declines would shift within one or two decades to fast fertility, and fast mortality, declines. But even under these conditions, large populations of 917.0 million and 936.5 million would exist by 2001 (8).

In brief, regardless of the route followed, India faces massive population problems over the next several generations.

## CHINA

### DEMOGRAPHIC TRENDS.

The People's Republic of China has the largest population of any country in the world. As noted in Appendix 1, in 1978 the Population Reference Bureau estimated China's population at 930 million, a number almost 300 million larger than that of the second most populous country, India. China today contains nearly one-quarter of the world's population.

When Mao Tse-tung assumed control of the government in 1949, population size was unknown, since a census had not been taken for many years. Following the 1953 census, the population was placed at approximately 583 million (1, 3). Its crude birth rate was estimated to be in the low to mid-40s, and its crude death rate in the low 20s (1:328). Although there is some discussion regarding the magnitude of the crude birth rate in the early 1950s, most demographers place the figure in the low to mid-40s (2, 4, 19).

In the past quarter-century, China's birth rate appears to have declined remarkably (see Fig. 17–1). The Population Reference Bureau estimates its 1978 crude birth rate to be 22. If correct, this would signify a reduction of more than twenty points in approximately 25 years, an extraordinary achievement.

During the course of the past quarter-century, however, China has not been characterized by a continuous and ongoing policy emphasizing birth control and family planning. Its first birth control campaign was not initiated until 1954 and lasted only 4 years. A second was initiated in 1962 and also lasted 4 years. The third campaign began in 1969 and continues to the present. Despite China's "on again, off again" policy on birth control, the country apparently has successfully reduced its birth rate significantly. To better appreciate the nature of population policy and the three birth control campaigns, China's specific stance on the issue of population, since 1949, will be discussed.

## CHINA'S CHANGING POPULATION POSITIONS AND THE BIRTH CONTROL CAMPAIGNS

### PERIOD OF DOCTRINAIRE MARXISM: 1949 TO 1954

When Mao Tse-tung and the leaders of the Chinese Communist Party assumed control of China in 1949, they maintained a strict Marxist position on population size and its control. According to Marxist doctrine, overpopulation is not a problem in socialist society. Indeed Marx was most critical of Malthus and his theory of overpopulation. According to Marx, the Malthusian explanation was contrived "to justify the use by capitalist societies of induced unemployment as a means of exploiting the workers. However, in socialist society, which placed the means of production in the hands of the workers, such manipulation would not occur, and hence there would be no unemployment and no surplus population" (1:222). The Marxists also held that state ownership tended to inspire socialist workers "to such hitherto unknown levels of productivity and inventive-

ness that economic adversity, including population problems, would soon be banished forever" (1:222).

Mao and the party leaders thus saw people as a precious commodity, and the means through which China would advance. This optimistic stance was reflected in a September, 1949, news release of Mao Tse-tung:

It is a very good thing that China has a big population. Even if China's population multiplies many times, she is fully capable of finding a solution; the solution is production. The absurd argument of Western bourgeois economists like Malthus that increases in food cannot keep pace with increases in population was not only thoroughly refuted by Marxists long ago, but also has been completely exploded by the realities in the Soviet Union and the Liberated Areas of China after their revolutions.... Of all things in the world, people are the most precious. Under the leadership of the Communist Party, as long as there are people, every kind of miracle can be performed.... We believe that revolution can change everything and that before long there will arise a new China with a big population and a great wealth of products, where life will be abundant and culture will flourish. All pessimistic views [i.e., about population and food] are utterly groundless (1:223).

In 1952 and thereafter, discussions became more intense in the highest circles of the Chinese Communist Party regarding the possibility of an imbalance between food and population. China conducted a census in 1953, and the data from the large rural areas suggested that its population would be much larger than had been estimated in 1949. These data stimulated even more discussion about population limitation, and ultimately led to the first family planning campaign.

### THE FIRST FAMILY LIMITATION CAMPAIGN: 1954 TO 1958

Even after the first census, the party leaders were not unanimously convinced of a population problem. Many took pride in the vast size of China's territory and population. A principal spokesman for population limitation recognized this pride when he observed, in 1954, that "it is a good thing to have a large population, but in an environment beset with difficulties, it appears that there should be a limit set" (1:227).

Discussions continued during 1954 and

1955, although a specific campaign was not introduced until mid-1956. By this time, an actual imbalance between food and population had occurred in the form of a famine, in the spring of 1956. In August of the same year the Ministry of Public Health ordered the local health departments to establish birth control clinics, train appropriate personnel, increase supplies, and develop contraceptive distribution strategies. The first campaign had finally been launched (1).

Mao himself placed a very high priority on this first birth control effort, as is evidenced by the remarks of a supporter:

At present the construction of our country is being carried out in a planned way and with leadership, but the birth of children is without plan and without leadership. It is very obvious that this is not suitable. Chairman Mao has criticized this situation and pointed out that a great effort should be made to promote birth control from now on (1:238).

Another supporter reported that Mao had warned the Supreme State Conference that China would be nearing extinction when it reached a population size of 6 billion. Although demographically implausible, these observations clearly indicate that Mao had assumed a Malthusian stance with regard to Chinese population problems, a complete reversal from his doctrinaire Marxist perspective of 1949 (1).

The impact of the first birth control campaign on China's birth rate is unknown. There was no effective birth registration system, and thus no possible way to ascertain annual fluctuations in birth rates, let alone the effects of a campaign. Aird has noted, however, that there is "no reason to believe that the efforts to promote birth control [during the years of this first campaign] had any perceptible effect on the national birth rate" (1:275).

The failure of the first campaign to affect the birth rate does not mean that it made no contribution. Its initiation alone suggests that some of the party leadership had begun to adjust their originally Marxist perspective on overpopulation, itself a contribution worthy of attention.

There was never any official notice that the first campaign was to be terminated, but by the spring months of 1958, virtually no discussion or news of the campaign appeared in the daily press, and by the second week of June, all mention ceased. National attention had shifted away from the population aspect of the population-food relationship, to the food aspect.

## THE "LEAP FORWARD" AND THE ENSUING FOOD CRISIS: 1958 TO 1962

In late 1957, the prospects for agricultural production apparently were poor. Some Chinese observed that unless production improved, conditions might deteriorate, because of population growth and the undeveloped nature of the rural economy. It was also felt that many peasants in the rural areas were "wavering" in their "allegiance to the cooperatives" (1:277). Unrest was stirring in the countryside (1).

Thus the Chinese embarked on their "leap forward" in agricultural production in the spring of 1958: "The plan involved a revolutionary struggle against nature to realize the great potential of agriculture by maximizing the advantages of the collective economy" (1:278).

By late 1958 it appeared to many that the "leap" was successful. Reports and statistics indicated substantial improvements in agricultural productivity. But in early 1959 the reality of the situation contradicted these statistics. Apparently the grain-production figures maintained by the State Statistical Bureau had been significantly inflated, and food shortages, rather than increases, were the rule in 1959 and the early 1960s. It was clear that the "leap" had fallen short, and attention reverted to the population side of the population-food relationship, during the early 1960s. The Chinese were not able to immediately establish another birth control campaign, because of the existing food crises. Aird notes that by the beginning of 1962, "when the first signs of significant improvement were in evidence, a new birth control campaign was instituted" (1:287).

## THE SECOND BIRTH CONTROL CAMPAIGN: 1962 TO 1966

The second campaign began as quietly as the first had ended. In January, 1962, Chinese customs officials announced that duty would no longer be imposed on imported contraceptives, and a few months later the major newspapers featured articles on birth control and late marriage. The emphasis on planned childbirth and smaller families was officially rationalized as advantageous "to the health of mothers and children, to the opportunities for work, and political progress for both parents, and to the economic welfare of the family and the state" (1:289). A major objective of the second campaign was to "make planned childbirth a new way of life in our society" (1:289).

One of the unique features of the second campaign was the gross exaggeration of the ill effects of early marriage and childbearing on the health of parents and children. Aird describes articles which said that

unrestrained indulgence of the sexual impulse not only prevents the young men from getting adequate rest and exercise after work, but results in "strong nervous stimulation" and "excessive dissipation of bodily fluid," "malfunctioning of the central nervous system," "sexual neurasthenia, low spirits, headaches, ... discomfort all over the body," emaciation, dizziness, tension, memory decline, premature old age, mental and physical pain and impotence. ... Only by marrying later when the cerebrum was "mature" could the "reckless sexual impulse" be controlled (1:289–290).

The interests of the Chinese Communist Party were also emphasized. Young people were encouraged to develop their careers prior to reaching the age of 30, instead of placing all of their efforts on family formation. It was suggested that

childbirth was "not altogether a personal matter" but also a legitimate concern of the State because of its relationship to the national economy and the economic welfare of the people. The State ... had to bear the burden of providing food, clothing, housing, transportation, schooling, and employment for all the children. Hence family planning had a bearing not only on the family but also on the "health and prosperity of the entire people and the socialist construction of the State" (1:293).

The second campaign appeared to be more directed to value change, particularly among women and the young, then to a frontal assault on the birth rate. The goals tended to be more long-term than immediate, and the entire campaign lasted less than 4 years. It has been suggested that urban birth rates were probably not affected at all by this campaign and that "the impact on rural birth rates must have been extremely slight" (1:304). The situation might have been different had the second campaign not been interrupted in 1966 by the "cultural revolution." Nevertheless, the

stage had been set for discussion and reflection; family planning and birth control were slowly becoming integrated into the people's way of life. These results were to eventually have an impact on a much larger scale. But the third campaign could not begin until after the "cultural revolution."

### THE "CULTURAL REVOLUTION" AND THE INTERRUPTION OF BIRTH CONTROL WORK: 1966 TO 1969

The cultural revolution originated in the reaction against Mao Tse-tung and his policies that had set in after the failure of the "leap forward." Following the food crises of the early 1960s, and the subsequent recovery, the administration and control of the party had passed to Liu Shao-ch'i and his followers. Mao and other loyalists later sought to remove Liu from control. The "cultural revolution" was the vehicle used by Mao in this struggle against Liu.

Since he had lost control of the party apparatus, Mao was not able to employ usual administrative procedures in his attempts to purge Liu. Mao and his followers were forced to form an independent arm of political power; the Maoists thus, Aird reports,

called upon youth faithful to Mao throughout the country by direct appeal via the mass media to form entirely new organizations as "Red Guards" and "Revolutionary Rebels." These were summoned to Peking to "see Chairman Mao," to "exchange experiences" in making revolution, and to participate in mass rallies in the Tien An Men Square. The rallies were intended to intimidate Mao's enemies and to fire the youths to a peak of fervor before they were dispatched to various localities to "drag out the power holders" who were opposed to Maoism (1:304–305).

More than nine million youths attended rallies in Peking in the summer and fall of 1966.

The young groups of revolutionaries were hastily organized, with little or no internal structure, and no external command organization. Not surprisingly, anarchism prevailed. Originally incited to remove the traces of the "old society," the young revolutionaries carried their activities to extremes by tearing down street signs and historic monuments, and by harassing Westerners, diplomats, foreign dignitaries, and all those in Western dress. Whenever possible, they seized teachers and government officials and as many of Liu's followers as they could find. These victims were, Aird explains,

subjected to such humiliation and physical abuse that some committed suicide, died of injuries and exhaustion, or were broken in body and spirit. [The mood of the Red Guards] was expressed in such battle cries as, "We will crush your dogs' heads" and "Rats are running across the street with everyone shouting 'Kill them! Kill them!' " (1:309).

Ironically, the Maoists had originally stimulated the youths to act as autonomous units above the control of the party because of the party's domination by Liu. They soon discovered that the Red Gaurds were also rejecting Maoist control (1) and were becoming increasingly difficult to control at all. Finally, by late 1969, Mao's position within the party had improved substantially. Simultaneously, the "Red Guard" and the revolutionaries were becoming an intolerable embarrassment to Mao, and they were therefore renounced. The military assisted the Maoists to drive the youths from the cities. Mao then turned attention to rebuilding the party. The leaders also reverted to family planning issues and another birth control campaign.

## THE THIRD BIRTH CONTROL CAMPAIGN: 1969 TO THE PRESENT

The third campaign, more so than the previous two, had the complete support of the government and of the party leaders. Indeed, Maoist phrases were used frequently to legitimate various aspects of the birth control program. Contemporary news reports, according to Aird, declared that

birth control work is "a major event bearing on the national economy" and "one of the most important tasks of socialist revolution and socialist construction." To promote birth control is to "carry out . . . Chairman Mao's instructions" and "to hold high" the "great red banner of Mao Tse-tung thought" (1:311).

The second campaign exhibited some of these justifications, but on nowhere near the grand scale of the latter. The third is *the* major campaign in terms of its ambition, comprehensiveness, commitment, and success. Despite certain ambiguities, there is no doubt "that a major birth control effort is under way in China, and it is probably having a significant effect on population growth" (2:226).

The campaign was initiated with extensive political rhetoric and discussion. Individuals who objected to the goals of planned births and late marriage were said to be under the "pernicious influence of that 'traitorous scab' Liu Shao-ch'i and his ubiquitous 'agents' " (1:311). During its first few years, the campaign proceeded within this narrow perspective, as the Maoists rebuilt the machinery of the party, and the country recovered from the "cultural revolution." However, it was not "until late 1972 or 1973 [that] a major drive was launched on a national scale" (2:237).

Local birth control committees were established at all levels, and the party was involved in short- and long-run participation. As in former campaigns, the key effort was to convince the population that traditional values and preferences for large families were no longer applicable in China and should be eliminated:

The campaign propaganda argues that lower infant mortality rates make it unnecessary to have many children to ensure that some survive; that the state provides social security for old age, obviating the need for many descendents; that the emancipation of women makes daughters as valuable as sons; that fewer children and longer birth intervals are in the interests of maternal and child health and of the economic well-being of the family, the community, and the state; and that in a planned economy the "anarchical" increase in population cannot be allowed to continue (2:238).

The campaign has specifically sought to delay marriages for men until 25 years of age, and for women until 23 years. It has also encouraged couples to limit their families to two children. And, as well as can be ascertained, the birth control technology available for meeting these goals includes "all modern methods of contraception, in the further development of which China is conducting an aggressive program of research; abortion in case of contraceptive failure; and sterilization, mainly of women and especially of those who exceed the two-child limit" (2:238–239).

Despite its previous "on again, off again" family planning policy, since 1969 the country has apparently concentrated maximum attention on birth control efforts. In the eyes of many experts, China today may well have the most comprehensive and determined fertility control policy of any country (2, 11). But since data are both sketchy and incomplete, and perhaps even biased, the Western observer is unable to determine with certainty the actual amount of influence that the Chinese birth control campaigns have had on reproductive behavior.

## CHINA'S DEMOGRAPHIC FUTURE

Despite a pre-demographic-transition birth rate in the 40s, when the Communist Party assumed control in 1949, China today appears to be achieving the status of a developed country. Berelson (4) has stated that China is one of ten countries with a "probable" chance of reaching a birth rate of 20:1000 by the year 2000. However, if the birth-rate data for China are reasonably accurate (a crude birth rate in 1978 of 22:1000—see Fig. 17–1), its prospects should be considered even better than "probable." Between 1975 and 1978, China apparently reduced its birth rate by four points! Given even a minor continuation of this trend, China would achieve a birth rate of 20:1000 even by the mid-1980s.

H. Y. Tien, a demographer specializing in Chinese population trends, has reported birth rates even lower than 22:1000 for some parts of the country. For example, data from Shanghai, in the early 1970s, suggested a total birth rate of 12:1000, and a rate of 7:1000 for its inner city. Crude birth rates below 10:1000 appear more than occasionally in some rural communities (33). These are very select data, but even if they are adjusted on the basis of reasoned expectations, they still suggest a rather marked decline in the country's fertility.

Unfortunately, social and economic development data are not available; consequently, it is difficult to estimate the country's position regarding the major socioeconomic factors presumed to influence fertility decline. As noted in Table 17–1, data are only available for China's nonagricultural labor force and its per-capita gross national product. On the basis of these two indices, China has not yet attained the threshold values expected. With data for the other indices, it would be easier to assess the likelihood of continuous fertility decline. Nevertheless, the Chinese birth rate is presumably very low today, particularly in view of its magnitude 30 years ago. Assuming that these data are reasonably valid, China will probably attain birth rates in the mid- to high teens by the year 2000, especially if the current population policy favoring planned fertility remains in vogue.

## THE UNITED STATES

### TRENDS IN FERTILITY AND POPULATION GROWTH

The United States's population has increased from about four million in 1790, the date of its first census, to an estimated 218 million in 1978 (25, 31). The 1800s and early 1900s were years of very high growth; the country was experiencing the demographic transition from high birth and death rates to low birth and death rates; the high growth rates resulted from a major imbalance between fertility and mortality, thus producing significant increases in population size. These birth- and death-rate trends from 1910 to the present are presented in Figure 17–2.

Unlike the other countries previously discussed, in the United States fertility has already declined to low levels. Also, an intriguing deviation in the long-term decline has occurred, as will be indicated later in the chapter.

In 1800, the crude birth rate was above 50:1000; consequently, by the time American women had completed their childbearing years, they had given birth to between eight and ten children each (31, 35). The birth rate fell to 32:1000 by 1900, and to about 18:1000, during the depression years in the 1930s (35). However, it began to rise at the close of World War II and continued to increase through the late 1940s and the 1950s, reaching a high of 25:1000 in 1957. The total fertility rate at that time was near 3800, a rather significant increase from the approximately 2400 in 1940 (35) (see Fig. 17–2).

In 1958, American fertility began to decline once again. By 1964, the total fertility rate had fallen to 3208; by 1970, to 2480; and by 1974, to 1856. The most recent information from the National Center for Health Statistics (36) places the 1975 total fertility rate at 1799. As portrayed in Figure 17–2, in a period of approximately 20 years, American fertility has dropped by almost two children per woman, a most remarkable decline.

It is particularly interesting that these fertility declines have occurred in the absence of a national, large-scale, federally sponsored family planning program. For decades, government leaders would not consider subjecting population growth to any measure of government control. For example, President Eisen-

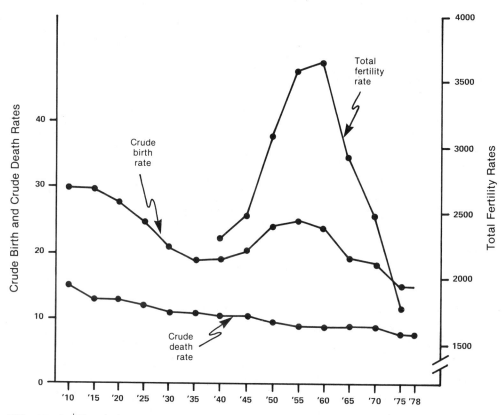

**FIG. 17–2.** Trends in crude birth and death rates, 1910–1978, and in total fertility rates, 1940–1975: United States. (Sources of data: [Birth and death rates through 1970]: U.S. Bureau of the Census: Historical Statistics of the United States. Washington, D.C., U.S. Government Printing Office, 1975. [Rates for 1975]: U.S. Bureau of the Census, Statistical Abstract of the U.S., 1977. Washington, D.C., U.S. Government Printing Office, 1977. [Rates for 1978]: Population Reference Bureau, World Population Data Sheet, 1978)

hower made the following statement at a 1959 press conference (12):

> I cannot imagine anything more emphatically a subject that is not a proper political or governmental activity or function or responsibility. . . . The government has no, and will not make, . . . as long as I am here, a positive political doctrine in its program that has to do with this problem of birth control. . . . That is not our business.

Although a wide range of birth prevention means was readily available to women at this time, there was no Congressional funding of family planning programs until the very late 1960s (38). Indeed,

> it was not until 1958 that the ban on prescribing contraceptives in public hospitals was lifted in New York City . . . [thus opening the way] for publicly financed health institutions to provide family planning services. [Moreover], it was not

until 1965, when the Supreme Court struck down the Connecticut statute barring the use of contraceptives, that a number of states repealed their restrictive laws (16).

## WHY THE RECENT FERTILITY DECLINES?

Despite the absence of a national population policy in the United States, fertility has declined, particularly since the late 1950s. Indeed the 1975 total fertility rate of 1799 is the lowest it has ever been (36). Although demographers do not fully agree about the causes of the decline, a compelling case may be made for one explanation. Since the late 1950s, American society has undergone significant change in its normative fabric dealing with family formation, fertility control, and the role of women. The country has internalized the values and norms of a modern fertility control society. The realization of equal opportunities between the sexes has become increasingly possible, and, in a very genuine sense, non-familial roles for females have become a realistic option.

These normative changes and rapid fertility reduction were both a product of the market availability of oral contraceptives in the early 1960s and their rapid diffusion. The rate at which they were adopted was clearly unprecedented. Although the rate is difficult to measure precisely, because of the ambiguous nature of the population considered to be at risk of becoming pregnant, the diffusion of the pill may be estimated by defining the risk population broadly to include all married women under age 35, with husband present. Three per cent of this risk population used oral contraceptives in 1961, and 29 per cent used them in 1970 (30). The pill's high acceptance rate was probably due to its noninterference with coitus and the significantly improved levels of contraceptive protection which it provided. After the development of the oral contraceptive, "significant proportions of the population came to expect fertility control to be both complete and unobtrusive," (6:67) and that efficacy brought about a "revolution in fertility." Bumpass has observed that

the essential characteristic of this revolution is that child bearing now may be voluntary in a radically different sense than ever before. Under the previous fertility regime, women could not confidently plan a lifetime of childlessness, nor even the prevention of unwanted fertility (6:67).

Although the pill set this revolution in motion, it is a mistake to refer to these changes as resulting solely from the introduction of efficient contraception. As Bumpass has noted, although the revolution in the norms and values resulted at least in part from the revolution in birth control, its impact on fertility decline ultimately overshadowed that of contraception (6).

When the intrauterine device (IUD) was introduced in 1965, it experienced an equally rapid diffusion among the risk population. The percentage of women using the IUD increased from 0.7 per cent in 1956 to 6 per cent in 1970 (30). Furthermore, in the 1960s and 1970s there were rather dramatic changes in the attitudes and behaviors of the American population concerning male and female contraceptive sterilization. By 1970, nearly two-thirds of the population who intended to have no more children (i.e., the risk population) had either been sterilized or were seriously considering sterilization for contraceptive reasons (29).

Public attitudes regarding abortion have also changed dramatically since the mid-1960s. Between 1965 and 1970, the number of American wives approving abortion for couples who could not afford, or did not want, a child rose by 14.3 per cent. During the same period, the number approving abortion for unmarried mothers rose 19.8 per cent (17). These changes are as much a result of the changes in fertility-control values as a response to concerns "about the role of accidental pregnancy in limiting the achievement of women," and a concern with the poor health consequences occurring with illegal abortions (6:68). It must be remembered that proabortion attitudes developed prior to the Supreme Court decision of 1973 which legalized the procedure. In other words, this very receptive climate for abortions existed when abortions were still illegal. As Bumpass notes,

the potential for complete fertility control makes childbearing—when and if—a matter of choice in an ultimate sense that never before existed. For the first time, motherhood itself is fully a matter for rational evaluation. Since it [no longer must] be rationalized because it is inevitable, costs as well as virtues must be weighed. . . . Obviously, childbearing roles offer much that is rewarding, but these rewards are not likely to be experienced equally by all women. [The events of the fertility control revolution have thus placed motherhood] more squarely in competition with other social roles (6:68).

In the past, pregnancy was inevitable for most women, and, therefore, society developed norms expecting women to remain in the home, expecting husbands to be the prime, if not sole, "breadwinners" in the family. These expected behaviors (norms) are no longer as influential and operational in American society as they were in past years.

## THE POPULATION COMMISSION OF PRESIDENT NIXON

Despite the United States's fertility decline in the virtual absence of a federally sponsored population policy, in 1969 President Richard Nixon proposed that Congress create a commission to study population growth and the American future and "to make recommendations on how the Nation can best cope with the impact" of its growth in the future (9: preface). The following section reviews the commission's work and the reaction to it by President Nixon.

### THE COMMISSION AND ITS RECOMMENDATIONS

*The Report of the Commission on Population Growth and the American Future* (9) was a landmark in the American stance regarding population growth. "For the first time in the history of our country, the President and the Congress have established a Commission to examine the growth of our population" and its impact (9: preface). The Population Commission was comprised of appointees representing a broad spectrum of American life. The commission included two senators and two representatives, businessmen, students, housewives, and many specialists in population matters. The commission heard more than 100 witnesses in hearings across the country. The Executive Director, Charles Westoff, and the Deputy Director, Robert Parke, Jr., two eminent and respected demographers, assembled an impressive staff and solicited a wide range of outside research reports. The resultant six volumes provide an unprecedented survey of current thinking on United States population; they are a compendium which will be useful for many years.

The actual report sent to the President was a most impressive document. *The New York Times* best expressed it editorially, calling the report

a model of courage, candor and clarity. The Commission has tackled head on such sensitive issues as sex education, genetic research, abortion, and the dissemination of contraceptive information and services. In every case it has taken a forceful stand for open discussion and freedom of individual choice (23).

The commission concluded that "no substantial benefits would result from continued growth of the nation's population" (9:1). Accordingly, it urged that "the nation welcome and plan for a stabilized population" (9:192). Aside from its attention to stabilization, the commission made a number of additional recommendations which largely were unheralded

by the popular press. Noting that the United States is emerging as an almost totally urban society, it urged the promotion of "high quality urban development in a manner and location consistent with the integrity of the environment and a sense of community" (9:212). In another important series of recommendations, it boldly decried discrimination based on sex:

We believe that increasing the freedom of women to seek alternative roles [to childbearing] may reduce fertility, [but] this change is not sought on demographic grounds alone. The limitations on the rights and roles of women abridge basic human liberties that should be guaranteed to all, regardless of the future course of population growth (9:152).

There were other recommendations—sixty-two in all—equal in their importance and degree of relevance to those discussed here. The commission recommended stabilizing our present immigration levels, argued against discrimination against illegitimate children, and urged the implementation of adequate child-care services for all.

### PRESIDENT NIXON'S RESPONSE TO THE REPORT

President Nixon's response to the report was, unfortunately, unusually limited and selective. Aside from a ritualistic expression of appreciation to commission members, he had no comments on which recommendations he found valuable, nor did he indicate the manner in which his administration would act on the commission's suggestions. Instead, he singled out two of the recommendations—those dealing with abortion and the availability of family planning services to minors—for explicit repudiation. A response of this type may well be interpreted as more guided by an election-year strategy (the 1972 presidential election would occur later that year) than by concern with population and the American future. Indeed the rejection of these two recommendations appeared to imply a rejection of, or at best, a lack of concern for, the other recommendations (5).

### THE UNITED STATES AND POPULATION POLICY

To this day, the United States is without an explicit and federally sponsored population policy. Yet its birth rate continues to decline. Apparently, even in the face of government inactivity, it is possible for the birth rate to decline, "if individuals see small families as being most advantageous to them" (38:297). As observed in an earlier section, the United States may be characterized as a *modern* fertility-control society: its norms and values encourage small, rather than large, families. And the declining birth rate may be interpreted in large part as a response to these normative and belief structures.

Despite government inactivity regarding population policy, it would be a mistake to believe that there has been no activity at all. Federal funding for national family planning services was first provided by the Congress in 1967 (see Chap. 10). The United States Supreme Court, in a landmark 1973 decision, essentially legalized abortion on demand during the first trimester of fetal life (see Chap. 9). Moreover, the Congress provides extensive support for research and training in the population field to the National Institute of Child Health and Human Development. President Carter's 1979 budget earmarked $37 million for this purpose.

# REFERENCES

1. Aird JS: Population policy and demographic prospects in the People's Republic of China. In People's Republic of China: An Economic Assessment. Washington DC, Joint Economic Committee, Congress of the United States, 1972
2. Aird JS: Fertility decline and birth control in the People's Republic of China. Pop Dev Rev 4:225, 1978
3. Aird JS: Recent provincial population figures. China Q 73:1, 1978
4. Berelson B: Prospects and programs for fertility reduction: what? where? Pop Dev Rev 4:579, 1978
5. Browning HL, Poston DL Jr: Population and the American future: a discussion and introduction to a review symposium. Soc Sci Q 53:445, 1972
6. Bumpass LL: Is low fertility here to stay? Fam Plann Perspect 5:67, 1973
7. Cassen R: Welfare and population: notes on rural India since 1960. Pop Dev Rev 1:33, 1975
8. Cassen R, Dyson T: New population projections for India. Pop Dev Rev 2:101, 1976
9. Commission on Population Growth and the American Future, Population and the American Future: The Report of the Commission on Population Growth and the American Future. New York, New American Library, 1972
10. Davis K: The Population of India and Pakistan. Princeton, Princeton University Press, 1951
11. Demerath NJ: Birth Control and Foreign Policy: The Alternatives to Family Planning. New York, Harper & Row, 1976
12. Eisenhower, President DD: Press Conference, December 2, 1959
13. El Colegio de Mexico, Centro de Estudios Economicas y Demograficos, Dinamica de la Poblacion de Mexico. Mexico, D.F.: El Colegio de Mexico, 1970
14. Goodstadt LF: Official targets, data, and policies for China's population growth: an assessment. Pop Dev Rev 4:255, 1978
15. Hernandez FA: La Poblacion de Mexico. Mexico, D.F.: El Colegio de Mexico, 1976
16. Jaffe F: Toward the reduction of unwanted pregnancy. Science 174:119, 1971
17. Jones EF, Westoff CF: Attitudes toward abortion in the United States in 1970 and the trends since 1965. In Westoff CF, Parke R Jr (eds): Demographic and Social Aspects of Population Growth, Commission on Population Growth and the American Future, Research Reports, Vol 1. Washington DC, USGPO, 1972
18. Mamdani M: The Myth of Population Control. New York, Monthly Review Press, 1972
19. Mauldin WP: Patterns of Fertility decline in developing countries, 1950–75, Stud Fam Plann 9:75, 1978
20. McCoy TL: The Dynamics of Population policy in Latin America. Cambridge, Ballinger, 1974
21. Mitra A: National population policy in relation to national planning in India. Pop Dev Rev 3:297, 1977
22. Nagel JS: Mexico's population policy turnaround. Population Bulletin 33, December, 1978
23. New York Times, March 17, 1972, p 40:1
24. Nortman DL: India's new birth rate target: an analysis. Pop Dev Rev 4:277, 1978
25. Population Reference Bureau, World Population Data Sheet, 1978. Washington DC, 1978
26. Portillo JL: Address to the International Union for the Scientific Study of Population. Pop Dev Rev 3:347, 1977
27. Poston DL Jr: The fertility control revolution and the future of working women. In Gerrard M (ed): Women in Management. Austin, School of Social Work, The University of Texas at Austin, 1976
28. Potter JE, Ordonez M, Measham AR: The rapid decline of Colombian fertility. Pop Dev Rev 2:509, 1976
29. Presser HB, Bumpass LL: The acceptability of contraceptive sterilization among US couples: 1970. Fam Plann Perspect 4:18, 1972
30. Ryder NB: Time series of pill and IUD use: United States, 1961–1970. Stud Fam Plann 3:233, 1972
31. Select Committee on Population, US House of Representatives, World Population: Myths and Realities. Washington DC, USGPO, 1978
32. Solis L: La Realidad Economica Mexicana: Retrovision y Perspectivas. Mexico, D.F., Siglo Veintinno, 1970
33. Tien HY: Fertility decline via martial postponement in China. Mod China 1:447, 1975
34. Urquidi V: On implementing the world population plan of action. Pop Dev Rev 2:91, 1976

35. US Bureau of the Census, Historical Statistics of the United States. Washington DC, USGPO, 1975

36. US Department of Health, Education and Welfare, Public Health Service, National Center for Health Statistics, Vital Statistics of the United States, 1975, Vol 1, Natality. Hyattsville, National Center for Health Statistics, 1978

37. Visaria P, Jain AK: Country Profiles: India. New York, Population Council, 1976

38. Weeks JR: Population: An Introduction to Concepts and Issues. Belmont, Wadsworth, 1978

# Anthropological and Sociological Perspectives

# IV

Building on concepts and theories presented in Part Three, such as the demographic transition and the contribution of economic development to fertility control, this section deals with the influence of family type, sex roles, religion, rural or urban residence, socioeconomic status, and various social-psychological factors on fertility.

Chapter 18 questions traditional interpretations of the demographic transition, proposing that the slow growth rates of pretransitional societies can be attributed to fertility control in response to moderate mortality rates, rather than to a precarious balance between births and deaths. Chapter 19 describes the change from relatively stable population growth to accelerated rates, viewing it as a product of the agricultural revolution, feudalism, and colonialism. Evidence is further presented to show that stable low rates of population growth are likely to follow economic modernization only if the benefits of such changes accrue to the masses as well as to the elite, and if the costs of raising children outweigh the benefits.

Chapter 20, which is written from a sociological perspective, describes various social structural factors that have been shown to be correlated with fertility, such as socioeconomic status, rural or urban residence, and religion. The application of social, and social-psychological, concepts to the implementation and operation of family planning programs is also addressed.

Chapter 21 describes ways in which traditional female roles encourage high fertility and explores highly valued nondomestic roles as incentives to fertility control. The influence of education and employment are particularly stressed because they provide women with opportunities to achieve status outside the maternal and domestic sphere. The influence of the male role, particularly machismo, on fertility, is also addressed. Related to this, Chapter 22 considers the relationship between fertility, family types, and conjugal unions. Chapter 23 addresses the cultural acceptability of contraceptive delivery systems and fertility-regulating methods and emphasizes the importance of adapting techniques and services to the needs of client populations.

# 18

# Population Growth and Regulation from a Cross-cultural Perspective

**Rochelle N. Shain**
**Rebecca A. Lane**

Although human population growth is accurately described as having been "gradual" until recent times, such a description masks the variability in growth among synchronic populations and the variability in growth of a single population through time. If one objective of population studies is to understand factors affecting fertility, then it is precisely the variability that must be examined. The present chapter examines population growth and regulation from a cross-cultural perspective. An appreciation of existing variability results in interpretations of fertility and mortality patterns alternative to the traditional demographic-transition model.

## COMPLEXITIES IN POPULATION CONCEPTS AND ANALYSIS

### DISTINGUISHING UNITS AND LEVELS OF ANALYSIS

Perhaps the most basic observation that can be made about *Homo sapiens* is that human groups are not randomly distributed over all available space but tend to be localized in the more habitable regions. Such nonrandom clusters have both a spatial and a temporal dimension. Each cluster has in demographic terms, a structure that can be partially described in terms of its distribution, size, and its sex and age composition. The structure is the result of biological and cultural processes, and also of the unique biological and cultural *history* of the particular group. The structural description of a population is a static view: it is valid for one moment in time and space. However, to the degree that biological and cultural processes are understood and the unique history of a group is known, its observed structure can be explained. Observed structure is thus the result of past processes and of history; demographic parameters estimated from it describe factors which are the partial determinants of its future structures. Viewed in this way, observed structures can provide a dynamic view of populations.

The most immediate problem in population studies is to determine meaningful units of analysis. Between the individual and the species there are a multitude of levels of integration that are referred to as *populations*. In fact, human population concepts are multidimensional. They possess not only both spatial and temporal aspects, but involve a variety of other dimensions, such as political, ethnic, and socioeconomic characteristics. Delimitation of an analytical unit ultimately depends on the theoretical basis upon which analysis proceeds. Thus the defined population of a geneticist may be very different from the population of an anthropologist, even though some of the individuals included in both groups may be identical. Lastly, whereas defined populations are composed of individuals, it is important to distinguish between individual and population levels of analysis (for further discussion, see Chaps. 14 and 22).

Given multidimensional population concepts and the distinction between individual and population levels of analysis, it is not surprising to find a great deal of debate and confusion in discussions of human population growth. We suggest that some debate, and much confusion, can be rendered moot when analytical unit and level distinctions are made. Such distinctions are especially important in discussions of "demographic transitions" and population growth.

## DEMOGRAPHIC TRANSITION: FROM EMPIRICAL GENERALIZATION TO THEORY

A large volume of demographic data has been amassed for historic and extant human populations. Based on these empirical observations, three basic patterns of fertility and mortality have been discerned: high fertility accompanied by high mortality, high fertility with degrees of lower mortality, and low fertility with low mortality. Such patterns are merely descriptions of the way things are, or of how they appear to be; they do not provide underlying reasons. Explanations depend on theory: as Hempel (39) emphasizes, "scientific hypotheses and theories are not derived from observed facts, but are invented in order to account for them." One theory devised to explain observed fertility and mortality patterns is that of demographic transition. Although not rigorously formulated, the theory is based on a concept of industrialization as a process. Basically it states that as a nation industrializes, general conditions improve and declines in the death rate precede those of the birth rate. The lag in time between the decline in the death and birth rates accounts for rapid population growth. (see Chap. 15 for further discussion.) "Stages" in the demographic transition have been characterized as follows (10, 17):

Stage I. Pretransitional—little regulation or control of death rates or birth rates, both of which are presumed to be high

Stage II. Transitional—reduction of birth and death rates

A. Early transitional—death rates reduced, but birth rates remain high

B. Mid-transitional—both rates being reduced, but birth rates still higher than death rates

C. Late transitional—death rates low, while birth rates are moderate to low, or fluctuating

Stage III. Posttransitional—both birth rates and death rates are low

It is clear that the theory of the demographic transition is macroanalytic—that is, its generalizations about fertility and mortality patterns apply only to an aggregate unit of analysis. More important, it should be realized that a large-scale perspective is assumed which does not necessarily correspond to the natural, nonrandom clustering of human populations through time. Rather it assumes a diachronic scale that includes all aggregates which share a similar degree of "industrialization." It also defines the relationship between fertility and mortality in the pretransitional stage by the *lack* of certain conditions related to industrialization as a process, namely the technology of birth and death control, and in the posttransitional stage by the *presence* of certain conditions related to industrialization as a process, namely economic development.

In its general outline, the theory of demographic transition does describe population trends in many European countries. However, since we do not adequately understand industrialization as a process, and, furthermore, since the process cannot be demonstrated to be a necessary and sufficient cause of population growth, the ability of the theory to predict future trends is very low (52). Moreover, some of its implications or assumptions have been seriously questioned, as follows:

(*1*) The premise that birth and death rates in pretransitional societies have always been high, and that they explain characteristic low rates of growth, has been challenged. Critics argue that slow rates of population growth in preindustrial times reflect population control. The debate has often been argued in terms of estimated mortality and fertility rates based on archaeological remains and simulation models. However, the significance of the debate is whether population growth was deliberately regulated prior to the Industrial Revolution.

(*2*) The ordered sequence of fertility and mortality patterns in the theory have also been questioned. Critics maintain that moderate rates of mortality and fertility were likely to have characterized the preindustrial era. High rates of fertility in some transitional populations may be partially explained as a product of Westernization.

(*3*) The theory predicts that stable low rates of population growth are a consequence of economic modernization. Critics argue that low growth rates are a likely consequence only if economic benefits accrue to the masses, as well as to the elite, and if the economic costs of raising children outweigh the benefits.

These arguments are examined within this and the following chapter.

## PREHISTORIC FERTILITY AND MORTALITY PATTERNS

We suggest that it is more useful to think in terms of demographic transition*s* than in terms of *the* demographic transition (52, 64). With this alternate perspective, the study of variability of human population growth facilitates the investigation of causes and consequences of growth.

Variability in fertility and mortality patterns at any stage in the demographic transition model becomes evident by simply changing the spatial scale to smaller aggregates. It is beyond the present development of macroanalytic theory to fully explain such variability in terms of different characteristics of populations or in terms of the relationships between their structural differences. Anthropological studies have focused on small-scale populations that have a greater degree of social and biological cohesiveness than do larger and more developed societies. Thus they provide potentially significant analytical units for exploring the relationship between demographic system structures and processes and aspects of social and biological systems. However, it should be emphasized that such small-scale societies cannot be considered representative samples of past or current large-scale aggregate groupings. Further, most analyses of small-scale societies have been focused at the microanalytic level, that is, they have focused on individual characteristics, decisions, or behaviors at various stages in the life cycle, and their relationships to individual survival and fertility (52).

## MORTALITY

At the macroanalytic level, with a large aggregate scale and sufficient temporal depth, human mortality is a remarkably predictable and regular process. Extensive studies have resulted in the development of "model life tables" that make possible the analysis of the *central tendencies* of the mortality experience in human populations (16, 82) (see Chap. 14). Mortality curves plotted for each age have a *U*-shape, representing relatively high rates in the first year of life, with a rapid decline in the second and third years, until age nine, then remaining low until middle age, with an increasing rate during older years (10). The character of the mortality curve is much the same for all large aggregate groups, regardless of the degree of economic development: the primary differences involve the actual rates at all ages. Given an extensive understanding of mortality as a process, models can be constructed that relate mortality with various levels and patterns of fertility, resulting in predictions of population growth. Thus it is possible to examine the implications of presumed high fertility, high mortality rates in prehistoric populations.

By assuming that prehistoric populations fall within the known range of physiological variables affecting fertility and age-specific susceptibility to death, several researchers have constructed models to estimate potential growth rates under high fertility, high mortality regimes (37, 38, 64, 75). Table 18–1 presents estimates of various parameters included by Hassan (38) to compute the average maximum potential of population growth in Paleolithic groups (hunters and gatherers). Given no birth control—that is, assuming that the groups were reproducing at the biological maximum, Hassan estimated annual growth rates ranging from 0.7 to 1.7 per cent. Under an exponential model of growth, a population with this rate could double its size in under 50 years. These large growth rates are obtained despite child mortality estimates of 40 to 50 per cent, maternal mortality estimates of 10 per cent, and assumptions of high incidences of sterility and fetal mortality. Given these estimated rates, about 23 to 35 per cent of all potential offspring would need to be removed to achieve slow growth. Thus Hassan argues, as does Polgar (64) that slow growth rates of human populations (based on archaeological

**Table 18–1. Estimated Parameters Included in Hassan (1975) Model for the Study of Maximum Potential Growth in Paleolithic Populations**

| Parameters determining birth interval: | |
| --- | --- |
| Amenorrhea | 10 months |
| Interval before conception | 3 months |
| Interval from conception to birth | 9 months |
| Total birth interval | 22 months |
| **Parameters determining live-birth interval:** | |
| Birth interval | 22 months |
| Fetal death rate | 12% |
| Sterility rate | 12% |
| Resultant live-birth interval | 27.3 months |
| **Reproductive parameters:** | |
| Age at menarche | 15 years |
| Adolescent sterility | 1 year |
| Age at ability to conceive | 16 years |
| Adult female longevity | 29 years |
| Reproductive span | 13 years |
| **Mortality parameters:** | |
| Maternal mortality | 10% |
| Infant mortality | 40–50% |

(Adapted from Hassan FA, In Polgar S (ed): Population, Ecology, and Social Evolution. The Hague, Mouton, 1975, p 27)

studies and estimated from .0007 per cent to .003 per cent per year prior to the agricultural revolution) must reflect fertility control.

Models constructed to examine growth potential of Paleolithic populations assume a large aggregate scale, and thus incorporate typical age-patterns of death. Aberrant mortality patterns for prehistoric populations have been suggested, such as low mortality during breastfeeding, with high mortality at weaning. However, as demographic data are amassed, it is clear that deviations from the central tendencies of mortality experience decrease when the quality of demographic data is improved (41). Although small populations may experience atypical age-patterns of death at a given point in time, the age-specific properties of death appear to be deeply rooted in the biology of the human species. Individuals have had little influence over mortality rates until modern times; for most of human history, then, mortality has been the control variable in population dynamics.

Given its importance in understanding growth, attempts have been made to empirically investigate the mortality experience of preindustrial populations. The method most commonly employed is the construction of life tables, based either on the age and sex distribution of extant groups or on skeletal remains. There are several methodological problems in either approach that have been discussed in a number of critiques (1, 3, 36, 53, 76, 80, 83). With skeletal data, there are problems regarding establishing the age and sex of remains, the relationship of the age-distribution of remains deposited through time to the age distributions of the specific populations from which they were derived, and the underenumeration of infants. In extant groups, migration is a confounding process. Observed age structures may primarily reflect migration effects, rather than fertility and mortality effects. Perhaps the most serious source of error in either approach is simply small population size. Stochastic fluctuations can result in significant deviations from predictions based on stable population theory, since the theory is based on a population of infinite size (7, 48, 49, 53, 54, 77, 85).

Although the empirical approach to the study of mortality in preindustrial societies is limited by inadequate data and methods that are often inappropriate for available data, studies of extant populations have provided an ecological perspective on general health conditions. The pattern which is emerging consists of various endemic diseases and generally excellent nutritional status (4, 21, 22, 44, 59, 62). Since ecological setting greatly influences disease patterns, it is expected that mortality rates in preindustrial societies would vary among different settings. Based on studies of extant hunting-and-gathering populations, Howell (41) suggests that mortality rates would be expected to vary between moderate levels, in favorable environments, and higher levels, in less favorable environments. Higher mortality rates than those that can be offset by fertility imply extinction for the group involved. The suggested range of mortality experience implies an expectation of life at birth, ranging from around 18 to 20 years to about 35 or 40 years, as is observed among the Kalahari Bushmen. It is believed that populations like the Bushmen which experience moderate mortality levels must resort to fertility-reducing behavior, since they do not evidence rapid population growth.

The criticisms discussed thus far of the characterization of pretransitional populations as having high fertility, high mortality rates have concentrated on mortality experience. However, it is important to explore factors other than mortality which affect the fertility of such populations.

## FERTILITY

In general, in all populations, the fertility curve by age for females has an inverted *U*-shape. Fertility is low during the mid-teens, but rises sharply toward the late teenage category. It is highest for women in their twenties, then declines slowly for women past thirty until menopause. There are a number of factors that affect the magnitude of age-specific fertility rates, but this general pattern reflects the biological basis of reproduction.

### ECOLOGICAL CONSTRAINTS

Studies of extant hunting-and-gathering populations have provided a perspective on ecological constraints affecting fertility behavior. Of primary importance in these nomadic groups is the relationship between child transport and birth spacing, a critical factor recognized over half a century ago (14, 45). Given the difficulty of a woman's carrying more than a single child along with her normal baggage, models have been constructed which show the adaptive advantage of birth spacing at both the individual and population level (46, 75). Birdsell (9) has estimated a minimum of 3 years between offspring, while data from extant groups indicate intervals of from 3 to 5 years (21, 46). Additionally, it has been observed in extant hunting-and-gathering

groups that there is an absence, or insufficient quantities, of suitable soft foods to allow weaning before 2½ to 3 years of age (21).

Assuming that these constraints operated on all hunting and gathering societies, it is clear that the population could not reproduce at the level of the biological maximum. That does not mean that *individuals* could not reproduce at a high rate. The requirements of child transport and infant rearing do not force individuals to space births; rather, they limit *the age interval between surviving offspring*. It is important to make the distinction between population and individual levels of fertility.

### FERTILITY REGULATION

It is clear from studies of extant nonsedentary populations that intervals between siblings are longer than they would be if mothers were reproducing at maximum rates and all natalities survived. However, the mechanisms that actually affect these intervals are not clear. Considerable demographic and ethnographic evidence indicates that infanticide may be a primary mechanism (9, 42, 45, 57, 59, 60). Demographic evidence is based on sex-ratio imbalances in the population, indicating a sex preference in infanticide (generally for the female). For example, Birdsell (9) reported a male sex ratio of 150 among Australian aborigines, and Neel (59) reported a male sex ratio of 128 among the Yanomama. Neel estimated that infanticide involved 15 per cent to 20 per cent of all live births in this group. Of course it must be remembered that such ratios are based on short-term observation in small populations. Thus, ratios could be skewed by other unobserved processes, or could reflect stochastic fluctuations.

Ethnographic evidence is based on practices of extant populations. For example, the practice of infanticide, with no preference as to sex, is admitted in the Dobe !Kung Bushmen, although at low rates (42). There are problems in collecting such data, since the practice may be treated with secrecy, and there are cultural differences in the recognition of what constitutes a live birth. Dumond (21) suggests that infants subjected to infanticide may be regarded as stillbirths by the Dobe !Kung. Thus it is difficult to assess the importance of infanticide for maintaining long intervals between sibs.

A proposed physiological mechanism for

the maintenance of long birth intervals is the suppression of ovulation due to long lactation. Breast-feeding for periods of 2.5 to 3.5 years has been observed in extant hunting-and-gathering groups (21, 46). The relationship between lactation and ovulation in nonsedentary societies is difficult to study directly. There is a developing literature on this relationship, however, in other populations, (11, 12, 32, 43, 66, 72) and in natural populations of nonhuman primates (2). Leridon (47) has estimated levels of natural fertility by a "Monte Carlo" simulation model which includes postpartum sterility due to breast-feeding. Although the model was not constructed to examine effects in hunting-and-gathering societies, it does reflect distributions of lactational amenorrhea estimated from studying populations with low, medium, and high incidences of natural sterility. Estimated numbers of live births (natural fertility) are presented in Table 18-2 for populations with no, low, and medium sterility, and under the conditions of no breast-feeding and breast-feeding for 24 months. The mean duration of lactational amenorrhea, if the infant survives to 1 year of age, is 15.3 months.

The simulation did not consider maternal mortality rates, but infant mortality was taken into account through the distribution of the duration of postpartum sterility. If the distribution were changed to reflect higher infant mortality rates, the number of live births would increase, since amenorrhea is assumed to cease when lactation is interrupted.

The large numbers of live births evident in Table 18-2 suggest that known distributions of postpartum sterility due to lactation probably cannot account for the rather low average completed fertility observed in extant hunting-and-gathering groups. For example, women over 49 years of age averaged 4.7 live births in the Dobe !Kung, with first births occurring around 19.5 years of age (42). It is possible that the distribution of lactational amenorrhea in hunting-and-gathering populations is different from that in modern populations. Lee (46) believes that the suppression of ovulation from lactation in the Bushmen is evident "to a greater degree than [in] other populations," suggesting phenotypic adaptation from genotypic selection. While intriguing, this hypothesis is untestable on a numeric basis alone. However, it is possible, through simulation, to derive the distribution of lactational amenorrhea, under various regimes of infant mortality, needed to account for observed low completed fertility. If the means of derived distributions fall within the range of known duration of postpartum sterility, a strong case can be presented for the effectiveness of prolonged lactation as a mechanism of birth spacing.

## DELIBERATE VERSUS NONDELIBERATE REGULATION

The physiology of reproduction is complex, and our understanding of individual variability is far from complete. Variability does exist, and it is not unreasonable to expect it in the distributions of physiological parameters among populations. There is increasing evidence that variability in fecundity, both at the population and individual levels, can be significantly explained by variability in nutrition (15, 18, 25–31, 34). Such studies have indicated that nutrition critically affects onset of menses, the duration of adolescent sterility, irregularity or cessation of menstrual function, spontaneous abortion, lactational amenorrhea, and onset of menopause.

At the macroanalytic level, variability in physiological distributions implies variability

**Table 18–2. Number of Live Births for Fecund Women, 15 to 45 Years, in the Absence of Mortality**

| Population sterility | Length of breast-feeding | Number of live births, with: | |
|---|---|---|---|
| | | Marriage at 15 | Marriage at 19 |
| None | None | 17.5 | |
| Low | None | 15.2 | 12.8 |
| | 24 mos. | 10.0 | 8.4 |
| Medium | None | 13.5 | 11.4 |
| | 24 mos. | 8.7 | 7.4 |

(Adapted from Leridon H: Human Fertility. Chicago, Univ. of Chicago Press, 1977)

in the degree to which physiological mechanisms affect birth intervals. Given this variability within a subsistence adaptation that includes strong ecological constraints on *population* fertility, it is expected that a variety of mechanisms may be deliberately adopted to effect birth or survivorship intervals. The cross-cultural study of extant and historic societies confirms the existence of a variety of fertility-regulating methods in preindustrial societies; some of these methods will be examined in a subsequent section of this chapter.

To this point, we have reviewed arguments suggesting that the traditional view of fertility and mortality in preindustrial societies is, at best, superficial, and certainly inadequate as a basis for understanding population growth. Although it is conceivable that individual fertility was high, effective birth rates at the population level could not have been so. The concept of *effective* birth rates is not standard to demography, and perhaps it is the key to understanding the debate. The concept is based on survivorship intervals between sibs rather than number of live births per female. Survivorship intervals may, in fact, be affected by the manipulation of infant mortality, i.e., infanticide, rather than by fertility control. The significance of the debate is not whether fertility and mortality, sensu stricto, were high, but whether such rates were *deliberately regulated.* Critics argue that control of population growth is a key development in human history (59), and one which occurred prior to the economic development evident in industrialized societies (21, 63–65). It is believed that many preindustrial societies base their use or nonuse of fertility-regulating methods on their immediate needs and goals. Therefore, before examining fertility-regulating methods, we shall review some population policies in preindustrial contemporary societies.

## FERTILITY CONTROL IN CROSS-CULTURAL PERSPECTIVE

### FERTILITY GOALS IN CONTEMPORARY PREINDUSTRIAL SOCIETIES

It has been argued that individuals in every society have goals related to fertility, whether these are implicit or explicit; that is, the size family that is preferred conforms to available resources and cultural values (70, 78, 79). What is important for the present discussion is

not whether these goals favor low, moderate, or high fertility, but the fact that they represent rational responses to a given priority system.

Satisfactory population levels are sometimes maintained through nondeliberate practice of fertility-regulating methods, such as cultural restrictions on intercourse at various times, or prolonged periods of lactation (55, 56, 67). In the absence of such automatic regulation, population control is often deliberately encouraged and practiced. Even when governmental goals are pronatalist, as in many parts of Eastern and Western Europe and in Israel (24), people may limit family size when they perceive it to be in their best interest to do so. On the other hand, despite governmental goals of curbing population growth, as in many developing countries, individuals often perceive family limitation as antithetical to their interests and therefore refuse to employ contraception.

In this section, examples of population policies among relatively small and confined groups of people are presented, because in such societies relationships between fertility and immediate sociocultural situations are more readily discerned than in more complex groups. What may appear to us as irrational reproductive behavior will be shown to represent rational responses to individual needs and values given their economic constraints and culturally defined priorities.

### THE TAPIRAPE AND THE TENETEHARA

The important role played by fertility goals in preliterate societies is demonstrated by the Tapirape and Tenetehara reaction to Portuguese colonialism. Both people are Tupi-speaking tribes in Central and Northeastern Brazil, respectively. During precontact times, both were tropical forest horticulturists who supplemented their diet with hunting, fishing, and gathering of forest fruits. The Tenetehara had better access to fish, whereas the Tapirape had better access to game. Both groups had sufficient land, but were forced to periodically move to new villages when suitable garden sites were consumed through slash-and-burn techniques. Both tribes occupied similar physical environments and were at the same stage of technological development. Their ecological niche appeared to have limited each village to approximately 200 individuals, but there was no upper limit to the number of villages (79).

Despite these similarities, contact with the Portuguese affected these groups very differently. The Tenetehara have recovered their initial losses from warfare and disease, and are now a functioning, expanding society. The Tapirape, on the other hand, are on the verge of extinction. Wagley (79), the anthropologist who studied these tribes, does not believe that the differences in the contact situation explain the different modes of adjustment, particularly since the Tenetehara experienced considerably more violent contact than the Tapirape. He believes the explanation is primarily based on the different fertility goals and social structures of each society.

The Tenetehara value children and large families. Little birth control is consciously practiced, and infanticide is rare. The Tapirape value small families—a maximum of three live children, not all of the same sex. Infanticide is the primary means of population control. It is utilized under a variety of circumstances, such as at the birth of twins or of the third same-sexed child, and in the case of offspring from a mother who has had sexual relations with more than two men during her pregnancy—apparently not an uncommon occurrence.

These feelings toward population regulation originally "fit" the social organization of each tribe. The Tenetehara were, and still are, organized along lines of extended families which could readily move as a unit and form a new village when necessary. Social organization among the now disorganized Tapirape was much more complicated, and consisted of various cross-cutting social units upon which ceremonial life and subsistence activities were based. Individuals belonged to various associations. Since no one group was self-sufficient, it was very difficult for splinter groups to successfully form. Whereas the flexible Tenetehara social structure was conducive to expanding population, that of the Tapirape was not. Individual fertility goals reflected this difference.

In addition to factors related to social structure, cultural values help explain the persistence of small family size among the Tapirape even in face of possible depopulation. The Tapirape base their fertility goals on economic factors. They state that they do not want their children to be hungry or thin, and add that meat is scarce during the rainy season. In addition, a complicated set of food taboos, which allows young children to eat only certain meats, and women others, makes the task of supplying meat to the family very difficult. Wagley notes, however, that there is no real hunger among the Tapirape, and that being "hungry" means being hungry for meat. Moreover, in Tenetehara villages meat is also scarce, and during the rainy season fish is in short supply, but the Tenetehara do not limit population growth in the manner of the Tapirape. Wagley concludes that whereas the ecological situation is important, culturally derived values, along with social structure, are in this case the determinants of population size. "In other words, although family limitation among the Tapirape has a basis in subsistence, it does not derive from a minimum starvation situation. Family limitation seems to be related to a desire for a specific food, which the organism needs, but which is also selected by Tapirape culture as particularly desirable" (79:275). Values which encourage drastic measures of population limitation remain rigid, even in the face of decimation. As irrational as this behavior may be on a societal level, given the *culturally defined priorities,* it makes "sense" for the individual.

### THE RENDILLE

The Rendille of Kenya rely on a diet of meat and milk produced by their herds of sheep, goats, and camels. Camels are their most valued resource and form the basis of their prestige system. Fertility goals in this group are based upon the limitations imposed by the size herd that can support each family, and the knowledge that people multiply faster than camels. The Rendille cope with their population problems through emigration, primogeniture, late age at marriage, and infanticide at given times, such as in the case of births which occur on Wednesays (20).

### THE TIKOPIA

The Tikopia occupy an island in the Pacific 700 miles away from the nearest big island. Because their resources are limited, their fertility goal is steady replacement. They limit their families to two, or at most three, offspring by use of abortion, contraception, and infanticide (20, 23).

The Tikopians live on fish, root crops from their gardens, and tree crops, including coconuts, from their orchards. Food is plentiful, and cereal and root crops are readily shared. Members of this society, however, told anthropologist Firth, who studied them in 1929 and 1952, that they were very concerned about the availability of food during times of famine, which occur approximately once in 20 years. Insight into this society obtained through fieldwork during times of famine led Firth to believe that these people were primarily concerned with their supply of coconuts: there was a sufficient supply of naturally growing foods to avoid mass starvation, and, in fact, very few deaths during times of famine were actually attributed to starvation. On the other hand, coconuts are very valuable in this society, and men will fight over orchard lands, but never over garden lands. The milk of the coconut is used to make all other foods palatable. Feasting lies at the core of their social and religious ceremonies; without coconut milk they would not enjoy feasts; and without feasts their social and religious life would come to a standstill. Firth therefore concluded that Tikopian fertility goals were not based on actual biological survival, but on sociological survival (20, 23).

## THE NAMBUDIRI BRAHMINS

The Nambudiri Brahmins belong to one of the richest landowning castes in South India. They are rich and exclusive. They maintain their social advantages by not dividing their estates—only a family's eldest son, and one daughter, are allowed to marry. The eldest son inherits and administers the estate on behalf of his brothers. While the remaining brothers can console themselves with women of lower castes, the daughters are secluded and remain childless all their lives. In this case, population control is not employed by a given caste because of basic subsistence needs; rather, small family size allows Nambudiri individuals to retain their economic hegemony, which, in turn, provides them with their primary source of prestige (20).

## THE ONOTOA

Fertility goals among the Onotoa in the Gilbert Islands, in the Pacific, are based upon shortage of land. Each family's holdings are divided into a number of plots for the sons and the eldest daughter. Couples determine how many sons they reasonably can provide for; the wife is encouraged to subsequently abort

all pregnancies following fulfillment of this quota. Landless daughters are usually ineligible to marry. They consort with men, but any offspring of such unions are considered illegitimate, with no rights to land, unless formally recognized by the father. In the absence of such recognition, landless women resort to abortion (33).

## THE PEOPLE OF MANIPUR

This final example from a village in India illustrates how low fertility goals and population control are a rational response for some castes, but not for others (50).

In Manipur, the lower caste Indians never used the fertility-regulating devices they so obligingly accepted from their donors during a six-year project, the Khanna Study. To do so would have been an irrational response, from their point of view. Families belonging to agricultural castes required many sons to work the land. Moreover, as a result of agricultural expansion, demands for such labor increased. Members of traditional nonagricultural service sectors were also dependent upon their sons' work, and this dependence grew as a consequence of technological innovation. For example, as the sewing machine became widely distributed, tailors were deprived of business. Blacksmiths, with their traditional skills, could not repair the new, complicated farm machinery, and thus were forced out of this line of work. Many middle-aged parents were too unskilled to train for new occupations; moreover, they were prevented from doing so by the potential wrath of higher caste individuals, who began relying upon them for such menial tasks as carrying messages. Parents in such situations depended on their children's labor for survival. Sons began to work outside the home at the age of ten, or younger. Part of their wages were used for daily sustenance. The remainder was often saved to educate one son in a modern vocation, so that he could start a new economic enterprise. Upon completion of this training, the chosen son would train his brothers in the family business. Many sons were consequently seen as the only means to present survival, and future viability in old age (50).

Large families with many able-bodied men also had an advantage in confrontations with other families, and in emergency situations, when a great deal of manpower was needed to complete a task. For example, a large family could easily rebuild a home destroyed by a monsoon; a small one would have to pay to have it done (50).

Despite governmental goals of stemming runaway population growth, villagers never really believed that the purpose of the family planning project was family planning. To them, such a purpose made no sense. Their reproductive goal was to increase their number of sons, not to limit them (50).

The Brahmin class, on the other hand, limited the size of their families, even before family planning became widely available. Although they were not well-off financially, they valued education for their offspring and disdained agricultural labor. They did not hire out their sons until they were approximately sixteen and could work in shops. As a result, children often cost more to raise than they produced. The rational response for Brahmins, with respect to fertility control, was not the rational response for the rest of the population (50).

In summary, individual reproductive goals and behavior, even in preindustrial societies, can be viewed as rational responses to *socioeconomic situations* and *culturally defined priorities*. Such priorities most commonly involve economic factors, ranging from providing basic subsistence to maintaining and improving a given life-style—that is, enjoying the "oysters and champagne" (20) of life. The following section describes types of fertility-regulating methods used by preliterate and preindustrial people when population limitation has been their goal.

## FERTILITY-REGULATING METHODS IN PREINDUSTRIAL SOCIETIES

The literature on fertility-regulation among preindustrial groups (5, 8, 19, 35, 40, 56, 74) indicates that birth control has been utilized throughout recorded history, and in societies representing all levels of socioeconomic development. Birth planning is not an invention of modern times, but is as old as mankind (40).

### INFANTICIDE

Infanticide and abortion have been the most prevalent methods of effective fertility-regulation utilized throughout history (5, 40). Infanticide has not been restricted to a given area or period. It has been commonly used in Australia, North America, Africa, Asia, and South America. In addition to its use in population-regulation, it has been employed to dispose of children in various categories—those who are sickly and deformed, or the products of illegitimate, incestuous, or adulterous unions, or who are members of an undesired sex; of a child of mixed blood, a sib in a set of twins, or a child born before an elder sibling is either weaned or mobile, or born on an unlucky day (5, 40, 74).

Sometimes, as among the natives of the Murray Islands in the Torres Straits, equal sex ratios among offspring are desired. Consequently, in case of an overproduction of one sex, children of that sex are destroyed (74). More commonly, elsewhere, infanticide has been practiced preferentially, with regard to one sex. Female infanticide is the most common form, and has been practiced when women are considered a burden, with no compensatory benefits either in warfare or subsistence (8).

The Netsilik Eskimos, for example, destroy many of their female infants because of the adult sexual division of labor. These people live in a harsh environment, with exceedingly limited resources, and are entirely dependent upon hunting for survival. Because women do not hunt, they are seen as consumers of vital resources without a complementary role in production (6, 20). In Tahiti, girls were preferentially killed because they were considered useless in warfare, religious ceremonies, fishing, or navigation (74). Preferential female infanticide was widely practiced in pre-Communist China and is still known to occur in India, where girls are valued much less than boys (57, 61, 74). Even when Indian girls are not deliberately killed, they are still frequently neglected and undernourished, often perishing, whereas their brothers thrive (8, 50, 78, 84, 87). A similar form of female neglect has been found in Ecuador (69, 70). Another variant of female infanticide is practiced by the natives in a northern Mayan community. Women in this group practice infanticide so as to provide sufficient breast milk for one child at a time. If they are suckling a son and give birth to a daughter, they will kill the daughter. If they are suckling a daughter and give birth to a son, they will allow the newborn infant to live at the expense of the daughter (58).

Preferential male infanticide also occurs, but is reported much less frequently. It appears to occur in those societies where women are valued for the brideprice they eventually bring to their families when they marry. This type of population control has been practiced, for example, in the Banks Islands and in what was formerly British New Guinea (74).

## ABORTION

Abortion is as widespread as infanticide. Devereux, in his study of abortion, found (denials to the contrary) that "there is every indication that abortion is an absolutely universal phenomenon, and that it is impossible even to construct an imaginary social system in which no woman would ever feel at least impelled to abort" (19:98). Women throughout history have either performed their own abortions or have sought help from community practitioners, friends, or relatives. Techniques of abortion are extremely varied, including strenuous physical effort; jolts to the body; heat applied externally; skin irritants; bleeding; starvation; and the use of abortifacients, magic, and mechanical methods such as constriction, instrumentation, and insertion of foreign bodies into the uterus (5, 19).

The following examples attest to how strongly women have desired to control their fertility, in the absence of effective contraception. Among the Miriam, in the Torres Straits, women climb a coconut palm, bumping their bellies against the trunk as they are ascending and descending (19). In Alor, Melanesia, and Papua, women jump from high objects such as rocks and trees (19). Among the Kroe of Sumatra, hot ashes are placed on the female's abdomen. A similar technique is practiced by the Kalmuck, where hot coals wrapped in an old shoe sole are placed on the female's belly immediately above her uterus (19). Pima women of North America strain themselves, whereas Kgatla of Africa and Bukaua women bleed themselves, either by incision, or by the use of leeches. Women among the Manus of New Guinea, the Hottentots of South Africa, and those inhabiting Eddystone Island in Melanesia use belts to tightly constrict their abdomens (19).

Devices such as sticks, hooks, and bent wires have been used, respectively, by the Fijians, the Persians, and the Mescalero Apache (19). A thinly carved rib of walrus is used by certain Eskimo tribes, whereas the Mangbettu of the Congo insert a sliver of ivory into the uterus (5). Sheikh Muslim practitioners insert either medicinal herbs or a thin stick into the vagina

of women seeking to terminate their pregnancies (56).

Yap women either drink boiled, concentrated sea water, which induces vomiting and cramping, or insert a thin, rolled plug of hibiscus leaves into the cervix. The leaves expand when moistened, thus dilating the cervix. The women then injure and scratch the cervix with a stick or other sharp object until bleeding ensues (68).

Abortifacients range from the seemingly innocuous to the toxic. Substances such as writing ink, potassium permanganate, purgatives, turpentine, castor oil, quinine, horseradish, ginger, epsom salts, ammonia, mustard, and opium have been reported. The more toxic are indirectly effective—that is, they either poison or irritate the woman's body, expelling the fetus as a side effect (5, 35). The more innocuous are often accompanied by magic ritual. For example, some Algerian Arab women drink water from a cup in which sacred words were written and their ink dissolved, simultaneously reciting a magic formula (19).

Various herbal abortifacients are a part of folk culture and are handed down from generation to generation. For example, marjoram, thyme, parsley, and lavender, used in tea form, are part of old German folk medicine, both as abortifacients and as contraceptives (35, 40). Some of these appear to be mild emmenagogues, stimulating menstruation (35).

Some of the more "exotic" folk abortifacients used in preliterate societies have also been found to be potentially effective. For example, the foam from a camel's mouth is eaten by pregnant women in the Siwa Oasis, and the Taulipang consume a paste of pounded ants which had been standing outdoors overnight (19). The sputum apparently contains irritant properties, and the ants, formic acid. The latter would certainly be lethal to the fetus, and perhaps even to the mother. The Menomini of North America chop the tail hairs of the black deer and mix it in bear fat. When consumed, this mixture causes gastric irritation and perhaps uterine contractions. The Menomini attribute its effectiveness to the tiny bodies of hair, which they believe act like magic arrows searching out and destroying the fetus (19).

## CONTRACEPTIVE METHODS

Although methods of contraception have been utilized in all parts of the world, in ancient as well as modern times, they are not believed to be as prevalent as abortion and infanticide (5, 40). Sexual behavior has not, however, been the subject of much research, nor has it been reported by most ethnographers. Consequently, contraception has probably been practiced to a much greater degree than the limited data would indicate (40).

Abstinence. Abstinence during the fertile period has been reported (40, 56). Sometimes timing is accurate with respect to preventing conception, but more often it is not. The Tallensi of Africa believe that women cannot conceive in the period immediately following menstruation. On the other hand, the Masai of Africa believe a woman is most likely to conceive during the first four or five days following menstruation (56).

Because it requires no knowledge of the relationship between fertility and the menstrual cycle, postpartum abstinence is usually a more effective method of contraception, providing its restrictions are properly adhered to. Postpartum abstinence lasts anywhere from several weeks to more than two or three years (55, 56, 67). It has been documented in Subsahara and North Africa; the Mediterranean area; East Eurasia; the Insular Pacific; and in North, South, and Central America (67). Practice of particularly long periods of postpartum abstinence is prevalent in Subsahara Africa (55, 67).

In analyzing the available data, Nag has found positive correlations between prolonged postpartum sexual abstinence and reduced fertility. However, actual causality has not been demonstrated: because the period of lactation usually corresponds with the period of postpartum abstinence, it is a confounding variable (56). It also must be noted that information is not always available with respect to the purpose of postpartum abstinence. Although in many cases it is consciously practiced for birth spacing, that reason cannot be generalized to all, or most, instances of the practice (13).

Coitus Interruptus. Coitus interruptus, or withdrawal, is the most prevalent method of contraception used specifically for fertility regulation. It is used extensively throughout South, Central, and East Africa, Europe, Oceania, and India, and by Islamic cultures (8, 35, 51). Coitus interruptus may take various forms. Among the Kgatla of Africa, for example, there are two varieties. In one, the

male takes responsibility for withdrawal at the appropriate time. Should the male be negligent, however, the woman moves her hips, so that the penis is withdrawn and semen is ejaculated onto her side, or she may quickly turn to her side, pushing the man off (56).

Variants of coitus interruptus have also been noted. For example, in what was formerly German East Africa, *coitus inter femora,* that is, ejaculation of semen between the partner's legs, is reported (40). *Coitus obstructus,* that is, applying pressure on the testicles to force the ejaculate into the bladder, to be passed into the urine, is described in medieval Indian and Islamic texts (40). *Coitus reservatus,* that is, the complete avoidance of ejaculation, has been utilized by the Hindus (35).

Expulsion of Semen. Various methods of attempting to expel semen following coitus have been reported. For example, the Kavirondo women of Africa stand up after intercourse and shake their bodies in quick, jerking rhythm, to rid themselves of the semen. The Kgatla turn over on their abdomens, or urinate, immediately after coitus. Some Bengali and Yap women wash the vagina with water, and bathe. Zande women of Africa repeatedly strike the base of the back (56). The native women of Port Darwin, in Australia, try to avoid impregnation by Caucasians by making violent abdominal movements, following intercourse with white men (40).

Magic and Symbolism. The least effective of all methods of folk contraception are those which rely solely on magic and symbolism. Although these methods are medically ineffective, their existence indicates people's pervasive desire to regulate fertility. Several examples will suffice.

Knots, a widespread symbol of infertility, are often tied as a magical way of warding off pregnancy (35, 40). For example, in East Africa, Yao women seek the services of a specialist in knot-tying to prevent conception. This specialist, or "fundi," locates two kinds of bark and twists them into a cord, into which he rubs the yolk of an egg. He then ties three knots, simultaneously reciting an incantation against fertility. The cord is worn by the woman for as long as she wishes to remain sterile. When she desires to conceive, she unties the knots, submerges the cord in water, drinks the water, and throws the cord away (40).

The Ait Sàddĕn, of Morocco, believe that a

corpse has a sterilizing effect on a woman who wishes to avoid impregnation. Such a woman is encouraged to remain behind a burial party and step three times over the grave, in the same direction (40).

The use of magic to avoid conception is not confined to preliterate peoples. Roman and German peasants believed that a tea made from the seeds of barren willow trees could protect them against pregnancy (5). Serbian and Bosnian peasant women have traditionally, and in some cases still, make magical gestures with their fingers to signify the number of years they wish to be free of pregnancies. One account reports that while riding in their wedding coaches, women would sit down on the appropriate number of fingers. Another describes women as placing the desired number of fingers in a child's first bath. Still another variation is reported for the Bosnians, who insert the appropriate number of fingers into their girdles, in the process of mounting a horse (40).

### Barrier Methods and Spermicidal Agents.
Various forms of intravaginal plugs, pessaries, and spermicidal agents have been reported cross-culturally. Some of these are quite ingenious, and potentially effective. Perhaps the most unique is the female vegetable condom used by the Djukas, in what was formerly Dutch New Guinea. These women snip one end from an okralike seedpod, which is approximately 5 in. long, and insert it into the vagina, with the intact end resting against the cervix or in the posterior fornix (40).

Vaginal plugs come in many forms. The Dahomey crush a tubercled root and use it as an intravaginal plug (40). Several tribes in the Kasai Basin, in Central Africa, plug the mouth of the uterus with rags of finely chopped grass. Unfortunately, this technique has been reported to have serious consequences, such as retention of urine, with incontinence, uremia, and infection of the genital organs and kidneys (40). Before having sexual relations with foreign sailors, the native women of Easter Island block their cervixes with algae or seaweed (40). The ancient Jews who lived by the sea used sponges intravaginally. Sponges were, in fact, recommended in birth control clinics as late as 1930 (35). The Achehnese of Sumatra introduce a pill-like black mass intravaginally before coitus. This mass was found to contain tannic acid, which is a potent spermicide (40).

Another potentially effective spermicide is utilized by the Negro women of Guiana and Martinique, a mixture of lemon juice and the extract from mahogany husks. Provided enough is used, lemon juice immobilizes sperm; moreover, the extract of mahogany appears to have an astringent effect (40).

In ancient writings there are many "recipes" for vaginal suppositories, which were intended to block or kill spermatozoa. One of the oldest texts which contains such information is the *Petrie Papyrus* of 1850 B.C., a medical manual. It recommends one of three bases: crocodile dung, a mixture of honey and natural sodium carbonate, and a type of gum. Because of their consistency, all of these substances could effectively block the passage of sperm (35). The use of dung as a pessary is not confined to Egypt but is found in Indian, African, and Islamic sources (35).

The *Ebers Papyrus* (1550 B.C.) recommends a suppository consisting of lint, honey, and acacia. The latter plant contains lactic acid, an effective spermicide. Other potentially effective spermicides have been recommended in other ancient sources. Rock salt is suggested in Islamic and Sanskrit medical sources; rock salt and oil are recommended by an Indian source from the first century B.C. Rock salt would disrupt the sperm's ionic balance, thus destroying its viability. Oil would help to clog the cervix and impede sperm mobility (35). According to Marie Stopes, an early advocate of contraceptive use in the United States, the 2,000 patients whom she encouraged to use a contraceptive of oil had a zero rate of pregnancy (35, 73).

### Drugs and Potions.
Medicinal potions designed as contraceptives or abortifacients are mentioned in ancient writings and in ethnographic literature almost as frequently as magical rites. A good summary statement describing these medicinal brews is provided by Himes: "A considerable variety of leaves, herbs, and roots, as well as all manner of odd and obnoxious substances are pulverized, liquified, swallowed. It almost seems the less palatable the substance the greater the faith in its effectiveness" (40:54). Many, if not most, of these potions have been judged to be ineffective (40). However, most have not been subjected to scientific analysis (56).

When tested, some substances have been found to possess potential contraceptive or abortifacient value. For example, German women, and Baholoholo women from Africa who drink the water from the smithy's fire buckets are consuming iron sulfate, an emmenagogue (5). The plant *Lithospermum ruderale* is used by the Indian tribes of Nevada. "It has been found to reduce the number of estrous smears and inhibit the action of gonadotrophins on the ovary of rats" (56:134). The Lesu are Melanesian people who occupy an island near the Fijian chain. They are convinced that they have efficacious methods of contraception and abortion in the form of several varieties of plants. The leaves are chewed, the juice swallowed, and the pulp spit out. Powdermaker, the anthropologist who studied these people, had seven varieties analyzed. Two were found to have constituents which might make them useful as emmenagogues. One is *Acanthacae,* which contains a bitter alkaloid, and the second is *Curcuma,* which contains a volatile oil (40). Radcliffe-Brown attempted to have some of the roots, berries, and bark used by New Guinea tribes analyzed. He learned that at least one of these plants produced shrinking of the breast within a few days (40). This substance may, consequently, contain an antiestrogen or antiprogesterone. Their contraceptive effect, however, remains uncertain.

The possible contraceptive or abortifacient value of at least some herbs and other substances used by preindustrial peoples is attested to by the World Health Organization's (WHO) Task Force on Indigenous Plants for Fertility Regulation. WHO has identified from 3000 to 4000 plant species which have been used as fertility-regulating agents. In 1976, 116 species were selected for further investigation. It is not, however, anticipated that any will be available for clinical testing before 1980 (86), since the active agents must first be isolated and synthesized on a large-scale basis and then further developed and tested on animals.

WHO is pursuing other projects in the same area—specifically, isolating and characterizing the active agent in substances where preliminary pharmacological data already exist. Plants used either as contraceptive agents or abortifacients in Mexico, Paraguay, Hong Kong, Bangladesh, and India are currently being studied. Some preliminary results appear quite promising. For example, the Central Drug Research Institute in Luchnow, India, had successfully screened extracts from

plants used as antifertility agents in that country. Fourteen of the more than 100 tested demonstrated "greater than 60 per cent antifertility in rats; eight of these were also active in hamsters" (86:73). These results must be confirmed before isolation of the active ingredient can begin. Similar antifertility activity has been found in the crude extracts of Haitian plants. Lastly, preliminary screening of uterotonic activity in 25 Chinese plants has recently begun in Hong Kong. Extracts from three plants have been tested and all show activity (86). It thus seems possible that not only have preliterate and preindustrial people desired to curb their fertility by using abortifacients and antifertility agents; they have utilized substances which, in at least some cases, have effectively helped them to achieve their goal.

If the motivation and, in some instances, techniques for fertility control have always existed, why do many populations presently grow at alarming rates? In order to answer this question, changes in growth patterns beginning with an alteration in subsistence adaptation during the Neolithic age will be examined in the following chapter. It will be shown that low-to-moderate birth rates increased as a result of the agricultural revolution, feudalism, and colonialism.

## REFERENCES

1. Acsadi G, Nemeskeri J: History of Human Lifespan and Mortality. Budapest, Akademiai Kiado, 1970
2. Altmann J, Altmann SA, Hausfater G: Primate infant's effects on mother's future reproduction. Science 201:1028, 1978
3. Angel JL: The basis of paleodemography. Am J Phys Anthrop 30:427, 1969
4. Angel JL: Paleoecology, paleodemography and health. In Polgar S (ed): Population, Ecology, and Social Evolution. The Hague, Mouton, 1975, p 167
5. Aptekar H: Anjea: Infanticide, Abortion and Contraception in Savage Society. New York, 1931
6. Balikci A: The Netsilik Eskimos: adaptive processes. In Lee RB, DeVore I (eds): Man the Hunter. Chicago, Aldine/Atherton, 1968
7. Bartlett MS: An introduction to stochastic processes with special reference to methods and applications. Cambridge, Cambridge University Press, 1955
8. Benedict B: Population regulation in primitive societies. In Allison A (ed): Population Control. Baltimore, Penguin Books, 1970, p 165
9. Birdsell JB: Some predictions for the Pleistocene based on equilibrium systems among recent hunter-gatherers. In Lee RB, DeVore I (eds): Man the Hunter. Chicago, Aldine, 1968, p 229

10. Bogue DJ: Principles of Demography. New York, John Wiley & Sons, 1969
11. Bonte M, Van Balen H: Prolonged lactation and family spacing in Rwanda. J Biosoc Sci 1:97, 1969
12. Buchanan R: Breast-feeding: aid to infant health and fertility control. Pop Rep, Series J, No. 4, 1975
13. Caldwell JC: The economic rationality of high fertility: an investigation illustrated with Nigerian survey data. Pop Stud 31:5, 1977
14. Carr-Saunders AM: The Population Problem. Oxford, Clarendon Press, 1922
15. Chen LC, Ahmed S, Gesche M, Mosley WH: A prospective study of birth interval dynamics in rural Bangladesh. Pop Stud 28:277, 1974
16. Coale AJ, Demeny P: Regional model life tables and stable populations. Princeton, Princeton University Press, 1966
17. DeJong GF: Patterns of human fertility and mortality. In Harrison GA, Boyce AJ (eds): The Structure of Human Populations. Oxford, Clarendon Press, 1972, p 32
18. Delgado HL, Lechtig A, Yarbrough C, Martorell R, Klein RE, Irwin M: Maternal nutrition—its effects on infant growth and development and birthspacing. In Moghissi KS, Evans TN (eds): Nutritional Impacts on Women. New York, Harper & Row, 1977, p 133
19. Devereux G: A typological study of abortion in 350 primitive, ancient and preindustrial societies. In Rosen H (ed): Abortion in America. Boston, Beacon Press, 1967, p 97
20. Douglas M: Population control in primitive groups. Br J Soc 17:263, 1966
21. Dumond DE: The limitation of human population: a natural history. Science 187:713, 1975
22. Dunn FL: Epidemiological factors: health and disease in hunter-gatherers. In Lee RB, Devore I (eds): Man the Hunter. Chicago, Aldine, 1968, p 221
23. Firth R: We the Tikopia, 2nd ed. Boston, Beacon, 1957
24. Friedlander D: Family planning in Israel. J Marr Fam 35:117, 1973
25. Frisch RE: Weight at menarche, similarity for well-nourished and undernourished girls at differing ages, and evidence for historical constancy. Pediatrics 50:445, 1972
26. Frisch RE: Critical weight at menarche, initiation of the adolescent growth spurt, and control of puberty. In Grumbach M, Grave G, Mayer F (eds): Control of the Onset of Puberty. New York, Wiley, 1974, p 403
27. Frisch RE: Critical weights, a critical body composition, menarche and the maintenance of menstrual cycles. In Watts E, Johnston F, Lasker G (eds): Biosocial Interrelations in Population Adaptation. The Hague, Mouton, 1975
28. Frisch RE, McArthur JW: Menstrual cycles: fatness as a determinant of minimum weight for height necessary for their maintenance or onset. Science 185:949, 1974
29. Frisch RE, Revelle R: Variation in body weights and the age of the adolescent growth spurt among Latin American and Asian populations, in relation to calorie supplies. Hum Biol 41:185, 1969
30. Frisch RE, Revelle R: Height and weight at menarche and a hypothesis of critical body weights and adolescent events. Science 169:397, 1970
31. Frisch RE, Revelle R: Height and weight at menarche and a hypothesis of menarche. Arch Dis Childh 46:695, 1971
32. Ginsberg RB: The effect of lactation on the length of the postpartum anovulatory period: an application of a bivariate stochastic model. Theor Pop Biol 4:276, 1973
33. Goodenough WH: Social implications of population control. Expedition 14:11, 1972
34. Gopalan C, Naidu AN: Nutrition and fertility. Lancet 2:1077, 1972
35. Gordon L: Woman's Body, Woman's Right. New York, Grossman, 1976, p 26
36. Green S, Green S, Armelagos GJ: Settlement and mortality of the Christian site (1050–1300 A.D.) of Meinarti (Sudan). J Hum Evol 3:297, 1974
37. Hassan FA: On mechanisms of population growth during the Neolithic. Curr Anthrop 14:534, 1973
38. Hassan FA: Determination of the size, density, and growth rate of hunting-gathering populations. In Polgar S (ed): Population, Ecology and Social Evolution. The Hague, Mouton, 1975, p 27
39. Hempel CG: Philosophy of Natural Science. Englewood Cliffs, Prentice-Hall, 1966
40. Himes NE: Medical History of Contraception. New York, Gamet Press, 1963
41. Howell N: The feasibility of demographic studies in "anthropological" populations. In Crawford MH, Workman PL (eds): Methods and Theories of Anthropological Genetics. Albuquerque, University of New Mexico Press, 1973, p 249
42. Howell N: The population of the Dobe Area !Kung. In Lee R, Devore I (eds): Kalahari Hunter-Gatherers: studies of the !Kung San and Their Neighbors. Cambridge, Harvard University Press, 1977
43. Jain AK, Hsu TC, Freedman R, Chang MC: Demographic aspects of lactation and postpartum amenorrhea. Demography 7:255, 1970
44. Kolata GB: !Kung hunter-gatherers: feminism, diet and birth control. Science 185:932, 1974
45. Krzwicki L: Primitive Society and its Vital Statistics. London, Macmillan, 1934
46. Lee RB: Population growth and the beginnings of sedentary life among the !Kung bushmen. In Spoone B (ed): Population Growth—Anthropological Implications. Cambridge, MIT Press, 1972
47. Leridon H: Human Fertility. Chicago, University of Chicago Press, 1977
48. Leslie PH: The properties of a stochastic model for two competing species. Biometrika 39:363, 1958
49. Lotka AJ: The structure of a growing population. Hum Biol 3:459, 1931
50. Mamdani M: The Myth of Population Control. New York, Monthly Review Press, 1972
51. Mandelbaum DG: Human Fertility in India: Social Components and Policy Perspectives. Berkeley, University of California Press, 1974
52. Matras J: Populations and Societies. Englewood Cliffs, Prentice-Hall, 1973
53. Moore JA, Swedlund AC, Armelagos GJ: The use of life tables in paleodemography. In Swedlund AC (ed): Population Studies in Archaeology and

Biological anthropology. Soc Am Arch Memoir 30, 1975, p 57

54. Morgan K: Computer simulation of incest prohibition and clan proscription rules in closed, finite populations. In Dyke B, McClure J (eds): Computer Simulation in Human Population Studies. New York, Academic Press, 1974, p 15

55. Murdock GP: Ethnographic atlas: a summary. Ethnology 6:109, 1967

56. Nag M: Factors affecting human fertility in nonindustrial societies: a cross-cultural study. Yale University Publications in Athropology, No. 66. Reprint. New Haven, Human Relations Area Files Press, 1968

57. Nag M: Population anthropology: problems and perspectives. In Fried MH (ed): Explorations in Anthropology: Readings in Culture, Man and Nature. New York, Thomas and Cromwell, 1973, p 254

58. Nations JD: Imbalanced sex ratios and the male supremacist complex: an alternative hypothesis. Paper presented at the 2nd Annual Meeting of the CIBOLA Anthropological Association, Austin, Tx, 1978

59. Neel JV: Lessons from a "primitive" people. Science 170:815, 1970

60. Neel JV, Chagnon NA: The demography of two tribes of primitive, relatively unacculturated American Indians. Proc Natl Acad Sci USA 59:680, 1968

61. Pakrashi K: On female infanticide in India. Bull Cult Inst. 7:33, 1968

62. Polgar S: Evolution and the ills of mankind. In Tax S (ed): Horizons of Anthropology. Chicago, Aldine, 1964

63. Polgar S: Culture, history and population dynamics. In Polgar S (ed): Culture and Population. A Collection of Current Studies. Carolina Population Institute, No. 9, Cambridge, Schenkman, 1971, p 3

64. Polgar S: Population history and population policies from an anthropological perspective. Curr Anthrop 13:203, 1972

65. Polgar S: Population, evolution and theoretical paradigms. In Polgar S (ed): Population, Ecology and Social Evolution. The Hague, Mouton, 1975, p 1

66. Potter RG, Wyon J, New M, Gordon J: Applications of field studies to research on the physiology of human reproduction (lactation and its effects upon birth intervals in eleven Punjab villages). J Chron Dis 18:1125, 1965

67. Saucier JF: Correlates of the long post-partum taboo: a cross-cultural study. Curr Anthrop 13:238, 1972

68. Schneider D: Abortion and depopulation on a Pacific island. In Paul B (ed): Health, Culture and Community. New York, Russell Sage, 1955, p 211

69. Scrimshaw S: Culture, Environment, and Family Size: A Study of Urban In-Migrants in Guayaquil, Ecuador. Columbia University Doctoral Dissertation, 1974

70. Scrimshaw S: Cultural values and behaviors related to population change. Institute of Sociology, Ethics and the Life Sciences, UCLA, 1977

71. Sengel RA: Discussion of "On mechanisms of population growth during the Neolithic" by Hassan FA. Curr Anthrop 14:540, 1973

72. Sharman A: Ovulation in the post-partum period. Int J Fertil 12:14, 1967

73. Stopes M: Positive and negative control of conception and its various technical aspects. J State Med (Lond) 39:354, 1931

74. Sumner WG: Folkways. New York, New American Library, 1940

75 Sussman RW: Child transport, family size, and increase in human population during the Neolithic. Curr Anthrop 13:258, 1972

76. Swedlund A, Armelagos GJ: Une recherche en Paleodemographie: La Nubie Soudanaise. Annales Economies—Societies—Civilisations 6, 1969

77. Sykes ZM: Some stochastic versions of the matrix model for population dynamics. Am Stat Assoc J 72:111, 1969

78. Tinker I, Reining P, Swidler W, Cousins W: Culture and Population Change. Washington DC, American Association for the Advancement of Science, 1976

79. Wagley C: Cultural influences on population: a comparison of two Tupi tribes. In Vayda AP (ed): Environment and Cultural Behavior. New York, American Museum of Natural History, 1969, p 268

80. Weiss KM: On the systematic bias in skeletal sexing. Am J Phys Anthrop 37:239, 1972

81. Weiss KM: A method for approximation of age-specific fertility. Hum Biol 45:195, 1973

82. Weiss KM: Demographic models for anthropology. Soc Am Arch Memoirs 27, 1973

83. Weiss KM: Demographic disturbance and the use of life tables in anthropology. In Swedlund AC (ed): Population Studies in Archaeology and Biological Anthropology. Soc Am Arch Memoir 30, 1975, p 46

84. Winikoff B: Nutrition, population and health: some implications for policy. Science 200:895, 1978

85. Wobst HM: Boundary conditions for paleolithic social systems. Am Antiq 39:147, 1974

86. World Health Organization: Special Programme of Research, Development and Research Training in Human Reproduction, Sixth Annual Report. Geneva, 1977

87. Wyon JB, Gordon JE: The Khanna Study: Population Problems in the Rural Punjab. Cambridge, Harvard University Press, 1971

## ACKNOWLEDGMENTS

Grateful acknowledgment is made to Drs. Thomas C. Greaves, Eugene A. Hammel, and Nancy Howell for having reviewed this chapter.

# 19

# Accelerated Population Growth: The Agricultural Revolution to Present Prospects

**Rochelle N. Shain**
**Rebecca A. Lane**

In the preceding chapter, various assumptions and implications of the demographic-transition theory were seriously questioned. It was concluded that slow rates of population growth characteristic of pretransitional societies may be attributed to the use of some form of population control in response to moderate mortality rates, rather than being interpreted as the result of a precarious balance between births and deaths. Such a perspective suggests that accelerated growth rates should be examined in terms of changes in, and effects on, fertility behavior, rather than changes in mortality rates. This is a departure from the theory of the demographic transition, which suggests that accelerated growth results from changes in mortality levels alone.

The present chapter examines growth patterns beginning with the agricultural revolution. It will be shown that although rates of population growth increased at this time, they were nonetheless relatively low. Population growth generally did not assume its accelerated pace until the disruptive effects of Westernization—in the form of colonialism—were felt. It will also be shown that stable low rates of population growth will not necessarily follow economic modernization—another assumption of the demographic-transition theory. Slow growth rates are a likely result only if the benefits of economic modernization accrue to the masses as well as to the elite, and if the costs of raising children outweigh the benefits.

## THE AGRICULTURAL REVOLUTION

A detectable acceleration of population growth rates occurred with a shift in the basic subsistence adaptation from hunting and gathering to cultivation and domestication of plants. There are two basic perspectives regarding the development of agriculture: one views innovation in agriculture as resulting in population increase, and the second views the exploitation and development of additional food sources as a result of population pressures.

Since population size and density are strongly correlated with the carrying capacity of a given ecological niche, the first approach maintains that additional food sources must have been developed prior to increases in population size. It is believed that people relied more heavily at first on concentrated local resources, such as fish. With the development of sendentary agriculture, groups were able to expand their size because of the increased availability of food (6, 21, 35, 59, 69, 71).

The second view maintains that the shift in economic mode must have been the result of population pressure on society (5, 9, 10, 13, 14, 34, 67, 75). It is believed that the primary benefit from a shift to agriculture is a higher output of food per area of land exploited (51). The quality of the diet, however, may have decreased in terms of quantity and quality of protein (assumed to be predominantly derived from cereals), and workloads may have increased.

Regardless of which viewpoint is adopted, there is no doubt that there is a significant relationship between population growth and agriculture. Carneiro and Hilse (11) have estimated annual growth rates between 0.08 per cent and 0.12 per cent during the Neolithic period, the time of the agricultural revolution. Although these rates are low, they are significantly above those of the Paleolithic period.

## CHANGES IN FERTILITY PATTERNS

Studies of extant groups have revealed changes in fertility rates concomitant with a shift to sedentary agriculture. A detailed study of Nunamiut Eskimo demographic history has demonstrated that population growth occurred coincidentally with sedentism (4). Further, the population approached "transitional" growth levels through a rise in the birth rate, rather than through a decrease in the death rate. Results of a recent study of the Sudan (37, 38) indicated that nomads have lower fertility than settled agriculturalists. The latter's fertility rate is almost twice that of the former. As nomadic populations in the Sudan become sedentary and improve their socioeconomic conditions, particularly through stabilization of food supplies, their fertility tends to rise considerably. For example, one group of cultivators in the Sudan raise animals, are relatively sedentary, but depend on rain, rather than irrigation, for cultivation. Their fertility lies, correspondingly, between that of the nomads and the more stable agriculturalists (37, 38).

Several researchers have argued that the relative sedentariness of agriculturalists is sufficient to explain increased population growth. The argument is based on the reduced mobility of the population, and, hence the relaxing of child-transport requirements critical in their effects on birth intervals (20, 45, 69). For example, the mean birth interval among hunting-and-gathering Bushmen is 4 years. However, among Bushmen who have settled down, lower birth intervals—33 to 36 months—have been observed (39, 43, 45). It has also been noted that a shift in food base may have resulted in the availability of softer foods for earlier infant weaning (45) and may have affected the physiology of reproduction (65, 88). Frisch (26) has concluded that the onset and maintenance of regular menstrual function are dependent on the achievement and maintenance of a minimum weight in proportion to height, apparently representing a critical level of fat storage. If all of these factors were operative, they not only could shorten the live-birth interval but could also modify mechanisms of, and the need for, the regulation of the survivorship interval between sibs.

It is unrealistic to suggest, however, that the effects of sedentariness and nutritional changes on population growth are thoroughly understood. For example, the implications of a change in diet are not clear. Diets which are predominantly grain may lead to amino acid malnutrition, which can not only affect infant mortality rates, physical development, and resistance to infectious diseases (19), but can also directly interfere with reproduction (44, 53). Hassan (36) argues that it must be assumed that the effect of a change toward a diet consisting primarily of cereals is disadvantageous for rapid population growth. Therefore he maintains that the dietary advantage of cereals, based on high caloric content, high yield, storability, and transportability (24) could not have been realized without the concomitant innovations of animal domestication and cultivation of legumes. Thus, the relationship between agricultural and population growth is much more complex than is implied by the effects of fat storage or quantity of protein intake on age at menarche.

Similarly, the relationship between sedentariness and population growth is much more complex than is implied by models examining workloads, child transport, and birth intervals, since the role of migration in population growth during this period of prehistory must also be considered. The evidence for migration in this period is the diffusion of agriculture. Archaeological evidence has firmly established the spread of farming from an area of origin in the Near East throughout Europe (1). The spread was slow and regular, starting about 9000 years ago and ending about 5000 years ago.

The spread of agriculture may have occurred by the diffusion of farmers themselves (demic diffusion), diffusion of the technology to preexisting populations of hunters and gatherers (cultural diffusion), or by both methods. Archaeological evidence favoring demic diffusion, or migration, has been supported recently by a study of the geographic distribution of genes (52). The genetic consequences of demic and cultural diffusion are distinct, and maps of the distributions of gene frequencies show clines (gradients) in remarkable agreement with those expected for demic diffusion.

The detection of migration at the genetic level partially depends on the ratio of migrants to the indigenous population and on patterns of differential reproduction among coexisting groups. That mass migration is apparently detectable suggests its importance not only to population growth within a given area, but also as a mechanism to regulate population size. That is, the primary mechanism to control population size among early agriculturalists appears to have been migration.

## EFFECTS OF MIGRATION ON GROWTH

The effects of migration on growth are more significant than the net number of migrants —that is, the resultant gain or loss in the total number of individuals within a given area. Although little empirical data exists on migratory movements in different kinds of societies, it is intuitively clear that mass migration can drastically affect the age structure of populations both at the site of origin and at the destination. If the immigrant population is composed of young individuals, the age structure of the destination population could become younger. The destination population would have an increased reproductive potential because of the resultant younger age structure. Conversely, the reproductive potential of the origin population would decrease, an effect that could be evident for a long period of time.

The effects of migration on population growth may not be limited to impacts on demographic structure. It has been suggested that genetic dissimilarities between migrants and destination populations may have a long-term effect on population fertility. A study of the demographic and socioeconomic evolution of an isolate population in Quebec, Canada, suggests that an increase in the fertility of the isolate, in the course of time, is partially explained by the increased fecundity of a genetically dissimilar group of migrants (56). The study reports higher heritability values for fecundity and postpartum sterility than have been reported in other studies (23, 40, 55, 74). Although little is actually known about the heritability of fertility factors, the possibility that gene frequencies which affect fecundity may be different for migrants and non-

migrants introduces an additional dimension to the impact of migration on population fertility.

## EFFECTS OF ECONOMIC AND SOCIAL ORGANIZATION ON GROWTH

There are other reasons for increased population size within an agricultural subsistence pattern. As discussed later in this chapter, in rural sectors, children, from relatively young ages, are able to share in productive efforts and often produce more than they consume. Moreover, the responsibility for economic and affective support of offspring is shared by the extended family. (See Chap. 22 for a detailed discussion of the effects of family structure on fertility.) This type of family structure is in itself a product of sedentary agriculture (20). However, despite increases in population growth during the Neolithic period, fertility rates among preindustrial agricultural peoples have not been excessively high.

An extensive review of ethnographic data relating to fertility demonstrates that in societies with maximum fertility—that is, where no mechanisms are employed to curb growth—each woman produces an average of 6 to 8 live births, with a mean of 7.45 (46). With child mortality rates estimated at 45 to 50 per cent among sedentary nonindustrial agricultural peoples, 3 to 4 children could reach maturity, and thus double the population of each generation (69). Since growth rates were not this high during the preindustrial era, it would therefore appear that fertility was being restricted at this time. For example, there is evidence that fertility was being controlled in areas such as Northwestern Europe, or in island situations where land was scarce. Mechanisms such as primogeniture, restriction of marriage to only those who inherited land or emigrated, sexual continence, fertility-regulating practices (particularly coitus interruptus), and late age of marriage were employed. In fact, in some areas of Europe, half of the eligible females remained unmarried and childless (17, 31, 32).

### FEUDALISM AND COLONIALISM

During the feudal era, peasants did not own the sources of their livelihood; high fertility was thus indirectly encouraged. Because vassals were responsible to overlords who demanded heavy taxation, it was to the peasants' advantage to produce many children to work the land and thus decrease the burden of work. The cost of these children was less than the benefit derived from their labor (58, 71). Growth rates during this period are judged to have ranged from 1.5 to 4.0 per 1000. They would have been considerably higher had it not been for the offsetting effects of pandemics (58).

Initial colonial contact had drastic demographic consequences for indigenous populations. In the New World, the first effects of Western expansion were large increases in mortality among indigenous populations, due to introduction of new diseases, slavery, and the intensification of warfare. Polgar (57, 58) believes indigenous people began to deliberately increase their fertility as a defense against decimation.

After the period of initial contact, growth rates were effectively increased by the missionaries' opposition to indigenous antinatalist practices, such as polygyny (discussed in relation to fertility in Chap. 22), infanticide, and abortion, and by their advocacy of early marriage (22, 57). More indirect pronatalist effects of Westernization included the reduction of long periods of postpartum abstinence and lactation, and the loosening of prohibitions against widow remarriage (57).

Colonialism abetted population growth through other processes as well. Mortality was eventually decreased through famine relief, by the introduction of new food products, improved transportation systems (and, thus, better distribution of food), and, more recently, by measures of public health. Better nutrition not only decreased mortality, it contributed to higher levels of fertility by decreasing age at menarche. The consistent decline of age at menarche during the past 150 years in developed nations is believed to be related to improved nutrition (27-29, 71). Consequently, in societies where age of marriage followed shortly after menarche, the result would be to increase the reproductive period (71).

Lastly, and perhaps most importantly, the imposition of taxation, usually in the form of produce, and the introduction of cash crops, made it advantageous for peasants to bear many offspring. A large number of working offspring decreased the amount of labor each individual would have to expend for taxation purposes, and increased the cash flow into the family (58, 71).

The colonial situation was very similar to that of the feudal era, with several basic exceptions: absence of major pandemics and famines, improved nutrition, the erosion of indigenous practices which had served to curb high rates of population growth, and, finally, improved public health. The result is the currently high rate of growth in the developing world today (57, 58).

## THE MODERN ERA

Four projections of the world's demographic future were discussed in Chapter 13. It was suggested that, depending on when replacement-level fertility is reached, the world's population will minimally reach 6.4 billion by the year 2100 and maximally will continue growing beyond 2150, attaining a size larger than 15.1 billion. It was concluded that world population growth will be significantly influenced by the developing countries.

Considerable efforts and monies have consequently been directed toward family planning. As discussed at length in Chapter 16, it is being argued that the course of world population growth is being affected by the size, quality, and spread of family planning programs (49, 72). On the other hand, it is also being argued that the critical determinant of reduced fertility is economic development, as opposed to organized family planning efforts (50). Some aspects of the economic development and fertility relationship were discussed in Chapter 17. Further elaboration is presented in the remainder of this chapter.

## ECONOMIC DEVELOPMENT AND FERTILITY

Advocates of traditional demographic-transition theory, as well as government officials in many parts of the world, often consider economic development as a panacea for stemming runaway population growth. Cross-culturally, most priority systems do in some way involve economic goals. Consequently, economic development could, in fact, serve as the mechanism by which to curb rampant population growth. Economic development, however, takes many forms, which have differential effects on birth rates.

In this section, data are presented to demonstrate that population growth is most likely to be negatively affected by economic development if *1*) benefits of modernization accrue to the masses of people as well as to the elite, and *2*) children become more of an economic liability than an asset.

## EQUITY IN RESOURCE DISTRIBUTION

It is generally accepted that high fertility contributes to reduced per-capita income: the amount of national product allocated to capital investment is necessarily reduced, because increasing resources must be diverted to basic subsistence needs such as food, health, and education. Recent studies, however, have demonstrated the reverse: whereas a more equal distribution of resources is correlated with decreases in birth rates, economic development within an economy characterized by grossly unequal distribution of resources is correlated with relatively high birth rates among the poor (3, 15, 31, 41, 42, 60, 61, 62, 63, 64, 66, 70, 71, 76).

## THE ENGLISH AND FRENCH EXPERIENCE

Goldscheider was one of the first demographers to affirm that industrialization does not automatically result in reduced fertility. In a now classic comparison, he delineated those characteristics which contributed to high fertility in England, despite industrialization, and those which favored low fertility in France before the advent of industrialization (31).

Birth rates remained high in England for at least 50 years following major transformations in that country's economy. One of the primary factors which accounted for this phenomenon was that the urban proletariat was very poor—that is, their standards of living were not sufficiently high to be in conflict with large family size.

Moreover, despite the improvement in overall economic growth as a result of industrialization, wealth in England was concentrated in the hands of the few. The majority of urban working class England probably did not feel the improvement in living standards until the 1860's or 1870's. Hence, the lack of actual improvements in living standards combined with the absence of a base for rising aspirations conspired to retain constant high fertility in the early decades of the English Industrial Revolution. Moreover, only those who have experienced rising real incomes and the social and economic benefits that such personal economic increases bring could be sensitive to the disadvantages of a large family size. Thus it was

only the generation after average real incomes moved decisively upward (in England in the 1870's and 1880's; in other areas around 1850) that began to deliberately restrict the size of their families. (31:154)

The evidence which Goldscheider presented to explain why fertility declined in France in the late eighteenth and early nineteenth century provides additional support for the relationship between equity in resource distribution and small family size. In contrast to England, equity in land distribution, along with equal distribution of property among heirs, characterized France even before the French Revolution. The latter event merely replaced the remaining "vestiges of feudalism" with the "exceptional phenomenon within Europe, peasant proprietorship" (31:157). Moreover, economic resources were much more evenly dispersed. New aspirations of social and economic mobility were not restricted to the upper classes. Economic opportunities were open to all, and, in turn, allowed for greater social advancement. French peasants had less incentive and less opportunity to migrate to the cities than people from the rural areas of England. Consequently, they had to choose between large family size and maintaining, or increasing, their levels of living. They chose the latter.

## CONTEMPORARY SOCIETY

Similar examples are found among contemporary societies. Despite large-scale efforts at economic modernization, fertility declines have not occurred in many countries. The reason may be that only the rich have benefitted from economic development. Most developmental policies have concentrated upon improving overall rates of economic growth, usually measured in terms of Gross National Product (GNP). Unfortunately, despite good growth rates in many countries, the status of the poorer classes has either remained stationary or has deteriorated. In many instances, such as in Brazil, Pakistan, Indonesia, the Philippines, and India, income distribution has become more uneven. For example, the average per-capita income in Brazil increased approximately 35 per cent from 1960 to 1970, whereas that of the poorest half of the population remained almost stationary (64, 66).

A similar situation is found in the Philippines, and is particularly striking in contrast to that of Taiwan. Both countries had similar per-capita incomes in the 1960s—that is, $246, and $235, respectively. There was, however, a large discrepancy in income distribution. The wealthiest 10 per cent in the Philippine population were much richer than their counterparts in Taiwan, whereas the poorest 20 per cent of the Taiwanese were twice as well off as their counterparts in the Philippines. Moreover, whereas income distribution had become significantly more equal in Taiwan, the reverse was true for the Philippines. The great fertility declines in Taiwan are attributed, at least in part, to a greater proportion of the population having reached a sufficiently high level of socioeconomic development to make small family size decline attractive (64). Although Taiwan has had a strong family planning program, it is important to note that fertility began to decline before its establishment (16, 18, 42).

In addition to growing disparities in income distribution between the rich and the poor in many parts of the world, unemployment among the poorer classes has soared, exacerbating all existing problems. For example, in Pakistan, Ceylon, Malaysia, the Philippines, and Bangladesh, 15 per cent or more of the labor force is now unemployed. Moreover, in India 100,000 new applicants seek employment each week (64). It is thus evident that traditional approaches to economic development do "not necessarily lead to the reduction of poverty or malnutrition within the lowest economic groups" (64:23).

The poorer classes in most developing countries, living without the benefits of social and economic development, continue to exhibit high fertility. They still do not have a future worth planning for, and thus have nothing to gain from restricting family size. Moreover, they greatly benefit from children's labor, as explained in the following section. It is the elite, those who are receiving the direct benefits of economic growth, who are regulating their fertility (15, 64, 70).

In countries such as China, Cuba, South Korea, Taiwan, Ceylon, Barbados, Mauritius, Hong Kong, the Indian States of Kerala and Punjab, Singapore, parts of Egypt, Costa Rica, Argentina, and Uruguay, developmental policies have stressed equity in resource distribution. Fertility has correspondingly dropped, in most cases, prior to the institutionalization of large family planning programs (16, 41, 42, 60, 61, 62, 63, 64). Detailed

information on the Indian state of Kerala follows.

Kerala is unique in India in that what little it has, in terms of socioeconomic resources, is equally distributed. In sharp contrast to the rest of the country, it has successfully redistributed income throughout the state, through land reform, high wages for both agricultural and industrial laborers, intersectorial mobility, and employment legislation to insure retirement pensions for all individuals employed in industry, agriculture, services, and government. It has also allocated educational resources, so that the poor majority benefit instead of the elite. Consequently, universal primary education and mass literacy characterize the state. Compared to 29 per cent of all Indians, 60.2 per cent of Kerala citizens are literate. Third, again in sharp contrast to the rest of India, limited health resources are equally distributed. Kerala's utilization rate of health facilities is the highest among Indian states for which data are available. Fourth, political power and participation are not concentrated in the hands of a few. In fact, because of high levels of political consciousness on the part of the poor majority, the government has been impelled to maintain, and even increase, its progressive stance. Unions and other peasant organizations have, moreover, insured that certain laws, such as minimum wage and child labor legislation, are not ignored or that health resources are not distributed with favoritism toward the rich (60).

Concomitant to resource redistribution, Kerala has enjoyed a very rapid decline in both mortality and fertility. Life expectancy at birth and the crude death rate are now 60.9 years and 9.2:1000, respectively, compared to 46.5 years and 16.9:1000, respectively, for India in general. The latest crude birth rates for Kerala are 27:1000. In fact, two of its nine districts have achieved birth rates of 20:1000. The corresponding rate for India at large is 34:1000 (60).

Family planning projects are not given primary credit for this fertility decline. Kerala ranks only fifth among all Indian states with respect to the proportion of its population served by family planning program methods. Both mortality and fertility declines are attributed to improved quality of life among the masses, particularly to education and widespread employment opportunities for women, higher wages, and general economic security. The combination of economic security and enforcement of child labor laws has also caused a shift in the cost-benefit ratio of children, so that they have become more of a liability than an asset (60).

## CHANGE IN THE ECONOMIC VALUE OF CHILDREN

Family planning programs sometimes meet with failure because potential clients are not motivated to limit family size. Children in South Asia, Africa, and many parts of Latin America are valuable assets for present and future economic security and are primary sources of prestige (2, 8, 47, 48, 54).

For example, in the aforementioned Indian village of Manipur, children begin working between the ages of four and six, caring for their younger siblings. Children's domestic tasks include cleaning, grazing, milking, and providing drink for animals, taking buffalo dung out to the dung pots, washing clothes, making tea, and carrying water. Children also wait hand and foot on their fathers when they return home from work. The young child will massage his father's head and feet, or his body, if it aches. He brings water for a bath and makes lemonade, on hot days (47). Additionally, as soon as they are old enough, male children work their father's fields or are hired out to work in consumer services or to perform hard physical labor. Often they are the primary source of their parents' economic viability and the only source of their old-age security. Because daughters always leave their parents' village upon marriage and there are stringent restrictions against accepting anything free from them, including shelter, sons are much more highly valued than female offspring (47).

The situation is very similar in many parts of Africa. African children are very highly valued and are often considered equivalent to wealth (7, 8). Among the Ashanti, as in many other tribal societies, farmers team together and work their respective fields in rotation. A man with many children is in the strongest position. Among the Fante, in Southern Ghana, a child is instructed in agricultural technology as soon as he is old enough to handle tools, such as a cutlass. Among coastal fishermen, sons are given oars and sail off with their fathers at age six or seven. Children in Taleland join in all activities from building to farming. Ga boys carry tools and tackle as soon as they can walk. When they are ten, they

make a substantial economic contribution by spreading the sails and fishing lines to dry, and preparing them for the next day's work (30).

Among the Yoruba of Nigeria, children begin to work at age five, starting with simple tasks, such as housework and carrying messages. They proceed to cooking, marketing, farming, food processing, and bearing heavy objects such as firewood. These contributions increase with age. Moreover, even among urban Yoruba, older children make considerable contributions to the household by remitting part of their salaries from employment, such as office and governmental work, to their extended families. Children who have moved from village to city continue to make substantial contributions to their family's welfare and are often the vehicle by which major debts are paid, latrines built, farming technology bought, and the careers of siblings advanced. The importance of children as an investment is clearly seen:

> There are two essential elements in maximizing the chance of success. One is a kind of "lucky-dip" principle or the backing of many horses: with a large number of children there is a good chance that at least one will do well, and one elite salary will outweigh the earnings of a string of children working in traditional or poor urban occupations and will make up for expenditure on several educations. The other is the value of a sibling chain of assistance. The child who breaks through first into extended education and the jobs that this secures almost invariably helps his siblings (usually, but not always, younger ones). . . . The successful investment buys security. . . . There are, in fact, few other competitive sources of investment for rural populations. . . . The most comfortably off old man will be he who has some nonmigrant children helping him locally and other migrant ones channelling the new forms of wealth from afar (8:20, 24).

Because of the long-established and thoroughly reinforced tradition of filial piety and mutual obligations, children in many African tribes feel obligated to support their kin in their old age (7, 8, 30).

Given the extended family structure of the Yoruba and of other African societies, which appears to facilitate what Caldwell calls the "flow of wealth" from children to parents as opposed to parents subsidizing children, motivation exists for large families. (See Chap. 22 for further discussion of the flow of wealth.) The adjusted total fertility ratio for all surveyed women between 1973 and 1975 was 7.4. This motivation, however, is expected to diminish with the encroachment of Western influence. There are already signs that indicate change: the flow of resources is slowly being directed toward children, and the costs of educating and maintaining offspring is rising. Eventually, these changes will make a large family prohibitively expensive (8).

The determinative role played by the economic value of children is sometimes most evident following periods of change. A recent study of Massachusetts during the period from 1680 to 1800 provides this type of evidence. During the early part of this period, children worked for their parents on farms until they married. Because sons did not usually marry until age 27, their contribution was substantial; parents thus benefitted from large family size. As land became increasingly scarce, children emigrated to less populated areas of Vermont and New Hampshire. Moreover, as opportunities for wage employment developed, the amount of work parents could expect from their children diminished significantly. This created the motivation to limit family size (25).

A decrease in the economic value of children is closely related to economic development, provided there is equality in resource distribution. In fact, such a decline can be viewed as one of the mechanisms by which social and economic equality motivate low fertility. If the benefits of economic modernization, in terms of health, education, employment, and social security, are felt by the masses in addition to the elite, individuals do not have to rely on large numbers of children, particularly sons, to work with them as an economic unit or to assist them in times of need, particularly in old age. Children become costly to raise and educate, and parents soon begin to perceive the increased expenses, and costs in loss of opportunity, of raising many offspring. This phenomenon has, in fact, occurred in Kerala.

Land reforms have provided literally millions of couples with the opportunity to invest in land rather than children as a long-term security investment. Wages have been increased, and job security for the landless has been legislated; and the need to rely upon children to fulfill welfare functions has been diminished. Finally, opportunities for child labor have been virtually eliminated due to enforcement of minimum wage and child labor laws. And when the value of children as employable economic assets declines, so does fertility. (60:40)

## POLICY IMPLICATIONS

New approaches in developmental strategy are being advocated, since the more traditional models focusing on GNP have not had the desired effect. The essence of these recommendations is to distribute the benefits of progress more evenly, so that a large majority of families will reach a level of living sufficiently high to be conducive to fertility regulation. Emphasis is being redirected from aggregate rates of growth to the meaning or content of this growth:

Development goals must be defined in terms of progressive reduction and eventual elimination of malnutrition, disease, illiteracy, squalor, unemployment and inequalities. We were taught to take care of our GNP as this will take care of poverty. Let us reverse this and take care of poverty as this will take care of the GNP. In other words, let us worry about the *content* of GNP even more than its rate of increase (73:12, cited in 64:23).

Today, developing countries are being advised by population specialists in demography, economics, and anthropology to increase health benefits, meaningful educational opportunities, real wages, social security, and employment for the poor. They are also being urged to couple industrialization efforts with increasing agricultural productivity. This should stem unwieldy rural-to-urban migration and have an immediate impact on the lifestyles of the poor (3, 12, 33, 42, 50, 58, 60, 61, 62, 63, 64, 71, 76).

It has also been recommended that population experts join forces with those involved in economic development. Economic efforts undoubtedly affect fertility. Consequently, these programs should be designed with population issues in mind, so that their effects on fertility will have the desired result (33, 76).

As discussed in Chapter 16, recent analyses of declines in high fertility rates in most developing countries suggest that family planning programs may have a direct effect on fertility reduction (49, 72). Direct-intervention programs may result in more rapid fertility reduction than might occur by economic and social development alone (72). However, family size limitation will not improve the lot of the poor in the absence of realistic efforts to improve their quality of life. Family planning projects are extremely important facilitators of fertility decline provided the necessary *motivation for birth planning* already exists (58, 76). Arguments over whether concentration upon modern methods of birth control or upon developing a given country's economy is the best means to attain fertility decline may thus be futile. What is needed is an increase in the availability and accessibility of contraceptive services—in addition, not to economic development per se, but to providing the poor with the social and economic benefits of modernization.

## REFERENCES

1. Ammerman AJ, Cavalli-Sforza LL: Measuring the rate of spread of early farming in Europe. Man 6:674, 1971
2. Benedict B: Population regulation in primitive societies. In Allison A (ed): Population Control. Baltimore, Penguin Books, 1970, p 165
3. Bhattacharyya AK: Income inequality and fertility: a comparative view. Pop Stud 29:5, 1975
4. Binford LR, Chasco WJ Jr: Nunamiut demographic history: a provocative case. In Zubrow EBW (ed): Demographic Anthropology. Albuquerque, University of New Mexico Press, 1976, p 63
5. Boserup E: The Conditions of Agricultural Growth. Chicago, Aldine, 1965
6. Bronson B: The earliest farming: demography as cause and consequence. In Polgar S (ed): Population, Ecology, and Social Evolution. The Hague, Mouton, 1975, p 53
7. Caldwell JC: Toward a restatement of demographic transition theory. Pop Dev Rev 2:321, 1976
8. Caldwell JC: The economic rationality of high fertility: an investigation illustrated with Nigerian survey data. Pop Stud 31:5, 1977
9. Carneiro RL: Slash and burn agriculture among the Kuikuru and its implications for cultural development in the Amazon Basin. In Wilbert J (ed): The Evolution of Horticultural Systems in Native South America. Caracas, Sociedad de Ciencias Naturales La Salle, 1961
10. Carneiro RL: A theory of the origin of the state. Science 169:733, 1970
11. Carneiro RL, Hilse DF: On determining the probable rate of population growth during the Neolithic. Am Anthro 68:171, 1966
12. Chen L, Chaudhury RFH: Demographic change and food production in Bangladesh. Pop Dev Rev 1:201, 1975
13. Cohen MN: Population pressure and the origins of agriculture: an archaeological example from the coast of Peru. In Polgar S (ed): Population, Ecology, and Social Evolution. The Hague, Mouton, 1975, p 79
14. Cohen MN: The Food Crisis in Prehistory: Overpopulation and the Origins of Agriculture. New Haven, Yale University Press, 1977
15. Cowgill G: On causes and consequences of ancient and modern population changes. Am Anthrop 77:505, 1975
16. Davis K: Population policy: will current programs succeed. Science 158:730, 1967
17. Davis K: The theory of change and response in modern demographic history. In Ford TR, de-Jong GE (eds): Social Demography. Englewood Cliffs, Prentice-Hall, 1970
18. Demerath MJ: Birth Control and Foreign Policy. The Alternatives to Family Planning. New York, Harper & Row, 1976
19. Dubos R: Man Adapting. New Haven, Yale University Press, 1971
20. Dumond DE: The limitation of human population: a natural history. Science 187:713, 1975
21. Faris JC: Social evolution, population, and production. In Polgar S (ed): Population, Ecology, and Social Evolution. The Hague, Mouton, 1975, p 235
22. Firth R: We, the Tikopia, 2nd ed. Boston, Beacon, 1957
23. Fisher RA: The Genetical Theory of Natural Selection, 2nd rev ed. New York, Dover Publications, 1929
24. Flannery KV: Origins and ecological effects of early domestication in Iran and the Near East. In Ucko PJ, Dimbleby GW (eds): The Domestication and Exploitation of Plants and Animals. Chicago, Aldine, 1969, p 73
25. Folbre N: The politics of reproduction: Hampshire County, Massachusetts, 1680–1800. Paper presented at the Annual Meeting, Population Association of America, Atlanta, 1978
26. Frisch RE: Demographic implications of the biological determinants of female fecundity. Soc Biol 22:17, 1975
27. Frisch RE: Population, food intake, and fertility. Science 199:22, 1978
28. Frisch RE, McArthur JW: Menstrual cycles: fatness as a determinant of minimum weight for height necessary for their maintenance or onset. Science 185:949, 1974
29. Frisch RE, Revelle R: Height and weight at menarche and a hypothesis of critical body weights and adolescent events. Science 169:397, 1970
30. Gaisie SK: Fertility levels among the Ghanian tribes. In Ominde SH, Ejiogu CN (eds): Population Growth and Economic Development in Africa. London, Heinemann, 1972
31. Goldscheider C: Population, Modernization, and Social Structure. Boston, Little, Brown, 1971
32. Goodenough WH: Social implications of population control. Expedition 14(3):11, 1972
33. Green M: New directions in US foreign assistance for population programs. Pop Dev Rev 3:319, 1977
34. Harner MJ: Population pressure and the social evolution of agriculturalists. S W J Anthrop 26:67, 1970
35. Hassan FA: Determination of the size, density, and growth rate of hunting-gathering populations. In Polgar S (ed): Population, Ecology, and Social Evolution. The Hague, Mouton, 1975, p 27
36. Hassan FA: Reply to "On mechanisms of population growth." Curr Anthrop 16:289, 1975
37. Henin RA: Nomadic fertility as compared with that of rain cultivators in the Sudan. International Population Conference, London, 1969, Vol 1, p 792. Liege, International Union for the Scientific Study of Population, 1971
38. Henin RA: The level and trend of fertility in the Sudan. In Ominde SH, Ejiogu CN (eds): Popula-

tion Growth and Economic Development in Africa. London, Heinemann, 1972

39. Howell N: The population of the Dobe Area !Kung. In Lee R, DeVore I (eds): Kalahari Hunter-Gatherers: Studies of the !Kung San and Their Neighbors. Cambridge, Harvard University Press, 1977

40. Imaizumi Y, Nei M, Furusho T: Variability and heritability of human fertility. Ann Hum Genet 33:251, 1970

41. Karush G: Plantations, population, and poverty: the roots of the demographic crisis in El Salvador. Paper presented at the Annual Meeting of the Population Association of America, Atlanta, 1978

42. Kocher JE: Rural Development, Income Distribution, and Fertility Decline. New York, The Population Council, 1973

43. Kolata GB: !Kung hunter-gatherers: feminism, diet, and birth control. Science 185:932, 1974

44. Leathem JH: Reproductive Physiology and Protein Nutrition. New Brunswick, Rutgers University Press, 1959

45. Lee RB: Population growth and the beginnings of sedentary life among the !Kung Bushmen. In Spoone B (ed): Population Growth—Anthropological Implications. Cambridge, MIT Press, 1972

46. Lorimer F: Culture and Human Fertility. Paris, UNESCO, 1954

47. Mamdani M: The Myth of Population Control: Family, Caste, and Class in an Indian Village. New York, Monthly Review Press, 1972

48. Mandlebaum DG: Human Fertility in India: Social Components and Policy Perspectives. Berkeley, University of California Press, 1974

49. Mauldin WF, Berelson B: Conditions of fertility decline in developing countries. Stud Fam Plann 9(5). Population Council, New York, 1978

50. Mauldin W, Choucri N, Notestein F, Teitelbaum M: A report on Bucharest. Stud Fam Plann 5:357, 1974

51. Meiklejohn C: Review of "The food crisis in prehistory." Am J Phys Anthrop 49:286, 1978

52. Menozzi P, Piazza A, Cavalli-Sforza L: Synthetic maps of human gene frequencies in Europeans. Science 201:786, 1978

53. Millen JW: The Nutritional Basis of Reproduction. Springfield, IL, C C Thomas, 1962

54. Nag M: Factors Affecting Human Fertility in Nonindustrial Societies: A Cross-cultural Study. Yale University Publications in Anthropology No. 66. Reprint. New Haven, Human Relations Area Files Press, 1968

55. Neel JV, Schull WJ: Differential fertility and human evolution. In Dobzhansky T, Hecht MK, Steere WC (eds): Evolutionary Biology. New York, Appleton-Century-Crofts, 1972, p 363

56. Philippe P, Yelle L: Heritability of fecundity and post-partum sterility: an isolate-based study. Hum Biol 50:1, 1978

57. Polgar S: Culture, history and population dynamics. In Polgar S (ed): Culture and Population. A Collection of Current Studies. Carolina Population Center Monograph 9. Cambridge, Schenkman, 1971, p 3

58. Polgar S: Population history and population policies from an anthropological perspective. Curr Anthrop 13:203, 1972

59. Polgar S: Population, evolution, and theoretical paradigms. In Polgar S (ed): Population, Ecology, and Social Evolution. The Hague, Mouton, 1975, p 1

60. Ratcliffe JW: Poverty, politics, and fertility: the anomaly of Kerala. Institute of Society, Ethics and the Life Sciences, Hastings Center Report, Feb, 1977

61. Repetto R: The interaction of fertility and the size distribution of income. Manuscript, 1974

62. Repetto R: Inequality and the birth rate in Puerto Rico. Evidence from household census data. Cambridge, Harvard Center for Population Studies, Research Paper No. 14, 1976

63. Repetto R: Economic development and fertility decline in the Republic of Korea. In Repetto R (ed): Economic Equality and Fertility in Developing Countries. Baltimore, Johns Hopkins Press, 1979

64. Rich W: Smaller Families through Social and Economic Progress. Washington DC, Overseas Development Council, 1973

65. Sengel RA: Discussion of "On mechanisms of population growth during the Neolithic" by Hassan FA. Curr Anthrop 14:540, 1973

66. Singer P: Population and economic development in Latin America. Int J Health Serv 3:731, 1973

67. Smith PEL, Young TC: The evolution of early agriculture and culture in greater Mesopotamia: a trial formulation. In Spooner B (ed): Population Growth: Anthropological Implications. Cambridge, MIT Press, 1972

68. Stephens CD: On mechanisms of population growth. Curr Anthrop 16:288, 1975

69. Sussman RW: Child transport, family size, and increase in human population during the Neolithic. Curr Anthrop 13:258, 1972

70. Taylor CE: Economic image of the poor and population control. Am J Pub Health 67:660, 1977

71. Tinker I, Reining P, Swidler W, Cousins W: Culture and Population Change. Washington DC, American Association for Advancement of Science, 1976

72. Tsui AO, Bogue DJ: Declining world fertility: trends, causes, implications. Population Bulletin, Vol 33 (4). Washington DC, Population Reference Bureau, 1978

73. ul Haq M: Employment in the 1970's: a new perspective. Int Dev Rev 13(4), 1971

74. Williams LA, Williams BJ: A re-examination of the heritability of fertility in the British peerage. Soc Biol 21:225, 1974

75. Wright GA: Origins of food production in Southeastern Asia: a survey of ideas. Curr Anthrop 12:447, 1971

76. Zeidenstein G: Testimony before the Select Committee on population. Washington DC, House of Representatives, April 20, 1978

## ACKNOWLEDGMENTS

Grateful acknowledgment is made to Drs. Thomas Greaves, Eugene A. Hammel, and Nancy Howell for having reviewed this chapter.

# Social and Social-psychological Correlates of Fertility

## Sue Keir Hoppe

While birth rates have declined in Western industrial societies, current levels of fertility remain high in developing societies, though there is recent evidence of a "slight slowing in the overall rate of population growth" in these countries (75:83; 109). Even in countries with low fertility, various segments of the population show wide and systematic differences in fertility. The most important social factors affecting fertility both within countries and cross-culturally are socioeconomic status, rural or urban residence, religion, and the employment status of women, the latter of which will be addressed in Chapter 21. In addition, social-psychological factors are important, though many questions concerning the role of such factors remain largely unanswered. In this chapter, major fertility differentials related to socioeconomic status, rural or urban residence, and religion are briefly described, and the various theories which have been put forth to explain them are reviewed. The application of social and social-psychological concepts to the implementation and operation of family planning programs is also addressed.

## DIFFERENTIAL FERTILITY

As each of the major fertility differentials is discussed here, the relationships may seem deceptively simple. However, the factors that influence fertility are so numerous and complex in their interrelation that Thomlinson (107:174) has concluded, "Unfettered repro-duction is a chimera." Most research has understandably focused on a limited part of the complex whole. This makes cautious interpretation of the findings essential, so as not to construe an observed difference as unequivocally due to one variable rather than to some other(s) closely associated with it. For example, whether the high fertility of certain religious groups may simply be a reflection of lower socioeconomic status or of rural background must be questioned. Similar issues will frequently confront the reader in succeeding pages.

Various schemes have been suggested to classify the many social and social-psychological variables related to fertility. Davis and Blake (20:211), in a seminal article entitled "Social Structure and Fertility: An Analytic Framework," outlined eleven "intermediate variables" through which "social factors influencing the level of fertility must operate." The following classification of intermediate variables is quoted from Davis and Blake's article:

I. *Factors Affecting Exposure to Intercourse*

    A. Those governing the formation and dissolution of unions in the reproductive period.

        1. Age of entry into sexual unions.

        2. Permanent celibacy: proportion of women never entering sexual unions.

        3. Amount of reproductive period spent after or between unions.

a. When unions are broken by divorce, separation, or desertion.
b. When unions are broken by death of husband.

B. Those governing the exposure to intercourse within unions.

4. Voluntary abstinence.
5. Involuntary abstinence (from impotence, illness, unavoidable but temporary separations).
6. Coital frequency (excluding periods of abstinence).

II. *Factors Affecting Exposure to Conception*

7. Fecundity or infecundity, as affected by involuntary causes.
8. Use or non-use of contraception.
   a. By mechanical and chemical means.
   b. By other means.
9. Fecundity or infecundity, as affected by voluntary causes (sterilization, subincision, medical treatment, etc.).

III. *Factors Affecting Gestation and Successful Parturition*

10. Foetal mortality from involuntary causes.
11. Foetal mortality from voluntary causes.

Davis and Blake (20:213) make no attempt to classify the social factors, or "conditioning variables," which affect fertility, but they argue that the scheme offers an "approach to selecting and analyzing" them. Age of entry into sexual union clearly affects fertility, but reasons for early or late marriage must be sought in the realms of sociology (norms regarding the "proper" age at marriage), economics (the cost of marriage), and social psychology (the "feeling of being a family").

Though they will not be reviewed here, the reader is also referred to classifications set forth by Hill, Stycos, and Back (52), and Freedman (34). Such schemes are useful in helping to organize and clarify our thinking, and, importantly, they underscore the fact that the explanation of fertility is dependent upon unraveling a complex process, and that our understanding of this process is limited by the influence of as yet undefined factors. The problem is not simply in the discovery of causal variables, but in the adequacy of their measurement, as well—problems to be discussed in a subsequent chapter.

## SOCIOECONOMIC STATUS AND FERTILITY

As demographers studied the long-term fertility decline which began in the industrial nations in the mid- to late nineteenth century, evidence accumulated that different socioeconomic strata were not contributing equally to changes in the birth rate. In almost all countries, families of higher socioeconomic status, whether measured by income, education, or occupation, had fewer children than those of lower status. Three factors were thought to be responsible for this phenomenon. First, the average age at marriage was higher in the upper than in the lower socioeconomic strata (120). Second, some argued that changes in physiological reproductive capacity were occurring, with persons in the upper socioeconomic strata becoming sterile or subfecund (33; 37:21), an interpretation which found little empirical support. A third, more plausible explanation was the spread of the practice of contraception to limit family size, which was first adopted by members of the upper class and gradually diffused to those below (1). Although there is convincing evidence for the third explanation, it is not in itself, a "satisfying explanation" for the observed trends, because it does not specify the "conditions, presumably personal or social, that give rise to increasing but differential practice of family limitation" (10:362). The need for a satisfying explanation of class differentials in fertility in developed nations has been met by two other suppositions, which are discussed below: the social-mobility hypothesis, and the utility-cost theory. The latter bears some resemblance to the argument advanced in Chapter 19 that the reproductive behavior of individuals in pre-industrial societies can be viewed as a rational response to their economic situation. The hypothesis that rising levels of education result in lower fertility in developing countries will also be addressed.

### THE SOCIAL-MOBILITY HYPOTHESIS

As early as 1890, class differences in fertility in developed societies were related to social mobility, or the change in status or occupation in either an upward or downward direction. Arsène Dumont (114:30), a French demographer, wrote that "just as a column of liquid has to be thin in order to rise under the force of capillarity, so a family must be small in order to rise in the social scale." Lower fertility is a prerequisite to upward mobility, he reasoned, since large families tend to inhibit career success.

Two versions of the basic hypothesis have been formulated: the "strong form" proposes that all differences in fertility among social classes can be explained in terms of mobility, lower fertility in the higher social classes being due to the presence of upwardly mobile couples with few children and the departure of couples with relatively more children, and vice versa. It implies that the fertility of nonmobile couples does not differ by social class (10:414). Fisher (33), who is often mentioned in connection with this version of the mobility hypothesis, further suggested that "hereditary influences" were an important cause of fertility differentials among social classes, with natural selection promoting subfecundity and sterility among the upper classes. The "strong" form of the mobility hypothesis has found few other proponents and little empirical support. Berent (7), for example, demonstrated that upwardly mobile couples in Britain have higher fertility than the nonmobile in the class into which they rise, contradicting Fisher's selective infertility hypothesis. And Blau and Duncan (10:374) demonstrated that the average fertility of nonmobile American couples in each social class varies, contradicting the hypothesized uniformity.

The "weak form" of the mobility hypothesis, which has been more widely advanced, proposes that social mobility is not the only variable, but one of several associated with differences in fertility (10:368; 108:114; 114:30–31). Empirical tests of this version of the mobility hypothesis compare the fertility of mobile individuals with that of nonmobile individuals of comparable status, seeking to demonstrate that the family size of upwardly or downwardly mobile couples varies significantly from that of couples who remain in the same social class. In general, such tests of the weak form of the mobility hypothesis have failed to confirm it. Rather, they suggest that the additive effects of present social status and social origin are more important than the experience of mobility per se in influencing fertility. Since a mobile couple experiences life in more than one social class, their fertility is something of a composite, reflecting "maintenance of the social characteristics of the class of origin as well as . . . acquisition of the fertility habits of the social class subsequently reached" (7:252). Upwardly mobile individuals typically have fewer children than those who are downwardly mobile, with the nonmobile having an intermediate number (7, 10, 13, 32, 55).

## THE UTILITY-COST THEORY

While the relationship between socioeconomic status and fertility is thought to have been positive in primitive societies (46:114–120; 68; 84:313–342), with high fertility accompanying high status, the pattern reversed as countries underwent the demographic transition. Until World War I, birth rates in different social classes diverged widely and rapidly. Since then, class differentials have tended to diminish, as contraceptive knowledge and practice have diffused throughout the class structure (120). Some argue that the final stage in this transformation will be a return to a positive relationship between high socioeconomic status and high fertility in the more developed societies, since affluent couples can better afford large families (46).

Whether this pattern is in fact emerging is the subject of contention. Debate centers on recent attempts to explain socioeconomic fertility differentials in terms of the classical economic theory of consumer behavior, which assumes that an individual, faced with a variety of goods and services from which to choose, will apportion his or her income so as to maximize utility (satisfaction), in accordance with personal tastes and current market prices. Thus, high-income families are expected to purchase more cars or refrigerators, of higher quality, than low-income families. Becker (4) applied this model to fertility, arguing that children are a "commodity" that generates consumer satisfaction in the form of psychic reward and are an "investment" as well. Because there are costs involved in having children, the satisfaction gained by having a child will be balanced against available resources. At least among couples with contraceptive knowledge, high-income families are expected to have more children, and spend more per child, than low-income families.

Becker's economic theory of fertility has been widely criticized. Blake (9:24), its most outspoken critic, argues that the model unrealistically presupposes rational decision-making in an area of human behavior which, in many instances, is conspicuously nonrational. She notes, "Were poor people economically rational and informed in their reproductive preferences, 'the rich would get richer, and the poor wouldn't even get children.' " Further, obviously there are significant differences between material goods and children, though the analogy is admittedly heuristic: the number of children a couple has is not subject to the credit constraints imposed in the acquisition of material goods—that is, there is no single "purchase price" for a child, and parents are not prevented from overextending themselves by having to show evidence of ability to provide, before having a child. In addition, "quality" is impossible to anticipate, and the freedom to substitute or exchange, as Blake (9:16) argues, is "sociologically absurd when applied to children."

It is also believed that Becker failed to take into account social factors which influence fertility. For example, social norms regarding family size are important, for, as Blake (9:18) reasons, "poor parents as well as rich ones will view the only-child unit as a deprived one. Hence, two children, and not one, become the minimum for the avoidance of childlessness." In other words, there is a lower threshold below which even the fertility of couples in the lower socioeconomic strata will not drop, in spite of their economic situation. Thus, the relationship between income and number of children may be "inelastic" within certain culturally determined ranges (42; 61:115–118). This is illustrated by the findings of Whelpton, Campbell, and Patterson (118:36–37), who asked couples in the United States how many children they would want to have if they could live their lives over again. Only 2 per cent of the wives chose no children at all; 2 per cent chose one child.

The utility-cost theory of fertility has been criticized as a middle-class model, ill-suited to explain the behavior of couples in the lower socioeconomic strata, because it assumes that "each family has perfect control over both the number and the spacing of its births" (4:210). Even in countries where family planning is widely practiced, the ability to control conception varies by socioeconomic status and race. Bumpass and Westoff (14:1179), for example, estimate that in the United States, be-

tween 1960 and 1965, one-fifth of all births, and one-third of births to black women, were unwanted. The proportion of unwanted births was twice as high for families in the lower classes as for those in the upper classes. Finally, child "quality" and the direct and indirect costs of children are not uniform, as Becker assumes, but tend to be positively associated with socioeconomic status. Direct costs are the usual expenses of maintaining a child until he or she is self-supporting, and these, like the indirect costs (those incurred when such opportunities as the wife's employment, or leisure activities, are foregone as a result of having children) may be increased by social pressure. For example, couples in the higher socioeconomic strata are expected to spend more than others on their offspring (9; 22:233–234).

Thus, a positive relationship between income and fertility has not been generally evident, because various intervening factors—the cost of children being one—tend to offset the positive effect of higher income. This does not mean that economic resources are irrelevant. When couples in the United States were asked why they did not want or expect more children, or why they used contraceptive techniques, the most frequently given reasons were financial (118). Moreover, a sense of economic well-being, or security, has been found to be positively correlated with family size (65). And among couples who were asked how much change they expected in their income in the next 10 years, and the extent to which the change would affect their standard of living, those who anticipated a significant increase in income and change in lifestyle expected a larger family size (35).

Easterlin (26, 27) has advanced the notion of "tastes" (or aspirations) as a significant intervening variable in the relationship between income and fertility. He argues that "relative" income (the ratio of achieved income to expected living standards, or aspirations), rather than income per se, explains fertility behavior. The basic hypothesis is that the changing balance between earning potential and desired level of living influences fertility:

If young men—the potential breadwinners of households—find it easy to make enough money to establish homes in the style desired by them and their actual or prospective brides, then marriage and childbearing will be encouraged. On the other hand, if it is hard to earn enough to support the desired style of life, then the resulting economic stress will lead to deferment of marriage and, for those already married, to the use of contraceptive techniques to avoid childbearing, and perhaps also to the entry of wives into the labor market (26:181).

## EDUCATION

In general, parents with more education have fewer children and are more likely than others to use contraception (48, 63). In the United States, the fertility of married women between 15 and 44 years of age declines consistently as number of years of schooling increases—from an average of 3.4 children, for women with less than 8 years of school, to 1.6 for those who have completed 4 or more years of college. The inverse relationship is particularly strong among women married for 2 years or less, reflecting the indirect but significant effect of education on postponement of marriage and first birth (54:158).

In developing countries, where inverse relationships between other components of socioeconomic status and fertility are less consistent, differentials associated with the educational achievement of women are strong. In Puerto Rico, for example, the average number of children born to married women aged 45 and over with no formal schooling was 7.4 in 1960; the average number born to those with 1 to 4 years of primary schooling was 6.9; to those with 1 to 3 years of secondary schooling, 3.4; and to those with at least some college, 1.9 (103). In urban areas of Thailand, the average number of children born to women aged 15 and over, with less than 4 years of education, was 4.9 in 1970; those with more than 4 years of education had an average of 3.4 children (67:84). World Fertility Survey data indicate that use of contraception among currently married, nonpregnant women in five Asian countries varies with level of education—from 27 per cent of those with no education, to 48 per cent of those with at least some secondary schooling, in Thailand; and from 2 per cent to 46 per cent for women in those educational categories, respectively, in Nepal (115:11).

Education, which exhibits a "stronger and more consistent relationship to fertility than does any other single variable" (54:156), is thought to influence fertility in "indirect" as well as "direct" ways. For example, it delays age at marriage; facilitates the acquisition of information about contraception; increases aspirations for upward mobility; increases prospects for the employment of women outside the home; reduces the perceived economic utility of children; and imparts a sense of self-reliance, control over one's own fate, and trust in science and technology which encourage the use of contraception as a rational means of controlling the size of one's family. As Holsinger and Kasarda (54:154) note, "Belief in the universality and invariant nature of [the inverse relationship between education and fertility] has invested formal education with substantial promise as the major social institution amenable to policy manipulation that can help solve the problem of rapid population growth in less developed nations" (see Chap. 21 for further discussion).

## RURAL OR URBAN RESIDENCE AND FERTILITY

In North and South America, and in Europe, fertility tends to be higher in rural than in urban areas. Robinson (92:292) notes that "urban fertility 30 per cent or more below rural fertility can be described as common" in these parts of the world, though differences are becoming less pronounced. For example, in 1970, the average number of children born to women 45 to 49 years old in the United States was 2.5 in urbanized areas (cities of 50,000 or more population and their suburbs) and 3.4 among farm residents (112). In Cuba and Panama, urban gross reproductive rates are one-half the rural rate; in Puerto Rico and Brazil, about two-thirds; and in Mexico, three-quarters (104:274). There is now considerable evidence that rural-urban fertility differentials are emerging in the high-fertility countries of Africa and Asia (73:51; 92). For example, in Ghana, in 1965/1966, the average number of children born to women 40 to 49 years old was 4.9 in urban, and 6.4 in rural areas (86:838).

### URBANISM

Rural-urban fertility differentials have been interpreted as a function of the differences between economic and social organization of towns and cities, and of rural areas. Urbanization—the proportion of population living in cities, or the change in this proportion—is closely associated with economic development, industrialization, and the process of modernization, which have profoundly changed the structure and functions of family organization across cultures. In rural areas, children are economic assets because they are productive members of a family; in urban areas, their economic value is lowered by widespread compulsory education, which removes them from the potential labor force. Urbanization has been conducive to the decline of traditional bases of social solidarity, has weakened kinship bonds, and decreased the social significance of the family, with joint and extended families being replaced by nuclear ones, as a result of factors which tend to push or pull kin to different industrial areas or geographic locations (119). Urbanization has been called the greatest social revolution in history, but according to Davis (18:3), "neither the recency nor the speed of this evolutionary development is widely appreciated." He continues, "Before 1850 no society could be described as predominantly urbanized, and by 1900 only one—Great Britain—could be so regarded. Today, only 65 years later, all industrial nations are highly urbanized." By the year 2000, more than one-half of the world's population is expected to be living in urban areas.

Sociologically, urban life is described as consisting mainly of "secondary," as opposed to "primary," relations: in contrast with rural communities, where social relationships ordinarily persist through life, urban contacts are characterized by greater impermanence and anonymity. They tend to be more impersonal, less intimate, more formal, and less emotional. Urbanism is thought to reduce fertility because women are more likely to be employed, marriage tends to be postponed, and fewer people marry, so that the proportion of single and unattached persons is greater in cities (49:50); levels of income and education are higher, and birth control is more available in urban than in rural areas. In addition, urbanism is said to influence fertility through its impact on personality. Individuals raised in urban environments have been observed to be more competitive; more open to change; more rational (they are not dominated by tradition, but presumably collect adequate information about an issue and make a choice based on it); more time-conscious and future-oriented; and more confident than individuals in rural environments of the human ability to control

events, that is, they tend to be less fatalistic (56, 70), and thus more likely to practice contraception.

### MIGRATION AND GENERATIONAL STATUS

Several special features of rural-urban fertility differences have attracted the interest of demographers in recent years. One is the paradoxical nature of the fertility of those who migrate from rural to urban environments. The case of black fertility in the United States illustrates this paradox:

> Crude birth rates for the Negro population in the United States indicate that fertility declined while Negroes remained in the South and then climbed in the last twenty-five years as Negroes became urbanized.... Negro fertility has risen despite the urbanization of Negroes and improvements in their socioeconomic characteristics (29:188).

Between 1947 and 1957, the fertility of blacks increased substantially; white fertility actually declined during the first 3 years of the decade, and then increased, but not as dramatically as that of blacks. Explanations for the racial difference include: *1*) the increased fecundity of blacks after World War II, due to the decline of venereal disease; *2*) the large-scale migration of blacks from the rural South to urban places in the North where general health conditions were better; and *3*), despite urban residence, the fact that blacks were not being assimilated as previous migrants had been (29:202). Blacks migrated to urban areas because "economic, political, and social pressures forced them out." Not being a self-selected group, well equipped for urban jobs and ways of life, they remained essentially rural in their "orientation, experience, and outlook": their "fertility patterns in this circumstance remained more rural than urban, except that improved medical care may have increased the general level of their fecundity" (61:101–102).

Petersen (84:476) notes that similar patterns of urbanization are occurring in less developed countries, where populations are doubling every 25 to 30 years. Their large cities, however, are doubling in size every 10 to 15 years, while the urban slums, or shanty towns, that house the rural migrants double in population every 5 to 7 years. It is estimated that 80 per cent of the low-income urban population of the developing countries, more than one-half of the world urban population, will soon be living in such slums (87). In Brazil, for example, 80,000 to 100,000 migrants from the "backlands" arrive in Rio de Janeiro each year. They come to the *favela,* or slum, already with large families, and there they bear more children, an average of 5.1 per couple. The *favela* is a crowded "island" in the city. In one sense, it protects the migrant, because it retains some of the values of the old life, but it also preys on them: Brazil has one of the highest infant mortality rates (110 deaths per 1000 live births) and one of the highest estimated illegal abortion rates in the world (79). But people continue to migrate, in Brazil as elsewhere, because they perceive that there are opportunities in the city not available on the farm, and this excites hope for a better life.

The speed with which rural migrants accommodate to urban standards of fertility varies. Goldberg (38:214) and Duncan (23) indicate that lowered fertility as a result of acculturation in an urban environment occurs after about two generations, while Hutchinson (55) suggests that the process is complete in a generation. Others have shown that the fertility of migrants is lower than, or at least equal to that of nonmigrant urban couples (40, 72, 80, 98, 105). Such contradictory evidence indicates that urbanization alone does not unequivocally explain the differences in fertility. To be considered also are birthrates in the community of origin, cultural patterns, levels of health, the strength of social networks, and the age and sex selectivity of migration. For example, in 1960, there had been almost no reduction in family size among second- and third-generation Mexican Americans: among ever-married women who had completed childbearing, the foreign-born averaged 4.6 children; the second-generation, 4.5; and those with native-born parents, 4.4 (110:33–34). While the majority of Mexican Americans live in urban areas of the United States (80%, in 1960), their "mere presence in a modern, urban milieu has only a limited impact upon reproductive behavior." Future trends in Mexican-American fertility, Uhlenberg (110:36–38) has concluded, will depend upon how rapidly upward social mobility and greater involvement in mainstream society are achieved.

## RELIGION AND FERTILITY

Religious preference is thought to influence fertility in several ways: *1)* through particular church doctrines or religious norms about birth control and family size; *2)* through religious norms with specific but unintended effects on fertility; and *3)* as simply a reflection of the socioeconomic status or rural or urban background of the various religious groups. Most empirical research on religion and fertility has dealt with differences between Roman Catholics and other major religious groups, primarily Protestants and Jews, because of the Catholic church's well-known opposition to birth control and the traditionally higher fertility of Catholics in the United States. It is less often recognized that other religious groups exhibit fertility rates which, in general, far exceed those of Catholics. Moreover, most Protestant denominations, until only recently, opposed contraceptive practices, including abortion and sterilization.

The Hutterites, a communalistic anabaptist sect now residing in the western United States and Canada, have the highest documented fertility of any religious group. The Hutterites believe that birth control is "murder" and that its practice will lead to eternal damnation. A study of one Hutterite colony revealed that the mean number of children born to women who were between 45 and 54 years of age in 1950 was 10.6, despite the fact that the women first married at an average age of more than 20 years. The period gross reproduction rate of all Hutterite women from 1946 to 1950 was 4; the crude birth rate in 1948 was 45.9:1000 population (28:220, 225, 244).

The birth rate among Moslems is similarly high, although Islamic doctrine permits birth control. Responding to demographers who have "stressed the absence of specific prohibitions on contraception in other major religions," Kirk (64:561, 579) wrote that "Islam has been a more effective barrier to the diffusion of family planning than Catholicism" because of "distinctive Islamic attitudes and practices in family life." Birth rates have declined somewhat in the last decade in countries with large Moslem majorities, but they are almost universally high, ranging from the mid- to high 30s, e.g., in Egypt and Turkey, to the low 50s, e.g., in Niger and Senegal in West Africa. Roman Catholic countries, as Kirk stressed, display considerably greater variability than Moslem countries in birth rate: for example, birth rates in Catholic countries currently range from about 13, in Belgium, to 43, in Mexico. Birth rates in countries which are predominantly Hindu and Buddhist, (religions which, like Islam, are generally supportive of family planning) are similarly high, but variable—ranging from 19, in Japan, to 50, in Bangladesh (111).

## MINORITY-GROUP STATUS

In explanation of the apparent contradiction presented by such extreme variability in fertility among Catholic nations, Day (21) hypothesized that fertility is highest among Catholics who are in a minority position and are subject to social discrimination or political persecution by non-Catholic groups. He argues that high Catholic fertility is partly a function of religious proscriptions on birth control, and partly a function of the extent to which one's faith provides support, and is thus emphasized, in a "spiritually hostile culture." Goldscheider (39), pursuing Day's hypothesis, explains the fertility levels of certain religious (and ethnic) groups in this way: alienation, and the insecurity of minority status, engender group integration and strong identification with the prevailing normative system. When the normative system prohibits, or discourages, birth control and encourages large families, as with Catholics, then minority-group status increases fertility; when it does not prohibit birth control or encourage large families, as with American Jews (and segments of the black population), fertility is depressed below majority levels.

## SOCIOECONOMIC STATUS, RURAL OR URBAN BACKGROUND, AND RELIGION

A question frequently posed about religious differentials in fertility concerns the extent to which such differences simply reflect the socioeconomic status or rural or urban background characteristic of each religious group. For example, though there is some evidence that income patterns among the major religious groups in the United States have reversed (41:72), researchers still ask whether Catholics have higher fertility than Protestants or Jews because their average educational attainment or occupational status is lower. Similarly, do

Moslems in India have higher fertility than Hindus because they are less literate, and is the lower fertility of the Parsis due to the fact that they are the most literate, the most urban, and probably the wealthiest of all religious groups in India (19:80, 185, 193; 73:44–46; 77; 122)? The evidence is not clear: some argue that while religious affiliation "may have some bearing on fertility rates ... the operative forces seem to be more economic and educational than directly religious" (73:44; 84:536); others argue that the "factor least dependent upon socio-economic status and yet strongly related to tastes for children is that of religious affiliation" (47:98; 117:191).

The fervor with which these opposing views have been advanced and the often different interpretations given data are at least in part related to underlying attitudes about the significance of religion in society. Following Durkheim (25), who stressed the uniquely commanding role of religion in the life of primitive people, the pervasiveness of religion in underdeveloped societies today is generally recognized. In most Moslem and Hindu countries, religion and traditional values, attitudes, and ways of life are so thoroughly fused that it is difficult to separate their independent effects on fertility. For example, religious prescriptions often coincide with economic necessity: conditions of labor-intensive agriculture and high mortality create the need for survival of sons. In addition, religious practices with unintended but important effects on fertility, such as those favoring the early remarriage of widows and divorcees and the subordinate role of women in these societies, foster large families.

A narrow role is often associated with religion in more modern, economically developed societies. "Contrary to what might have been expected," however, "religion has remained a vigorous and influential institution," whose "influence extends to the very core of social behavior, attitudes, and values" (39:270). This is so, at least in part, because, as Durkheim argued, religion—in one form or another—is an eternal part of human existence. It serves to reduce the uncertainties of life, to satisfy a sense of dependence, and to assuage feelings of hopelessness and powerlessness. In a study of Detroit residents, Lenski (69) found that religion was as important an influence on many kinds of social behavior (including fertility) as socioeconomic status.

Of the three major religious groups in the United States, Catholics have the highest fertility, Jews the lowest, with Protestants in an intermediate position. Compared to Protestants and Jews, Catholics expect, desire, and have larger families; though the gap between Catholic and non-Catholic contraceptive practice is narrowing (116), Catholics tend to use less effective contraceptive methods and to have more unplanned pregnancies, with shorter intervals between births. Jews, at the other extreme, tend to marry later, have smaller families, use more effective contraceptive measures, have fewer unplanned pregnancies, and, because they are more likely to plan the number and spacing of children, have longer birth intervals (118). Although there appear to be important differences within these religious groups, fertility differences remain when socioeconomic status is controlled (97, 118).

Though Catholics exhibit a generally higher birth rate than other Christians or those expressing no religious preference, not only in the United States but in other countries as well (39:277), the evidence is contradictory in Latin America (104:180–182; 105:75ff.). Thus, the precise mechanism(s) by which religion affects fertility is an unresolved issue. Catholic differences cannot be wholly explained in terms of the differential use of contraception and abortion, which are proscribed by church doctrine: the incidence of abortion, for example, in Chile, is similar in Catholic and non-Catholic groups (94). Another anomalous finding is that while Catholics in the United States have generally larger families than non-Catholics, they appear to become effective contraceptors when desired family size is attained (96). As Teper (106:203) notes, this could reflect many factors:

The couple could always have wanted that number of children, that number could have emerged as experience of the partnership and parenthood was gained, economic considerations may have supervened, opportunities may have occurred outside the family unit which were preferable to additional children. Any of these factors would make effective contraceptive behaviour desirable at a particular stage of the family building process. The fact that Catholics become efficient contraceptors may result from a belief that the dogma on family size has been satisfied by four children; or that Catholics cease becoming "good" Catholics at that point in the family cycle; or that Catholic norms are used in the early stages

of marriage to justify non-contracepting behaviour which subsequently becomes untenable in the light of the real-world pressure imposed on couples by large families.

## PERSONAL MOTIVATIONS AND SOCIAL-PSYCHOLOGICAL CONSIDERATIONS

Up to this point, social-psychological factors have been discussed only as they affect fertility incidentally or indirectly, through other variables. Such factors will now be considered more explicitly, following Freedman (34:31), who divides them into two broad classes: *1*) those concerned with the process by which reproductive norms are learned, and *2*) those concerned with social attitudes or personality traits which affect the norms or the actual level of fertility. Interest in the impact of social-psychological variables, such as norms and values, on fertility behavior is recent, and the major efforts to document a relationship have been "rather unsuccessful" (34)—that is, the associations so far established between fertility and socioeconomic status, rural or urban residence, and religious preference have been more revealing than those involving psychological factors (101:743). Despite this, population researchers have continued to pursue social-psychological predictors of fertility "tenaciously in the face of rather consistently negative evidence" (45:99). They do so at least partly because observed relationships between various structural variables and fertility, while perfectly satisfactory from a logical point of view, are "informatively unsatisfying." For example, as Hawthorn (47:54) notes: when "we say that working mothers *cause* low fertility we can only make the statement intelligible . . . by hypothesizing an intervening mechanism"—"the mental states of the women" and their "feelings about their roles." While Hawthorn may be more liberal in attributing causation than the available evidence warrants, one can agree that social-psychological factors are important "intervening mechanisms" in the explanation of fertility behavior, not only because "common sense inclines us" to believe this, but also because there "is a very good argument that this must be the case" (47). The norms, values, and ways of feeling, thought, judgment, and behavior learned by individuals in a society—what is called *culture*—are indispensable to understanding human behavior:

From the very beginning of life, one's inter-action with others is normatively bounded, nor-matively inspired, and normatively main-tained. . . . Strictly speaking, everything we find in man's behavior in society that is not the direct product of his biological structure is culture. That is, it has been learned through some process of so-cialization in the social order (82:222–223).

## THE SOCIALIZATION OF REPRODUCTIVE NORMS

Socialization is the process of learning by which members of a society acquire the beliefs and behaviors defined as appropriate to their social position or role, and the norms and values that support those beliefs and behav-iors. In early childhood, the primary agent of socialization is the family. It is during this time that basic values are acquired or "inter-nalized." While socialization is a continuous process that occurs over the life span, many theorists of personality are convinced of the decisive importance of the experiences of early life in the formation *and persistence* of patterns of motivation. As this relates to fertility, two main trends are evident: first, the origin of the wish for a child has been traced to an early stage of development in women and is carried into adulthood as sex-role behaviors are rein-forced in later stages (121). This trend will be dealt with in greater depth in the next chapter. Second, the values acquired in childhood about life and human nature in general influ-ence notions about family size and contracep-tion.

### VALUES

According to Kluckhohn, certain basic value orientations exist which grow out of the efforts of all human groups to solve five common problems: defining the relation of man to na-ture and to time, and understanding the na-ture of sex, of human activity and work, and of human relations (66). Each value orientation constitutes a conceptual continuum, with "traditional" and "modern" orientations being the polar types (17, 60), and each is theoretically associated with different proba-bilities of expected family size, birth control effectiveness, and actual fertility. In other words, low fertility is thought to be associated with:

modern orientations of mastery over the outcome of events, long-range rational planning, behavior directed toward the realization of objective goals and primacy of goals of the conjugal pair and mu-tual gratification from sex relations.

In contrast, high fertility is thought to be as-sociated with:

traditional orientation of fatalistic resignation, in-ability to link immediate experiences with future consequences, primacy of goals and welfare of the extended family group, perception of sex as a duty, and so on (17:186).

Empirical tests of the hypothesis relating fer-tility to values have demonstrated only mod-est predictive power, or have altogether failed to confirm it (17, 89). The area of investigation is new, however, and the problems involved in measuring values—or approximating them through the measurement of norms and atti-tudes—are great. Moreover, norms vary in the degree to which they are accepted and in their moral force, though individuals often make fertility decisions in "pluralistic ignorance," mistakenly assuming that everyone else is ob-serving the norms. This phenomenon was ob-served by Hill, Stycos, and Back (52), who found that Puerto Rican men desired smaller families than their wives, contrary to the norm of *machismo,* according to which men are ex-pected to want large families, especially sons, as proof of their masculinity.

### SIZE OF FAMILY OF ORIENTATION

If fertility is viewed as a product of early de-velopmental interactions, an obvious question is whether individuals who grow up in large families are likely to have about the same number of children as their parents did. Sev-eral studies have addressed this question, and, in general, the number of an individual's sib-lings and the number of his or her own chil-dren tends to be positively correlated (8, 24, 62). The effect of size of family of orientation appears to operate in two ways. First, women from large families tend to leave school earlier, marry younger, and begin childbearing at an earlier age than those from small families (24:514). Thus, selectivity with respect to length of exposure to risk of pregnancy may be associated with size of family of orientation. Second, individuals may attempt to create in their own family an environment similar to the one in which they were raised, especially if they consider their childhood as happy or satisfying (24, 50), or if they were first-born (59). The value of children, that is, the functions they served, or the needs they fulfilled, for an individual's parents, affects his or her own motivation to have children. These values, several of which are mentioned elsewhere in this chapter, include love and affection, the feeling of being a family, stimulation and fun, expansion of self, and economic utility, among others (53; 85:48ff.).

## PERSONALITY TRAITS, AND ATTITUDES

In the broader area of motivation, personality traits and attitudes, developed either in the process of socialization or as a result of situational factors, influence reproductive behavior. One of the pioneering inquiries in this area was the Indianapolis Study, which was conducted in the United States in 1941. In addition to social and demographic variables, measures of various "personality" characteristics were included: feeling of personal inadequacy; feeling that children interfere with personal freedom; ego-centered interest in children; fear of pregnancy; tendency to plan; interest in religion; adherence to tradition; and conformity to group patterns. The results of the survey were published between 1946 and 1958 in a series of articles in the *Milbank Memorial Fund Quarterly,* and in collected volumes. The Indianapolis Study had a number of conceptual and methodological shortcomings, and the data failed to reveal significant correlations between psychological factors, and contraceptive use and size of planned family, but in "historical context" it "contributed provocatively" to the area of fertility analysis, particularly in its emphasis on motivational and psychological factors as determinants of fertility (30:32). In the 1950s, two similar projects were initiated, the Growth of American Families (GAF) surveys (36, 118) and the Princeton Study (117). The main personality measures included in the Princeton Study were generalized manifest anxiety; need for nurturance; compulsiveness; tolerance of ambiguity; cooperativeness; and need achievement. Like the Indianapolis Study, these surveys yielded largely negative findings with respect to personality variables. Bardwick and others (54:167) speculate:

Assuming that psychological characteristics *are* important, one may hypothesize that the relevant psychological variables were not measured. While people seem to be able to talk about sex, family size, or contraception, in our experience the explanatory or predictive variables seem to be the use of denial, the level of sexual anxiety and/or guilt, the level of interpersonal dependence and passivity, and the origins of vulnerability or self-esteem. These variables are not generally observable at the conscious interview level (2:275, [italics added]).

While relationships to fertility are still modest, a degree of success has been achieved with indices or measures of "alienation" (3, 43, 44), "fatalism" (31; 104:128), and "internal-external control" (71). These attitudes or aspects of personality, which are conceptually quite similar, seem to indicate that individuals who want and are able to limit family size are less fatalistic, less alienated, and more "internal" than others, that is, they are "psychologically organized to carry out a planful course of action" (100:13ff.). They perceive the outcomes of their behavior as under their own control, rather than that of fate, chance, or powerful others. Rainwater's (90, 91) studies of middle- and working-class whites and working-class blacks in the midwestern United States describe, in detail, fatalism and similar psychological states as preconditions to ineffective contraception. The earlier work of Hill and his coworkers (52), also documents lack of "planfulness" as a psychological force that *deflects* the effective implementation of decisions about family size reached by lower-class Puerto Ricans. As Hill (51:5) notes, Puerto Rican couples are extremely conscious of optimum family size, almost uniformly preferring two or three children, yet bearing six, on the average. Both authors describe women who, although lacking knowledge about physiological processes, attempted to control pregnancies, but in a sporadic and ineffective manner. A sense of powerlessness and low self-esteem appeared to discourage effective discussion of family planning and the cooperation among partners necessary for the control of conception.

## KNOWLEDGE AND THE DIFFUSION OF BIRTH CONTROL

Knowledge alone is not sufficient for successful contraception, but it is closely associated with motivation. Specific knowledge about contraception will be focused upon here, though literacy and education, knowledge about the anatomy and physiology of reproduction, and knowledge of population as a demographic problem, are also relevant. The primary mechanisms by which contraceptive knowledge has been assessed are the Knowledge-Attitudes-Practice (KAP) Surveys, more than 400 of which have been conducted around the world, and the World Fertility Survey (WFS), an international research program in which more than 50 developing, and developed, countries currently participate (113). KAP data have shown that women typically desire a smaller family than they are likely to have by the end of their reproductive period and that those in developing countries have little knowledge of contraceptive methods, but express interest in learning about them (83:10ff.). Initial results of WFS research in five Asian countries confirm an almost universal desire by women aged 45 to 49 for fewer children than they actually have (16:4). Unwanted fertility, for example, ranges from an average of 1.2 children for ever-married women in Thailand and Malaysia to 3.4 in Nepal. Knowledge of specific contraceptive methods appears to have increased: more than 90 per cent of ever-married women in Korea, Malaysia, and Thailand have heard of some method; however, only 22 per cent of those in Nepal have, a "remarkably low level of knowledge for a country in which a family planning program has been in existence since 1966" (115:12–13).

At one time, it was widely held that the major problem in reducing fertility was "ignorance, rather than failure to act on information already acquired" (11:507; 102:11). KAP studies and other research had shown that awareness of methods of birth control varied directly with urban residence and levels of education and income (15, 78). However, even in large cities, many individuals were uninformed about how and when conception takes place, and unaware that fertility control is possible (11:507). For example, almost two-thirds of the urban population, and more than 85 per cent of the rural population, in India in the 1950s did not know that fertility control was possible.

On the basis of such evidence, early education in family planning in developing countries was guided by the "classical diffusion

model," which describes the process by which an innovation (a new idea, practice, or object) is communicated through certain channels over time to members of a group (93). The model specified that the adoption of an innovation such as birth control proceeds by four stages: *1*) knowledge, or awareness; *2*) persuasion, or the formation of a favorable or unfavorable attitude toward the innovation; *3*) decision-making, or evaluation, which leads to adoption, rejection, or trial and discontinuation; and *4*) confirmation, or seeking reinforcement for the decision which was made. Bogue (12:4ff.) argues that the model was applied with great usefulness between 1961 and 1971, but that today, as a result of massive family planning campaigns, most couples of childbearing age, including those in the developing countries, have "already been through this process." Almost all are aware that family planning is available and a majority can name and describe how several of the modern methods of contraception work. While knowledge is high (in most developing countries, 60 per cent to 90 per cent of adults have completed the adoption process), "vast segments of the population have . . . arrived at a negative evaluation of the family planning methods currently available," either deciding not to try family planning or trying it, only to discontinue after a brief time.

The striking disparity between knowledge and use of family planning—the so-called KAP-gap—has been explained in two ways. One explanation is based upon a "cultural-motivational" approach, which views declines in fertility as resulting only from broad social changes involving economic development, increased literacy, a rising standard of living, and modern orientation (76). A second explanation argues that motivation to reduce fertility is a prerequisite, rather than a consequence, of modernization and that it is wrong to assume that radical social change must occur before family planning is accepted (6, 12, 74). For example, as was noted earlier, a couple which aspires to higher status realizes that a large number of children limits the possibility. The "availability," or "accessibility," approach, as this second view has been called, maintains that there are more immediate obstacles or barriers than social structural ones to the practice of family planning. Research findings suggest that the difficulties of those in need of family planning are due in large part to a lack of realistic opportunities to achieve genuinely held aspirations for small families. Worldwide, there were nearly 560 million women at risk in 1976, a number which has risen at the rate of 2.3 per cent annually since 1971; of these, about 360 million—two out of three—use no birth control methods at all (88). Proponents of the "availability" approach advocate the development of family planning programs in such a way as to "alter the opportunity structure," creating services where none exist, or minimizing problems of accessibility to existing services, such as distance, crowding, eligibility requirements, fees, scheduling, lack of accurate information, and the often depersonalized manner in which services are delivered (58:169–170).

The first family planning programs in developing countries used a medical, clinical approach, patterned after Planned Parenthood services in the United States prior to 1960. Most often, they relied on a single method of contraception and a single means of distribution (the doctor in the clinic), ignoring particular sociocultural conditions and local motivations for child limitation. After providing clinic facilities, contraceptives, and doctors to distribute them, "family planning staffs sat back and waited for the clients to come in. A few did so, but most did not" (93:86).

A more active approach to family planning, based on the classical diffusion model, was initiated in the mid-1960s, in many countries. Clinics were still used to distribute contraceptives, but efforts to provide information and motivation were primarily the responsibility of "change agent aids," indigenous workers whose credibility derived both from their social homophily with clients and, in some cases, from their prior adoption of a method of contraception. The persuasive influence of the latter is illustrated by the vasectomy "canvasser" in India, who, by showing his scars to a client, in essence communicated, " 'Look here, I've adopted this family planning method; I know what I'm talking about' " (93:89).

Many of the important principles in the diffusion of birth control information which were developed in this "field era" are being usefully applied today. These include mobile clinics, postpartum recruitment, offering family planning at the work site, and various strategies for avoiding distribution of contraception by physicians (57, 81, 95, 99, 123). In designing services, these approaches consider the social and cultural circumstances, perceptions, needs, and motivations of target audiences. Efforts to reduce fertility have more recently been linked to attempts to raise the legal age of marriage, to enhance the roles of women, and to provide such monetary incentives as tax breaks for small-sized families. Berelson refers to these efforts to broaden the scope of family planning, from that of just providing contraceptive services to changing institutional and social structures in antinatalist directions, as "beyond family planning" (5).

In summary, this chapter has described the major social factors which influence fertility, and has attempted to link them to social-psychological variables. Progress toward empirically establishing the relationships between these factors or variables and fertility has been limited, and there are many remaining gaps in our knowledge. Nevertheless, examination of such theories sensitizes the reader to the general relevance of social factors in reproductive behavior. By locating groups in a society which have different levels of fertility, it is possible to make inferences about the factors which will eventually be isolated as determinants of fertility. As noted, the mechanisms which connect socioeconomic status, urbanization, and religion with individual action, as expressed in fertility decline, cannot yet be precisely defined. There is reason to believe, however, that the relationship is mediated by changes in education, increased mobility and expanding opportunities, the availability of family planning programs, and the emergence of new attitudes and aspirations, and new modes of family decision-making, which make people more aware of the future consequences of present action.

## REFERENCES

1. Banks JA: Prosperity and Parenthood: A Study of Family Planning Among the Victorian Middle Classes. London, Routledge and Kegan Paul, 1954
2. Bardwick J: Psychological factors in the acceptance and use of oral contraceptives. In Fawcett JT (ed): Psychological Perspectives on Population. New York, Basic Books, 1973, p 274
3. Baumann KE, Udry R: Powerlessness and regularity of contraception in an urban Negro male sample: a research note. J Marr Fam 34:112, 1972
4. Becker GS: An economic analysis of fertility. In National Bureau for Economic Research, Demographic and Economic Change in Developed

Countries. Princeton, Princeton University Press, 1960, p 209

5. Berelson B: Beyond family planning. Science 163:533, 1969

6. Berelson B: An evaluation of the effects of population control programs. Stud Fam Plann 5:2, 1974

7. Berent J: Fertility and social mobility. Pop Stud 5:244, 1952

8. Berent J: Relationships between family size of two successive generations. Milbank Mem Fund Q 31:39, 1953

9. Blake J: Are babies consumer durables? A critique of the economic theory of reproductive motivation. Pop Stud 22:5, 1968

10. Blau PM, Duncan OD: The American Occupational Structure. New York, John Wiley & Sons, 1967

11. Bogue DJ: Some tentative recommendations for a 'sociologically correct' family planning communication and motivation program in India. In Kiser CV (ed): Research in Family Planning. Princeton, Princeton University Press, 1962, p 503

12. Bogue DJ: Twenty-five Communication Obstacles to the Success of Family Planning Programs. Chicago, Community and Family Study Center, University of Chicago, 1975

13. Boyd M: Occupational mobility and fertility in metropolitan Latin America. Demography 10:1, 1973

14. Bumpass L, Westoff CF: The 'perfect contraceptive' population. Science 169:1177, 1970

15. Caldwell JC: Fertility differentials as evidence of incipient fertility decline in a developing country: the case of Ghana. Pop Stud 21:23, 1967

16. Cho LJ: Family preferences in five Asian countries. Int Fam Plann Perspect Dig 4:2, 1978

17. Clifford WB, Ford TR: Variations in value orientations and fertility behavior. Soc Biol 21:185, 1974

18. Davis K: The urbanization of the human population. Sci Am 213:3, 1965

19. Davis K: The Population of India and Pakistan. New York, Russell and Russell, 1968

20. Davis K, Blake J: Social structure and fertility: an analytical framework. Economic Development and Cultural Change 4:211, 1956

21. Day L: Natality and ethnocentrism: some relationships suggested by an analysis of Catholic-Protestant differentials. Pop Stud 22:27, 1968

22. Duesenberry JS: Comment. In National Bureau of Economic Research, Demographic and Economic Change in Developed Countries. Princeton, Princeton University Press, 1960

23. Duncan OD: Farm background and differential fertility. Demography 2:240, 1965

24. Duncan OD, Freedman R, Coble JM, Slesinger DP: Marital fertility and the size of family of orientation. Demography 2:508, 1965

25. Durkheim E: The Elementary Forms of the Religious Life. Swain JW (trans). New York, Free Press, 1947

26. Easterlin RA: Relative economic status and the American fertility swing. In Sheldon EB (ed): Family Economic Behavior: Problems and Prospects. Philadelphia, JB Lippincott, 1973, p 170

27. Easterlin RA: The conflict between aspirations and resources. Pop Dev Rev 2:417, 1976

28. Eaton JW, Mayer AJ: The social biology of very high fertility among the Hutterites: the demography of a unique population. Hum Biol 25:206, 1953

29. Farley R: Recent changes in Negro fertility. Demography 3:188, 1966

30. Fawcett JT: Psychology and Population: Behavioral Research Issues in Fertility and Family Planning. New York, Population Council, 1970

31. Fawcett JT, Bornstein MH: Modernization, individual modernity, and fertility. In Fawcett JT (ed): Psychological Perspectives on Population. New York, Basic Books, 1973, p 106

32. Featherman DL: Marital fertility and the process of socioeconomic achievement: an examination of the mobility hypothesis. In Bumpass LL, Westoff CF (eds): The Later Years of Childbearing. Princeton, Princeton University Press, 1970, p 104

33. Fisher RA: The Genetical Theory of Natural Selection, 2nd ed. New York, Dover 1958

34. Freedman R: The Sociology of Human Fertility: An Annotated Bibliography. New York, Irvington, 1975

35. Freedman R, Coombs L: Economic considerations in family growth decisions. Pop Stud 20:197, 1966

36. Freedman R, Whelpton PK, Campbell AA: Family Planning, Sterility, and Population Growth. New York, McGraw-Hill, 1959

37. Gini C, Nasu S, Kuczynski RR, Baker OE: Population: Lectures on the Harris Foundation, 1929. Chicago, University of Chicago Press, 1930

38. Goldberg D: The fertility of two-generation urbanities. Pop Stud 12:214, 1959

39. Goldscheider C: Population, Modernization, and Social Structure. Boston, Little, Brown, 1971

40. Goldstein S: Interrelations between migration and fertility in Thailand. Demography 10:225, 1973

41. Greeley AM: Ethnicity, Denomination, and Inequality. Beverly Hills, Sage, 1976

42. Griffith J: Social pressure on family size intentions. Fam Plann Perspect 5:237, 1973

43. Groat HT, Neal AG: Social psychological correlates of urban fertility. Am Soc Rev 32:945, 1967

44. Groat HT, Neal AG: Alienation antecedents of unwanted fertility: a longitudinal study. Soc Biol 22:60, 1975

45. Hauser PM, Duncan OD: Demography as a body of knowledge. In Hauser PM, Duncan OD (eds): The Study of Population: An Inventory and Appraisal. Chicago, University of Chicago Press, 1959, p 76

46. Hawley AH: Human Ecology: A Theory of Community Structure. New York, Ronald Press, 1950

47. Hawthorn G: The Sociology of Fertility. London, Collier-Macmillan, 1970

48. Heer DM: Economic development and fertility. Demography 3:423, 1966

49. Heer DM: Society and Population. Englewood Cliffs, Prentice-Hall, 1968

50. Hendershot GE: Birth order and fertility values. J Marr Fam 31:27, 1969

51. Hill R: The significance of the family in population research. In Liu WT (ed): Family and Fertility: Proceedings of the Fifth Notre Dame Conference on Population, December 1–3, 1966. Notre Dame, In University of Notre Dame Press, 1967, p 3

52. Hill R, Stycos JM, Back K: The Family and Population Control: A Puerto Rican Experiment in Social Change. Chapel Hill, University of North Carolina Press, 1959

53. Hoffman LW, Hoffman ML: The value of children to parents. In Fawcett JT (ed): Psychological Perspectives on Population. New York, Basic Books, 1973, p 19

54. Holsinger DB, Kasarda JD: Education and human fertility: sociological perspectives. In Ridker RG (ed): Population and Development: The Search for Selective Interventions. Baltimore, Johns Hopkins University Press, 1976, p 154

55. Hutchinson B: Fertility, social mobility and urban migration in Brazil. Pop Stud 14:182, 1961

56. Inkeles A: The modernization of man. In Weiner M (ed): Modernization: The Dynamics of Growth. New York, Basic Books, 1966, p 138

57. Isaacs SL: Nonphysician distribution of contraception in Latin America and the Caribbean. Fam Plann Perspect 7:158, 1975

58. Jaffe FS, Polgar S: Family planning and public policy: is the "Culture of Poverty" the new cop out? J Marr Fam 30:228, 1968

59. Johnson NE, Stokes CS: Family size in successive generations: the effects of birth order, intergenerational change in lifestyle, and familial satisfaction. Demography 13:175, 1976

60. Kahl JA: The Measurement of Modernism: A Study of Values in Brazil and Mexico. Austin, University of Texas Press, 1968

61. Kammeyer KCW: An Introduction to Population. San Francisco, Chandler, 1971

62. Kantner JF, Potter RG Jr: Social and psychological factors affecting fertility. XXIV. The relationship of family size in two successive generations. Milbank Mem Fund Q 32:294, 1954

63. Kasarda JD: Economic structure and fertility: a comparative analysis. Demography 8:307, 1971

64. Kirk D: Factors affecting Moslem natality. In Berelson B (ed): Family Planning and Population Programs: A Review of World Developments. Chicago, University of Chicago Press, 1966, p 561

65. Kiser CV, Whelpton PK: Social and psychological factors affecting fertility. XI.The interrelation of fertility, fertility planning, and feeling of economic security. Milbank Mem Fund Q 29:41, 1951

66. Kluckhohn C: Values and value-orientations in the theory of action: an exploration in definition and classification. In Parsons T, Shils EA (eds): Toward a General Theory of Action. Cambridge, Harvard University Press, 1961, p 388

67. Kunstadter P: Child mortality and maternal parity: some policy implications. Int Fam Plann Perspect Dig 4:75, 1978

68. Leibenstein H: Economic Backwardness and Economic Growth: Studies in the Theory of Economic Development. New York, John Wiley & Sons, 1957

69. Lenski G: The Religious Factor. New York, Doubleday, Anchor Books, 1961

70. Lerner D: The Passing of Traditional Society: Modernizing the Middle East. New York, Free Press, 1965

71. MacDonald AP Jr: Internal-external locus of control and the practice of birth control. Psychol Rep 27:206, 1970

72. Macisco JL Jr, Bouvier LF, Renzi MJ: Migration status, education and fertility in Puerto Rico, 1960. Milbank Mem Fund Q 47:167, 1969

73. Mandelbaum DG: Human Fertility in India: Social Components and Policy Perspectives. Berkeley, University of California Press, 1974

74. Mauldin WP: Assessment of national family planning programs in developing countries. Stud Fam Plann 6:30, 1975

75. Mauldin WP: Patterns of fertility decline in developing countries, 1950–75. Stud Fam Plann 9:75, 1978

76. Mauldin WP, Choucri N, Notestein FW, Teitelbaum M: A report on Bucharest. Stud Fam Plann 5:357, 1974

77. Mazur DP: Fertility among ethnic groups in the USSR. Demography 4:172, 1967

78. Morsa J: The Tunisia survey: a preliminary analysis. In Berelson B (ed): Family Planning and Population Programs: A Review of World Developments. Chicago, University of Chicago Press, 1966, p 581

79. Mundigo AI: Brazil's changing family planning policy: a first step? Int Fam Plann Perspect Dig 4:18, 1978

80. Myers GC, Morris EW: Migration and fertility in Puerto Rico. Pop Stud 20:85, 1966

81. Neumann AK, Bhatia JC: Family planning and indigenous medicine practitioners. Soc Sci Med 7:507, 1973

82. Nisbet RA: The Social Bond: An Introduction to the Study of Society. New York, Alfred A Knopf, 1970

83. Nortman D: Changing contraceptive patterns: a global perspective. Population Bulletin 32. Washington DC, Population Reference Bureau, 1977

84. Petersen W: Population. New York, Macmillan, 1961

85. Pohlman E: The Psychology of Birth Planning. Cambridge, Schenkman, 1969

86. Pool DI: The rural-urban fertility differential in Ghana. International Population Conference, Vol 1, London, 1971. Liege, International Union for the Scientific Study of Population, 1971

87. Population Information Program: Twenty-two dimensions of the population problem. Population Reports, Series J, No. 11, J–177, 1976

88. Population Information Program: Filling family planning gaps. Population Reports, Series J, No. 20, J–369, 1978

89. Poston DK Jr, Singlemann J: Socioeconomic status, value orientations, and fertility behavior in India. Demography 12:417, 1975

90. Rainwater L: And the Poor Get Children. Chicago, Quadrangle Books, 1960
91. Rainwater L: Family Design: Marital Sexuality, Family Size, and Contraception. Chicago, Aldine, 1965
92. Robinson WC: Urbanization and fertility: the non-western experience. Milbank Mem Fund Q 41:291, 1963
93. Rogers EM: Communication Strategies for Family Planning. New York, Free Press, 1973
94. Romero H: Chile: the abortion epidemic. In Berelson B (ed): Family-Planning Programs: An International Survey. New York, Basic Books, 1969, p 134
95. Rothenberg L, McCalister D: Family planning in hospital and non-hospital settings. In McCalister DV, Thiessen V, McDermott M (eds): Readings in Family Planning: A Challenge to the Health Professions. St. Louis, CV Mosby, 1973, p 128
96. Ryder NB: Contraceptive failure in the United States. Fam Plann Perspect 5:133, 1973
97. Ryder NB, Westoff CF: Reproduction in the United States 1965. Princeton, Princeton University Press, 1971
98. Scrimshaw SC: Families to the city: a study of changing values, fertility and socioeconomic status among urban in-migrants. In Nag M: Population and Social Organization. Chicago, Aldine, 1975, p 309
99. Silver MA, Singletary M: Offering family planning at the work site. Fam Plann Perspect 7:180, 1975
100. Smith MB: A social-psychological view of fertility. In Fawcett JT (ed): Psychological Perspectives on Population. New York, Basic Books, 1973, p 3
101. Stolnitz GF: Population composition and fertility trends. Am Soc Rev 21:738, 1956
102. Stycos JM: Obstacles to programs of population control—facts and fancies. Marriage and Family Living 25:5, 1963
103. Stycos JM: Education and fertility in Puerto Rico. In Proceedings of the World Population Conference, Belgrade, 1965, Vol 4. New York, United Nations, 1967
104. Stycos JM: Human Fertility in Latin America: Sociological Perspectives. Ithaca, Cornell University Press, 1968
105. Stycos JM, Back KW: The Control of Human Fertility in Jamaica. Ithaca, Cornell University Press, 1964
106. Teper S: Social theory and individual fertility behavior: some issues of research orientation. Soc Sci Med 9:195, 1975
107. Thomlinson R: Population Dynamics: Causes and Consequences of World Demographic Change, 2nd ed. New York, Random House, 1976
108. Tien HY: Social Mobility and Controlled Fertility: Family Origins and Structure of the Australian Academic Elite. New Haven, College and University Press, 1965
109. Tsui AO, Bogue DJ: Declining world fertility: trends, causes, implications. Population Bulletin 33, Washington DC, Population Reference Bureau, 1978
110. Uhlenberg P: Fertility patterns within the Mexican-American population. Soc Biol 20:30–39, 1973
111. United Nations Demographic Yearbook, 1975. New York, United Nations, Department of Economic and Social Affairs, 1976
112. US Bureau of the Census. United States Census of Population, 1970, PC(2)-3A, Women by Number of Children Ever Born. Washington DC, Government Printing Office, 1973
113. Vaessen M: World fertility survey: the current situation. Int Fam Plann Perspect Dig 4:73, 1978
114. Westoff CF: The changing focus of differential fertility research: the social mobility hypothesis. Milbank Mem Fund Q 31:24, 1953
115. Westoff CF: The unmet need for birth control in five Asian countries. Int Fam Plann Perspect 4:9, 1978
116. Westoff CF, Jones EF: The secularization of U.S. Catholic birth control practices. Fam Plann Perspect 9:203, 1977
117. Westoff CF, Potter RG, Sagi PG, Mishler EG: Family Growth in Metropolitan America. Princeton, Princeton University Press, 1961
118. Whelpton PK, Campbell AA, Patterson JE: Fertility and Family Planning in the United States. Princeton, Princeton University Press, 1966
119. Wirth L: Urbanism as a way of life. Am J Soc 44:1, 1938
120. Wrong DH: Trends in class fertility in Western nations. Can J Econ Pol Sci 24:216, 1958
121. Wyatt F: Clinical notes on the motives of reproduction. J Soc Issues 23:29, 1967
122. Yaukey D: Fertility Differences in a Modernizing Country: A Survey of Lebanese Couples. Princeton, Princeton University Press, 1961
123. Zatuchni GI: The post-partum program: a new approach. In Berelson B (ed): Family-Planning Programs: An International Survey. New York, Basic Books, 1969, p 157

# 21

# The Influence of Sex Roles on Fertility

Rochelle N. Shain
Victoria H. Jennings

An individual in a social system occupies a status, that is, she or he has a certain rank vis-à-vis others in that system. A person's status is either *achieved* or *ascribed.* Status is said to be achieved when a position is attained by successfully engaging in those activities deemed appropriate by the particular culture; ascribed status derives from relationships to other persons (for example, parents, spouses, political leaders). In virtually all societies until recently, and in some today, the status of most men and women was ascribed, dependent on age, sex, and the rank of one's family. Modernization and industrialization, however, have allowed many males to achieve a relatively independent position in society through their accomplishments. The status of women has been slower to change. Blake (10) argues that with industrialization, women's status became increasingly ascribed, as basic economic production was transferred from the home into factories and cities. Consequently, women normally attain their social positions not through their own achievements, other than bearing and rearing children, but through those of their family. It is also argued that in many instances economic development has accelerated this process by concentrating resources on male agricultural pursuits and ignoring, even undermining, those of the female (12–14).

## THE FEMALE ROLE: PUBLIC AND PRIVATE SPHERES

In this section we will assess the contention that illiterate, unemployed, generally low-status women have more children than educated, employed, high-status women, and to examine why and how female status in public and private spheres is related to fertility.

Common indicators of women's status in the public sphere are education and employment. High levels of female participation in formal schooling and in the labor force generally are acknowledged to reflect relatively high status, and vice versa. To assess women's status in the private sphere, it is necessary to examine their role within the family.

## TRADITIONAL ROLES

In those societies which have not been affected by modernization and/or by female aspirations for greater role independence, the female is often wholly dependent upon having children to attain a favorable position in society, and thus a positive self-image. According to Blake, "Children are the instrumentalities for achieving virtually prescribed social statuses . . . [,] the almost exclusive avenues for feminine creativity and achievement. . . ." (7:1174). Since most individuals want to feel valued, it is not surprising that high birth rates often characterize those societies with traditionally defined female roles. Having a large number of children is the only manner in which these women can prove to themselves and to society that they are worthy (8, 12, 24, 28, 33, 45, 51–53, 63, 64, 96, 97).

The way in which the traditionally defined female role supports high fertility rates is exemplified by the status and roles of women in many Latin American communities. Most of these women, particularly those living outside of Argentina, Chile, and Uruguay, have little education, do not belong to secular voluntary associations, have few or no career aspirations, desire a relatively large number of children, and appear to subordinate themselves to their husbands' wishes and demands. Moreover, the few middle- and upper-class women who do work outside the home are careful to subordinate their work interests to the needs of their families. Additionally, they have access to servants who maintain their households. Lower-class women do not aspire to work outside the home, but some must, in order to help support their families. These women engage in low-status, menial tasks which provide little satisfaction and usually are quite compatible with reproduction and child-rearing (16, 19, 69, 80, 83).

Although the traditionally defined dichotomy between male and female roles, where the male is seen as overtly virile, dominant, and sexually aggressive, and the female as passive and wholly submissive, is either a myth or at best an ideal, many individuals model their behavior after these stereotypes. Stevens (83) argues that many mestizo women conform to and actually encourage these stereotypes because they are able to manipulate them to their advantage. She notes that whereas girls learn very early in life that they are inferior to their brothers, they also observe the enormous veneration with which their father treats his mother and the respect bordering on religious awe accorded their mother by their brothers. They also observe and master the techniques by which the female members of the household manipulate the males in order to attain their objectives. By playing on role stereotypes in which the woman is seen as patient, saintly, and even as a martyr to the sinfulness of men, women usually are the winners in most internal struggles for power. However, in order for a woman to achieve the position she desires, she must have a large number of adult sons who will pay her homage. Her status is thus absolutely contingent upon motherhood.

Similarly, it has been argued that the highly romanticized Mexican courtship patterns, in which the future bride is the center of attention, admiration, and respect, make the woman's inferior position within the marital unit all the more evident and poignant. Married men and women usually are not companions, nor are they lovers in the real sense, since wives are expected to be pure and disinterested in sex. Consequently, passionate love is often reserved for less "pure" women outside the household, whereas true love is saved for "momma" (55, 66). The young wife thus feels alone, socially isolated, and even betrayed. She consequently turns to childbearing and child-rearing to reestablish her status, regain feelings of self-worth, and, eventually, become the object of her sons' adulation. Since many of these women usually have no alternative sources of status and/or satisfaction, it would be difficult to convince them that it is advantageous to limit their family size to two children (55).

Female status in parts of South Asia and Africa is also dependent upon childbearing. In many areas of India, for example, a woman's current welfare and future destiny depend upon her procreative role (51, 52). The typical Indian woman marries shortly after menarche. She resides with her husband's family, to whom all of her allegiances are transferred. She is expected to submissively satisfy her new kin's demands, to become pregnant as soon as possible, and subsequently to bear as many children as she can. Sons are more highly valued than daughters; daughters leave home upon marriage, taking a dowry with them, and cultural restrictions often prevent parents from accepting anything from their married daughters. Therefore a woman's status depends primarily upon the number of sons she produces. The pressure placed upon women is very clear. For example, when a young bride enters her husband's house in the village of Manipur, she touches her mother-in-law's feet with her fingers, signifying obedience and respect. Her mother-in-law responds with, "May you have seven sons." As she greets her husband's relatives, they each say, "Bathe in milk and you will have lots of sons" (51:139).

Failure to fulfill procreative obligations results in social ostracism and an uncertain future. Severe penalties are imposed upon barren women and upon those who fail to bear male offspring: they are treated as a disgrace to the family, sometimes are regarded as witches who can harm children, and are thus prevented from attending the birth of a child, or its celebration, and frequently cannot attend many other family celebrations. Divorce or polygyny may be the ultimate result of childlessness (51, 52).

In traditional societies, women without

sons, moreover, have no security in their old age. Approximately 50 per cent of Indian women who live to age 50 to 59 are widowed (68). In the absence of their fathers, sons (unlike sons-in-law), are obligated to care for their mothers. Consequently, women with neither husband nor sons live a pitiable existence, impoverished and neglected. Because of high child mortality, a woman must bear many sons to insure that a few survive to adulthood (52).

Women in many African tribes face similar situations. For example, among the Ashanti, prolific childbearing is honored. A mother of ten is given a public ceremony of congratulations. On the other hand, barren women are at best ignored or pitied, and at worst regarded with contempt (28, 33).

## CHANGES IN FEMALE ROLES

The traditionally defined female role is undergoing gradual modification, primarily as a result of modernization, urbanization, and industrialization. More women are educated and are more likely to work outside the home in positions of moderate status, such as in factories, offices, and schools. They consequently are beginning to think of themselves in a different light, as capable and competent human beings in other than family-related matters, and are taking advantage of the increasing number of opportunities for self-expression. Research conducted within the past 15 years indicates that to the extent to which women redefine their sex roles, receive education, and/or work outside the home, fertility rates usually decrease correspondingly (6, 24, 26, 34, 38, 47, 64, 69, 70, 90, 97).

As this discussion suggests, for women to be motivated to reduce their fertility, there must be highly valued nonmaternal roles available to them. This leads us to an examination of education and employment, both of which provide women with opportunities to achieve status outside their traditional role as mothers.

### EDUCATION

The relationship between fertility and education is not a simple one. Most empirical evidence suggests that on both the individual and aggregate levels, this relationship usually is inverse. In most societies, women who have more education have fewer children than those with less education; in societies characterized by high levels of female education, fertility levels are correspondingly low (4, 8, 17, 26, 31, 37, 40, 57, 64, 67, 70, 72, 74). Eastern European and Scandinavian countries, the Soviet Union, Germany, Britain, Japan, Canada, and the United States are characterized by very low birth rates (some are below replacement level) and very high levels of education. In Third World countries as well, low birth rates are associated with high levels of education, for women as well as men (64, 72). For example, results of a recent study in Jordan indicated that education was the factor most strongly correlated with fertility level. There was a high correlation between level of education and attitude toward family planning: eighty per cent of the women who disapproved of family planning were illiterate, less than 1 per cent of the disapprovers had attended secondary school, and none had attended college. Moreover, 79 per cent of the respondents who had attended a university, 69 per cent of those who had attended secondary school, 44 per cent of those who had attended primary school, and only 20 per cent of the illiterate had ever attempted to control their fertility. Cumulative fertility for each of these groups, 2.7, 4.0, 5.9, and 6.4 children, respectively, reflected these differences. An inverse relationship between fertility and education was also found when respondents were classified according to their husbands' level of education (72).

### MITIGATING FACTORS

Several factors influence the strength of the relationship between fertility and education, including levels of socioeconomic development, rural or urban residence, and pronatalist pressures.

In Europe, the United States, Canada, Australia, and New Zealand, the negative effect of education on fertility has diminished over the past several decades. In these countries, many educated women are married to men who earn high incomes, and they themselves are often unemployed, a situation which probably contributes indirectly to their relatively high fertility (22, 26, 35). In addition, the amount of education required to influence fertility is affected by the level of socioeconomic development. For example, in the 1960s, in India, the critical number of years of schooling appeared to be between 7 and 11; in Puerto Rico, it occurred after completion of elementary school; in the United States, women who completed 17 years of schooling exhibited a sharp drop in fertility (23, 25, 67, 74, 87).

Rural or urban residence also affects the relationship of education and fertility. Cultural pressures toward high fertility in rural areas may be strong enough to obliterate entirely the effect of several years of school on reproductive behavior. For example, Stycos and Weller (89) found that in the rural areas of Turkey, women with primary level, or higher, education did not have smaller families on the average, whereas in urban areas, family size varied clearly by the level of female education. Finding a similar situation in Latin America, Stycos suggested that a certain amount of urbanization may be necessary to "activate the effects of education on fertility" (88:269).

Strong pronatalist pressures (institutionalized features of a society's value system which strongly favor large numbers of children) also can weaken the relationship between education and fertility. Newland (64), describing Hull's work in Indonesia (43), notes that among Indonesian women, education is associated with high income, and thus with increased fertility (64:8):

At all economic levels, the traditional Indonesian society values large numbers of children, but only the relatively well off can afford to put the ideal into practice—just as it is only the relatively well off who can afford to keep their daughters in school. The relationship between education and fertility is so closely entangled with the income-fertility link that the direct influence of education is obscured. Within a single income class, however, the difference in birth rates for women of different educational levels seems to follow the expected pattern: the more education, the fewer children.

In the United States, strong pronatalist pressures have considerable negative impact on women's desire to excel academically, to continue their education beyond a certain level, and to use their education within a career. Blake (9) explains that in the United States, parenthood is the most important marker of adult status in general, and of feminine status in particular, a condition which makes even many highly educated women reluctant to choose childlessness or even parenting single children. She notes that the content of education which many young women receive, as well as the values perpetuated by educators, parents, and peers, encourages early marriage and motherhood.

Several empirical studies demonstrate the impact of pronatalism on young women in the United States. In the early 1950s, Komarovsky (48) found that college women believed their peers and parents were discouraging them from high levels of academic achievement by labeling it "unfeminine" and encouraging the more feminine activities of marriage and motherhood. Goldsen and his coworkers (36) demonstrated that both male and female students at Cornell University believed that women should have careers only insofar as their jobs did not interfere with maternal responsibilities. Education for women was viewed as necessary only to make them more interesting companions for educated men, and better mothers. It was not regarded as a substitute for more traditional activities. Blake's more recent study (9) showed that although college students in the 1970s prefer fewer children than did their counterparts in previous decades, not many want fewer than two offspring. She concluded that pronatalist values still encourage traditional beliefs regarding the purpose and value of women's education.

## FACTORS WHICH MEDIATE THE EFFECTS OF EDUCATION ON FERTILITY

Clearly, it is important to explore the means by which education directly affects fertility. Education may influence family size by keeping women in school and delaying the age at which women marry and/or bear their first child. Because most births occur within marriage or, at least, within a relatively stable union, delayed marriage is likely to decrease the number of children a woman bears (2, 62, 73). Differences in average age at first marriage between groups of women with varying levels of education may be the most important factor affecting their fertility (4, 15, 17, 30, 34, 92). Minkler (57), who compared the fertility of two groups of working women in India, found that education and fertility were negatively related. He attributed this to the fact that the educated women married 7.4 years later than the uneducated. However, in other studies in which a control for age (or age at first marriage) has not been used, education has often been found to exert an independent effect on family size (59).

Another way in which education can directly affect fertility is by facilitating acquisition of contraceptive information. In most societies, illiterate women have less access than literate women to information about birth control—where and how to obtain, and use, contraceptives. Indeed, education provides women with basic skills that enhance their ability to take advantage of family planning services, and with information conducive to positive attitudes regarding their use (47, 64).

Education can also influence fertility indirectly by providing women with the requisite skills needed to enter the labor force (implications of employment for fertility are discussed elsewhere in this chapter), by changing their self-images, and by increasing their ambitions for themselves and their children.

Regarding the effect of education on women's self-images, Blake and Komarovsky (9, 48) suggest that in the face of strong pronatalist pressures, education has little impact on women's ideas about motherhood and family size. Others, however, have found that education provides women with "new images of femininity," furnishing them with an arena in which they can achieve success and feelings of self-worth (80). In India, for example, where pressures for high fertility are strong and where most women live with their husband's parents, education has played an important role. According to Mandlebaum (52:54–55),

An educated woman is usually less closely confined, physically and psychologically, within her husband's family and its narrow familial concerns than is the woman who is brought into their home as an uneducated girl shortly after her menarche. Village elders commonly tell you, and they are probably right, that a young wife who has been to high school or college is not as duly submissive to her mother-in-law as is a less educated daughter-in-law, nor will she brook the kind of social restraints that the strict tradition requires. She is more likely to feel that she can do something about certain conditions of her life, including the condition of pregnancies in close succession or conceiving during her later reproductive years. Her schooling has commonly disclosed to her more leeway in her *karma*, more alternatives in her *dharma* than an uneducated woman can know. Her horizons of information are wider, if only from being able to read a newspaper; her network of communication is likely to be broader, if only to school friends beyond the confines of household

kin. These differences are not, of course, direct results of her having studied algebra or learned to read another language, but they are potent consequences that help her shape her life and are likely to induce her to limit her fertility. Both educated and uneducated brides still know well that they have to prove themselves by bearing children, but the educated wife is not as likely to want to keep proving herself through obstetrical channels throughout the whole reproductive span of her life.

Education can also give women a desire for a higher standard of living for themselves as well as their children (26). This increases the cost of raising children, and the new life style is thus incompatible with large family size (34).

Higher standards of living usually involve a good education for one's offspring. There are several costs, both direct and indirect, associated with educating children. Therefore, when parents value education, they may base their decision about family size on the number of children they think they can afford to educate. Even when parents believe their children will provide security for them in their old age—a belief which often is associated with high fertility—they may choose to limit family size to improve their children's chances of success; they have as many as they can afford to educate to the extent necessary for achieving success in the job market (64). For example, Kunii and Katagiri (49) found that most of the Japanese wives they studied based their reproductive decisions on the number of children they believed they could afford to educate.

## FEMALE PARTICIPATION IN THE LABOR FORCE

The correlation between female participation in the labor force and reduced fertility is well documented (20, 21, 32, 35, 50, 56, 58, 71, 95). For example, as early as 1959, Freedman, Whelpton, and Campbell (32) reported that among a representative sample of currently married American Caucasian women between the ages of 18 and 39, fertility and expected fertility were lower among working women than among nonworking wives. Working women had an average of 2.88 children, compared to an average of 3.94 children for nonworkers. This relationship persisted when such variables as duration of marriage, educational attainment, wife's religion, and husband's income were controlled. The authors concluded that the wife's employment history is of fundamental importance in the analysis of fertility.

Participation in the labor force is a significant fertility differential in other countries as well, such as Denmark, Norway, England, Wales, Switzerland, Czechoslovakia, Hungary, Brazil, India, Japan, France, and in many parts of Latin America (21, 27, 35). In representative samples of approximately 2000 women, aged 20 to 50, in Rio de Janeiro, Panama, and San Jose, nonworking women averaged 3.5, 2.5, and 3.7 live births respectively, but working women averaged only 3.0, 1.8, and 1.9 births (60). However, despite the prevalence of positive correlations between female participation in the labor force and reduced fertility, it should be noted early in this discussion that causality has not been proved. This issue will be discussed in greater detail later in this chapter.

### CONDITIONS WHICH STRENGTHEN THE WORK-FERTILITY RELATIONSHIP

Some studies have demonstrated that the strength of the inverse association between female participation in the labor force and fertility is dependent upon type of employment (usually white collar, professional, or managerial, as opposed to blue-collar work) (1, 65, 71, 86, 94); duration of employment (32, 71); percentage contribution of female salary to family income (71); compatibility of work with motherhood (89, 94); reason for employment (95); and strength of the woman's commitment to her job (74–76).

Whelpton and his coworkers (95) reported that fertility rates of women who work only because of financial need were higher than those of women who worked because of the satisfaction they obtained from their jobs. Safilios-Rothschild (74–76) found that Greek women who worked because they wanted to work, and planned to continue working regardless of their husbands' financial situation, tended to have fewer children than those who would stop working under more favorable economic conditions. Stycos also reported that the fertility of Peruvian women engaged in white-collar employment was markedly lower than that of domestic workers (86). In a similar vein, Reed and Udry (71) found that among black and white United States women, white-collar workers had lower fertility than blue-collar employees. This type of research has helped delineate those conditions in which employment is most likely to be inversely related to family size.

### CAUSE AND EFFECT

Participation in the labor force may depress fertility in various ways. First, it can reduce the proportion of women marrying, or postpone the age of marriage and thus shorten the childbearing period. Work participation provides an alternative to early marriage by enabling a woman to become self-supporting (20). Secondly, it can reduce the fertility of married women by providing alternative sources of emotional satisfaction and status outside their homes and children. Not only are increasing numbers of women able to feel fulfilled and valued without having large numbers of offspring; they are becoming more aware of the costs in terms of lost opportunities involved in bearing and raising a large family. Thirdly, except where servants are widely available or an extended family network provides babysitting services, having additional children is incompatible with employment outside the home. Women would be deprived of needed income and the sense of accomplishment and satisfaction which they gain from their work, or the financial ability to seek other forms of satisfaction that compete with those derived from the family (20, 39, 56, 89, 94).

Participation in professional or white-collar work may be particularly conducive to diminished fertility because the higher salaries, prestige, fulfillment, and educational requirements involved in such work act as greater incentives to family size limitation. Women employed in these positions have more to lose, if forced to forfeit their jobs to raise children. On the other hand, the greater demands made by this work on women's time and psychic energy make it more difficult for them to combine employment and domestic roles.

Fourthly, it has been suggested that employment contributes to a woman's self-confidence, knowledge, and power within her own family, and that this newly gained status directly affects fertility-reduction (67, 93). (See Chap. 22 for a detailed discussion of conjugal relationships and fertility.) Weller's work in Puerto Rico (93) demonstrates that employed women are more likely to successfully resist their spouses' desire for more offspring. The negative correlations between fertility and female employment are, however, greater in female-dominated and equalitarian family structures and weaker in male-dominated households.

Despite apparent correlations between female participation in the labor force and reduced fertility, there are inconsistencies in the data, and the relationship between family size and female employment is not maintained under all conditions, in all countries, or in all sectors of the same country (3, 5, 26, 27, 44, 54, 57, 65, 67, 87, 89, 90, 94). For example, data from rural Japan (44), Poland (3), Italy (27), and Egypt (5) demonstrate that female agricultural workers have the same, or even higher, fertility than housewives. Further, it has been shown that work performed by women at home, particularly that which is unpaid, has no effect on family size (21, 44, 90).

The issue is even less clear in developing countries (26, 89). The employment–fertility relationship is, for example, not substantiated in urban and rural Turkey (89); Lima, Peru (86); India (57); or in Lagos, Nigeria (65). In Lima, Peru, Stycos (86) found that white-collar employment was negatively related to fertility, although blue-collar and domestic work were not. White-collar workers had 43 per cent fewer children than housewives, but since they constituted a minimal part of the labor force, work in general was not found to be correlated with reduced fertility. Similar results were found in West Africa by Ohadike (65). The most prevalent explanation offered for the nonassociation of fertility and female participation in the labor force is the absence of role incompatibility in most jobs in these countries (5, 39, 89, 90, 94). In the rural setting, for example, most women can combine work with childbearing and child-rearing. Their two roles are viewed as complementary, rather than as mutually antagonistic.

Most critically, even in situations where significant correlations between fertility and employment have been established, the direction of causality has not yet been substantiated. Consequently, it is impossible to determine whether reduced fertility is a consequence or a determinant of female employment status; whether both variables are simultaneously consequences and determinants of one another; or whether both are consequences of other variables, such as economic development and industrialization (26, 58, 67, 71, 89).

Research has not yet provided evidence that female participation in the labor force actually induces lower fertility.

The employment–fertility relationship has, moreover, been seriously questioned by the work of Reed and Udry (71). Despite their demonstration of an inverse relationship between current parity and various dimensions of labor-force participation among white and black females, they were unable to find, with certain exceptions, a significant association between employment status and regularity of contraceptive use. These authors concluded that the relationship between reduced fertility and employment status cannot be explained by a deliberate attempt on the part of working women to control their fertility. They suggested that subfecund women may self-select into the labor force, or that participation in the labor force itself in some unexplained manner reduces fecundity.

## THE COMPOSITE PICTURE

The issue of exactly which element of female status affects fertility is highly complex. It is likely that opportunities for both education and employment, in conjunction with each other and with other factors such as cultural milieu and availability of mother surrogates (to free mothers to work), directly contribute to reduced family size. However, it also is as likely that both of these factors effect other changes, such as increases in self-confidence and aspirations for individual achievement and higher standards of living, which, in turn, significantly affect fertility. Although it is easier to "measure" changes in employment or educational status of women and relate them to family size than to consider the complex interraction of factors, it is important to bear this interaction in mind.

## INTERACTION OF EDUCATION AND EMPLOYMENT

A detailed example from Puerto Rico illustrates this point (80). Scott chose Mountain Town to study the relationship between social change, women's status, family structure, and fertility, because the community was undergoing industrial, demographic, educational, and ecological expansion. The town was originally a typical example of most Latin American communities: rural, male-dominated, with low literacy rates, a belief in innate female inferiority, and a limited social or work life outside the home for women. As the town became increasingly urbanized and industrialized, and as more opportunities for female education and employment were provided, these features began to change. In fact, the socioecological changes in the town affected women more than they did men. For example, between 1950 and 1960, ten factories were established which hired mostly women, because of their supposed superiority in sewing and other "delicate" skills. By 1960, five times as many women as men were employed in manufacturing, and professional women outnumbered professional men. Governmental agencies, transportation, communication, and eating facilities purposely catering to females were established. Women were thus given the opportunity to socialize outside the home and to redefine their self-image in the direction of greater independence, self-reliance, and equality.

Scott hypothesized that such effects of the new social and economic conditions would be reflected in more equalitarian family patterns and in lower fertility rates of those women most involved in these experiences of change. His results corroborated his hypotheses. In every age-grouping, fertility rates showed significant negative correlations with the woman's education and employment status. Moreover, high education and employment, combined, were consistently related to the equalitarian, or nearly equalitarian, type of family organization, whereas low education and employment combined were consistently related to the patriarchal type of family organization. Families of the equalitarian type had the lowest fertility rates, and families of the patriarchal type, the highest.

Scott's description of the direct, indirect, and interacting effects of employment and education bears repetition (80:527–528):

In the open competition with males for prestige, power, grades, scholarships, girls begin to acquire new images of femininity which contrast sharply with the traditional images. Winning leadership positions in school and winning scholarships, or even seeing other girls do so, gradually has the effect of changing the traditional self-idea of females from the idea of inferiority to equality, or at least near equality. The girls discover that in social competition education itself is an "equalizer." They also discover that systematic knowledge and skill are more important in seeking employment in the modern factories than maleness or femaleness. . . .

By leaving home for outside employment and earning as much or more than their husbands, a near-independent status can be achieved. Once the females start working in the factories side by side with the males, where they cannot ask for any "breaks," nor give any "breaks," especially where piecework is involved, the idea of equal worth is tested in reality. As it happens, on payday, many women line up at the pay window and take home more than their male counterparts. At this time the cognitive idea of equality receives a reinforcement as never before. Personal worth is financially measurable now, and out of this experience they conclude that money and productivity are also more valued than maleness or femaleness, in fact money and productivity, like education, are objective measures of individual worth; they become ways by which women and men alike can compare themselves to one another. . . .

With participation in school, females acquire a new degree of personal freedom of mobility, new social interests, and new memberships in clubs designed for ego expansion and diversion. After marriage, these conditioning experiences typically result in a broadening social life, especially when combined with the work plant's encouragement of social life through its worker associations, parties and recreation programs.

The combination of employment and educational achievement not only affects female motivation to curb fertility, but facilitates effective use of contraceptive methods. As previously mentioned, better-educated women are more knowledgeable and sophisticated with respect to contraceptive techniques. The perceived risks of contraceptive failure, particularly for employed women, may be considerably more grave than for women with traditional roles. Consequently, women with more modern roles and self-images are less likely to be careless in their contraceptive behaviors (56, 79).

## SEX-ROLE DEFINITIONS

Some social scientists believe that the effects of increasingly available opportunities for rewards outside the domestic sphere, particularly occupational pursuits, influence fertility by changing female sex-role definitions. Modern self-concepts are related to participation in the labor force, but are not believed to be entirely dependent upon it (77–79). For example, Clarkson and his coworkers administered a self-evaluative personality test to 60 women (18). Those females who ranked themselves in the "high competency" cluster had significantly fewer children than those who considered themselves less competent. There was virtually no difference in the mean number of children borne by women ranked high in competency, who had worked 7 years or less, or 8 years or more (3.12, versus 3.13). However, among low-competency women, employment status made a significant difference. Those mothers who had worked 7 or fewer years had an average of 4.43 children, whereas those who had worked 8 or more years had an average of 3.30 offspring. The data not only suggest that women with more traditional views of themselves tend to have more children than their more modern counterparts, but also that more modern self-concepts outweigh the effect of employment status on fertility (18, 79).

The effect of sex-role definition may be mediated, in part, through the differential value of children for traditional and modern women. Data from a national survey indicate that women who have few outside activities value children more than those with more modern orientations. The factor that best explains this differential response is that women who define the female role as that of housewife have less access to alternative sources of activity and rewards; children thereby play a more central and vital role in their lives than in those of their less traditional counterparts (42).

## WOMEN'S OVERALL POSITION IN SOCIETY

The impact of a woman's general cultural and economic situation, as opposed to her education and employment level alone, on fertility is further attested to by results of a study on female fertility and status in 17 countries. In this study, 11 variables were used as indicators of women's position. Societies which were controlling their population growth most successfully were characterized by the following indicators: freedom of women to choose whom and when they will marry, freedom to move about the community at will, freedom and opportunity to participate politically, and absence of a double standard with regard to premarital sexual relations (91).

In summary, although employment and educational opportunities for women are related to reduced fertility, other elements in women's status, interacting with these two major variables, are also significant. It is consequently important to consider many elements of women's status, as opposed to focusing on only one or two factors (6, 26, 34, 64, 91).

## MALE SEX ROLES AND FERTILITY

Research on the correlation between sex roles and fertility has focused primarily on women; they are, after all, the actual bearers of children. However, it also is important to consider men in this equation, since they also influence choices about child-bearing.

### THE ROLE OF MACHISMO

In 1952 Stycos first proposed that high fertility rates in Puerto Rico were partially attributable to machismo, or more specifically, to the male's need to prove his virility by siring a large number of offspring (84). Since that time, the existence of machismo in other than ideal or mythical terms has been questioned, and its supposed influence upon fertility behavior is not widely accepted. Many researchers in the field of family planning, including Stycos himself (41), now discount the role of machismo, particularly the need to prove one's sexual potency.

Misra (61), studying fertility attitudes among urban black males in Chicago, found no evidence of machismo; neither did Kay, (46) working with Mexican-American males in Arizona. In fact, Kinzer (47), deplores the attention given to machismo in studies of fertility behavior and states that the primary variables affecting fertility rates are female employment status and level of educational achievement.

The issue is still unresolved. Some men do object to limiting family size. Studies conducted by Weller (93) and Scott (80) in Puerto Rico demonstrate that fertility rates are highest in partriarchally-oriented family structures, in which the husband has the ultimate say on most issues, including birth planning. Moreover, although machismo may, in fact, be only a myth or an ideal (41), ideals affect behavior. In the 1950s, Puerto Rican women may not have taken appropriate measures to curb family size because of their unrealistic views of their husbands' need to procreate (41).

Men affected by the ideal of machismo may not aspire to a large number of children to demonstrate their sexual potency, but they may be influenced by the traditionally patriarchal definition of the male role, which directly or indirectly encourages large family size. For example, Stycos (85) reported that Puerto Rican males often objected to family planning because they wanted to keep a firm reign over their wives in order to preserve their fidelity and felt that a large number of children would serve this purpose. Some men objected to their wives' utilization of contraceptives because they felt it undermined their authority in the sexual sphere.

Other men may not necessarily object to limiting family size, but may feel threatened by a major antecedent of reduced fertility rates—that is, modernization of the female role. For example, the role of Cuban women has been purposely modernized to encourage rapid expansion of the national labor force to meet the needs posed by rapid economic and social development. Widespread employment of women, creation of day-care centers for children, and general modernization of female roles have apparently met with considerable male resistance (69). Results of a study of male workers who immigrated from Cuba to the United States indicate that a primary cause for migration was the challenge to male self-esteem presented by this change in traditional female roles. These men felt their familial power was weakened and that their wives were not caring for their needs as well as they did when they were unemployed. They also feared loss of respect from their children (29). Since role modernization is related to reduced fertility, by objecting to such changes, males may indirectly encourage large family size.

## FERTILITY AS COMPENSATION

The male role may be related to fertility in another way. The human need to attain a favorable position in society and a positive self-image recognizes no sexual boundaries. It is possible that men, like women, may compensate for inferior social positions through producing many offspring.

Men have traditionally proved themselves through their work. Even in the equalitarian and communal environment of the Israeli kibbutz, males are more dominated by work interests than females. On one Kibbutz studied intensively, men were primarily concerned with their work, and with work-related ambitions. Their greatest sources of conflict were related to their employment; their worth as human beings appeared dependent upon their worth as workers. On the other hand, although kibbutz women worked 8 hours a day and were concerned with their performance, their primary concerns were family-related. The greatest degree of male despondency resulted from being obligated to work in unsatisfying, menial, and unimportant tasks, whereas women suffered most from family instability, loss of a family member, etc. (81, 82).

The need for a man to work to prove his worth is not confined to the kibbutz. In most societies, it is the prerogative and the responsibility of the male to support his family, and, in so doing, earn social status for himself and members of his family. The sexual division of labor whereby women are assigned child-rearing, domestic, or subsistence work near the home, and men are assigned what the given society considers the more important tasks (hunting, mechanized farming, executive positions, etc.), is an almost universal phenomenon, perhaps second only to the incest taboo in its pervasiveness (81, 82). However, what is important to consider here is that assigning males the task of family support does not necessarily presuppose that the means for fulfilling this obligation is available. Although males in many communities can theoretically achieve their position in society through their own accomplishments, whereas female status is ascribed, economic and social conditions often interfere with their doing so. Men cannot always obtain the necessary training or find satisfactory employment that provides an acceptable position in society and a positive self-image (81). Under these circumstances, men as well as women may be expected, among other things, to turn to a large family for both emotional satisfaction and a feeling of accomplishment that they could not derive elsewhere.

A similar point of view is presented by Blau and Duncan (11). They argue that low-status workers have larger families than high-status workers, so as to compensate for their inferior social and economic position. A large family provides them with alternative rewards. Unsuccessful male workers may compensate for their lack of authority in their jobs by exercising control over a large number of offspring. The authors also believe that one of the reasons that women with modern self-concepts have fewer children than their more traditional counterparts may be that the former tend to be highly educated themselves and to marry highly educated men. These men have greater access to social and economic opportunities than do poorly educated ones. Consequently, they may have less need for a large family, either as a source of emotional satisfaction or as a means by which to validate their position in society.

Whether or not Blau and Duncan's view is valid, improvements in education and socioeconomic opportunities should raise men's as well as women's aspirations for individual achievement and higher levels of living, and thus foster small family size.

In summary, in societies where the traditionally defined female role prevails, high fertility is encouraged, because bearing and raising children are women's only sources of status and satisfaction. In more modern societies, which favor greater female independence and offer opportunities for women to achieve rewards outside the domestic sphere, particularly in education and employment, low fertility is encouraged. Although the male sex role in fertility behavior has not been extensively investigated, it is suggested that men may also compensate for inferior social positions through siring many offspring. Consequently, it is expected that increased education and employment opportunities for males, as well as for females, will be associated with reduced family size. Negative correlations between fertility and general levels of literacy and economic opportunities, discussed in Chapter 19, support this conclusion.

## REFERENCES

1. Anicic Z: Certain indicators of recent fertility trends of Yugoslav population. In International Population Conference, London, 1969, Vol 1, p 495. Liege, International Union for the Scientific Study of Population, 1971
2. Baldwin CS: Policies and realities of delayed marriage. The cases of Tunisia, Sri Lanka, Malaysia and Bangladesh. PRB Report 3(4):1, 1977
3. Berent J: Some demographic aspects of female employment in Eastern Europe. In International Population Conference, London, 1969, Vol 3, p 1572. Liege, International Union for the Scientific Study of Population, 1971
4. Bhatnagar NK: Status of women and family planning in India. J Fam Welfare 18:21, 1972
5. Bindary A, Baxter CB, Hollingsworth TH: Urban-rural differences in the relationship between women's employment and fertility: a preliminary study. J Biosoc Sci 5:159, 1973
6. Birdsall N: Women and population studies. Signs: J Women Cult Soc 1:699, 1976
7. Blake J: Demographic science and redirection of population policy. J Chron Dis 18:1181, 1965
8. Blake J: Family size in the 1960's—A baffling fad. Eugen Q 14:60, 1967
9. Blake J: Coercive pronatalism and American population policy. In Parke R Jr, Westoff C (eds): Aspect of Population Growth Policy. US Commission on Population Growth and the American Future, Vol 6, p 85. Washington DC, Government Printing Office, 1972
10. Blake J: The changing status of women in developed countries. Sci Am 231:136, 1974
11. Blau PM, Duncan OD: The American Occupational Structure. New York, Wiley, 1967
12. Blumberg RL: Fairy tales and facts: economy, family, fertility, and the female, In Tinker T, Bramsen MB, Buvinic M (eds): Women and World Development. New York, Praeger, 1976, p 12
13. Boserup E: Woman's Role in Economic Development. London, George Allen and Unwin Ltd, 1970
14. Bossen L: Women and economic underdevelopment: when are babies like bananas. Paper presented at the annual meeting of the American Anthropological Association, Mexico City, 1974
15. Caldwell J: Some factors affecting fertility in Ghana. In International Population Conference, London, 1969, Vol 1, p 751. Liege, International Union for the Scientific Study of Population, 1971
16. Chaney EM: Old and new feminists in Latin America: the case of Peru and Chile. J Marr Fam 35:331, 1973
17. Chung BM, Palmore JA, Lee SJ, Lee SJ: Psychological perspectives: family planning in Korea. Seoul, Hollym Corporation, Korea, 1972
18. Clarkson FE, Vogel SR, Broverman IK, Broverman DM: Family size and sex role stereotypes. Science 167:390, 1970
19. Cohen LM: Woman's entry to the professions in Colombia: selected characteristics. J Marr Fam 35:322, 1973
20. Collver OA: Women's work participation and fertility in metropolitan areas. Demography 5:55, 1968
21. Collver OA, Langlois E: The female labor force in metropolitan areas: an international comparison. Econ Dev Cult Change 10:367, 1962
22. Council of Europe. Second European Population Conference, Strasbourg, 1971
23. Dandekar K: Effect of education on fertility. World Population Conference, Belgrade, 1965, Vol 4. New York, United Nations, 1966
24. Day LH, Day AT: Family size in industrialized countries: an inquiry into the socio-cultural determinants of levels of childbearing. J Marr Fam 31:242, 1969
25. Dinkel RM: Education and fertility in the United States. World Population Conference, Belgrade, 1965, Vol 4. New York, United Nations, 1966
26. Dixon RB: Women's rights and fertility. Reports on Population/Family Planning, No. 17, New York, The Population Council, 1975
27. Federici N: The influence of women's employment on fertility. In Szabady E (ed): World Views of Population Problems. Budapest, Akademiai Kaido, 1968, p 77

28. Fortes M: Kinship and marriage among the Ashanti. In Brown R, Forde D (eds): African Systems of Kinship and Marriage. London, Oxford University Press, 1950, p 262

29. Fox GE: Honor, shame and women's liberation in Cuba. In Pescatello A (ed): Female and Male in Latin America: Essays. Pittsburgh, University of Pittsburgh Press, 1973, p 273

30. Freedman R, Hermalin A, Sun TH: Fertility trends in Taiwan: 1961–1970. Taiwan Population Studies Working Paper No. 15. Ann Arbor, Population Studies Center, University of Michigan, 1971

31. Freedman R, Takeshita J: Family Planning in Taiwan. Princeton, Princeton University Press, 1969

32. Freedman R, Whelpton PE, Cambell AA: Family Planning, Sterility and Population Growth. New York, McGraw-Hill, 1959

33. Gaisie SK: Fertility levels among the Ghananian tribes. In Ominde SH, Ejiogu CN (eds): Population Growth and Economic Development in Africa. London, Heinemann, 1972, p 84

34. Germain A: Status and roles of women as factors in fertility behavior: a policy analysis. Stud Fam Plann 6:192, 1975

35. Gille H: Summary review of fertility differentials in developed countries. In International Population Conference, London, 1969, Vol 3, p 2011. Liege, International Union for the Scientific Study of Population, 1971

36. Goldsen RK, Rosenberg M, Williams RM Jr, Suchman EA: What College Students Think. Princeton, Princeton University Press, 1960

37. Goldstein S: The influence of labour force participation and education on fertility in Thailand. Pop Stud 26:419, 1972

38. Hall R: The demographic transition: stage four. Curr Anthrop 13:212, 1972

39. Hass PH: Maternal role incompatibility and fertility in urban Latin America. J Soc Issues 28:111, 1972

40. Heer DM: Educational advance and fertility change. In International Population Conference, London, 1969, Vol 3, p 1903. Liege, International Union for the Scientific Study of Population, 1971

41. Hill R, Stycos JM, Back KW: The Family and Population Control. Chapel Hill, University of North Carolina Press, 1959

42. Hoffman LW, Thornton A, Mannis JD: The value of children to parents in the United States. J Pop 1(2):91, 1978

43. Hull VJ: Women in Java's rural middle class: progress or regress? Paper prepared for the Fourth World Congress for Rural Sociology, Torun, Poland, 1976

44. Jaffe AJ, Azumi K: The birth rate and cottage industries in underdeveloped countries. Econ Dev Cult Change 9:52, 1960

45. Karush GE: Plantations, population, and poverty: the roots of the demographic crisis in El Salvador. Paper presented at the annual meeting of the Population Association of America, Atlanta, 1978

46. Kay M: The ethnosemantics of Mexican American fertility. Paper presented at the annual meeting of the American Anthropological Association, Mexico City, 1974

47. Kinzer NS: Priests, machos and babies: Or, Latin American women and the Manichaean heresy. J Marr Fam 35:300, 1973

48. Komarovsky M: Women in the Modern World: Their Education and Their Dilemmas. Boston, Little, Brown, 1953

49. Kunii C, Katagiri T (eds): Basic readings on population and family planning in Japan. Japanese Organization for International Cooperation in Family Planning, Tokyo, 1976

50. Kupinsky S: Non-familial activity and socio-economic differentials in fertility. Demography 8:353, 1971

51. Mamdani M: The Myth of Population Control: Family, Caste, and Class in an Indian Village. New York, Monthly Review Press, 1972

52. Mandelbaum DG: Human fertility in India: Social components and policy perspectives. Berkeley, University of California Press, 1974

53. Marsden LR: Human rights and population growth—A feminist perspective. Int J Health Serv 3:567, 1973

54. Mazur P: Birth control and regional differentials in the Soviet Union. Pop Stud 22:319, 1968

55. McGinn N: Marriage and family in middle-class Mexico. J Marr Fam 28:305, 1966

56. Michel A: Working wives and family interaction in French and American families. Int J Comp Soc 11:157, 1970

57. Minkler M: Fertility and labour force participation in India: survey of workers in Old Delhi area. J Fam Welfare 17:31, 1970

58. Miro CA: Some misconceptions disproved: a program of comparative fertility surveys in Latin America. In Berelson B, (ed): Family Planning and Population Programs: A Review of World Developments. Chicago, University of Chicago Press, 1966, p 615

59. Miro CA, Mertens W: Influences affecting fertility in urban and rural Latin America. Milbank Mem Fund Q 46(Pt 2): 89, 1968

60. Miro CA, Rath F: Preliminary findings of comparative fertility surveys in three Latin American cities. Milbank Mem Fund Q 43(Pt 2): 36, 1965

61. Misra BD: Correlates of males' attitudes toward family planning. In Bogue D (ed): Sociological Contributions to Family Planning Research. Chicago, Community and Family Study, 1967

62. Muhsam HV: Education and demography. In International Population Conference, London, 1969, Vol 3, p 1867. Liege, International Union for the Scientific Study of Population, 1971

63. Nag M: Factors affecting human fertility in non-industrial societies: a cross-cultural study. New Haven, Yale University Publications in Anthropology, No. 66. New Haven, Reprinted by Human Relations Area Files Press, 1968

64. Newland K: Women and population growth: choice beyond childbearing. Worldwatch Paper 16, 1977

65. Ohadike P: The possibility of fertility change in modern Africa: a West African case. In International Population Conference, London, 1969, Vol 1, p 801. Liege, International Union for the Scientific Study of Population, 1971

66. Penalosa F: Mexican family roles. J Marr Fam 30:680, 1968

67. Piepmeier KB, Atkins TS: The status of women and fertility. J Biosoc Sci 5:507, 1973
68. Poffenberger T: Motivational aspects of resistance to family planning in an Indian village. Demography 5:757, 1968
69. Purcell SK: Modernizing women for a modern society: the Cuban case. In Pescatello A (ed): Female and Male in Latin America: Essays. Pittsburgh, University of Pittsburgh Press, 1973
70. Ratcliffe JW: Poverty, politics and fertility: the anomaly of Kerala. Hastings Center Report, February, 1977, p 34
71. Reed FW, Udry JR: Female work, fertility and contraceptive use in a biracial sample. J Marr Fam 35:597, 1973
72. Rizk H: Trends in fertility and family planning in Jordan. Stud Fam Plann 8:91, 1977
73. Ryder NB, Westoff CF: Reproduction in the United States, 1965. Princeton, Princeton University Press, 1971
74. Safilios-Rothschild C: Sociopsychological factors affecting fertility in urban Greece: a preliminary report. J Marr Fam 31:595, 1969
75. Safilios-Rothschild C: The influence of the wife's degree of work commitment upon some aspects of family organization and dynamics. J Marr Fam 32:681, 1970
76. Safilios-Rothschild C: The relationship between work commitment and fertility. Int J Soc Fam 2:64, 1972
77. Scanzoni J: Sex Roles, Life Styles and Childbearing: Changing Patterns in Marriage and Family. New York, Free Press, 1975
78. Scanzoni J: Gender roles and the process of fertility control. J Marr Fam 38:677, 1976
79. Scanzoni J, McMurry M: Continuities in the explanation of fertility control. J Marr Fam 34:315, 1972
80. Scott JW: Sources of social change in community, family and fertility in a Puerto Rican town. Am J Soc 72:520, 1967
81. Shain RN: The Functional Nature of the Sexual Division of Labor on an Israeli Kibbutz. Ph.D. dissertation, University of Calif, Berkeley, 1974
82. Shain RN: The functional nature of the sexual division of labor on an Israeli Kibbutz. Presented at the annual meeting of the American Anthropological Association, Houston, 1977
83. Stevens EP: The prospects for a woman's liberation movement in Latin America. J Marr Fam 35:313, 1973
84. Stycos JM: Family and fertility in Puerto Rico. Am Soc Rev 17:572, 1952
85. Stycos JM: Birth control clinics in crowded Puerto Rico. In Paul B (ed): Health, Culture, and Community. New York, Russell Sage Foundation, 1955, p 189
86. Stycos JM: Female employment and fertility in Lima, Peru. Milbank Mem Fund Q 43:42, 1965
87. Stycos JM: Education and fertility in Puerto Rico. World Population Conference, Vol 4, 1965. New York, United Nations, 1966
88. Stycos JM: Human Fertility in Latin America: Sociological Perspectives. Ithaca, Cornell University Press, 1968
89. Stycos JM, Weller RH: Female working roles and fertility. Demography 4:210, 1967
90. Tien HY: Employment and education of women in China: implications for fertility change. In International Population Conference, London, 1969, Vol 3, p 1974. Liege, International Union for the Scientific Study of Population, 1971
91. Tinker I, Reining P, Swidler W, Cousins W: Culture and Population Change. Washington DC, American Association for the Advancement of Science, 1976
92. United Nations: Study on the interrelationship of the status of women and family planning: report of the special rapporteur. E/Cn.6/757 (November), 1973
93. Weller R: The employment of wives, dominance and fertility. J. Marr Fam 30:437, 1968
94. Weller RH: The employment of wives, role incompatibility and fertility: a study of lower and middle-class residents of San Juan, Puerto Rico. Milbank Mem Fund Q 46:507, 1968
95. Whelpton PK, Campbell AA, Patterson JE: Fertility and Family Planning in the United States. Princeton, Princeton University Press, 1966
96. Youseff NH: Differential labor force participation of women in Latin America and Middle Eastern countries: the influence of family characteristics. Soc Forces 51:135, 1972
97. Zeidenstein G: Including women in development efforts. World Development 6, (7) 1978

# 22

# Family Structure and Fertility

**Rochelle N. Shain**
**Victoria H. Jennings**

Although many factors affect fertility, it is within the family that actual fertility decisions are made—or not made. For purposes of this discussion, a *family* is defined as "a married couple or other group of adult kinsfolk who cooperate economically and in the upbringing of children, and all or most of whom share a common dwelling" (16:760). Family-related variables which appear to have considerable influence on fertility are type of family unit, form of marriage, and the nature of the conjugal relationship.

## FAMILY TYPE:
## THE EXTENDED FAMILY VERSUS
## THE NUCLEAR FAMILY

Most families can be broadly categorized as either *nuclear* or *extended*. Nuclear families include a husband, wife (or wives), and their children. The nuclear family prevails in hunting-and-gathering societies, and in most industrialized nations today. However, in many agricultural societies, both past and present, the extended family has been the dominant form. Extended families can be either "horizontal" (consisting of siblings, their spouses, and their children), "vertical" (consisting of parents, married children, and their children), or a combination of the two. Extended families include groups of relatives living in the same household, as well as networks of kin living in different households.

It generally has been assumed, but never proved, that women in nuclear families have smaller numbers of children than those in ex-

tended families. In nuclear families, parents usually have the sole responsibility for providing and caring for their children, and young married couples are relatively free to make their own childbearing decisions. On the other hand, in extended families the cost and burden of children are shared, and young couples are often constrained in their fertility decisions by family pressure (often intensified by religious and moral strictures) to have as many children as soon as possible. Elders appear to encourage the younger generation to marry young, so that the family may establish links with other households, thereby increasing their networks of mutual assistance and obligation. Young couples are motivated to have children in order to strengthen these links, and to enhance their status within the household (2–5, 8, 15, 20, 27, 29).

Using demographic data from pre- and post-revolutionary France, Goldschieder explains that domination by the kin group encouraged high fertility during the former period, while an emphasis on equal family rights and obligations, engendered by the postrevolutionary period, was conducive to lower fertility (15).

## THE INFLUENCE OF RURAL AND URBAN ENVIRONMENTS

The influence of rural and urban conditions, particularly the presumably greater economic value of children in rural environments, may contribute to fertility differences between family types (see Chap. 20 for further discussion).

In modern industrial societies, where the nuclear family prevails, the workplace is removed from the home. Child-labor laws exist and prevent children from working. Fertility is usually low, although both age at marriage and family size are strongly influenced by general economic and cultural conditions, and by individual desires and capabilities (20).

In agricultural societies, extended families usually function as units of production and distribution, as well as of reproduction and socialization. Regardless of age or sex, almost all family members work to maximize family resources. Unless there are considerations of land distribution, children are seen as economic assets, and high fertility is encouraged. Examples of the economic value of children in various agricultural societies abound (see Chap. 19). Thus, the differences in fertility between nuclear and extended families may be a product, at least in part, of their overall environment.

## THE INTERGENERATIONAL FLOW OF WEALTH

Caldwell (4–6) has observed that in order for parents and other kin in extended family structures to benefit from high fertility, members of the younger generation must be willing, and even feel an obligation, to aid the older generation. The flow of resources must be from children to parents and other relatives, not vice versa, as Caldwell explains in commenting on this social pattern in Nigeria:

The essential factor in the system is the retention of the traditional system of assistance and of the direction in which that assistance flows, a system which developed in huge rural compounds where four generations of the lineage often lived together. A Nigerian research worker contrasted, with some surprise at the extent of the difference, his survey sample of the new elite in Nigeria's Western State, where 97 per cent of employed children with living parents assisted their parents financially, irrespective of the level of the parents' income or health, with a study of an American New-England population where a similar proportion of parents emphasized that they would not accept help from children even though most had spent massively on the children up until the time of their employment (5:19).

When the flow of wealth is from children to parents, fertility is encouraged, even during the society's transition to urbanization. Fertility, however, is expected to decline in the urban environment when the nuclear family supercedes extended kin structures, particularly with respect to patterns of expenditure and obligation, and when emphasis is placed on what parents owe children, rather than on what children owe parents (5).

## METHODOLOGICAL PROBLEMS

Whereas factors such as urban or rural conditions and the direction of the flow of wealth may contribute to fertility differences between family types, there is no conclusive evidence that a positive correlation between fertility and family types per se actually exists. Studies focusing specifically on this relationship have been conducted in India, Taiwan, Bangladesh, and Guatemala. Unfortunately, most of the data are contradictory and inconclusive: in some studies, nuclear families demonstrate higher fertility and in others, extended families do (2, 3, 13, 18, 23, 26, 29, 31, 44). Most of these studies have serious shortcomings (2, 3, 29). Sample size is small, and family types are not uniformly defined. Common residence, as opposed to kin interaction, is usually defined as the basis of extended-family structure; this may be problematic in that people may reside separately, but participate in a system of mutual obligation which reinforces high fertility (2–5, 29). In most studies of fertility and family structure, cumulative fertility is related to family type at the time of investigation, rather than at the time when children were born. This can produce confusing results. Finally, theoretical analyses of family type and fertility have used aggregate units of analysis, comparing fertility in societies characterized primarily by either nuclear or extended families. Empirical studies, on the other hand, have focused upon individual women, comparing fertility in nuclear and extended families within a given society, primarily because it is difficult to identify the predominant family type in a given society. Since an association between the two variables on one level of analysis does not necessarily imply an association on another, the conclusions of the theoretical and empirical studies are not comparable. In a given population, extended families may be associated with high fertility; on the other hand, nuclear families may predominate, and thus the society would exhibit lower aggregate fertility (2, 3, 29).

Despite these shortcomings, the available data do question the prevalent assumption that extended families encourage high fertility. For example, in a study of 1018 married couples in Calcutta, controlled for duration of marriage and social class, women in nuclear families had higher cumulative fertility than those in extended structures, except in the very lowest class (31). A study in Taiwan indicated that whereas women in nuclear families wanted fewer children than those in extended families, there were no clear differences in mean number of live births (13).

Nag tested the association between high fertility and extended-family structure on a societal level by comparing the fertility of 41 nonindustrial societies. His results do not support the association, but he cautions that the sample size was small and the data for some societies were incomplete or unclear. Moreover, the influence of family structure on fertility is affected by many other factors for which there was no information (29).

Previous assumptions regarding the relationship of family structure to fertility need further cross-cultural study, with adequate sample sizes, appropriate controls, clear definitions of family type, and considerations of changes in family structure over time. Attention should also be given to the role of "direction of flow of wealth" within a family. This may be the aspect of family organization which most significantly affects fertility, with extended-family structure merely facilitating the process.

## FORM OF MARRIAGE: POLYGYNY VERSUS MONOGAMY

Besides the nuclear and extended-family distinctions, families, or, more appropriately, marriages, may also be classified according to the number of husbands or wives included within the union. It has been assumed thus far in this discussion that marriage consists of a sanctioned union between a male and a female—that is, monogamy. Some societies, however, permit polygamy. In these cases, a sanctioned union may include one female and more than one male (polyandry), or one male and more than one female (polygyny). Polyandry, as an ideal or approved form of marriage, is very rare, and fertility data are available for only two societies in which it is practiced, the Toda and Jaunsari of India (27, 29). Both societies are characterized by low fertility; however, nonpolyandrous marriages within these

groups also have low fertility (27, 29, 42). Because of insufficient information on this type of society, the present discussion is limited to monogamy and polygyny.

It is difficult to quantitate the incidence of polygyny. In most polygynous societies, a man must provide a brideprice for his wife. Although polygyny may be the culturally preferred form of marriage, very few men may actually be able to afford more than one brideprice (27, 29).

Despite such problems, the anthropological literature suggests that most societies are characterized by a mixture of monogamy and polygyny (29). Polygyny is most prevalent in Africa, where three-fourths of the societies found in the Human Relations Area File are characterized by that form of marriage (7, 29).

The relationship between fertility and form of marriage has been discussed at length by Nag. He believes that the average number of children born to men in polygynous unions is apt to be greater than that born to those in monogamous ones. Also, in societies where women outnumber men, the potential loss of fertility is alleviated by polygyny. What is most important, however, Nag believes, is to determine whether polygynous societies exhibit higher overall fertility than monogamous ones, and whether the fertility of polygynously married women in a given society is higher than that of monogamously married women within that society (29).

Most studies have concentrated on the second issue and have been conducted in Africa (29). The majority indicate that polygyny has a slightly depressing effect on female marital fertility (24, 25, 27, 29, 30, 43). For example, among the Bedouin of the Negev, the number of children between the ages of 0 and 4, per 1000 women of all ages, was 735.8 in polygynous marriages, and 1076.6 in monogamous ones (25). Table 22–1 presents an overview of the literature on this issue.

Most of these studies suffer from various shortcomings. Some did not control for age at, or duration of, marriage, and all are based on the form of marriage at the time of study, which may be problematic, because the women may have experienced different forms of marriage prior to the study period. Also, because of differences in the fertility measures used and in the types of women considered (some studies consider all women, some only

**Table 22–1. Summary of Selected Polygyny-Fertility Studies**

| Author | Conclusion | Fertility Measure | (N) | Control Variables |
|---|---|---|---|---|
| Culwick and Culwick (1939) | PF* slightly but not significantly greater than MF† | Births per 1000 women (married) | 237 monogamous, 235 polygynous | Place, age of wife |
| Busia (1954) | PF not significantly different from MF | Indeterminable | Indeterminable (several thousand) | None |
| Muhsam (1956) | PF less than MF but only slightly | Living coresident children, 0–4 years and 5–9 years | 240 | Age, childlessness |
| Olusanya (1971) | MF same as PF | Average number of live births | 2742 | Date of first marriage, duration of marriage, age, childlessness, urbanicity |
| Pool (1969) | MF same as PF | Average number of live births | Approximately 2000 | Age, urbanicity |
| Ohadike (1968) | MF same as PF | Number of living children | — | Urbanicity |
| Brebant (1954) | PF less than MF | Registered live births to women 15–45 years | Six areas | None |
| Brito (1952) | PF less than MF | Mean number of children | Several hundred | Childlessness |
| Van de Walle (1968) | PF significantly less than MF | Age-specific fertility rates | Over 1000 | None |
| Dorjahn (1958) | PF significantly less than MF | Live births and living children per wife | 507 | Age at marriage, duration of marriage |
| Ivins (1956) | PF significantly less than MF | Completed fertility | 6700 women | None |

* Fertility of women in polygynous unions.
† Fertility of women in monogamous unions.
(Smith JE, Kunz PR: Population Studies, 30: 467)

married women, etc.) many of these investigations are not comparable (29, 43).

A comprehensive investigation of the Upper Volta, conducted in 1967 (24), compared the cumulative fertility of two groups of women: those who had always been monogamously married, and those who had at some point experienced a polygynous union. Controlling for age, length of exposure to risk of pregnancy, education, religion, and other sociocultural factors, the study found a correlation between polygyny and lower fertility.

A recent study (43) which utilized genealogy records of Mormons from 1907 to 1913 indicated that 72.4 per cent of married men had only one wife at any given time in their lives. Polygynists with two wives constituted 19.4 per cent of the population, and those with three or more wives accounted for 8.2 per cent. Wives in monogamous marriages had an average completed fertility of 7.82, compared to an average of 7.46 for wives in polygynous unions. Interestingly, the first wife, in two-wife polygynous marriages, exhibited the highest fertility, that is, 9.2 births. Moreover, the birth interval between marriage and first birth was similar for first wives, but somewhat longer for second wives, and longest for third wives. Smith and Kunz (43) speculate that a decline in male fecundity as the husbands aged accounts for this. Finding a similar situation in Nigeria, Okaegbu (30) attributes it to increasing age differences between a polygynist and his subsequent wives.

There is only one study (27) in which societal fertility, as opposed to the fertility of women in different types of marriages within one society, is compared. A significant problem in this type of research is the selection of criteria by which to deem a given society as monogamous or polygynous. Labelling a society as high in polygyny if 20 per cent or more of married women were polygynous, Nag compared 45 nonindustrial societies and found no significant relationship between polygyny and reduced fertility. However, because of incomplete data, this study is not conclusive.

If polygyny is indeed related to lower fertility within a given society, what explains this? Dorjahn (10, 11) suggested that polygyny may be associated with a lower frequency of coitus, a wider age span between spouses, and higher frequencies of divorce or separation, postpartum abstinence, and childlessness (or infertility). These are five of the eleven "intermediate variables" proposed by Davis and Blake (9) as mediators of cultural effects on fertility (see Chap. 20).

It has been suggested that although coital frequency is higher for polygynously than monogamously married men, the reverse is true for women. Despite intricate rotational systems of coupling that exist in some polygynous societies, favorite wives receive more attention. Moreover, only older men can usually afford the brideprice required in most polygynous societies. Since older men usually engage in sexual relations less frequently than younger men, a lower frequency of coitus per polygynously married woman is assumed (10, 11, 27). Furthermore, Nag suggests that even if frequency of coitus were the same for polygynously and monogamously married women, fertility probably would still be lower for the former because of a decreased sperm count concomitant with high frequencies of intercourse (12, 27). This possibility may, on the other hand, be partially offset by other factors: for example, avoiding coitus with a menstruating, pregnant, or lactating wife is likely to increase coital frequency with more fecund wives. Secondly, polygynously married women usually engage in extramarital affairs more frequently than monogamously married ones (27). The case for diminished coital frequency in polygynous marriages remains uncertain, because of insufficient data (27, 29).

A similar conclusion is drawn with respect to age differences between spouses in polygynous unions. It is assumed that because only older men can usually afford the brideprice, they marry young second or third wives, thus depriving younger men of women of assumed higher fecundity. Young men are often forced to remain celibate for long periods of time, or to marry older widows, or separated women of diminished fecundity. Consequently, there may be a potential loss of fertility in both monogamous and polygynous marriages in polygynous societies (27). There are, however, no good data upon which to test these assumptions. Moreover, Nag finds no support for the positive association between polygyny and the other factors suggested by Dorjahn (10, 11)—divorce or separation, postpartum abstinence, and childlessness—as mediators of reduced fertility (27, 29).

In sum, although the majority of studies support a positive association between polygyny and reduced fertility, little is understood regarding the "mechanisms through which the reduction occurs" (29:19).

## FERTILITY AND CONJUGAL RELATIONSHIPS

Most fertility research has concentrated on two aspects of conjugal relationships: *1)* the type of union, and *2)* the nature of the interpersonal relationship.

## TYPE OF UNION AND FERTILITY

Studies of marriage in different societies reveal three basic types of conjugal unions: *1)* legal marriage, *2)* common-law or consensual unions, and *3)* visiting relationships. Although legal marriage usually is viewed as the most desirable form, both common-law or consensual unions and visiting relationships occur frequently, occasionally as predecessors to legal marriage. In such countries as Jamaica, Barbados, and Granada, legal marriage typically is not attained until a person is in his or her late 20s, while other unions begin much earlier (29, 37).

Of these three types of unions, legal marriage is thought to be the most stable. It is usually more expensive, involves a public declaration of commitment, and requires legal action for its termination. Consensual unions generally are also relatively stable: they often result from the inability to afford a marriage celebration or the accoutrements deemed necessary for a legal union. Visiting unions, on the other hand, tend to be less stable. In these, the woman either lives by herself or with her family, and is visited periodically by the man. Visiting unions are found primarily in the Caribbean, but they exist in parts of Latin America and Africa (29).

Most studies report that legal marriage tends to be correlated with higher fertility, whereas the other types of union are correlated with lower fertility (29, 36, 37, 45, 46). The major shortcoming of these studies is that they reflect cumulative fertility at the time of investigation (29). Therefore, it is not known if a married woman's children were born during her marriage or while she was involved in a visiting or consensual relationship. An investigation of Indians in East Trinidad (38) tried to minimize this difficulty by comparing completed fertility according to 15 patterns of union change. These comparisons involved *1)* initial type of union, *2)* type of union at the end of the reproductive period, and *3)* differences between, or consistency in initial and final types of unions. Depending on the type of comparison, women in either legal or consensual unions exhibited the highest fertility. The only consistent conclusion was that women in visiting unions had the lowest fertility (29, 38).

The probable explanation for this finding is that women in such unions tend to have less frequent sexual contact than those in either legal or consensual ones. Women in stable marriages (legal or common-law) have considerable opportunity for intercourse, but women in visiting unions often spend a significant period of time between relationships, thus reducing their frequency of sexual contact (1, 28, 29, 37, 45). There is also the possibility that the type of union is affected by fertility. In Jamaica, for example, high fertility appears to encourage union stability, whereas low fertility may facilitate the maintenance of unstable unions (29, 46).

Few explanations have been offered for fertility differences between women in legal and consensual unions. As a result of an extensive fertility survey in Latin America, Miro and Mertens (22) determined that live births were lower for consensually than for legally married women in Buenos Aires, Santiago, Bogota, and San Jose, whereas the reverse was true in Rio de Janeiro, Mexico, Caracas, and Panama. They tentatively concluded that fertility for the consensually married tends to be higher in those cities with a high incidence of common-law marriage, and that further research is necessary to differentiate among the various kinds of common-law relationships.

## THE NATURE OF INTERPERSONAL CONJUGAL RELATIONS AND FERTILITY

Changes in women's roles, discussed in the previous chapter, have resulted in alterations in the dynamics of marital relationships, allowing women to have a more equal voice in family decisions, especially with respect to fertility. It may be partially through the influence on the husband–wife relationship that female education and employment affect fertility decisions and behavior (32, 47).

Theoretical discussions of the relationship between the nature of conjugal relations and fertility suggest that as the status of the woman rises, in comparison with that of the man, communication between spouses improves, and the wife plays a more active role in decision-making processes. It is believed that the wife generally has a stronger desire to limit family size than does her husband. As a result, couples characterized by an "equal-partner" relationship are likely to have fewer children than ones in which the wife has a "junior-partner" status (40).

In empirical studies as well, greater equality between husband and wife appears to be associated with lower fertility. Research in predominantly urban areas in developing, and developed, countries indicates that equality in division of labor and decision-making in marriage is correlated with communication about sex, family-size desires, and birth planning; desires for small families; and practice of effective contraception (14). In research on gender-role norms and the use of fertility control, Scanzoni (40) found that American couples with more egalitarian relationships desired smaller families and had fewer children than couples in which the husband was dominant and the wife subordinant. Nonegalitarian couples desired larger families and practiced contraception less often, and less effectively. In a study of lower- and middle-class residents of San Juan, Puerto Rico (47, 48), and of working and nonworking women in Mountain Town, Puerto Rico (41), reduced family size was also found to be associated with more equal husband-and-wife relationships. Similar conclusions are reported for Brazil (39).

These findings support the results of Hill, Stycos, and Back's pioneering work in Puerto Rico (17), and those of Rainwater in the United States (34, 35). For example, Rainwater found that social class, with husband-and-wife relationship as the significant intervening variable, was a very important factor explaining fertility differentials among contemporary urban couples in the United States. Specifically, lower-class couples tended to have highly "segregated" conjugal relationships, in which communication, including that related to fertility decisions and family-size desires, was extremely limited. Furthermore, in such units, fertility-control measures were believed to be relatively unreliable, and difficult to use effectively. Higher-class couples, on the other hand, tended to have "joint," or "intermediate" relationships, which involved more communication and co-

operative decision-making. In addition, these couples had more confidence in contraceptive methods and in their own ability to use them (34, 35).

A particular type of relationship is not limited to one social class, nor are all marriages in a given social class characterized by a particular type of relationship. Nonetheless, Rainwater's research indicates that social class may be associated with different types of marital relationships, which are, in turn, related to differences in both desired and completed family size. His work also indicates that within a family the type of conjugal relationship is significantly related to family planning behavior.

Other empirical evidence is less decisive. Results of a study of Hong Kong families, who ostensibly wanted no more children, indicated that wives with greater decision-making influence were more likely to contracept than wives with little influence; nonetheless, when a husband and wife differed in their desire for children, the desires of the husband usually prevailed (21). In a study of Cebu City, in the Philippines, the degree of communication between husband and wife had no apparent effect on contraception or fertility (19). Similar results were found in Turkey, particularly in urban areas (33).

Several researchers have noted that fertility control can be a highly sensitive issue in a conjugal relationship—that is, that an ability to communicate about other topics does not necessarily mean an ability to communicate about sex, and sex-related issues, regardless of whether or not the husband-and-wife relationship is otherwise egalitarian.

As Liu and Hutchison explain,

Communications about, and decisions on, issues dealing with instrumental and impersonal problems, such as family purchases and leisure-time activities may be quite different from communications about sex. The latter are deeply embedded in the nonverbal aspects of interpersonal relations. In some cultures, there are rare opportunities for a child to learn how to *communicate* about sex. Marriage ceremonies may only make appropriate the discussion of sex between conjugal couples; they do not, however, provide the necessary skills nor even the vocabulary for the communication. Sex, to paraphrase W. C. Fields, may not be the greatest thing in life or it may not be the smallest thing in life, but there is *nothing exactly like it.* Social scientists who wish to compare communication about interaction involving sex with other areas of conjugal decision-making may find themselves in quite a bind. Most cultures have never been very rational in dealing with sex, although in every known society there are ways to control it. Thus, while the proposition that the family's effectiveness as a planning unit is a function of its communication system may be plausible in many ways, it becomes less certain when planning involves conception *and* sex (19:35).

Although type of conjugal relationship and communicativeness may be related to fertility control in some societies, in others it may play an insignificant role, or none at all. More sophisticated research is required to determine the relationship between these variables.

In general, few firm conclusions can be drawn with respect to family structure and fertility. The extended, as opposed to the nuclear family; the monogamous, as opposed to the polygynous, unit; the legal and consensual union, as opposed to the visiting one; and husband-dominant, as opposed to egalitarian, conjugal unions, appear to be associated with higher fertility. However, because of methodological shortcomings, inadequate data, and the complexity of the problem at hand, these generalizations do not always hold true; moreover, even when they do, as of now, we still do not adequately understand the underlying mechanisms.

# REFERENCES

1. Blake J: Family Structure in Jamaica. Glencoe, Free Press, 1961
2. Burch TK, Gendell M: Extended family structure and fertility: some conceptual and methodological issues. J Marr Fam 32:227, 1970
3. Burch TK, Gendell M: Extended family structure and fertility: some conceptual and methodological issues. In Polgar S (ed): Culture and Population: A Collection of Current Studies. Carolina Population Center Monograph 9. Cambridge, Schenkman, 1971, p 87
4. Caldwell JC: Toward a restatement of demographic transition theory. Pop Dev Rev 2:321, 1976
5. Caldwell JC: The economic rationality of high fertility: an investigation illustrated with Nigerian survey data. Pop Stud 31:5, 1977
6. Caldwell JC: A theory of fertility: from high plateau to destabilization. Pop Dev Rev 4:553, 1978
7. Clignet R: Determinants of African polygyny. In Goody J (ed): Kinship. Baltimore, Penguin, 1971, p 163
8. Davis K: Institutional patterns favoring high fertility in underdeveloped areas. Eugen Q 2:33, 1955
9. Davis K, Blake J: Social structure and fertility: an analytic framework. Econ Dev Cult Change 4:211, 1956
10. Dorjahn VR: Fertility, polygyny and their interrelations in Temne Society. Am Anthrop 60:838, 1958
11. Dorjahn VR: The factor of polygyny in African demography. In Bascom WR, Herskovits MJ (eds): Continuity and Change in African Cultures. Chicago, University of Chicago, 1959, p 87
12. Farris EJ: Human Fertility and Problems of the Male. White Plains, Author's Press, 1950
13. Freedman R, Takeshita J, Sun TH: Fertility and family planning in Taiwan: a case study of demographic transition. Am J Soc 70:16, 1964
14. Germain A: Status and roles of women as factors in fertility behavior: a policy analysis. Stud Fam Plann 6:192, 1975
15. Goldscheider C: Population, Modernization and Social Structure. Boston, Little, Brown, 1971
16. Gough K: The origin of the family. J Marr Fam 33:760, 1971
17. Hill R, Stycos JM, Back KW: The Family and Population Control. Chapel Hill, University of North Carolina Press, 1959
18. Liu PKC: Differential fertility in Taiwan. In Contributed Papers, Sydney Conference, 1967. International Union for the Scientific Study of Population, p 363
19. Liu WT, Hutchison IW: Conjugal interaction and fertility behavior: some conceptual problems in research. In Tien HY, Bean FD (eds): Comparative Family and Fertility Research. Leiden, The Netherlands, EJ Brill, 1974, p 27
20. Lorimer F: General theory. In Lorimer F (ed): Culture and Human Fertility. Paris, UNESCO, 1954, p 15
21. Mitchell RE: Husband-wife relations and family planning practices in urban Hong Kong. J Marr Fam 34:139, 1972
22. Miro C, Mertens W: Influences affecting fertility in urban and rural Latin America. Milbank Mem Fund Q 46:89, 1968
23. Mosena PW, Stoeckel J: Correlates of a desired family size in a rural area of Bangladesh. Comp Stud 3:207, 1972
24. Munson ML, Bumpass LL: Determinants of cumulative fertility in Upper Volta, West Africa. Working paper 73–76, mimeographed manuscript, Madison, Wisconsin, University of Wisconsin, 1973
25. Musham HV: The fertility of polygamous marriages. Pop Stud 10:3, 1956
26. Nag M: Family type and fertility. In Proceedings, World Population Conference, Vol 2, 1965. New York, United Nations, 1967
27. Nag M: Factors affecting human fertility in nonindustrial societies: a cross-cultural study. New Haven, Yale University Publications in Anthropology, No. 66. New Haven, Reprinted by Human Relations Area Files Press, 1968
28. Nag M: The influence of conjugal behavior, migration and contraception on natality. In Polgar S (ed): Culture and Population: A Collection of Current Studies. Carolina Population Center Monography 9. Cambridge, Schenkman, 1971, p 105
29. Nag M: Marriage and kinship in relation to human fertility. In Nag M (ed): Population and Social Organization. The Hague, Paris, Mouton, 1975, p 11
30. Okaegbu AO: Fertility of women in polygynous unions in rural eastern Nigeria. J Marr Fam 39:397, 1977

31. Pakrasi K, Malaker C: The relationship between family type and fertility. Milbank Mem Fund Q 45:451, 1967

32. Piepmeier KB, Atkins TS: The status of women and fertility. J Biosoc Sci 5:507, 1973

33. Prather OE: Family planning and husband-wife relationships in Turkey. J Marr Fam 38:379, 1976

34. Rainwater L: And the Poor Get Children. Chicago, Quadrangle Books, 1960

35. Rainwater L: Family Design: Marital Sexuality, Family Size and Contraception. Chicago, Aldine, 1965

36. Roberts GW: Emigration from the island of Barbados. Soc Econ Stud 4:245, 1955

37. Roberts GW: Some aspects of mating and fertility in the West Indies. Pop Stud 8:199, 1955

38. Roberts GW, Braithwaite L: Fertility differentials by family type in Trinidad. Ann NY Acad Sci 84:963, 1960

39. Rosen BC, Simmons AB: Industrialization, family and fertility: a structural psychological analysis of the Brazilian case. Demography 8:49, 1971

40. Scanzoni J: Gender roles and the process of fertility control. J Marr Fam 38:677, 1976

41. Scott JW: Sources of social change in community, family and fertility in a Puerto Rican town. Am J Soc 72:520, 1967

42. Sen DK: Some notes on the fertility of Jaunsari women. East Anthrop 10:66, 1956

43. Smith JE, Kunz PR: Polygyny and fertility in nineteenth century America. Pop Stud 30:465, 1976

44. Stoeckel J, Choudhury MA: Differential fertility in a rural area of East Pakistan. Milbank Mem Fund Q 47:189, 1969

45. Stycos JM: Human Fertility in Latin America: Sociological Perspectiveness. Ithaca, Cornell University Press, 1968

46. Stycos JM, Back KW: The Control of Human Fertility in Jamaica. Ithaca, Cornell University Press, 1964

47. Weller RH: The employment of wives, dominance and fertility. J Marr Fam 30:437, 1968

48. Weller RH: The employment of wives, role incompatibility and fertility: a study of lower and middle-class residents of San Juan, Puerto Rico. Milbank Mem Fund Q 46:507, 1968

# 23

# Acceptability of Contraceptive Methods and Services: A Cross-Cultural Perspective

Rochelle N. Shain

Many factors are involved in an individual's decision to use a given contraceptive method or family planning clinic. One of the most important is the compatibility of the method or clinic setting with cultural beliefs, values, and norms. Emphasis is now being placed on research into the cultural acceptability of contraceptive delivery systems and fertility-regulating methods. Its goal is to understand client perceptions of methods and services so as to ultimately modify negative perceptions through education, and to make necessary changes to fit clients' needs. In cross-cultural perspective, the "perfect" contraceptive and delivery system do not, and probably never will, exist. Even if such ideal conditions prevailed, not all individuals at risk could be recruited, because of competing high fertility goals. Nonetheless, research on acceptability is of great value in maximizing the effective use of currently available techniques and in developing the most culturally acceptable contraceptive innovations.

Despite the long-standing tradition of market research in the development and/or promotion of consumer products, similar studies of the acceptability of contraceptive programs and methods are a relatively recent phenomenon. The impetus for such work emerged with the establishment of the World Health Orga-

nization (WHO) Task Force on the Acceptability of Fertility Regulating Methods in 1973/1974. This organization was mandated to undertake social-science research to gain fundamental understanding of existing and potential contraceptive methods from the perspective of client populations, in order to provide guidance to biomedical scientists engaged in developing new methods and improving existing ones (22, 50, 51). In 1978, task force activities were broadened to include the psychosocial aspects of family planning behavior, including motivation to plan births (51). Because the new projects are in incipient stages of development and the focus of this chapter is contraceptive and service acceptability, discussion of WHO activities is limited to the task force's initial role.

To date, there is not an abundance of "hard data" on method or service acceptability, either from WHO-sponsored studies or from other sources. Consequently, this chapter focuses upon 1) the conceptual and methodological framework of WHO studies, 2) current research conducted or coordinated by WHO, with available findings, and 3) the results of other investigations which are relevant to the acceptability of contraceptive methods or modes of service delivery from a cross-cultural perspective.

## STUDIES SPONSORED BY THE WORLD HEALTH ORGANIZATION

### CONCEPTUAL AND METHODOLOGICAL FRAMEWORK

The WHO Task Force conceives of each fertility-regulating method as a cluster of qualities or attributes. Some of the more important attributes concern: gender of user, duration of action, effectiveness, route of administration (oral, injection, or intravaginal insertion), frequency and convenience of use, coitus-relatedness, main action (either abortifacient or contraceptive), mode of action (chemical, mechanical, surgical), and side effects (20, 22, 30). The importance and meaning of each attribute varies among different cultural groups, and what is regarded as desirable in one may be undesirable in another. For example, people in one culture may believe that sterilization increases physical strength by conserving sperm, and in another culture that sterilization decreases strength; individuals in other groups may not conceive of sterilization in either of these terms. In one culture amenorrhea may be accepted as a positive side effect of fertility-regulating methods, because menstrual bleeding imposes social and sexual restrictions on women. In another, amenorrhea may be considered dangerous or unattractive because it is thought to decrease a woman's femininity, lead to hemorrhaging, and/or because menstrual blood is considered impure and needs to be expelled from the body (20, 38–40). The condom, which is usually disliked in many cultures because it is coitus-dependent and is believed to decrease sexual pleasure, appears to have positive features for many Japanese, who consider its placement part of sexual foreplay (21, 24).

The ultimate acceptability of a given method depends on the user's evaluation of *all* of the attributes perceived as important, what has been referred to as the "mix" or balance (21, 30). The mix of attributes perceived as salient depends not only upon cultural factors, but also on the health, motivation to avoid pregnancy, age, and reproductive stage of the user. A woman in her forties who has completed childbearing will probably demand a highly effective method and will be less influenced by attributes of convenience or reversibility. A young, recently married woman who wants to space births may be satisfied

with a less effective method, but will insist on a reversible, convenient, and coitus-independent one (21, 30). In South Korea, the intrauterine device (IUD) and oral contraceptive are associated with serious side effects, but nonetheless rank relatively high in acceptability. Coitus-related methods are not associated with side effects, but are generally considered less reliable, inconvenient, and disruptive to sexual enjoyment. Moreover, if barrier methods are employed, contraceptive use cannot be kept secret from the male's mother, who sleeps in the same room as the couple (11). In sum, individuals are willing to trade disadvantages for advantages, depending upon what is personally perceived as important and culturally valued.

### TYPES OF RESEARCH

The WHO Task Force on acceptability is pursuing three complimentary types of research: field surveys on perceptions of methods and their attributes, studies in conjunction with clinical trials of new methods, and studies of preferences in free-choice situations. Though the three types of research are often used in combination, they will be discussed separately here. They differ with respect to their immediate objectives, advantages, and disadvantages (22, 49, 50).

In field surveys, researchers question knowledgeable sources and users or potential users of contraceptive methods, usually with regard to the acceptability of hypothetical methods and their attributes. This type of research is conducted outside of the clinic setting and thus allows for a representative sampling of the population in question. While this type of data is needed as a guide to future biomedical research, there is some question as to the reliability and validity of responses to descriptions of hypothetical methods (22). Knowledgeable sources are also queried with respect to attitudes and patterns of behavior exhibited by members of their communities. While these opinions may not always accurately reflect the behaviors in question, they do constitute a useful data base from which to construct interview schedules for further study (50).

Before any fertility-regulating agent can be marketed, it, like any other drug or medical device, must pass three sets of clinical trials (Phases I, II, III) so that its effectiveness and safety can be ascertained. During Phase I, studies seek preliminary information on a drug or treatment protocol that has not been previously used in human trials. These are pilot studies, which are not large either in scope or sample size, and are usually limited to a few investigators. During Phase II, studies are more far-reaching in scope than those in Phase I. They are designed to further define the activity of a drug and levels of responsiveness to the agent or treatment. Phase III clinical trials consist of large-scale testing of a drug or device which has already been tested in smaller, more select groups.

During the course of Phase I and II clinical trials, contraceptive methods are also tested for their acceptability. A sample of randomly selected volunteers (usually paid), on whom the new or modified method is tested, are asked to report on the advantages and disadvantages of the method as a whole, and on its various attributes. Although this type of research is based on real, as opposed to hypothetical agents or devices, the small group of volunteers is not normally representative of the population at large. Moreover, because they are closely monitored, their situation certainly does not represent that of a typical clinic patient. The forthcoming data are, nonetheless, very valuable in that they represent the first indicators of acceptability with regard to that particular fertility-regulating method (4, 22).

The third approach involves measuring individual preferences for various existing contraceptives. Clients in family planning clinics are provided with unbiased, standardized information about each method and then are offered a number of fertility-regulating agents from which to choose. After they have made their selection, they are interviewed to determine the reasons for their choice, as well as what they consider to be the salient attributes of all methods offered. This allows researchers to understand which attributes most heavily influence actual preferences, and the type of "contraceptive mix" (e.g., 70 per cent oral contraceptive, 25 per cent IUD, and 5 per cent diaphragm) selected by a given population, independent of preferences exhibited by clinic personnel (22, 50, 51). This type of approach is also being followed with respect to continuation and discontinuation of various methods.

Examples of the three major types of WHO acceptability research are presented in the following section.

## MULTINATIONAL FIELD SURVEYS

The task force is coordinating survey research in the following areas: acceptability of male fertility-regulating methods; patterns and perceptions of menstrual bleeding (these can affect contraceptive preferences); preferences for various routes of administration; and indigenous fertility-regulating methods (49–51).

## MALE METHODS

The study of potential demand for male antifertility agents and the acceptability of the attributes associated with male methods was begun in 1975 in Fiji, India, Iran, the Republic of Korea, Mexico, and the United States. Data for the latter country are not yet available. The first phase of the research consisted of interviewing "knowledgeable sources," including physicians, family planning field workers, and social scientists, regarding the acceptability of male methods to men in their communities. This information was utilized to develop interview schedules, in order to survey potential users during the second phase of the study. Three hundred and fifty men, representing rural areas, and both low and middle socioeconomic strata in urban areas, were interviewed at each site with respect to two existing methods, the condom and vasectomy, and two potential ones, the male daily pill and monthly injections (50).

Considerable willingness to participate in family planning and to use male methods, with the exception of vasectomy, was found. The pill was preferred to the injection in all cases, except among the Iranian rural and lower-class urban sample. Reasons offered in explanation include beliefs that the pill is less painful, more convenient, less embarrassing to obtain, and less prone to induce decreased sexual desire. In general, the two most unacceptable side effects in all countries studied were decreased sexual desire and irreversibility. Increased sexual desire was rated as neutral in acceptability. The most desired contraceptive attribute was self-administration. Approval of a given contraceptive method by one's wife was considered more important than that of close friends, in all countries but Korea. On the basis of this result, WHO researchers concluded that the wife's role should be considered in male-oriented contraceptive programs (50, 51).

### PATTERNS AND PERCEPTIONS OF MENSTRUAL BLEEDING

The study of patterns and perceptions of menstrual bleeding begun in 1975 in ten countries was undertaken to determine what constitutes normal bleeding patterns cross-culturally, and the extent of tolerable deviation from such patterns. This information will be used in the development of contraceptive agents which in some way affect menstrual bleeding. Although this project is not yet completed—analysis of data collected during Phase III is nearly finished—the following tentative results are available from Phase I: in all countries, knowledgeable sources believe that women are more upset by the unexpectedness of changes in vaginal bleeding than by the changes themselves. Experts from countries with liberal abortion policies think women notice a missed period earlier than sources from countries with more stringent policies (49, 50). Furthermore, as a result of interviewing approximately 6000 women (Phase II), many tentative hypotheses have been generated. The more salient of these include the importance of menstrual periods to women, both as an indication of their ability to become pregnant and as assurance that they are not pregnant; the ability of most women to predict relatively well the onset of menstrual periods; the belief that menstrual bleeding removes impure blood; the unacceptability of amenorrhea as a contraceptive side effect, in most developing countries; avoidance of sexual intercourse and other behaviors while menstruating; and misinformation regarding time of ovulation (50). Preliminary findings also indicate that the frequency and length of menstrual episodes are not similarly distributed throughout the world (51).

### ROUTES OF ADMINISTRATION

WHO (49, 50) undertook a pilot study of preferred routes of administration in Indonesia, Korea, Pakistan, the Philippines, and Thailand, in 1976. Its goal was to determine preferences and reasons for preferences among three routes of administration—oral, injection, and intravaginal. This information is intended to help biomedical researchers to develop contraceptive agents whose route of administration will be acceptable to potential users, and to provide information on how individuals perceive the different routes. This insight can

also help family planning workers dispel inaccurate beliefs and fears.

Preliminary results indicate that orally administered contraceptives are preferred by 68 per cent of the sample in the Philippines, and by 54 per cent in both Indonesia and Pakistan. In Korea, preferences are divided relatively equally among the three routes, and results are not yet available from Thailand (49, 50). (Interestingly, data from another WHO-sponsored study in Thailand (50) reveals that with respect to general medical treatment, women prefer injections to heal the sick and pills to strengthen those who are well; further study is being undertaken to determine if these attitudes extend to family planning). The intravaginal route was chosen least frequently in all four countries. Least expected was the relative popularity of the injection, particularly considering the women's lack of experience with that route of administration. In Korea, 34 per cent of the sample selected an antifertility agent administered via injection. Moreover, women in Korea, Pakistan, and Indonesia who had discontinued one or more methods tended to prefer the injection. However, the most significant finding of this research is that route of administration, in and of itself, is not as important as a determinant of contraceptive choice as effectiveness, side effects, and ease of use (49, 50).

### INDIGENOUS ANTIFERTILITY AGENTS

In 1974, WHO began to study the use and acceptability of indigenous antifertility agents. The first step consisted of surveying scientists engaged in this type of fertility research, in order to uncover previously unpublished data. Analysis of this information suggests that many traditional methods act to induce bleeding when menstruation is late (49). Thus, contraceptive methods involving forms of menstrual induction might be particularly acceptable in these communities.

WHO is also funding small-scale projects in this area. For example, preliminary findings from studies in two Egyptian villages indicate that indigenous antifertility methods are primarily contraceptive, rather than abortifacient in nature, and are used to space, rather than to limit, family size. They are accepted by the population because they can be used clandestinely, consist of natural ingredients, do not require clinic visits, do not interfere with lactation, and are not believed to increase menstrual bleeding or spotting, which would be unacceptable because of social and sexual restrictions placed on Muslim women during menstruation (49, 50).

Results from a third study, of Chinese in Malaysia, indicate that traditional methods act as abortifacients and are administered orally in the form of pills and herbal teas. On the basis of these results, the WHO Task Force believes that the most acceptable new method for these people would be an injection or pill which induces menstruation within 2 to 4 weeks of a missed period (50).

## STUDIES IN CONJUNCTION WITH CLINICAL TRIALS

In order to supplement the multinational surveys on the acceptability of hypothetical male infertility agents, WHO initiated acceptability studies of daily pills and monthly injectables in conjunction with clinical trials. (The agents in question involve steroidal suppression of pituitary function by the use of gestagen/androgen combinations). Prospective studies are being conducted in Bangkok and Santiago. Users are interviewed before, during, and after discontinuation of treatment, as well as monthly, to determine any change in sexual functioning. Results are not yet available (23, 49, 50).

Preliminary data from pilot studies in Manila and Alexandria on the acceptability of injectable contraceptives (depot-medroxyprogesterone acetate or norethisterone oenanthate) for women indicate that the most negatively perceived side effect is interference with normal menstrual bleeding. Eighty per cent of respondents at both sites preferred a fertility-regulating method which does not affect duration or amount of menstrual flow; less than 20 per cent of the subjects at each site would use a totally effective method which caused amenorrhea (50).

A study of prostaglandin vaginal suppositories in Stockholm suggests the potential acceptability of this method. Its nonsurgical character was perceived as a major advantage; however, abortion time was long and fraught with anxiety. Moreover, the prostaglandin group ($n=30$) also expected and experienced more pain, nausea, and bleeding than the vacuum-aspiration subjects ($n=30$). Nonetheless, the former still preferred abortion by supposi-

tory to vacuum aspiration, and many would be willing to attempt a self-abortion technique at home without the aid of medical personnel (50).

Investigations are also being conducted on the acceptability of the "paper pill," (see Chap. 6), and medicated vaginal rings (see Chap. 7) (23, 49, 51).

## PREFERENCE IN A FREE-CHOICE SITUATION, AND REASONS FOR DISCONTINUATION

Research on the contraceptive preferences of women was conducted in India, Korea, the Phillipines, and Turkey. Samples consisted of minimally 360 women in each site who had requested a contraceptive method. They were given a choice of the oral contraceptive, the IUD, or an injection, and were followed for 1 year (23, 50). If discontinuation occurred during that time, the subject was interviewed to determine the causes.

Preliminary results indicate an overall preference for the IUD. Interestingly, preferences vary significantly among clinics, even within the same city. In one Indian city, for example, two-thirds of the women in one clinic chose the IUD and only one-quarter selected it in another. A possible explanation is that one of the clinics, although within city limits, is heavily patronized by rural women; the differing preferences may reflect urban-rural variations. Another significant finding is that education, as opposed to age, years of marriage, age of youngest child, or number of living sons, is correlated with preferences. The relationship, however, varies among countries. In the Phillipines and Korea, the more highly educated women chose the IUD as opposed to the pill, whereas the least educated selected the injectable. The reverse pattern occurred in India (23, 51).

Research on discontinuation, both from clinical trials and national family planning programs, is currently being conducted in Bangkok, Santiago, and Mexico City. In Santiago and Bangkok, emphasis is being placed upon determining rates of discontinuation, reasons for discontinuation, and testing of research design and interview schedules. The Mexico City study focuses upon the relationship between short-term contraceptive continuation and anticipated and unanticipated menstrual changes. Husbands' influence on IUD continuation rates are also being investigated in Chile (51). Psychosocial research focussing directly upon providers of family planning services is being developed by the task force at the request of several countries. These studies will explore consumers' perceptions of clinic and nonclinic family planning workers, providers' views of their jobs and their clients, and the "culture of the clinics." (23, 51).

## OTHER RELEVANT STUDIES

### FERTILITY-REGULATING METHODS

#### THE RELATIONSHIP BETWEEN INDIGENOUS BELIEF SYSTEMS AND THE PERCEPTION OF SIDE EFFECTS

Side effects are considered to be the most important attribute affecting acceptance of any fertility-regulating method (13, 40). However, what consitutes a side effect, including its desirability and undesirability, varies cross-culturally, and is often dependent upon indigenous belief systems regarding human physiology and anatomy.

The IUD was unacceptable in the Indian village of Bunkipur because indigenous interpretation of its mechanism of action conflicted with cultural definitions of health. The people of Bunkipur operate within a cognitive system in which their world (food, religion, medical system, and other activities) is divided into "cold" and "hot." In order to maintain a state of well-being, states of cold and hot have to be maintained in relative equilibrium. Villagers believe that the IUD functions by "increasing the heat in a woman's genital region above the threshold at which conception could occur" (20:128). Normally, this would not constitute a physical hazard. However, should the woman contract certain disease states also characterized as "hot," such as smallpox, diarrhea, or a veneral disease, then the additional heat engendered by an IUD would be lethal. Consequently, the IUD was avoided (20).

In different forms, "hot and cold" cognitive systems exist in other cultures as well, where they do not necessarily interfere with IUD acceptance. For example, in a Mexican village, the IUD is interpreted as cold, and the uterus as hot. However, villagers believe that within approximately 3 months after insertion the IUD gradually takes on heat, thus becoming compatible with the uterine environment (38–40).

In Muslim and Orthodox Jewish cultures, menstrual blood is considered impure, and the menstruating woman "unclean." Many restrictions, including the proscription of sexual intercourse, are placed upon females at this time. Consequently, Orthodox women in general found it difficult to use the original low-dose oral contraceptive pills because they tended to cause breakthrough bleeding (8, 47). Moreover, Orthodox women in Ashquelon, Israel, had their IUDs removed five times more frequently than their nonreligious counterparts because they had difficulty coping with the increased bleeding and spotting (1, 47). Muslim women have similar reactions: a 3-month contraceptive injection was unacceptable to them because it increased spotting and irregular bleeding (7, 47).

Decreased sexual desire is frequently perceived as one of the most objectionable of possible contraceptive side effects (50). However, this does not automatically indicate that *increased* sexual desire and activity are desirable side effects. For example, some Indian males believe that vasectomy often results in heightened sexual needs (48). This outcome may be negatively perceived, because Hindus believe that semen is an important source of strength, not to be depleted by a high frequency of sexual intercourse (29). Increased sexual activity has even been offered as a reason for reanastomosis (48).

In order to retain good health while taking strong medication, such as the contraceptive pill, women in an Egyptian village felt it was necessary to consume large amounts of nourishing food, which they could ill afford. This decreased the pill's acceptability. Moreover, they also believed it was important to maintain a normal menstrual flow in order to be relieved of impure blood and its perceived associated symptoms of emotional distress, back pains, and headaches. Because the oral contraceptive decreased menstrual flow, it was associated with these negative conditions. The IUD was not acceptable either because it contributed to increased menstrual bleeding. In this culture, strength is directly related to the amount of blood in one's body; consequently, no one wanted to lose more than the normal amount of menstrual discharge (26).

#### MODES OF INTERVENTION

Response to various side effects is often based upon complex and even contradictory factors.

Once these are understood, it is often possible to find a culturally acceptable, medically effective contraceptive agent, as illustrated by research on indigenous fertility-regulating practices in a Mexican village. Results of this investigation indicate that amenorrhea, other than that which occurs during the postpartum period, is greatly feared. It is frequently believed to cause generalized ill health, hemorrhage, and tumors, and somewhat less frequently cancer, pain, death, and accumulation of blood into a hard mass in the throat, with resultant choking. Fear of hemorrhage, for example, is thought to be related to episodes of severe bleeding caused by spontaneous and induced abortions; fear of choking on blood, to the bloody sputum of tuberculosis, which is known to come from the lungs. Women in this village are so concerned with amenorrhea that they frequently resort to a variety of herbal teas and injectable medications to induce menstruation. Menstrual induction also serves as a test for pregnancy (38–40).

Given these beliefs and practices, any contraceptive agent inducing amenorrhea would probably not be acceptable (38). However, other culturally conditioned health beliefs predisposed villagers toward an injectable contraceptive administered every 3 months, despite possible amenorrhea. These people believe that conception occurs through the union of male and female blood or liquid. The medication contained in oral contraceptives and injectables is believed to act by either weakening the blood of one of the partners, thus preventing conception, or by destroying the joined male and female blood in the uterus. Individuals who believe that the medication weakens blood hesitate to employ oral contraceptives because weak blood is thought to cause ill health. Since the pill must be taken daily, it is believed to act in this capacity constantly, allowing no time for recuperation. A perceived side effect of the oral contraceptive is thus increased susceptibility to illness. On the other hand, because the injectable is administered once every 3 months, women believe there is sufficient time for their blood to regain its strength. These beliefs, along with a desire to curb family size, and effective instruction regarding the harmless effects of possible amenorrhea, account for the success of the injectable (39, 40).

This example also illustrates that fear of side effects can sometimes be mitigated when users are told exactly what changes to expect and the degree of their severity. It is, in fact, believed that one factor responsible for the nonacceptance of the IUD in India is that users were not adequately forewarned of side effects (30).

Sometimes indigenous anatomical beliefs must be understood so as to correct basic misconceptions about side effects. For example, Polgar was able to explain the refusal of some American women to use the diaphragm through the use of body-drawing techniques. The pictures which women drew of their reproductive areas generally depicted the vagina as being directly joined to the uterus, without a cervix. These women, because of their anatomical beliefs, feared that the diaphragm would get lost inside their uterus (10).

Similar anatomical misconceptions have been noted among women in Mexico and the Dominican Republic, who feared that the IUD would get lost, appear in various openings in their bodies, cause them to interlock with their mates during intercourse, etc. (28, 39, 40). Clinical personnel tried to allay these fears by illustrating the female reproductive system on a chart and assuring patients that an IUD could not move to another part of the body (28).

## ATTITUDES TOWARD OTHER CONTRACEPTIVE ATTRIBUTES

The ways in which attitudes toward contraceptive attributes other than side effects affect acceptance have not been considered at great length in the literature. One such attribute is the gender of the user. Male methods, such as the condom, and coitus interruptus, predominate in Europe, and the condom still is the most common method used in Japan (6). On the other hand, whereas male contraceptive methods are available in many parts of Latin America, they are not at all popular. Latin American women who were interviewed attribute the lack of acceptance of male methods to machismo and/or the belief that contraception is the woman's responsibility; however, additional research is needed to verify whether the women's perceptions are correct, and to determine the extent of male disapproval stemming from normative sex-role expectations as compared to other reasons for objection (13, 38, 40).

Marshall, after his study of cultural practices and beliefs in the Indian village of Bunkipur, suggested a hypothetical method which he felt would be the most acceptable form of contraception: a blue-colored contraceptive substance injected by hypodermic needle into the arms of females at 6-month intervals (20). The antifertility agent was directed to women because they appeared most aware of the health hazards and increased stress involved in having, and raising, large families. Although female control over contraception would concern the male, in that it would allow his wife to have clandestine affairs, this disadvantage was believed to outweigh the alternative, his own fear of impotence if he were the user (20).

The gender of the user may not necessarily involve the person to whom the agent is administered, but, in some cases, may primarily concern the individual within the family who oversees its use or administration. Interestingly, when viewed as women's responsibility, continuation rates for the oral contraceptive were very poor—12 per cent in 6 months—among lower-echelon military personnel in Iran. An alternative approach was attempted in this male-dominated society. Husbands were told to supervise pill-taking because their wives were "forgetful." The strategy worked, and at the end of another 6-month period, the continuation rate was excellent—93 per cent (6, 41).

Route of administration has also been the subject of investigation. In the previously mentioned study of contraceptive acceptability in the Indian village of Bunkipur, the injection was predicted to be the ideal route of administration for a variety of reasons: *1)* potential users had previous positive experience with antibiotics given in this form, *2)* it avoided exposure of one's genitals to medical personnel, and handling of one's own genitalia, *3)* it was coitus-independent, a highly desirable attribute, because of the lack of privacy in this society, *4)* it could be administered anywhere, and thus did not necessitate appearance in a clinic or hospital (inconvenient and threatening), and *5)* it could be administered by either a male or a female (20).

Research with Ecuadorian women also suggests that the injection, although still experimental, is preferred to the pill. Women are suspicious of the pill, dislike having to buy them each month and to take them each day. Injections are preferred because of their positive association with antibiotics administered

by this route, their convenience, and because women believe they work better than other methods (33). Injections are also reported to be preferred by women in Thailand, again because of their positive association with antibiotics (3).

Duration of action is also an important concern in contraceptive acceptability. With respect to the blue injection suggested for Bunkipur, administration every 6 months was considered ideal because it did not require continuous motivation; however, it allowed women who wanted to become pregnant soon again to do so (20).

This attribute appears to play a major role with respect to the acceptability of contraceptive sterilization. Surgical sterilization of both men and women is becoming increasingly popular. Data from the 1975 National Fertility Study indicate that among continuously married white women in the United States, 31.3 per cent of contracepting couples had been sterilized for contraceptive reasons (16.3 per cent opted for female sterilization and 15 per cent for vasectomy), compared to 22 per cent in 1973, 14 per cent in 1970, and 8.8 per cent in 1965 (46). Furthermore, among contracepting couples who want no more children, 43.5 per cent had been surgically sterilized by 1975, compared to 31.9 per cent in 1973, 20 per cent in 1970, and 13.7 per cent in 1965 (46). The oral contraceptive, in contrast, was adopted by only 24.1 per cent of these couples in 1975 (46). It is, however, believed that acceptance rates would be considerably higher in many parts of the world if reversible sterilization were available. Indian physicians feel particularly strongly in this matter (32). The low incidence of sterilization in Korea, 2 per cent, is attributed to its irreversibility (11). Moreover, researchers believe that even in countries such as Puerto Rico, where the rate of female sterilization is relatively high, acceptance would be greater if it were reversible (35). Analysis of preliminary data on the relative acceptability of permanent versus reversible sterilization among nonsterilized obstetrics and gynecology (including family planning) patients in San Antonio supports these beliefs. Twenty-one per cent of the sample reported that they intended to undergo tubal ligation sometime after completing child-bearing. This percentage increased to 57 per cent, in the case of reversible sterilization. The difference, representing an increase of 171 per cent, is statistically significant at $p<0.001$ and suggests a strong potential demand for reversible female sterilization (36). These data are supported by results of a larger study ($n=1074$) which was recently completed (37).

The cosmetic appeal of fertility-regulating methods, and their costs, have less influence on acceptability than other attributes, such as effectiveness, side effects, and route of administration. However, some research has dealt, either directly or indirectly, with these attributes.

Harvey found that a condom's color can affect its cosmetic appeal, and that color preferences vary by culture. Black and pale green are preferred in Sweden, blue and white in Kenya (black is disfavored), and pastels, in Japan (12). This type of information may prove useful in the manufacturing stage of development.

Color may have significance beyond cosmetic appeal, particularly for those cultures which operate within a "hot and cold" cognitive system. Regarding the blue, injectable contraceptive agent suggested as ideal for an Indian village, color was an important consideration. Marshall felt that the injectable should be given a distinct color to distinguish it from other injectable substances, and in order to dispel any fears on the part of villagers that they were being given contraceptives every time they received an injection. He also believed that the color should not be one that is considered particularly "hot" or "cold" Since injections are considered cold, and the substance itself would probably be considered cold, as is the pill, the most acceptable color would be one which conveys warmth (not heat), to balance the cold. Furthermore, the color should not be related to flesh or blood (red, pink, etc.), so as to make it acceptable to vegetarians (20).

The cost of family planning supplies can also play a role in contraceptive usage. If the costs are too high, that is, higher than the perceived cost of another child, individuals are not likely to engage in family planning. On the other hand, many family planning programs charge something, usually a token sum, for services and supplies, so as to enhance their value to the consumer (33). Schedlin observed that 46 per cent of her Mexican sample preferred to pay for contraceptive supplies, believing a product obtained at no cost might not be as effective as those for which some

payment is required, and might even be injurious to their health; only 18 per cent preferred to receive supplies at no charge; the remaining individuals expressed no preference (38).

## SERVICE DELIVERY

### FAMILY PLANNING CLINICS

The various components or attributes of contraceptive delivery systems, such as waiting time, convenience of location, crowding, etc., have various degrees of importance and significance within different groups of users. Because of inadequate data, it is difficult to compare cross-cultural perceptions of service-delivery attributes. Nonetheless, reference will be made to detailed studies of clinic procedures and reasons for discontinuation in various parts of the world to illustrate the types of factors which affect the use of family planning projects.

### WAITING TIME AND TREATMENT BY STAFF

In urban Mexico, Honduras, and Ecuador, clinics are overcrowded and waiting time is long. In Honduras, for example, the average waiting time for a new patient is about 2½ hours. A supply of pills demands a wait of 2 hours. The overall dropout rate for Honduran projects is approximately 40 per cent at the end of 6 months. The primary reason given for discontinuation is contraceptive side effects, but this reason does not account for difference in continuation rates among clinics (19 per cent to 44 per cent). Neither do age, education, and parity, since there is no difference between dropouts and active clients with respect to these characteristics. The researchers attribute dropout differences to the woman's experience at the individual clinics. In this regard, waiting time, poor performance in educating and reaching clientele, and poor treatment by staff are implicated (27).

Program dropout rates in Mexico City are considered high: only 60 per cent of clients remain active at the end of a 12-month period. Pressure of time is the most frequently cited reason (26%) for discontinuation, and in 75 per cent of these cases, waiting time at the clinic is either directly, or indirectly, implicated. Experience of negative side effects is the second most commonly mentioned reason (24%). Eight per cent of the clients also report mistreatment by staff, or failure to receive treatment. Women complain that they were often shamed by being lectured for tardiness in front of other patients, and consequently feared a return visit. Moreover, women sometimes were not served: they had either arrived late for an appointment or had not arrived at the appropriate time during the menstrual cycle, and did not understand why they could not be treated (16).

In order to alleviate some of these problems, particularly long waiting time, Stycos suggests maximizing the efficiency of clinic operations—for example, by assigning nurses some of the paperwork now handled by physicians (44). Physicians have long waits between patients and spend more time in completing forms than in examination and prescription. Data from the International Planned Parenthood Federation studies of family planning clinics in Brazil, Guatemala, Honduras, and Venezuela demonstrate that physicians in these countries see an average of only 1.1, 1.4, 1.0, and 0.9 new patients, respectively, each hour (44). Scrimshaw also suggests that examinations be conducted less frequently than several times a year, and that pills be resupplied every 3 months, as opposed to every month (33). Keller and his coworkers find that overall inefficiency in clinic organization, particularly inflexibility of client routes and staff activities, contribute to long waiting times (18).

Long waiting time does not, however, appear to be a problem among all cultural groups. Although women in Guayaquil, Ecuador, usually gather outside a clinic at 7:30 A.M., enter the clinic at 8:30 A.M., and do not begin seeing staff until as long as 1½ hours later, they do not mention waiting time as a problem (33).

### CONVENIENCE OF CLINIC LOCATION AND HOURS

Convenience of clinic location, either with respect to ease of transportation or proximity to a central gathering place, is important in some societies. In others, women prefer to attend clinics far from hubs of activity, in order to keep their attendance secret. For example, women in Barbados did not attend the clinic set up specifically for their village. They preferred attending a clinic an hour's bus ride away (33).

Clinic hours must also be considered in the success of any given family planning project,

because in some societies women routinely attend to household and other activities during a circumscribed part of the day. For example, a clinic established in a squatter settlement in Ecuador was open only in the morning. This clinic was underused, because women did not have any free time available until after the noon meal (33).

### EMBARRASSMENT

Lack of privacy is a major drawback to the success of public family planning clinics in Ecuador, and apparently in other countries as well. Results of a detailed family planning study in Guayaquil, Ecuador indicate that the combination of women's modest attitudes toward sexuality and the clinic situation, which violated this sense of modesty, was a major stumbling block to clinic use. Sexuality in the lives of Ecuadorian women is highly restrictive. Menstruation is not discussed, immodest dress is prohibited, and nudity even before one's husband causes great embarrassment. This cultural emphasis on modesty makes a gynecologic visit emotionally painful, under the best of circumstances (34).

Unlike visits to private physicians in Guayaquil, procedures in publicly supported family planning clinics exacerbate the patient's discomfort: *1)* women are interviewed by a receptionist within hearing distance of others; *2)* the physician's desk is in the same room as the examining table, and in most cases there are no partitions; *3)* women are asked questions which they find embarrassing and which, in the researcher's opinion, serve no purpose other than deterring their return; *4)* women are asked to remove their pants but to retain their dresses—they are not given a gown, and in most cases, not even a drape for their legs. In some clinics there is no privacy at all, while in others there is a screen, or a bathroom in which to undress (34).

In order to increase clinic attendance, Scrimshaw recommended the following changes: privacy during screening interviews and undressing, the use of drapes, visits every 3 months instead of monthly, and, whenever possible, use of female personnel. All women who were asked preferred female physicians. While the extensive use of women physicians is not possible, nurse midwives could be employed more extensively (27).

Feelings of embarrassment, or preference

for female physicians, have also been reported for India (19, 25), Puerto Rico (43), Honduras (27), and Brazil (15). Female personnel, specifically midwives and nurses, have been successfully inserting IUDs in many countries, such as Chile, the Republic of Korea, Barbados, Columbia, Trinidad, and Turkey (15, 50, 51). The situation in Mexico is less clear, probably because there is information on this topic from more than one source, and issues of female modesty undoubtedly vary by subcultural group, even within the same community. On the one hand, results from a Mexican village study indicate that women prefer female to male physicians, particularly with regard to IUD insertion (38, 40). On the other hand, results of a study of Mexico City family planning clinics suggest the reverse (16). In Mexico City, from 24 per cent to 54 per cent of patients (depending on the clinic) reported being nervous during visits. Nervousness is often interpreted as an indication of discomfort due to modesty (13). Nonetheless, female embarrassment is not construed as an issue here because the physicians in the two clinics with fewest deserters were male, and those in the three clinics with the highest dropout rates were female. Moreover, the highest rates of nervousness were generally reported for the female-run clinics.(16). Conclusions cannot be drawn, however, because of the small number of physicians involved (2 males and 3 females) and because at least two of the females took relatively little interest in their patients (17). The issue is obviously highly complex and requires further research.

## PATIENT EDUCATION

Clinic procedures sometimes cause, or exacerbate, patients' fear of side effects. In Guayaquil family planning clinics, pap smears were being taken during pelvic examinations without the patients' knowledge. Patients with positive results (normally not representing malignancies) were referred to the Cancer Institute. Women consequently associated family planning with cancer (33).

Explanation of the pap test, if done unthinkingly, can lead to similar fears. In Dominican Republic clinics, Mundigo and Stycos were witness to the following description of the pap test:

All of you have to have a Papanicolaou test, a vaginal test. The doctor inserts the speculum and takes a sample of the mucosity of the vagina and cervix. This is sent to Santa Domingo. I tell you this because the person who returns here after 10 days to find out that Santa Domingo reports she has cancer, did not get cancer from the pills or IUD—she already had it (28:45).

Lack of adequate information and explanation, particularly with regard to potential side effects, also contributes to discontinuation. Keller found that Mexican women who reported that they did not obtain information about side effects were more likely to discontinue clinic services than those who were forewarned, particularly if they actually experienced side effects (16).

Patients must be given adequate warning of both expected side effects and possible risks associate with use. Sometimes, however, risks are overemphasized to the point of terrifying clients. Explanations can also prove overtechnical, and scare techniques are sometimes used to ensure proper use of a method. For example, the following statement about the use of birth control pills from a Dominican Republic clinic certainly diminished the enthusiasm of potential contraceptors (28):

You cannot take them in a disorganized manner, or ever stop taking them, or lend them or borrow them because these pills are hormones and every one has a distinct function in the body and if you take them incorrectly, a tremendous lack of control will occur and it will be a long time before it is corrected. Ladies, do not stop taking the pills at any time. If you do stop, it will cause hemorrhaging (28:45).

Issues broader than clinic hours, convenience, and attention to feminine modesty are also being considered. For example, some experts in the field have advocated integrating family planning services within clinics for maternal and child-care, to increase their use (45). Fears, however, have been expressed that this approach may further minimize the impact of family planning programs by hiding them within the framework of larger programs (44).

## NONCLINICAL DISTRIBUTION OF CONTRACEPTIVES

Experiments with nonclinical distribution of contraceptives have been suggested (28, 44) and successfully implemented in many parts of Asia, Latin America, and Africa (2, 5, 9, 14, 15, 31, 50). These attempts have been promulgated, not so much to increase acceptability of service delivery, but so as to make it economically feasible to deliver contraceptive services to all individuals at risk, in all parts of the world.

Forms of community-based or commercial delivery systems vary from contraceptive supermarkets in Bangkok, to door-to-door condom saleswomen in Japan, to household or village distribution of oral contraceptives without prescription in countries such as Thailand, Bangladesh, the Philippines, Pakistan, Antigua, Brazil, and Colombia (2, 5, 9, 14, 42).

For example, a program in Brazil's northeastern state, Rio Grande do Norte, trains paramedical personnel and community leaders to distribute oral contraceptives at no charge to users. Follow-up and eduation are managed by teachers and other persons of stature in the community. Women reporting serious side effects are referred to the nearest health clinic or to one of 25 physicians employed by the private Brazilian family planning association. Women who want a method other than the pill are also referred to a clinic. This program has been deemed successful in bringing effective contraception to previously unreachable clients (5, 15).

Nonclinical distribution of contraceptive agents may prove not only most economical, but also most acceptable to clients. Results of a recent study of a sample of 83 community-based delivery programs in 35 countries indicate that acceptance rates range from 11 per cent to 44 per cent, compared to 6 per cent to 20 per cent for demonstration clinics (9, 31). The openness of community-based delivery conveys societal approval; women interact with their peers, whom they trust and respect; explanatory language is at their level; and problems with clinic hours, inconvenience of location, and feminine modesty are no longer issues. The only major concern is that of medical management of side effects and suitability of method to the health of the user.

## LIMITATIONS OF RESEARCH ON ACCEPTABILITY

When there is no motivation within a society to limit family size, understanding indigenous belief systems and adapting contraceptive agents or services to them may prove fruitless, as illustrated by research in an Egyptian village. An initial investigation indicated that women attributed their nonacceptance of both the oral contraceptive and the IUD to conflicts between perceived side effects and health beliefs.

While the reasons offered for nonacceptance of modern contraceptive methods were culturally valid, further study demonstrated that the primary reason was lack of motivation. Children were the only form of power and social security which women had; consequently, they had no desire to limit family size (see Chap. 21). In this case, even a contraceptive method with no undesirable side effects would not be used (26).

In summary, research is currently being directed toward understanding indigenous perceptions of fertility-regulating methods and of delivery systems and their attributes, so as to increase contraceptive acceptability. This type of endeavor should result in making contraceptive methods and services truly *accessible* to those who would use them, as opposed to being merely available. The practical application of study results are, however, limited by indigenous fertility goals. When there is *no* motivation to curb family size, adapting fertility-regulating methods and delivery systems to clients' belief systems is not expected to increase contraceptive use.

## REFERENCES

1. Bernard RR: IUD performance patterns—A 1970 world view. Int J Gynecol Obstet 8:926, 1970
2. Cuca R, Pierce CS: Experimentation in family planning delivery systems: an overview. Stud Fam Plann 8:302, 1977
3. Cunningham CE: Thai injection doctors. Soc Sci Med 4:1, 1970
4. Davidson AR: The psychological acceptability of contraceptive technology. In Gardner J, Wolff RJ, Gillespie D, Duncan GW (eds): Village and Household Availability of Contraceptives: Southeast Asia, 1976. Seattle, Battelle Memorial Institute, 1976, p 207
5. Davies PJ, Rodrígues W: Community-based distribution of oral contraceptives in Rio Grande Do Norte, Northeastern Brazil. Stud Fam Plan 7:202, 1976
6. Deys CM, Potts M: Factors affecting patient motivation. In Sciarra J, Markland C, Speidel JJ (eds): Control of Male Fertility. Hagerstown, Harper & Row, 1975, p 210
7. El-Mahgoub S, Karim M, Ammar R: Long term use of depot-medroxyprogesterone acetate as a contraceptive. Acta Obstet Gynecol Scand 51:251, 1972
8. Feldman DM: Birth Control in Jewish Law. New York, New York University Press, 1968

9. Foreit JR, Gorosh ME, Gillespie DG, Merritt CG: Community-based and commercial contraceptive distribution: an inventory and appraisal. Population Reports, Series J, No. 19: 1, 1978

10. Grossmith CJ: Body notions, family planning and natality. Unpublished manuscript, Department of Anthropology, University of North Carolina, Chapel Hill, 1972

11. Harding JR, Clement DC: Features affecting acceptability of fertility regulating methods in Korea. Paper presented at the Annual Meeting of the American Anthropological Assocation, Mexico City, 1974

12. Harvey PD: Condoms—A new look. Fam Plann Perspect 4:27, 1972

13. Hass PH: Contraceptive choices for Latin American women. Populi 3:14, 1976

14. Huber SC, Piotrow PT, Pott M, Chir B, Isaacs SL, Ravenholt RT: Contraceptive distribution—Taking supplies to villages and households. Population Reports, Series J, No. 5:69, 1975

15. Issacs SL: Nonphysician distribution of contraception in Latin America and the Caribbean. Fam Plann Perspect 7:158, 1975

16. Keller A: Patient attrition in five Mexico City family planning clinics. In Stycos JM (ed): Clinics, Contraception and Communication. New York, Appleton-Century-Crofts. 1973, p 25

17. Keller, A: Personal communication, 1979

18. Keller A, Villarreal FS, de Rodriguez AR, Correu S: The impact of organization of family planning clinics on waiting time. Studies in Family Planning 6:134, 1975

19. Marshall JF: Topics and networks in intra-village communication. In Polgar S (ed): Culture and Population: A Collection of Current Studies. Carolina Population Center, Monograph 9, Cambridge, Schenkman, 1971

20. Marshall JF: Fertility regulating methods: cultural acceptability for potential adopters. In Duncan G, Hilton EJ, Kraeger P, Lumsdaine AA (eds): Fertility Control Methods: Strategies for Introduction. New York, Academic Press, 1973, p 125

21. Marshall JF: Perceptions and attitudes towards fertility regulating methods and services. Paper prepared for the Economic Commission for Asia and the Far East, Expert Group Meeting on Social and Psychological Aspects of Fertility Behaviour, Bangkok, June 10–19, 1974

22. Marshall JF: Acceptability of fertility regulating methods: designing technology to fit people. Prevent Med 6:65, 1977

23. Marshall JF: Personal communication, 1979

24. Matsumoto YS, Koizumi A, Nohara T: Condom usage in Japan. Stud Fam Plann 3:251, 1972

25. Mencher J: Family planning in Chingleput District, Madras, India. In Polgar S (ed): Culture and Population: A Collection of Current Studies. Carolina Population Center, Mongraph 9, Cambridge, Schenkman, 1971

26. Moray S: Body concepts and health care: illustrations from an Egyptian village. Paper presented at the Annual Meeting of the American Anthropological Association, Houston, 1977

27. Mundigo AI: Honduras revisited: the clinic and its clientele. In Stycos JM (ed): Clinics, Contraception and Communication. New York, Appleton-Century-Crofts, 1973, p 98

28. Mundigo AI, Stycos JM: Information and education in perspective: The Dominican Republic family planning program. In Stycos JM (ed): The Clinic and Information Flow. Lexington, MA, Lexington Books, 1975, p 23

29. Nag M: Sex, culture and human fertility: India and the United States. Curr Anthrop 13:231, 1972

30. Polgar S, Marshall JF: The search for culturally acceptable fertility regulating methods. In Marshall JF, Polgar S (eds): Culture, Natality and Family Planning. Chapel Hill, Carolina Population Center, University of North Carolina, Monograph 21, 1976, p 204

31. Population Reference Bureau: Voluntary sterilizations soar, community-based distribution effectiveness grows. Intercom 6:2, 1978

32. Richart RM, Moderator: Discussion: reversible sterilization. In Richart RM, Prager DJ (eds): Human Sterilization. Springfield, IL, Charles C Thomas, 1972, p 229

33. Scrimshaw SC: Anthropology and population research: application in family planning programs. International Institute for the Study of Human Reproduction, Columbia University, New York, 1972

34. Scrimshaw SC: Women's modesty: one barrier to the use of family planning clinics in Ecuador. In Marshall JF, Polgar S (eds): Culture, Natality and Family Planning. Chapel Hill, Carolina Population Center, University of North Carolina, Monograph 21, 1976, p 167

35. Scrimshaw SC, Pasquariella B: Obstacles to sterilization in one community. Fam Plann Perspect 2:40, 1970

36. Shain RN: Acceptability of reversible versus permanent tubal sterilization: an analysis of preliminary data. Fertil Steril 31:13, 1979

37. Shain RN: Acceptability of reversible versus permanent tubal sterilization: a study of 1074 women. Report to the Rockefeller Foundation, 1979

38. Shedlin MG: Cultural factors relevant to the design and implementation of a community-based family planning program. Center for Population and Family Health, Columbia University, New York, 1975, Mimeo

39. Shedlin MG: Body image and contraceptive acceptability in a Mexican community. Paper presented at the Annual Meeting of the American Anthropological Association, Houston, 1977

40. Shedlin MG, Hollerbach PE: Modern and traditional fertility regulation in a Mexican community: factors in the process of decision making. Working Papers, Center for Policy Studies, Population Council, New York, 1978

41. Siassi I: The psychiatrist's role in family planning. Am J Psychiatry 129:80, 1972

42. Stokes B: Filling family planning gaps. Population Reports, Series J, No. 20:369, 1978

43. Stycos JM: Birth control clinics in crowded Puerto Rico. In Paul B (ed): Health, Culture, and Community. New York, Russell Sage Foundation, 1955, p 189

44. Stycos JM: Latin American family planning in the 1970s. In Stycos JM (ed): Clinics, Contracep-

tion and Communication. New York, Appleton-Century-Crofts, 1973, p 17

45. Taylor HC, Berelson B: Comprehensive family planning based on maternal/child health services: a feasibility study for a world program. Stud Fam Plann 2:22, 1971

46. Westoff CF, Jones EF: Contraception and sterilization in the United States, 1965–1975. Fam Plann Perspect 9:153, 1977

47. Whelan, EM: Attitudes toward menstruation. Stud Fam Plann 6:106, 1975

48. Wolfers H: The incidence of psychological complications after contraceptive sterilization. In Newman SH, Klein ZE (eds): Behavioral-Social Aspects of Contraceptive Sterilization. Lexington, MA, Lexington Books, 1978, p 137

49. World Health Organization (WHO): Special Programme of Research, Development and Research Training in Human Reproduction, Fifth Annual Report, Geneva, 1976

50. WHO: Special Programme of Research, Development and Research Training in Human Reproduction, Sixth Annual Report, Geneva, 1977

51. WHO: Special Programme of Research, Development and Research Training in Human Reproduction, Seventh Annual Report, Geneva, 1978

## ACKNOWLEDGMENTS

Grateful acknowledgment is made to Dr. Paula E. Hollerbach, Dr. John F. Marshall, Dr. Alan Keller, and Michele G. Shedlin for having reviewed this chapter.

# Social

# Science

# Methodology

# V

The more complex a phenomenon, the more difficult it is to design experiments or studies to elucidate it. Human fertility, at any level of analysis, is a complex phenomenon. Chapter 24 introduces three major research methods in the social sciences: the experiment, field research, and the sample survey. An understanding of the methods employed is basic to interpretation of research results. Methodological sources of variability—i.e., variability due to the method employed, have no doubt contributed to the contradictory interpretations of human reproductive behavior that are evident from comparing research results.

"If experimentation is the Queen of the Sciences, surely statistical methods must be regarded as the Guardian of the Royal Virtue" (M. Tribus). Chapter 25 introduces statistical terminology, notation, and description of variables measured at the nominal, ordinal, interval, or ratio level. Chapter 26 is concerned with two types of problems: estimation of population parameters, and hypothesis testing. These topics of statistical inference not only provide tools which formalize and standardize procedures of data interpretation, but are also essential for experimental design. Chapter 27 details two predictive and/or descriptive statistical methods: regression and trend analyses. The examples in Chapters 26 and 27 are based on data sets presented in Chapter 25.

# 24

# Methods and Problems of Measurement in Social Science Research on Fertility

## Sue Keir Hoppe

The purpose of this chapter is to introduce the reader to methods of social science research, and particular problems of measurement in studies of fertility and family planning. Three major research methods are described: the experiment, field research, and the sample survey. Their relative strengths and weaknesses are examined, as are the research topics to which they are appropriate. Examples of the use of each method are included, to reinforce an understanding of them and to convey the basic perspective of the social scientist who engages in fertility research.

Two caveats are in order. First, this chapter will be of relatively less interest to the veteran social scientist than to the beginning investigator, or to the biomedical scientist who wishes to expand his or her interest in fertility control into the area of social-science inquiry. Second, though "methodology" has come to refer not simply to techniques of data collection and analysis but to issues of problem selection and data interpretation as well, it is impossible in a chapter of this nature to comprehensively describe all of the methods of social science research and outline the various phases of each. The task of problem definition, the relationship between theory and research, and the issue of hypothesis formulation are not considered here, though they are important. Rather, the focus will be on three methods which play major roles in current efforts to understand reproductive behavior.

## THE EXPERIMENT

The experiment, which is frequently regarded as a model of the scientific method, is especially appropriate for social-science research which involves limited and well-defined concepts and hypotheses, and which is intended to explain, rather than to describe. Though many social scientists have tended to think of experiments as being conducted primarily in laboratories, the experimental method has been widely used in the study of fertility and family planning. This may be due to the fact that such research often involves collaboration with biomedical scientists, for whom the experiment is the most basic method of observation.

## THE CLASSICAL EXPERIMENT

Experiments involve taking action and observing the consequences of that action. In "classical" experimental design, the effects of an independent variable on a dependent variable are examined, using experimental and control groups. Typically, subjects in each group are measured in terms of the dependent variable under study; the experimental group is then exposed to a stimulus representing the independent variable; finally, both groups are remeasured in terms of the dependent variable. Differences between the two groups are attributed to the effect of the independent variable. (Controlling the variables in experiments in natural social settings presents special problems, however, as will be discussed under the "quasi-experiment.") Variations in the basic experimental design include increasing the number of variables and groups; increasing or decreasing the number of measurements of the dependent variable; and use of a "double-blind." The double-blind experiment is particularly useful in medical, and medically related, research because of the well-known "placebo effect," or the tendency of a patient to respond favorably to suggestion, apart from any specific effects of a drug or treatment. Since investigators are subject to the same tendency (i.e., they are more likely to think that they observe improvement in patients receiving a drug than in those receiving placebo), neither subjects nor investigators in a double-blind experiment know which is the experimental group and which is the control. It is understandable that not many double-blind (or placebo) studies have been conducted in the area of family planning, but there have been a few. Bakke (2), for example, reported a double-blind crossover study of oral contraceptives.

To assure external validity, or generalizability of findings, the comparability of experimental and control groups is critical, and is usually accomplished by random assignment, or by careful matching on the basis of relevant characteristics. In some cases, the assignment of subjects to experimental and control groups may be delayed until after initial measurement of the dependent variable (1). For example, a questionnaire might be administered to a particular group to determine level of acceptance of a particular method of contraception; then, experimental and control groups would be matched to assure similar levels of acceptability. Acceptability studies are usually conducted in conjunction with clinical trials, and involve a randomly selected sample of volunteers from the trials, as well as one or more control groups from the same clinic population, using a different method of contraception. All are interviewed regarding issues of acceptability before treatment, during treatment, and, if appropriate after discontinuation, during the first 12 to 18 months of their participation in the trial. Results of such studies, almost twenty of which have been sponsored by the World Health Organization in various countries, emphasize that careful consideration should

be given to identification of appropriately matched samples. For example, trial and control groups should have the same distribution of women who are using contraception to space births and those using it to permanently prevent pregnancy, since the latter appear more inclined to accept inconveniences and side effects of the methods (49:197 ff.).

## THE QUASI-EXPERIMENT

In natural social settings, conformity to classical experimental design is rare, because full experimental control is lacking; research in these settings is more accurately termed "quasi-experimental" (8). During a family planning experiment, for example, changes in the dependent variable can occur as a result of one or more extraneous factors not designed by the researchers: simple awareness of subjects that an experiment is taking place; the effect on subjects of a "pretest," to obtain baseline data; a change in socioeconomic factors or marital status of subjects during the experiment. Such factors jeopardize the *internal validity* of the experiment, or the certainty of concluding that the effect of the independent variable accounts for a change in the dependent variable. Campbell and Stanley (8) outline additional variables which may confound the effect of an independent variable and reduce internal validity:

*(1) Maturation,* or biological and psychological processes which systematically vary in subjects with time, independent of specific external events (e.g., fatigue, boredom, etc.).

*(2) Changes in observers or interviewers* due to learning or fatigue. If clinic flow is being studied, for example, an observer may be more skillful, or more blasé, the second time he or she observes. If clients are being interviewed, an interviewer's increasing familiarity with the questionnaire on succeeding occasions may produce changes.

*(3) Regression toward the mean,* or the imperfect test-retest correlation for groups selected on the basis of extreme scores. This result is not due to the effect of the independent variable or to test-retest practice, but to characteristics of the subject, or of the test, which encourage random response about a subject's long-term true mean. Thus, selection of a group of women for an experimental treatment based on a single test of desired family size will include some who randomly gave very low estimates (e.g., because of a recent argument with

their spouse) and some who randomly gave very high estimates at that time (e.g., because of recent contact with a cute baby). Retest of the former would probably yield a higher estimate; retest of the latter, a lower estimate, or one which regresses toward the true mean. Without random assignment to comparison groups, any change in a group selected because of its extremity may be mistakenly attributed to the effect of the independent variable.

(*4*) Bias resulting from *nonrandom selection* of respondents for the comparison groups; and

(*5*) *Experimental mortality,* or differential attrition of subjects from the comparison groups.

These validity criteria are mentioned to increase investigators' awareness of "residual imperfections" in social-science experiments that can suggest "competing interpretations" of data. As Campbell and Stanley (8) note, the "average student or potential researcher" reading the list "probably ends up with more things to worry about in designing an experiment than he had in mind to begin with." The list is not, however, intended to create a "feeling of hopelessness with regard to achieving experimental control [that] leads to the abandonment of such efforts." During the past two decades, experiments have been used extensively to determine effective ways of providing family planning services in developing countries. Cuca and Pierce (11) have summarized and evaluated these efforts. Although only 12 of the 96 experiments which they review can be considered "true experiments," they conclude that the method is generally valid and has had a "significant impact on the development of family planning delivery systems" (11). Experiments should be conducted with appropriate caution, recognition of their limitations, and with maximum efforts to consider the complexity of the social environment within which they take place. Whereas experiments do pose some unique problems, they are not too unwieldy to be useful. However, their results, like virtually all social-scientific findings, must be viewed with a certain amount of tentativeness.

## EVALUATION RESEARCH AND CONTROLLED STUDIES

As noted in Chapter 11, a family planning program may be organized and implemented like an experiment, permitting evaluation of

the program's effects, just as those of an experimental stimulus or independent variable would be assessed. Evaluation may be undertaken in a number of ways: fertility patterns or the use of various methods of contraception by clients, before, and after, a program is established may be examined; fertility patterns of individuals participating in the program may be compared with those who are not. In these instances, the evaluation is a "natural experiment," in that the investigator, once program goals have been specified, manipulates nothing, but merely observes. In other cases, more controlled experiments are executed. According to Cuca and Pierce (11:304–305), the latter generally test one or more specific aspects of the delivery system. The largest number of these have sought to determine the type of personnel that should be used to deliver family planning services and to motivate and recruit acceptors. In studies of postpartum sterilization by nurses, for example, women seeking a tubal ligation are randomly allocated to either a nurse or a physician for the procedure. Details of the operation are recorded, and follow-up is made at 5 days, and again at 6 weeks after the operation by an independent obstetrician-gynecologist who does not know which category of staff performed the original procedure (49:113 ff.). Experiments have also been used to study the effectiveness of mass media, integration of family planning with other services, intensive campaigns, monetary incentives, and various distribution schemes, in increasing the acceptance and practice of contraception (11:304).

A study by Stycos and Back (42) of the impact of three educational techniques on the fertility behavior and attitudes of Jamaican women in rural and metropolitan areas illustrates use of the experimental method outside clinic settings. The techniques included distribution of pamphlets, group discussion, and individual case visits. Each of these methods was used in one of three experimental groups, and a combination of all three techniques was used in a fourth group. A "preexperimental" interview was administered, and "postexperimental" interviews were given at 6 weeks, 8 months, and 3 years after exposure to a technique. Two kinds of control groups were used: one was similar to the experimental groups in every respect except that members were not exposed to an educational technique; a second received no preexperimental interview, but was exposed to an educational technique and postexperimental interviews. The purpose of the latter was to assess whether the preexperimental interview, "by the very nature of the questions asked, might have influenced the respondents in the direction of fertility control, or ... might have made them more receptive to the educational program" (42:194).

Assignment to experimental and control groups was made on the basis of geographic sampling areas, rather than by randomization or matching, because the "impact of each program on the whole community was considerable, and the Jamaican women were likely to discuss the program with each other" (42:192). Entire areas were assigned a specific technique, and within an area, all respondents who qualified (i.e., those with at least one pregnancy in the preceding 5 years, currently "mated," and not using contraception) were included. Problems encountered in carrying out the sampling design were significant, though Stycos and Back (42:207) note that "differences introduced by sampling are less serious than those by differential response after sampling has been completed; the loss of some of the selected respondents is certainly not random." Attrition, and related problems of nonresponse and refusal, will be addressed later.

## FIELD RESEARCH

Field research refers to methods used by social scientists who attempt to observe social phenomena in their natural settings. This approach includes methods of research sometimes referred to as "case studies" or participant observation. As Lazarsfeld (23:xi–xiii) notes, the methodology of field research is still very little developed, and we are often informed most by "careful scrutiny of successful work," and by experience. Early anthropological accounts of reproductive beliefs and customs and of the roles of men and women in various societies, such as Malinowski's *The Sexual Life of Savages* (25) and Mead's *Sex and Temperament in Three Primitive Societies* (30), are useful guides. More recent models of field research in fertility are described below.

## OBSERVATION AND CLASSIFICATION

Field methods are primarily qualitative, though it is sometimes possible to quantify observations; they involve going directly to a phenomenon and observing it as completely as possible over a period of time. This is accomplished in several ways (17:30–39): first, an investigator may participate in what is being studied, either as a genuine participant or by pretending to be one. This mode of observation, the latter of which is increasingly being questioned on ethical grounds, is thought to increase validity, since respondents are presumably more likely to be "natural" and candid if they do not know they are being studied. Second, an investigator may identify him- or herself as such, participating to various degrees in what is being studied.

Observations are generally recorded in a "field journal," which basically consists of a detailed, yet concise, chronological description of events, and an investigator's interpretation. Data collection and analysis are, thus, "interwoven processes in field research" (1:217), permitting greater flexibility than is typical of other research methods:

> The field researcher seldom approaches his task with precisely defined hypotheses to be tested. More typically, he attempts to make sense out of an ongoing process that cannot be predicted in advance—making initial observations, developing tentative general conclusions that suggest particular types of further observations, making those observations and thereby revising his conclusions, and so forth (1:195).

## USES AND LIMITATIONS OF FIELD RESEARCH

Because they are especially appropriate for studying "subtle nuances of attitudes and behavior, and for examining social processes over time" (1:219–220), field methods have been effectively used in fertility studies. Marshall (26), for example, lived for a year with the 570 residents of Bunkipur, India, before, during, and after their first exposure to a family planning program. When he arrived in the village, all of the adults had some knowledge of modern contraceptives; yet, the program which was established "had no immediate success in convincing a single villager to try a new contraceptive method" (27:125). Through the use of field research, Marshall provided an understanding that probably would not have been forthcoming had he conducted an experiment or a sample survey: the residents of Bunkipur were not "stupid intractable peasants refusing [contraceptive] innovations for irrational reasons." Rather, their decisions were "well-reasoned analyses of the perceived advantages and disadvantages of various techniques" (26:131). The depth of understanding gained by methods of field research is considered their chief advantage. Further, as Scrimshaw's (37) study of *pudor* (womanly modesty) as a barrier to family planning in Ecuador illustrates, the sensitivity, often circumspection, with which fertility-related issues must be raised in many contexts makes a flexible, unstructured approach to respondents desirable.

Field research has a number of weaknesses as well. There are two major types of possible error in data gathering: first, the investigators may affect what is being studied through their presence or participation in the process; second, the investigators' viewpoint may be biased, that is, they may fail to perceive facts correctly, or may perceive them selectively, "unconsciously observing only what they *expect* to find" (1:200). Some field researchers avoid such preparation as reviewing the relevant literature prior to data collecting, to reduce the risk of selective perception, but there is no precise guideline in this regard. Other weaknesses of field research relate to issues of intersubjectivity, or the extent to which different investigators studying the same phenomenon arrive at the same conclusions, and lack of generalizability, a problem which derives mainly from the fact that probability sampling is not usually possible, and may not be appropriate in such studies. For example, in early studies of primitive tribes, basic demographic information about a population (such as a census or vital statistics registration system) was nonexistent or unreliable. In many developing countries today, this is still a problem, though correction techniques designed to deal with incomplete and erroneous data sources make sampling such populations possible now (19).

With the gradual disappearance of truly primitive, isolated societies, methods of field research have increasingly been adapted to the study of literate populations. In these instances, more quantitative field approaches to the study of social phenomena, which often involve sampling procedures, are employed. Purposive, or "nonprobability" samples are most likely to be used—that is , an investigator samples among possible observations or categories of participants which she or he believes will yield the most comprehensive understanding of the phenomenon under study, based on an "intuitive 'feel' for the subject that comes from extended observation and reflection" (1:203). According to McCall and Simmons (29:64–67), three types of purposive sampling are appropriate to field research:

1. *Quota* samples, or the selection of respondents on the basis of specific characteristics (e.g., age, sex) in the same distribution in which they exist in the population being studied;

2. *Snowball* samples, in which respondents suggest additional individuals for interview or study; and

3. Selection of *deviant cases,* or those that do not conform to a typical pattern.

It is often useful to employ combinations of these sampling techniques. Cohen (10:292), for example, in a study of divorce in Africa, used what he called a "stratified judgmental sample." Local political authorities were asked to supply the names of 25 men and 25 women. The "men were to range across all ages equally, to have been married at least once, and to include eight 'rich' people, eight 'poor' people, and nine who were "not rich, not poor'—in the middle." The women were to be "married to or recently divorced from such men."

Though sampling is increasingly being used in field research, results of these studies are nevertheless regarded as suggestive, rather than definitive. Field research is weak in terms of its descriptive functions, but it serves an important exploratory or theory-generating role, especially when it is used in conjunction with more rigorously controlled research designs. In the area of fertility and family planning, field studies are valuable preliminary steps in the design of experiments and of large-scale, cross-cultural surveys. Smith and Radel (39:265) note that the "more constructive insights in [fertility] have not come from the hundreds of Knowledge-Attitudes-Practice (KAP) studies conducted around the world but from the intensive studies of small populations conducted by anthropologists." Further, the lack of understanding of social determinants of fertility in developing societies creates problems in the formulation of surveys, since it is "difficult to judge which social variables are critical and should be included." Field research often serves the purpose of identifying the relevant questions to be asked.

# SURVEY RESEARCH

Surveys, which typically involve the administration of a questionnaire to a sample of respondents selected from a given population, have been used for three major purposes in fertility research (13:30):

1. To identify social and psychological correlates of fertility;
2. To study fertility expectations and behavior, cross-sectionally and over a period of time, for the purpose of analyzing current fertility and of projecting future fertility; and
3. To provide baseline and change measurements for specific populations in connection with family planning programs.

Some fertility surveys have focused on only one of these objectives; others have been designed to serve more than one purpose. A majority have employed a cross-sectional design, collecting data about a phenomenon at a single point in time. A few longitudinal studies, which permit the analysis of change over the course of time, have been conducted. Longitudinal designs include trend studies in which a population is sampled for study at different points in time (4); cohort studies, in which a specific group, such as all women delivering in 1970, is sampled at several points in time (47); and panel studies, in which data are collected from the same sample over time (35, 36).

As the preceding discussion of field research suggests, survey approaches to the study of fertility—the KAP studies in particular—have often been criticized. An "overly structured" format, it has been asserted (39), makes it difficult to establish rapport with the person being interviewed, takes the form of an interrogation, provides insufficient response alternatives, and makes no allowance for explaining or qualifying an answer. Lazarsfeld (23:xi) notes, however, that critics of survey research "scoff at the use of questionnaires because they do not realize how much analytical thinking goes into the construction of a good instrument." Moreover, it is generally not recognized that many of the conventional techniques of field research have been profitably applied in surveys. For example, field studies have provided guidelines as to the questions to be asked in surveys and insight into such interviewing techniques as gaining rapport and

maintaining neutrality. Furthermore, questionnaires are frequently used in field research, and in experiments.

Survey research is especially appropriate for describing a population too large to observe directly, though surveys can be used for explanatory purposes as well. Collection of survey data requires less time, effort, and cost than the compilation of complete data. This is a substitution which introduces a potential for error, but with a questionnaire, information which might otherwise require hundreds of hours of direct observation can be acquired in a matter of minutes. Even if one could afford to spend a great deal of time observing an individual, it would be impossible, for practical reasons. Few people will subject themselves to sustained scrutiny over a period of time, especially regarding the private aspects of their behavior.

Certainty of results in survey research is achieved through probability sampling, the standardization of questionnaires, and recognition of nonsampling error. Though the survey researcher is confronted with numerous other theoretical and practical issues, the focus here will be on these three important ones.

## SAMPLING

One of the most critical steps in developing a sample survey is the selection of individuals to be interviewed. It is beyond the scope of this chapter, however, to consider in detail the procedures of survey sampling. The reader who contemplates a survey should consult the growing body of literature on sampling and should examine some of the published accounts of survey research. Here, basic sampling procedures are briefly described and the advantages of each are discussed. In addition, the issue of sample size is addressed.

Since the ultimate purpose of survey sampling is to select respondents in such a way that they are representative of the population from which they are drawn, probability samples are used. The basic principle of probability sampling is that every member of a population has an equal chance of being selected; this is achieved by random selection. It has been demonstrated that when probability sampling techniques are properly employed, it is possible to determine, with errors in most instances of only a few percentage points, the characteristics of a population of several million on the basis of interviews with as few as 600 individuals (1:136–138).

## TYPES OF SAMPLES

*Simple random sampling* is the most fundamental technique in probability sampling, though it is seldom used in large-scale survey research. Rather, *systematic sampling,* which involves selection from a total list (the "sampling frame"), at a fixed interval from a randomly chosen starting point, is more commonly employed. The selection of every fifth patient from a clinic log or every seventh house on a street illustrates the process of systematic sampling. The principle advantage of systematic sampling is the convenience with which it can be accomplished; the chief danger is periodicity, or the extent to which the elements in a list are arranged in a cyclical pattern that coincides with the sampling interval (1:155). For example, a systematic sample of houses in an area with the same number of houses on a block might result in only houses on northwest corners being selected. Or, a study of visits to a family planning clinic in Karachi during Ramadan, the month of fasting, when most Moslems remain indoors, might incorrectly conclude that clients are predominantly Christian in religious background. Keeping the sampling frame up to date and maintaining contact with the people in it present serious problems in fertility research. Movement of individuals and formation of households are closely related to marriage, pregnancy, and childbirth, key dependent variables in fertility surveys. For example, in many developing countries, pregnant women return to their mother's home to have a baby, remaining there until a few weeks after the birth. If such women are listed in a sampling frame and then visited several months later for interview, omission of those in the last stages of pregnancy, as well as of those with an infant (who were listed at their mother's home) will result in distortion of data (48).

*Stratified sampling* involves grouping members of a population into relatively homogenous categories prior to selection. It is used to increase representativeness, because it reduces the sampling error, which is an estimate of the probable magnitude of error resulting from reliance on data for only a sample of the total population. Choice of stratification variables is made on the basis of known or presumed correlation with the dependent variable or phenomenon under study. In fertility research, for example, stratification by age, and/or rural or urban residence, is common.

*Cluster sampling* is a more complex technique that is used when a list of all the members of a population does not exist, or is not adequate. A researcher turns instead to more or less permanent groupings, or natural "clusters," into which a population is divided, and which can be conveniently listed. Examples include the members of a church, residents of a city block, and patients in a clinic. A sample of clusters is selected; members of the selected clusters are then listed; finally, the list of members is sampled. Since this type of sampling is carried out in successive stages, it is also called "multistage cluster sampling"; when clusters at any stage consist of geographical units, it is described as "area sampling."

While cluster sampling provides an efficient way to study large populations, it is less representative than previously mentioned sampling procedures. This is due to the fact that members of a cluster are likely to be more homogeneous than the total population; thus, generalizability is reduced. To the extent that it is possible, therefore, the number of clusters selected should be maximized, while the number of members to be sampled within each should be decreased. Babbie (1:160) offers the following rule of thumb: "Aim for the selection of five households per census block." If, for example, a "total of 2,000 households are to be interviewed . . . aim at 400 blocks with five household interviews on each."

## SAMPLE SIZE

Sample size depends on three interrelated factors: *1)* the characteristics of the population which a sample is designed to represent; *2)* the "work to be performed by the sample," especially the number of subclassifications of data to be made; and *3)* cost constraints, which are an important practical issue, but irrelevant to sampling principles (31:389).

In general, the more heterogenous the population under study is judged to be, and the greater the number of subgroups about which generalizations are to be made, the larger the sample necessary to assure representativeness. Though survey samples are seldom, if ever, perfectly representative of the populations from which they are drawn, probability sampling makes it possible to estimate, by computation of the standard error, the probability that findings are the result of sampling error. The latter can include failure to adequately delineate or list the total population and/or failure to achieve randomness in selecting cases from it; the tendency of interviewers to select only certain types of respondents when it is left to their judgment; and self-selection by respondents (refusal, unavailability).

Procedures for estimating the standard error are numerous and vary according to the sample statistic (mean or percentage) and the nature of the sample (large or small, simple or stratified), as will be seen in Chapter 26. It is important to recognize, however, that the standard error is a function of sample size: as sample size increases, standard error decreases. As a general guide, it is useful to know the sample sizes necessary to attain particular degrees of accuracy in estimating a population proportion or mean (31:391). The width of the confidence interval, or the range of values within which the population parameter is estimated to lie, at a given level of confidence is one way of measuring such accuracy. At the 95 per cent level of confidence, a sample proportion or mean would be expected to differ from the population parameter by no more than one-half the width of the confidence interval. If, for example, the width of the confidence interval for a proportion at the 95 per cent level of confidence is 0.1, one-half the width is 0.05; thus, a researcher can be 95 per cent confident that the sample proportion will deviate from the population proportion by no more than 0.05 (see Chap. 26 for further discussion). Using this measure of accuracy, Table 24–1 shows the sample sizes necessary for selected levels of accuracy in the estimation of a population proportion.

The adequacy of a sample also depends upon the details of the analysis. If subclassification is important in a survey, then a sample size must be computed for the smallest subclass. Though it is desirable to determine sample size as precisely as possible, several general rules of thumb exist. Blalock and Blalock (5:286) state that the smallest subclass size can arbitrarily be set at 100. Similarly, Sudman (43:30) feels that a "sample should be large enough so that there are 100 or more units in each category of the major breakdowns and a minimum of 20 to 50 in the minor breakdowns."

## QUESTIONNAIRE DESIGN AND ADMINISTRATION

The success of a sample survey also depends greatly on the construction of the questionnaire or interview schedule. The most obvious considerations in questionnaire design are the wording of questions or "items" and the order in which they are asked, both of which affect the answers given. There are two basic types of questions: open-ended questions elicit an answer in the respondent's own words; closed-ended questions provide a set of exhaustive, mutually exclusive responses from which a respondent selects one. Closed-ended questions are easier to analyze than open-ended ones, but in prestructuring responses, potentially important categories may be overlooked. The use of statements as well as questions to obtain information is also desirable, since the combination makes a questionnaire more interesting. Statements are often used in attitude measurement; the responses of many follow a format developed by Likert, in which respondents indicate whether they "strongly agree," "agree," "are uncertain," "disagree," or

**Table 24–1. Sample Sizes Necessary to Reach Specified Degrees of Precision in the Estimation of a Population Proportion, Selected Assumptions About the Population**

| Population proportion | Maximum error allowable at the 95% level of confidence | | | |
|---|---|---|---|---|
| | 0.10 | 0.05 | 0.02 | 0.01 |
| 0.5 | 96 | 384 | 2400 | 9600 |
| 0.6 or 0.4 | 92 | 368 | 2300 | 9200 |
| 0.7 or 0.3 | 81 | 324 | 2025 | 8100 |
| 0.8 or 0.2 | * | 244 | 1525 | 6100 |
| 0.9 or 0.1 | * | * | 875 | 3500 |

* Sample size too small to justify use of the normal approximation
(Mueller JH, Schuessler KF, Costner HL: Statistical Reasoning in Sociology, 3rd ed., p 411. Copyright © Houghton Mifflin Company, Boston, 1977)

"strongly disagree" with a given statement (33).

Questions should be clearly and unambiguously phrased. While the use of short questions has been traditionally stressed, recent work indicates that longer questions help to facilitate recall, as well as give a respondent more time to think and speak (44:113). Negative terms such as "not" should generally be avoided, since they are often misinterpreted, as should wording that might suggest that there is a "right answer," or one which any self-respecting respondent should give (1:106 ff.). Furthermore, it is important that questions deal with issues with which respondents are reasonably familiar, since individuals tend to answer questions even if they know nothing about the matter.

The order in which questions are asked depends, in part, upon the method used to administer the questionnaire; this is an especially important consideration in fertility research because of the potentially sensitive nature of many questions. In self-administered questionnaires (those in which a respondent reads a question and enters his or her own answers), the "most interesting" questions are usually placed first, though it is not advisable to begin with questions about sexual behavior; requests for "duller demographic data" then follow (1:118). The opposite ordering of questions is usually appropriate in situations where questionnaires are adminstered by an interviewer: the interviewer can begin "quickly gaining rapport" by enumerating members of the household, collecting demographic data about each in a nonthreatening way. Figure 24–1, which shows the initial questions asked in the World Fertility Survey, illustrates this principle. Once rapport has been established, more sensitive attitudes and issues can be explored. An interview that begins with the question, "How often do you and your partner have intercourse?" will quickly end.

Before a questionnaire is used in a survey, it undergoes extensive pretesting to determine whether the questions are understood by the respondents and are asked in a logical and satisfactory order, and whether the answers given by respondents meet the survey objectives. In interview surveys, pretests are usually conducted by members of the investigator's staff and/or by experienced interviewers, who meet to discuss their experiences after interviewing a small, representative group of respondents.

The questionnaire may then be revised and retested.

Self-administered questionnaires are often used for mail surveys and surveys of groups of assembled individuals. Such studies are ordinarily less expensive and more quickly accomplished than interview surveys. Some feel that they are more appropriate than interviews for studies involving sensitive issues, since respondents may be reluctant to report "controversial or deviant attitudes or behavior in a face-to-face interview, but might do so more willingly in response to an anonymous self-administered questionnaire" (1:275). Others (24) doubt that respondents would necessarily be more willing to answer questions about taboo behavior. There is some evidence, however, that respondents are less likely to overreport "desirable" behavior, such as contraceptive use, in a self-administered questionnaire than in an interview. Questionnaires have not been as widely used as interviews in fertility research, partly because of the complicated nature of the information to be obtained and the low levels of literacy in the developing countries. Interviewers are able to observe a respondent's living conditions, manner of interaction, reaction to the survey, etc., aside from merely asking structured questions, and these observations often provide important clues to the phenomenon under study.

In addition, interviews produce fewer incomplete questionnaires, since "respondents may skip questions," and "interviewers are trained not to do this" (1:175). Moreover, response rates are generally higher in interview surveys than in studies involving self-administered questionnaires. Babbie (1:265, 268) feels that a return rate of "50 percent is *adequate* for analysis and reporting" with self-administered questionnaires, "60 percent is *good,*" and "70 percent or more is *very good.*" On the other hand, a response rate below 80 per cent to 85 per cent is generally unacceptable in interview studies. He concedes, however, as do others, that the response rate per se may not be as important a consideration as response bias, or the extent to which only certain types of respondents are interviewed, or return questionnaires.

The importance of training the interviewers, to the success of a sample survey, cannot be overemphasized; it is critical to insure standardization (i.e., that the wording of questions

Now we would like some information about the people who ordinarily live in your household, or are staying with you now.

| NAMES OF USUAL RESIDENTS AND VISITORS | RELATION-SHIP | RESIDENCE | | SEX | AGE | EDUCATION | | MARITAL STATUS: FOR THOSE AGED ___ AND OVER | | | FERTILITY: FOR ALL WOMEN AGED ___ YEARS AND OVER | | | | | | | | | | | FERTILITY RESPON-DENT: | ELIGIBILITY |
| | | | | | | | | | | | NUMBER OF LIVE BIRTHS | | | | | | | PARTICULARS OF HER MOST RECENT LIVE BIRTH | | | | | |
| Please give me the names of the persons who usually live in your household. | What is the relationship of th person to the head of the household? | Does this person usually live here? | Did this person sleep here last night? | Is this person male or female? | How old is the/ she? | Has (he/she) ever been to school? | IF YES: What was the highest level and year of schooling (he/she) completed? | Has (he/she) ever been married? | IF YES: (he/she) now married (M) widowed (W) divorced (D) or separated (S)? | Does she have any children of her own living with her? IF YES: How many sons and how many daughters? | | Does she have any children of her own who do not live with her? IF YES: How many sons and how many daughters? | | Has she ever given birth to a child who later died? IF YES: How many sons and how many daughters have died? | | Just to make sure I have this right, she has had ___ (SUM) births. Is that correct? IF NO: CORRECT RESPON-SES. | In what month and year did her last birth occur? | | Was that a boy or a girl? | Is that child still living? | GIVE LINE NUMBER OF PERSON ANSWER-ING COLUMNS 11 - 21 | TICK ALL WOMEN ELIGIBLE FOR INDIVI-DUAL INTERVIEW |
| | | | | | | | | | | | | | | | | SUM | MONTH | YEAR | B/G | Y/N | | |
| | | Y/N | Y/N | M/F | | Y/N | | Y/N | | S | D | S | D | S | D | | | | | | | |
| (1) | (2) | (3) | (4) | (5) | (6) | (7) | (8) | (9) | (10) | (11) | (12) | (13) | (14) | (15) | (16) | (17) | (18) | (19) | (20) | (21) | (22) | (23) |
| | | | | | | | | | | | | | | | | | | | | | | | 01 |
| | | | | | | | | | | | | | | | | | | | | | | | 02 |
| | | | | | | | | | | | | | | | | | | | | | | | 03 |
| | | | | | | | | | | | | | | | | | | | | | | | 04 |
| | | | | | | | | | | | | | | | | | | | | | | | 05 |
| | | | | | | | | | | | | | | | | | | | | | | | 06 |
| | | | | | | | | | | | | | | | | | | | | | | | 07 |
| | | | | | | | | | | | | | | | | | | | | | | | 08 |
| | | | | | | | | | | | | | | | | | | | | | | | 09 |
| | | | | | | | | | | | | | | | | | | | | | | | 10 |
| | | | | | | | | | | | | | | | | | | | | | | | 11 |
| | | | | | | | | | | | | | | | | | | | | | | | 12 |

Just to make sure I have a complete listing: 1. Are there any other persons, such as small children or infants, that we have not listed?

YES ☐ (ENTER EACH IN TABLE)    NO ☐

2. In addition, are there any other people who may not be members of your family, such as domestic servants, friends or lodgers who usually live here ?

YES ☐ (ENTER EACH IN TABLE)    NO ☐

3. Do you have any guests or visitors temporarily staying with you ?

YES ☐ (ENTER EACH IN TABLE)    NO ☐

IF CONTINUATION SHEET USED, TICK HERE: ☐

is followed exactly, and that similar, if not identical probing questions are used by different interviewers). Interviewers must interpret their task as one of eliciting information as accurately as possible. The fact that interviewers and respondents are strangers makes this a great deal easier, for under these circumstances, individuals are generally willing to divulge information which they would not give to acquaintances, or sometimes even to close friends. However, to create an atmosphere in which a respondent is willing to talk, interviewers must be trained to cultivate a professional and detached manner, at the same time appearing friendly and sympathetic to the views of the respondent. They must learn to feel confortable about asking sensitive questions, a particularly important consideration in fertility research. For example, in a study of Australian families, Caldwell and Ware (6:9) found that:

In spite of some local concern that the subject matter of the enquiry would prove to be so sensitive as to affect results . . . hardly any evidence for this could be detected. . . . The refusal rate for the question on the frequency of sexual intercourse between husband and wife was only 3 per cent, although in 8 per cent of interviews the interviewers felt unable to ask the question.

## NONSAMPLING OR RESPONSE ERROR

Although the use of probability sampling affords a basis for estimating the extent to which survey findings are the result of sampling error, "nonsampling" or "response" error is more difficult to appraise. Nonsampling error is an error made in giving or recording responses, rather than in sampling design. There are two sources of nonsampling error. First, respondents may give inaccurate answers because they are unable to recall information, are evasive or disinclined to tell the truth, or have misunderstood a question. Second, interviewers, though provided with a correct answer, may misunderstand, misinterpret, and wrongly classify the information, or make purely clerical errors in recording it. Since survey findings are dependent on the quality of inverviewing, as discussed in the previous

section, only the first source of error will be discussed here.

Accumulated experience is the best guide for reducing response error. Through many surveys, investigators learn that respondents tend to rationalize children already born, claiming that their births were desired even if they really were not; thus, unwanted fertility is often underestimated, and older women of high parity appear to "want" more children than younger women (21, 35). They learn that the total number of children born to a respondent may also be underestimated, particularly in the case of stillbirths and of children who have died, and that the omission is usually greater among older women and those in the lower socioeconomic strata (45:275). Experience may not solve problems of response error, but they can be anticipated and their magnitude estimated.

## CONCEPTUALIZATION AND OPERATIONALIZATION

Nonsampling error is often rooted in early stages of the research process, in faulty conceptualization, or inadequate specification of the empirical measures of theoretical concepts (operationalization). One of the most nagging issues in fertility research, the lack of correlation between attitudes about ideal or desired family size and actual fertility, illustrates this point. Especially in the developing countries, couples typically have more children than their stated desire. As a result of active research and theorizing in this area, there have been important recent changes in our understanding of this relationship: a need to identify social and social-psychological conditions which thwart fertility intentions has been recognized; and, perhaps more importantly, widely used measures of fertility attitudes and behavior have been questioned.

The failure of questions about ideal and desired family size to accurately predict actual fertility may largely be due to differences in wording among surveys, which has been shown to influence response. As George (16:357) notes, replies to the question, " 'If you were to live your life all over again, how many children would you like to have?' may be influenced by the number of children the re-

---

◀**FIG. 24–1.** Listing of persons in household to identify eligible women, World Fertility Survey. (World Fertility Survey: Basic Documentation: No. 3, Manual on Sample Design. The Hague, International Statistical Institute, 1975, pp. 72–73)

spondent has at present and therefore may not truly reflect the ideal." Further, at least 26 major variations of a question concerning ideal family size have been used (28). Blake (4:159, 162) argues that reliability, or the extent to which a given method of measuring a concept yields the same results on different occasions, is jeopardized when similar or identical questions about ideal family size are not used in different surveys, and that "greater precision is required in formulating the question . . . if its usefulness is to be maximized":

Clearly, any question regarding "ideal" family size which specifies no conditions or points of reference for the respondent to take into account leaves him free to answer in whatever terms seem relevant to him. . . . Is one respondent thinking of an "ideal" number of children who will appear under "ideal" conditions, whereas another is thinking of the best number under the stress of realistic limitations? . . . Are some respondents answering in personal terms and others in terms of some hypothetical "average man"?

Though there are no satisfying answers to such questions, some experimentation with the phrasing of single questions (14, 15), the construction of multiple-item indices and scales (18, 22, 32), and the use of projective tests (38) has been undertaken in an effort to improve the reliability of estimates of ideal and desired family size.

Doubts about the validity of the inquiries concerning family size or the extent to which they reflect the real meaning of ideas they are intended to measure, have been expressed as well. Particularly in developing countries, it has been argued that the concepts themselves make little sense to respondents, and hence the answers they provide have no intrinsic meaning (27, 40). Stycos (41:116) indicates that high proportions of Latin American women who state family-size preferences also admit that they had "never thought about this question before." A major difficulty in survey research is that simply raising a question structures the response; thus, although an individual may never have considered the "question of an ideal number of children, when specifically asked in these terms, a numerical reply can easily be made" (41:118). As the use of KAP surveys has proliferated in developing countries, questions on ideal or desired family size have been routinely incorporated into the interviews. Although 15 questions were used in a survey in Kenya to determine the ideal number of children per

family, it was found that the concept simply did not exist in the "indigenous philosophy": respondents insisted that they did not "waste their time on such useless projections; God (or Fate) does determine the number, and what is ideal for one time is not ideal for another" (39:279).

### EMPIRICAL ESTIMATES OF RESPONSE ERROR

Various internal and external checks can be used to empirically assess the reliability and validity of responses. Internal checks are predicated on the logic that the meaning and quality of a response can be inferred from its relation to some other response (20:151). They are incorporated into the design of a questionnaire and can include questions *1*) which require elaboration of an initial reply (e.g., open-ended questions, supplementary probes), providing a fuller context for interpreting the reply, or *2*) whose connections are not readily apparent to respondents. The former are not generally effective in detecting motivated or deliberate response errors, while the latter more frequently are. A third kind of internal check, a "sleeper," is intended to assess the "general trustworthiness" of a respondent, rather than the accuracy of a given response. In the course of an interview, for example, a respondent might be asked whether she or he has heard or read about a family planning clinic which does not exist. If the reply is "yes," the respondent's credibility is suspect. Fourth, a question can be posed in different ways, at separate points in an interview. For example, respondents sometimes falsify their age in response to the question, "How old are you?" An investigator might thus seek to elicit age twice during an interview, once by asking the usual question, and later by asking for the respondent's birthdate. Related to the fourth type of internal check, but considerably more expensive to employ, is the concept of "repeat reliability," which involves repetition of an item, not within the same interview, but after an interval of time, in a second interview (20:154). The postenumeration quality check (QC), recommended for use with World Fertility Survey projects, illustrates this procedure. It is based on partial repetition of the survey to a subsample of respondents at about a week following the main survey, to assess response reliability or "stability" (48:67 ff.).

A "husband's survey" (HS), which, like the

QC, is administered to a small subsample of households selected in the main World Fertility Survey, is primarily intended to assess congruity between husband's and wife's responses to the same item (since the wives were surveyed first). It plays the role of an external check. Results of such comparisons from the World Fertility Survey are not yet available, and other evidence on agreement between spouses is limited. Though Berelson (3:661) asserts that husbands and wives report similar attitudes about family size, others have demonstrated only low but variable agreement (16, 46). A detailed study of husband-wife agreement in contraceptive use was undertaken in Calcutta in 1956/1957, by Poti, Chakraborti, and Malaker (34). They found that husbands' reports were generally more accurate than those of wives. There was complete agreement in husbands' and wives' initial reports on contraceptive use in only 14 per cent to 22 per cent of the 1018 cases studied. If spouses' reports tallied, as frequently occurred among couples who stated that they had never used contraception, or had used it only since the last pregnancy, the information was taken as correct. In other cases, reconciliation of inconsistencies was attempted by editing or reinterviewing, resulting in agreement in 20 per cent to 76 per cent of the cases. Discrepancies were more frequent among couples in the lower social classes and those with several children. The most striking findings with methodological implications to emerge from the study include tendencies: *1)* by husbands and wives, to underreport the use of combinations of contraceptives; *2)* by wives, to underreport any contraceptive use, especially condoms; and *3)* by husbands, to underreport unplanned or "failure" pregnancies. Response errors among husbands were attributed primarily to problems of recall, whereas wives seemed to feel "too shy to report the use of contraceptives, particularly in large houseolds where it was difficult to hold the interview in privacy" (34:65).

Shyness of respondents, especially females, regarding such topics as sexual behavior, pregnancy, and childbirth is considered one of the most problematic elements in fertility surveys. Smith and Radel (39:271) note that survey results are fairly accurate when the method is used in the "cultural milieu for which it was originally designed." However, when it is "transported to other settings, especially traditional societies," validity of responses is at-tenuated by "unique cultural values and practices" related to fertility behavior. Asking such questions is equal to what Rogers termed "taboo communication." In addition, the culturally acceptable way to approach female respondents in many countries is by explaining to their husbands the kinds of questions to be asked in a survey, and why they are being asked, a convention often ignored by survey researchers. Questions regarding contraceptive practice were simply not asked in a 1959 survey in Santiago, Chile, because it was reasoned that "respondents might regard this as an inquiry of so intimate a nature as to be objectionable" (45:303). However, the extent to which respondents refuse to answer such questions appears to be exaggerated. Reports of significant refusal rates are few, often only on repeated follow-up and reinterview (7:168; 12:12). Especially in the United States, individuals are "more sensitive to answering questions about income than about sexual behavior." The "major barrier in obtaining such information" is the "timidity of the interviewers [and investigators] themselves" (27:98), a shortcoming further evidenced by the narrow context in which most fertility research is conducted, i.e., including only currently married women. A significant proportion of all first pregnancies are conceived outside of marriage. Only those which do not end in abortion or in a woman's becoming a single parent lead to marriage. Therefore conceptual frameworks which in the past have concentrated exclusively on marital fertility are no longer adequate. It should be recognized, however, that in many cultures it is still unacceptable to ask questions about contraceptives of young unmarried women or of those who are not currently married, but have been in the past (48).

Comparison with existing data, such as clinic records or the results of independent surveys on equivalent samples of the same population, constitutes another kind of external check on the accuracy of an interview response. Chen and Murray (9:246 ff.) suggest the use of baptismal records and "sibling-placement" and "peer-matching" techniques as external checks on age data in developing countries where most individuals do not know their exact age and "are not fundamentally interested in knowing" it. Other external checks include: *1)* splitting a sample into two equivalent groups and administering different questionnaires to each, to evaluate the effects of specific wording or order of questions on responses; and *2)* use of interviewers' ratings of respondents as honest, cooperative, etc., or of specific questions as "difficult to understand," "frequently evaded," etc. (20:163 ff.).

Though the focus here has been on sources of error in survey research, the discussion has important implications for experimental and field studies as well. Regardless of the method used, observations of social phenomena cannot be expressed without error. Vagueness in conceptualization, imprecision of operational definition, and limitations of human observers are compounded by the complexity and inconstancy of social behavior. Recognition of these problems does not mean that errors should be accepted. Rather, efforts should be made to identify and reduce them. The habit of critically questioning the accuracy of fertility data must be cultivated. Questions such as, "Are reported family size attitudes reliable?" and, "Do respondents merely state the number of children they have when asked about their family-size preferences, thereby rationalizing their fertility?" must be raised. These are questions which are now only infrequently raised, and less often put to empirical test. The tests will be best accomplished, not in the context of survey research alone, but through the combined use of experiments, field research, and sample surveys.

## REFERENCES

1. Babbie ER: The Practice of Social Research. Belmont, CA, Wadsworth, 1975
2. Bakke JL: A double-blind study of progestin estrogen combination in the management of the menopause. Pac Med Surg 73:200, 1965
3. Berelson B: KAP studies on fertility. In Berelson B (ed): Family Planning and Population Programs: A Review of World Developments. Chicago, University of Chicago Press, 1966, p 655
4. Blake J: Ideal family size among white Americans: a quarter of a century's evidence. Demography 3:154, 1966
5. Blalock HM Jr, Blalock AB: Methodology in Social Research. New York, McGraw-Hill, 1968
6. Caldwell JC, Ware H: The evolution of family planning in Australia. Pop Stud 27:7, 1973
7. Campbell AA: Design and scope of the 1960 study of growth of American families. In Kiser CV (ed): Research in Family Planning. Princeton, Princeton University Press, 1962, p 167
8. Campbell DT, Stanley JC: Experimental and Quasi-Experimental Designs for Research. Chicago, Rand McNally & Co, 1963
9. Chen K, Murray GF: Truths and untruths in village Haiti: an experiment in third world survey research. In Marshall JF, Polgar S (eds): Culture, Natality, and Family Planning. Chapel Hill, Carolina Population Center, 1976, p. 241
10. Cohen R: How to grow feet out of your ears when you land on your head: validity in an African survey. In Marshall JF, Polgar S (eds): Culture, Natality, and Family Planning. Chapel Hill, Carolina Population Center, 1976, p 288
11. Cuca R, Pierce CS: Experimentation in family planning delivery systems: an overview. Stud Fam Plann 8:302, 1977
12. Dandekar K: Family planning studies conducted by the Gokhale Institute of Politics and Economics, Poona. In Kiser CV (ed): Research in Family Planning, Princeton, Princeton University Press, 1962, p 3
13. Fawcett JF: Psychology and Population: Behavioral Research Issues in Fertility and Family Planning. New York, Population Council, 1970
14. Freedman R, Baumert G, Bolte M: Expected family size and family size values in West Germany. Pop Stud 13:136, 1959
15. Freedman R, Hermalin AI, Chang M: Do statements about desired family size predict fertility? The case of Taiwan, 1967–1970. Demography 12:407, 1975
16. George EI: Research on measurement of family-size norms. In Fawcett JT (ed): Psychological Perspectives on Population. New York, Basic Books, 1973, p 354
17. Gold RL: Roles in sociological field observations. In McCall GJ, Simmons JL (eds): Issues in Participant Observation: A Text and Reader. Reading, MA, Addison-Wesley, 1969, p 30
18. Goldberg D, Coombs CH: Some applications of unfolding theory to fertility analysis. In Milbank Memorial Fund (ed): Emerging Techniques in Population Research. New York, Milbank Memorial Fund, 1963, p 105
19. Howell N: Notes on collection and analysis of demographic field data. In Marshall JF, Polgar S (eds): Culture, Natality, and Family Planning. Chapel Hill, Carolina Population Center, 1976, p 221
20. Hyman H: Survey Design and Analysis: Principles, Cases and Procedures. New York, Free Press, 1955
21. Knodel J, Prachuabmoh V: Desired family size in Thailand: are the responses meaningful? Demography 10:619, 1973
22. Koch GG, Abernathy JR, Imrey PB: On a method for studying family size preferences. Demography 12:57, 1975
23. Lazarsfeld PF: Qualitative Analysis: Historical and Critical Essays. Boston, Allyn & Bacon, 1972
24. Locander W, Sudman S, Bradburn N: An investigation of interview method, threat and response distortion. J Am Stat Assoc 71:269, 1976
25. Malinowski B: The Sexual Life of Savages. New York, Harcourt, Brace and World, 1929
26. Marshall JF: Fertility regulating methods: cultural acceptability for potential adopters. In Rogers EM (ed): Fertility Control Methods: Strategies for Introduction. New York, Academic Press, 1973, p 125
27. Mauldin WP: Application of survey techniques to fertility studies. In Sheps MC, Ridley JC (eds):

Public Health and Population Change: Current Research Issues. Pittsburgh, University of Pittsburgh Press, 1965, p 93

28. Mauldin WP, Watson WB, Noe LF: KAP Surveys and Evaluations of Family Planning Programmes. New York, Population Council, 1970
29. McCall GJ, Simmons JL (eds): Issues in Participant Observation: A Text and Reader. Reading, MA, Addison-Wesley, 1969
30. Mead M: Sex and Temperament in Three Primitive Societies. New York, William Morrow, 1935
31. Mueller JH, Schuessler KF, Costner HL: Statistical Reasoning in Sociology, 3rd ed. Boston, Houghton Mifflin, 1977
32. Myers GC, Roberts JM: A technique for measuring preferential family size and composition. Eugen Q 15:164, 1968
33. Oppenheim AN: Questionnaire Design and Attitude Measurement. New York, Basic Books, 1966
34. Poti SJ, Chakraborti B, Malaker CR: Reliability of data relating to contraceptive practices. In Kiser CV (ed): Research in Family Planning. Princeton, Princeton University Press, 1962, p 51
35. Ryder NB, Westoff CF: Reproduction in the United States, 1965. Princeton, Princeton University Press, 1971
36. Ryder NB, Westoff CF: The Contraceptive Revolution. Princeton, Princeton University Press, 1977
37. Scrimshaw SC: Women's modesty: one barrier to the use of family planning clinics in Ecuador. In Marshall JF, Polgar S (eds): Culture, Natality and Family Planning. Chapel Hill, Carolina Population Center, 1976, p 167
38. Simmons A: Projective testing for ideal family size. In Stycos JM (ed): Ideology, Faith, and Family Planning in Latin America. New York, McGraw-Hill, 1971, p 339
39. Smith SE, Radel D: The KAP in Kenya: a critical look at survey methodology. In Marshall JF, Polgar S (eds): Culture, Natality, and Family Planning. Chapel Hill, Carolina Population Center, 1976, p 263
40. Stephan FF: Possibilities and pitfalls in the measurement of attitudes and opinions on family planning. Princeton, Princeton University Press, 1962, p 423
41. Stycos JM: Human Fertility in Latin America: Sociological Perspectives. Ithaca, Cornell University Press, 1968
42. Stycos JM, Back KW: The Control of Human Fertility in Jamaica. Ithaca, Cornell University Press, 1964
43. Sudman S: Applied Sampling. New York, Academic Press, 1976
44. Sudman S: Sample surveys. In Inkeles A, Coleman J, Smelser N (eds): Annual Review of Sociology, Vol. 2. Palo Alto, Annual Reviews, 1976, p 107
45. Tabah L, Samuel R: Preliminary findings of a survey on fertility and attitudes toward family formation in Santiago, Chile. In Kiser CV (ed): Research in Family Planning. Princeton, Princeton University Press, 1962, p 263
46. Westoff CF, Potter JR, Sagi PC, Mishler EG: Family Growth in Metropolitan America. Princeton, Princeton University Press, 1961
47. Whelpton PK, Campbell AA, Patterson JE: Fertility and Family Planning in the United States. Princeton, Princeton University Press, 1966
48. World Fertility Survey: Basic Documentation: No. 3, Manual on Sample Design. The Hague, Netherlands, International Statistical Institute, 1975
49. World Health Organization: Special Programme of Research, Development and Research Training in Human Reproduction, Sixth Annual Report, Geneva, 1977

# 25

# Basic Statistical Concepts and Techniques Useful for Family Planning Research and Management

**Harold D. Dickson**
**Rebecca A. Lane**

Statistics is the study and application of theory and methods of collecting, tabulating, and analyzing numerical data. Family planning administrators and researchers in fertility control utilize statistics for many and varied purposes: administrative data must be reduced and reported in a meaningful fashion; trends must be analyzed, in order to make predictions regarding clinic use or to evaluate effectiveness of services; researchers must design experiments so that results are indicative of more than random variation, and administrators and researchers must be able to critically evaluate the reports of colleagues.

This and the next two chapters present the basic terminology, approach, and methods of statistical description and analysis. The presentation is sufficiently complete to allow computation of basic statistical parameters and of several frequently used statistical tests. Further, the terminology and basic principles presented should enable the reader to pursue more sophisticated procedures in biostatistics or business statistics texts or to effectively communicate with a statistician about particular problems.

## BASIC CONCEPTS

The following questions are frequently posed to statisticians by family planning administrators and researchers:

1. How is a set of data succinctly and meaningfully described?
2. What can be inferred about a larger group from sample data?
3. What size of sample is required?
4. How can the effect of a given treatment or new program be measured?
5. When is it appropriate to use a chi-square calculation, as opposed to an analysis of variance; a one-tailed as opposed to a two-tailed test?
6. How can the independent impact of several variables be determined?
7. How can future family planning clinic activity be predicted from historical data?

This and the following chapters provide answers to these questions. Specific computations and analyses are based on three examples which represent typical data sets faced by either administrators or research scientists.

# EXAMPLES OF DATA SETS

### DATA SET 1: CASE OF THE DEPRESSED CLINIC MANAGER

A family planning clinic manager is concerned about persons who are discontinuing services. Prior to conducting a full-scale study, she or he decides to collect data from a *sample* of females who entered the clinic program during a specific 2-month period 2 years ago. The medical charts are reviewed, and selected variables are coded for each person in the sample; types of information collected include: *1)* status with respect to continuation; *2)* the desired number of children at the time of entry into the program; *3)* score on a family planning knowledge questionnaire administered at time of entry (maximum score of 100 points); *4)* the selected contraceptive method—including the pill, IUD, or foam and condom; *5)* preexisting hypertension, as de-

termined by three repeat blood pressure readings; *6)* age at time of entry, and *7)* parity at time of entry. The *observations* for each patient, or *variates* (individual measurements) for each variable, are coded in numerical form, as indicated in Table 25-1. Each row indicates a separate patient, and each column a different variable. The column headings also describe the number codes used to record patient data.

### DATA SET 2: THE CASE OF THE "HIGH" RABBITS

A researcher has been asked to investigate the possibility that marijuana use acts as a natural method of family planning. The researcher obtained 30 female rabbits, which were matched as closely as possible with respect to age and weight. Six of the rabbits were randomly designated as control subjects and were not subject to the injections. The other rabbits were injected with varying doses of tetra-

**Table 25–1. Data Set for the Case of the Depressed Clinic Manager**

| Patient no. | Group (1 = dropout, 2 = continuing) | Desired no. additional children when beginning program | Score on a family planning knowledge questionnaire | Method (1 = pill, 2 = IUD, 3 = foam and condom) | Has hypertension (1 = yes; 2 = no) | Age at entry | Parity |
|---|---|---|---|---|---|---|---|
| 1 | 1 | 2 | 100 | 1 | 1 | 25 | 1 |
| 2 | 2 | 0 | 50 | 2 | 2 | 30 | 3 |
| 3 | 2 | 1 | 30 | 1 | 1 | 25 | 1 |
| 4 | 1 | 0 | 75 | 3 | 2 | 32 | 2 |
| 5 | 1 | 1 | 55 | 1 | 2 | 27 | 1 |
| 6 | 2 | 1 | 60 | 2 | 2 | 22 | 2 |
| 7 | 2 | 2 | 30 | 2 | 1 | 20 | 0 |
| 8 | 1 | 3 | 25 | 3 | 2 | 18 | 0 |
| 9 | 1 | 1 | 80 | 3 | 2 | 22 | 2 |
| 10 | 2 | 2 | 85 | 1 | 2 | 15 | 0 |
| 11 | 2 | 0 | 100 | 3 | 2 | 31 | 2 |
| 12 | 1 | 0 | 85 | 3 | 1 | 32 | 2 |
| 13 | 1 | 1 | 99 | 1 | 2 | 26 | 1 |
| 14 | 2 | 0 | 85 | 2 | 2 | 27 | 2 |
| 15 | 2 | 0 | 95 | 1 | 2 | 25 | 0 |
| 16 | 1 | 1 | 60 | 1 | 2 | 27 | 1 |
| 17 | 1 | 2 | 50 | 2 | 2 | 21 | 1 |
| 18 | 1 | 1 | 50 | 3 | 1 | 20 | 1 |
| 19 | 2 | 2 | 65 | 3 | 2 | 16 | 1 |
| 20 | 2 | 1 | 75 | 1 | 2 | 25 | 1 |
| 21 | 1 | 0 | 90 | 3 | 2 | 28 | 2 |
| 22 | 2 | 1 | 88 | 1 | 2 | 23 | 2 |
| 23 | 1 | 0 | 76 | 3 | 1 | 29 | 2 |
| 24 | 2 | 2 | 84 | 1 | 2 | 21 | 0 |
| 25 | 1 | 1 | 96 | 1 | 2 | 23 | 1 |
| 26 | 1 | 2 | 91 | 1 | 2 | 20 | 0 |
| 27 | 1 | 0 | 98 | 3 | 2 | 28 | 2 |
| 28 | 2 | 8 | 90 | 1 | 2 | 15 | 0 |
| 29 | 2 | 2 | 81 | 1 | 2 | 22 | 1 |
| 30 | 2 | 1 | 87 | 1 | 2 | 25 | 2 |

**Table 25–2. Data for the Case of the High Rabbits**

| Rabbit no. | Weight (kg.) | Drug dosage (mg./kg.) THC | Peripheral plasma LH concentrations (ng./ml.) Precoital | Postcoital | Occurrence of ovulation | Number of corpora lutea | Number of implantations |
|---|---|---|---|---|---|---|---|
| 1 | 2.9 | 2.5 | <0.5 | 0.5 | No | 0 | 0 |
| 2 | 3.2 | 2.5 | <0.5 | 0.5 | No | 0 | 0 |
| 3 | 3.5 | 2.5 | <0.5 | 0.5 | No | 0 | 0 |
| 4 | 2.8 | 2.5 | <0.5 | 0.5 | No | 0 | 0 |
| 5 | 2.7 | 2.5 | <0.5 | 0.5 | No | 0 | 0 |
| 6 | 3.0 | 2.5 | <0.5 | 0.5 | No | 0 | 0 |
| 7 | 3.0 | 1.25 | <0.5 | 0.5 | No | 0 | 0 |
| 8 | 2.9 | 1.25 | <0.5 | 0.5 | No | 0 | 0 |
| 9 | 2.8 | 1.25 | <0.5 | 0.5 | No | 0 | 0 |
| 10 | 3.6 | 1.25 | <0.5 | 0.5 | No | 0 | 0 |
| 11 | 3.4 | 1.25 | <0.5 | 0.5 | No | 0 | 0 |
| 12 | 3.1 | 1.25 | <0.5 | 38 | Yes | 10 | 10 |
| 13 | 3.8 | 0.612 | <0.5 | 0.5 | No | 0 | 0 |
| 14 | 2.8 | 0.612 | <0.5 | 0.5 | No | 0 | 0 |
| 15 | 2.9 | 0.612 | <0.5 | 0.5 | No | 0 | 0 |
| 16 | 3.0 | 0.612 | <0.5 | 30 | Yes | 10 | 10 |
| 17 | 3.1 | 0.612 | <0.5 | 29 | Yes | 9 | 8 |
| 18 | 2.6 | 0.612 | <0.5 | 42 | Yes | 8 | 7 |
| 19 | 3.9 | 0.306 | <0.5 | 50 | Yes | 9 | 7 |
| 20 | 3.4 | 0.306 | <0.5 | 18 | Yes | 10 | 9 |
| 21 | 3.5 | 0.306 | <0.5 | 29 | Yes | 12 | 10 |
| 22 | 2.8 | 0.306 | <0.5 | 28 | Yes | 13 | 11 |
| 23 | 3.7 | 0.306 | <0.5 | 31 | Yes | 8 | 8 |
| 24 | 2.9 | 0.306 | <0.5 | 28 | Yes | 7 | 7 |
| 25 | 2.6 | Control | <0.5 | 35 | Yes | 9 | 9 |
| 26 | 3.0 | Control | <0.5 | 25 | Yes | 10 | 9 |
| 27 | 2.6 | Control | <0.5 | 23 | Yes | 8 | 6 |
| 28 | 2.9 | Control | <0.5 | 29 | Yes | 9 | 6 |
| 29 | 3.0 | Control | <0.5 | 33 | Yes | 11 | 10 |
| 30 | 3.1 | Control | <0.5 | 17 | Yes | 7 | 6 |

hydrocannabinol (THC), the psychoactive component of marijuana. Blood was drawn from each animal 30 minutes after injection of THC to determine luteinizing-hormone concentrations. One and one-half hours later, natural mating was allowed. Following another 1½ hours, blood was redrawn. Surgery was performed after an additional 18 hours to determine whether ovulation had occurred, and, if so, the number of corpora lutea and implantations. The results of these measurements and counts for each rabbit are presented in Table 25–2. The variables are found in each column, and the observations, or variates for each variable, in the rows.

**DATA SET 3: CASE OF THE CRYSTAL-BALL GAZER**

A budget for a family planning clinic must be prepared on the first of January for each quarter in the next calendar year. This requires accurate forecasting of quarterly activity (number of visits). The clinic manager inspects utilization statistics for the period from January, 1969, through December, 1978, which are found in Table 25–3. From this data an initial forecast is desired.

**MEASUREMENT LEVEL**

The variables in the example data sets contain variates, or observations, which are measured on different kinds of scales. The measurement scale determines the type of computations that can be performed.

Measurement is the process of assigning a value or a score to an observed phenomenon. The measurement process has been classified on the basis of the ordering (ranking) and distance properties of measurement rules (1). A traditional classification identifies four levels of measurement, presented in ascending order of refinement: nominal, ordinal, interval, and ratio (2).

*Nominal* data involves *classification,* the use of categories such as sex and marital status. No assumptions are made about ordering of the

**Table 25–3.  Data Pertaining to the Case of the Crystal-ball Gazer**

| Year | Months | No. visits | Year | Months | No. visits |
|------|--------|-----------|------|--------|-----------|
| 1969 | Jan.–Mar. | 50 | 1974 | Jan.–Mar. | 140 |
| 1969 | Apr.–Jun. | 80 | 1974 | Apr.–Jun. | 160 |
| 1969 | Jul.–Sep. | 70 | 1974 | Jul.–Sep. | 120 |
| 1969 | Oct.–Dec. | 75 | 1974 | Oct.–Dec. | 110 |
| 1970 | Jan.–Mar. | 100 | 1975 | Jan.–Mar. | 120 |
| 1970 | Apr.–Jun. | 110 | 1975 | Apr.–Jun. | 110 |
| 1970 | Jul.–Sep. | 90 | 1975 | Jul.–Sep. | 90 |
| 1970 | Oct.–Dec. | 60 | 1975 | Oct.–Dec. | 80 |
| 1971 | Jan.–Mar. | 60 | 1976 | Jan.–Mar. | 160 |
| 1971 | Apr.–Jun. | 80 | 1976 | Apr.–Jun. | 110 |
| 1971 | Jul.–Sep. | 50 | 1976 | Jul.–Sep. | 90 |
| 1971 | Oct.–Dec. | 70 | 1976 | Oct.–Dec. | 95 |
| 1972 | Jan.–Mar. | 50 | 1977 | Jan.–Mar. | 140 |
| 1972 | Apr.–Jun. | 70 | 1977 | Apr.–Jun. | 170 |
| 1972 | Jul.–Sep. | 70 | 1977 | Jul.–Sep. | 150 |
| 1972 | Oct.–Dec. | 80 | 1977 | Oct.–Dec. | 140 |
| 1973 | Jan.–Mar. | 110 | 1978 | Jan.–Mar. | 170 |
| 1973 | Apr.–Jun. | 130 | 1978 | Apr.–Jun. | 180 |
| 1973 | Jul.–Sep. | 120 | 1978 | Jul.–Sep. | 150 |
| 1973 | Oct.–Dec. | 110 | 1978 | Oct.–Dec. | 120 |

assigned categories or about distances between them. For example, the type of fertility-regulating method utilized by an individual is a nominal variable. Although it may be possible to order the categories according to frequency of use or according to user or method effectiveness, these are different concepts from "type of birth control method," and are not nominal data.

*Ordinal*-level measurement ranks categories of a variable in a meaningful sequence according to some criterion, which may be mathematical but does not have to be. Each category has a relative position in relation to every other category, but distances between them are not measured in equal units. Ranking contraceptive use according to the preference of users for various methods would be ordinal-level measurement. For example, person 1 might rank the pill as the first preference, while person 2 might rank the IUD as the first preference and the pill as the second preference. Then a researcher could report that a certain percentage of those questioned preferred the pill over the IUD, and a certain percentage preferred the IUD over foam and condom—but the researcher should *not* report an *average ranking* for each method and then compare the methods' acceptability.

Variables measured at an *interval* level have *fixed and equal distances* between categories. However, such measurement lacks an inherently determined zero-point. An obvious example would be temperature, measured by the Fahrenheit or the centigrade scale. Zero degrees, in either scale, does not imply total absence of heat. Thus interval-level measurement allows for study of differences, but not of proportionate magnitude: it is not meaningful to say that 90° is twice as hot as 45°. In contrast, measurement which includes an inherently defined zero-point allows proportionate comparisons between data. Such measures are called *ratio* level. For example, (referring to Table 25–2), it is meaningful to say that Rabbit 29 had 1.6 times the implantations of Rabbit 30, since a value of zero is the total absence of implantations.

Measurement level is an important criterion in determining the appropriateness of various statistical methods for a particular data set, since only certain arithmetic operations are permissible between observations at a given level. The arithmetic operations appropriate to each of the four levels of measurement are shown in Table 25–4. However, many statistical tests assume no more than an ordinal level of measurement, and "statistics developed for one level of measurement can always be used with higher-level variables, but not with variables measured at a lower level" (1:5) (with the ordering from low to high being: nominal, ordinal, interval, and ratio).

## DESCRIPTION OF DATA SETS

### NOMINAL AND ORDINAL-LEVEL DATA DESCRIPTION

*Statistical description of nominal- and ordinal-level data includes the number of observations in the data set*

**Table 25–4. Arithmetic Procedures That Are Possible with Various Measurement Scales**

| | Arithmetic procedures | | | |
|---|---|---|---|---|
| Scale | Equal to or not equal to ( =, ≠) | Greater than or less than ( >, < ) | Plus or minus ( +, − ) | Multiply or divide ( ×, ÷ ) |
| Nominal | √ | X | X | X |
| Ordinal | √ | √ | X | X |
| Interval | √ | √ | √ | X |
| Ratio | √ | √ | √ | √ |

Key: √, permissible; X, not permissible

**Table 25–5. Cross-tabulation of Clinic Status by Contraceptive Method**

| | | Method | | | |
|---|---|---|---|---|---|
| | | Pill | IUD | Foam & condom | Row total |
| Status | Drop | 6 0.40 0.40 | 2 0.13 0.33 | 7 0.47 0.78 | 15 0.5 |
| | Continue | 9 0.6 0.6 | 4 0.27 0.67 | 2 0.13 0.22 | 15 0.5 |
| | Column total | 15 0.50 | 6 0.20 | 9 0.30 | 30 |

Key for each cell:
$N$ = frequency
$P1$ = proportion of row total
$P2$ = proportion of column total

*and the proportion of each category in the variable.*

The depressed clinic manager (Data Set 1) could report that the data collected contained 30 females (number of observations or variates) and that 0.5 was the proportion of the group that had discontinued after 2 years. Although it is easier to use percentages, and to say that "50 per cent of the 30 females dropped out," the proportion, or relative frequency, is the statistical concept referred to in statistical methods.

Cross-tabulations of data are also useful in describing relationships among several nominal variables. For example, it could be reported from the clinic-manager data in Table 25–1 that 47 per cent of 15 dropouts used foam and condom, as compared to 13 per cent of 15 continuing patients. This would be shown in a "crosstab table" as illustrated in Table 25–5. In each cell of the "crosstab table," the number of persons fitting the categories indicated to the left and at the top is shown, followed by the portion that number is of the row total and

the proportion that number represents of the column total. For example, 7 persons who were dropouts used foam and condoms. This represents 47 per cent of the 15 dropouts and 78 per cent of the 9 foam and condom users.

## INTERVAL-LEVEL OR RATIO-LEVEL DATA DESCRIPTION

*The distance properties of interval-level and ratio-level measurement allow the entire data set to be summarized in terms of its central tendency and variability.*

### CENTRAL TENDENCY OF A VARIABLE

A set of data can be described in terms of its tendency to agglomerate about a central value. The simplest measure of central tendency is the *mode,* which is the single numerical value of an observation that occurs most frequently. A variable may have several modes. For example, drug dosage in the "high rabbits" has five modes, since the experiment was designed to give an equal number of rabbits one of five varying dosages. Since a variable can have more than a single mode, it is often not a useful description of central tendency.

A more useful measure is the *median*, defined as the value which has an equal number of variates above and below it when the data are arranged in ascending or descending numerical order. As an example, observe the ages for only the women who had discontinued clinic services in Data Set 1 (Table 25-1). In the original data they appear in the following order: 25, 32, 27, 18, 22, 32, 26, 27, 21, 20, 28, 29, 23, 20, 28. Arrayed in ascending order they appear as: 18, 20, 20, 21, 22, 23, 25, 26, 27, 27, 28, 28, 29, 32, 32.

The middle number in this array is 26, because there are seven numbers on each side of it. If there is an even number of observations, the median is the average of the middle two values in the ordered array. The median is especially useful in showing what much of the group is like when a data set includes several extreme values.

The most familiar description of central tendency is the *mean*, or the *average*. It is computed by summing all of the variates for a variable and then dividing the total by the number of variates. As an example of the computation of the mean, the average age for *all* women in the depressed clinic study will be computed. Each woman's age (a single observation from the variable called *age* in Table 25-1) is added. The total of 720 is then divided by 30 women to obtain an average of 24 years. A single very high, or low, value can distort an average so as to misrepresent the characteristics of most participants. Consequently, the median is used as a comparative measure of general location on the scale.

Whereas the mean age for all women in the study was 24 years of age, the mean age for women who *dropped out* is 25.2 years of age. The mean is slightly lower than the median of 26, because the 18-year-old weighs down the average. If a 12-year-old female were added to this group, the new mean would be 24.375, and the median, 25.5. While the average would be lower by a whole year, the median would only drop by half a year.

When the mean is considerably higher or lower than the median, the usual explanation is that one or two observations are causing the distortion, and that most of the individuals are closer to the median. Both the median and the mean should be reported. When the mean is higher than the median, there are a few persons with extremely high ages, but the majority of the group is probably closer to the median. An explanation of these outliers (those with extremely high ages) should be made by doing a short case study of the few with high ages. When the mean is lower than the median, there are one or two persons in the group who are extremely young. A case study should be done to describe these individuals.

## VARIABILITY OF A VARIABLE

When a mean age of 25 years is reported, it is clear that the group does not generally consist of teenagers or senior citizens. However, until the variability of the individual observations is known, very little can be said about the age composition of the group. Examination of Data Set 1 reveals a fairly even spread of ages between 18 and 32. As can be seen in this example, the description of a set of data in terms of central tendency is incomplete. Data not only tend to agglomerate, they tend to disperse. The *range* is a simple measure of dispersion, and is simply the numerical difference between the highest and lowest variates. For example, the range in desired number of additional children in Data Set 1 (Table 25-1) is 8 (a high of 8 minus a low of 0), although the average is only 1.26.

More useful measures of dispersion have been devised which describe the *variability* of the variable, showing how often the variates diverge from the measure of central tendency and the average distances (deviation) of the variates from it. The larger the deviation, the greater the dispersion of the data. However, when the mean is used as the measure of central tendency, the average of deviations from it *always* equals zero, regardless of the dispersion. (The average of deviations is expressed as

$$\left( \frac{[\Sigma (X_i - \bar{X})]}{n} \right)$$

where $\Sigma$ is the statistical notation for "sum of," $X_i$ is a specific variate of a variable $X$, and $\bar{X}$ is the mean.)

A statistical measure of variability that avoids the problem of summing deviation to zero is the variance ($\sigma^2$). The problem is avoided by squaring all deviations prior to summation. The variance is computed in the following steps:

(a) Subtract the mean from each observation;
(b) Square the difference obtained in step (a);
(c) Sum the squared values obtained in step (b);
(d) Divide the sum obtained in step (c) by the number of observations (in case of a *population set* of data) and by the number of observations minus one (in case of a *sample*). Assume for this paragraph that the data is from a population set. (The difference between population data and sample data is discussed in a later paragraph.) The result is called the variance ($\sigma^2$). An example of the computation of the variance is shown in Table 25–6.

The measurement unit of the variance is the *square* of the original variate measurement units. Thus the variance in Table 25–6 is expressed in years squared, rather than in years. For descriptive purposes, it is desirable that the measure of central tendency and the measure of dispersion be expressed in the same measurement units. For this reason, a related measure more commonly reported than the variance is the *standard deviation*. The standard deviation is simply the square root of the variance, and its unit of measurement is the same as that of the mean. Thus the standard devia-

tion in Table 25–6 is the square root of 17.8, or 4.23 years. This, the number 4.23 (years) is an *index* of the average deviations of the variates from the mean of the variable. Later it will be shown that statements can be made about the percentage of variates that fall between the mean plus or minus 2 standard deviations (that is, the mean number of years plus 8.46 years, and the mean minus 8.46 years). It is this kind of statement that makes it desirable to have the standard deviation in the same units of measure as the mean.

A distribution's relative variability may be quickly assessed by dividing the standard deviation by the mean. The ratio is called the *coefficient of variation*. If the result is less than 0.15, the variates are fairly concentrated around the mean of the variable. A value of 0.15 to 0.8 indicates moderate variability, and a value greater than 0.8 indicates extreme variability. When the ratio is greater than 1.2, the mean does not meaningfully represent the group, because there may be as many variates a large distance from the mean as there are close to the mean. A more thorough assessment of variability is discussed later in the chapter (see "Properties of the Normal Curve").

**POPULATIONS AND SAMPLES**

As already mentioned, the choice of computational formula used to measure the variance

**Table 25–6. Computation of Variance of the Ages of Clinic Dropouts from Table 25–1**

| Ages of the dropouts | (a) (Ages− 25.2*) | (b) (Ages− 25.2*)$^2$ |
|---|---|---|
| 25 | −0.2 | 0.04 |
| 32 | 6.8 | 46.24 |
| 27 | 1.8 | 3.24 |
| 18 | −7.2 | 51.84 |
| 22 | −3.2 | 10.24 |
| 32 | 6.8 | 46.24 |
| 26 | 0.8 | 0.64 |
| 27 | 1.8 | 3.24 |
| 21 | −4.2 | 17.64 |
| 20 | −5.2 | 27.04 |
| 28 | 2.8 | 7.84 |
| 29 | 3.8 | 14.44 |
| 23 | −2.2 | 4.84 |
| 20 | −5.2 | 27.04 |
| 28 | 2.8 | 7.84 |
| | (c) SUM = | 268.40 | $\dfrac{\text{SUM}}{N}$ = 17.893 years, squared = Variance |

* 25.2 = mean

depends on whether the data represent a population or a sample of a population. The distinction between data from a population and data from a sample is important, since sample data are used to *infer* quantitative characteristics (parameters) of the population from which they were derived. If a set of data is defined as including all possible variates *to be described,* it is *population* data. A *sample* is a subset of the population, and an estimate of a population parameter such as the population mean, based on a small sample of that population, is called a *statistic.* The determination of whether a particular set of data can be regarded as population data or as a sample depends on its use. For example, the time-series data in Data Set 3 (Case of the Crystal-Ball Gazer) is *population* data, in that the variates, or observations, are the numbers of *all* visits that occurred in the clinic. However, if the data are used for predictive purposes, they are a *sample* of all time, past and future. The data on the number of implantations in the rabbits, presented in Table 25-2, would be considered as a *sample,* because conclusions will probably be generalized to all rabbits.

If a given population were *repeatedly* sampled (although, in application, only one sample is taken), the average of the computed statistics (estimates from the samples) should be equal to the parameter (the true characteristic of the population), which would be found by a computation utilizing all the variates in a population variable. When a discrepancy occurs between the average of the statistics of repeated samples and the parameter, the statistics represent a *biased estimator* of the parameter.

Random sampling experiments have shown that if the variance of a sample were computed as

$$\frac{\sum\limits_{i=1}^{n} (X_i - \overline{X})^2}{n}$$

where $n$ is the sample size and $\overline{X}$ is the *sample* mean, it would be a *biased statistic:* the true variance of the population $(\sigma^2)$ is underestimated. To correct for this bias, $(n - 1)$ is substituted for $n$ in the denominator, as mentioned in step $(d)$ of the variance computation.

Random sampling experiments have shown that the sample mean, computed as

$$\frac{\sum\limits_{i=1}^{n} X_i}{n}$$

where $n$ is the sample size and $\Sigma X_i$ is the sum of the individual observations of the variable called $X$, is an *unbiased* estimator of the true population mean $(\mu)$.

Table 25-7 presents notation used in statistics, and formulas for the mean, variance, and standard deviation.

## GRAPHIC REPRESENTATIONS

In addition to numerical descriptions, a data set can be described by presenting an illustration of its distribution. A variable's distribution can be presented as a graph in which the horizontal axis contains the scale for the variable of interest (such as age, weight, and number of corpora lutea per rabbit) and the vertical axis indicates the frequency with which a particular value or range of values occurs.

An example of grouping data in preparation for graphical display is presented in Table 25-8. The ages are grouped into classes of equal span of years (column 1), and the number of persons within each age range is tallied (column 2). The total number of individuals in each age range is the absolute frequency (column 3). The absolute frequency in each class is divided by the total number of observations to derive the proportion, or relative frequency, in each age class (column 4).

Figure 25-1 presents graphs of the data in Table 25-8. These graphs illustrate the two aspects of a particular kind of graph called a histogram. The first aspect, illustrated in the first graph, is the determination of class boundaries on the $X$-axis (horizontal axis). In a histogram, the width of each bar is bounded by the lowest number in each class. The second graph illustrates that the height of the bar on the $Y$-axis is determined by class midpoints. (This graph is sometimes referred to as a frequency polygon.)

A spatial interpretation of frequency distributions allows visualization of its shape. Note that the relative frequency of any class is directly proportional to the area contained under its section of the histogram (the width of the bar times its height, $Y$). When the shape of a curve is symmetrical—that is, when it can be divided in half, and each side is a mirror image

**Table 25-7. Statistical Notation and Formulas for the Mean, Variance, and Standard Deviation**

## Notation

| | |
|---|---|
| $X_i$ | The individual variate, or observation $i$, for a variable $X$ |
| $N$ | Number in a population |
| $n$ | Number in a sample |
| $\Sigma$ | Greek letter capital sigma; summation |
| $\displaystyle\sum_{i=1}^{n} X_i$ | Sum of the $X$ values from $i = 1$ to $i = n$ |
| $\mu$ | Greek letter mu; mean of a population (a parameter) |
| $\sigma^2$ | Greek letter sigma (lowercase); variance of a population (a parameter) |
| $\bar{X}$ | Read "$X$ bar"; mean of a sample (a statistic) |
| $S^2$ | Variance of a sample (a statistic) |

## Formulas

| | Parameters | Statistics |
|---|---|---|
| Mean | $\mu = \dfrac{\displaystyle\sum_{i=1}^{n} X_i}{N}$ | $\bar{X} = \dfrac{\displaystyle\sum_{i=1}^{n} X_i}{n}$ |
| Variance | $\sigma^2 = \dfrac{\displaystyle\sum_{i=1}^{n} \left(X_i - \mu\right)^2}{N}$ | $S^2 = \dfrac{\displaystyle\sum_{i=1}^{n} \left(X_i - \bar{X}\right)^2}{n-1}$ |
| Standard deviation | $\sigma = \sqrt{\dfrac{\displaystyle\sum_{i=1}^{n} \left(X_i - \mu\right)^2}{N}}$ | $S = \sqrt{\dfrac{\displaystyle\sum_{i=1}^{n} \left(X_i - \bar{X}\right)^2}{n-1}}$ |

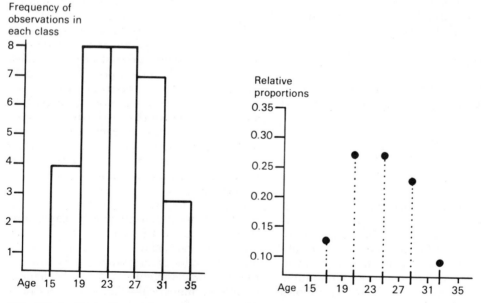

**FIG. 25-1.** Frequency and proportion histogram of ages of family planning patients, based on data in Table 25-9.

**Table 25–8. Distribution of Ages of Females in the Clinic Manager Example of Table 25–1**

| Ages (1) | Tally marks (2) | Frequency (3) | Proportion of the total frequency in the age class (4) |
|----------|-----------------|---------------|--------------------------------------------------------|
| 15–18 | 1111 | 4 | 4/30 = 0.13 |
| 19–22 | ++++ 111 | 8 | 8/30 = 0.27 |
| 23–26 | ++++ 111 | 8 | 8/30 = 0.27 |
| 27–30 | ++++ 11 | 7 | 7/30 = 0.23 |
| 31–34 | 111 | 3 | 3/30 = 0.10 |
| | Total | 30 | |

of the other, it may be, or approximate, a *normal distribution*. In such cases, it is easy to calculate areas under the curve.

## THE NORMAL DISTRIBUTION

The mathematical formula for relating the measurements of a variable ($X$) to the height of the graph ($Y$), or for determining the normal distribution, contains four basic terms: $\mu$, $\sigma$, $X$, and $Y$. The highest point on the graph of the normal distribution, i.e., the normal curve, is at the mean ($\mu$, read on the $X$-axis) as shown in Figure 25–2. In the normal distribution, the mean, median, and mode are equal. The variability of the curve is represented by the standard deviation $\sigma$. Any given point on the $X$-axis can be represented by $X$, that is, the $X$-axis is a *continuous variable*. The definition of a continuous variable and a discussion of the use of the normal distribution are given in the following sections.

## CONTINUOUS AND DISCRETE VARIABLES

Variables are *continuous* if the variates can logically assume any interval of measurement.

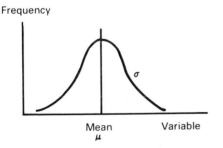

**FIG. 25–2.** General shape of a Standard Normal Distribution of a variable having mean $\mu$ and standard deviation $\sigma$.

In contrast, a variable is termed *discrete* if it can assume only fixed, predetermined values, such as the number of patient visits to a clinic: in this case, variates must be positive integers. Continuous variables are not exact, and their measurement is an approximation. Physical units, such as time and length, are continuous, since the value obtained is determined by the accuracy of measurement. For example, age can be measured by years; by years and months; by years, months, and days; by years, months, days, and hours; etc. The variable *age* can assume any interval of measurement and is therefore continuous.

## PROPERTIES OF THE NORMAL CURVE

The properties of the normal curve make it possible to calculate the proportions of the area lying between the mean and a given variate value by using the standard deviation. The relationship of $\sigma$ to the normal curve is such that

$\mu \pm \sigma$ contains 68.26% of all variates (see Fig. 25–3),

$\mu \pm 2\sigma$ contains 95.44% of all variates, and

$\mu \pm 3\sigma$ contains 99.74% of all variates.

It must be emphasized that these statements apply only to a set of data which is normally distributed. Other rules, which apply to different types of distributions, are discussed later (see the section "Distribution Other Than the Normal"). Areas under the normal curve have been compiled in table form. Since an infinite number of normal curves exist (one for each mean and standard deviation), empirically observed distributions are converted to the *standard normal curve,* in which $\mu = 0$ and $\sigma = 1$. Any normally distributed variate can be transformed to a variate in the standard normal curve by subtracting the mean from the variate and dividing by the standard deviation

$$X_i - \mu.$$

$$\sigma$$

The result is termed the *standard normal deviate,* and is denoted by $Z$. The standard normal deviate is the measure of the distance between a variate $X_i$ and the mean, in terms of the number of standard deviations which the variate is away from the mean.

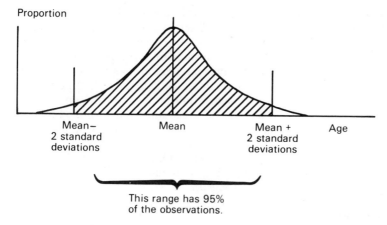

**FIG. 25–3.** Area under a normal curve covered by two standard deviations from the mean.

## USE OF Z-SCORES

Because the area under the standard normal curve has been constructed to sum to *one,* computation of the proportion of observations between any two specified areas is possible. For example, assume that an experimental group of 100 rabbits has a mean weight of 3 kg. and a standard deviation of 0.4 kg. If the weights are normally distributed, it is possible to determine the proportion or percentage of rabbits that weigh more than 3.6 kg. This area is diagrammatically represented as the shaded portion in Fig. 25–4. The following procedure is used to compute the proportion that weigh more than 3.6 kg. (or the probability of a rabbit's weighing more than 3.6 kg.):

*1.* Convert the value of interest to the Z-scale

$$Z = \frac{3.6 - 3.0}{0.4} = \frac{0.6}{0.4} = 1.5$$

This Z means that 3.6 kg. is 1.5 standard deviations above the mean.

*2.* Draw a picture of the distribution, and shade the area of interest as in Figure 25–4.

*3.* Refer to the standard normal table (Appendix 2–1) to determine the shaded proportion, i.e., the area equivalent to 1.5 standard deviations.

Table 25–9 presents a section of the standard normal table. Z-scores to the first decimal point are located on the left; the hundredths decimal of a Z-score is given across the top of the table. Tables vary. Some consider areas between a Z-score of 0 and the specified Z-score; this table indicates the area above the specified Z-score. Computations are similar, once it is recognized that the area above a Z of 0 equals 0.5. In this table, a Z of 0.10 has an area *above it* of 0.4602, while a Z of 0.12 has an area above it of 0.4522. A Z of 1.5 has an area of 0.0668, which is the proportion of the curve occupied by the shaded area in Fig. 25–4. This means that 6.7 per cent of the rabbits weigh more than 3.6 kg. It could also be stated that the probability of a rabbit, in the population

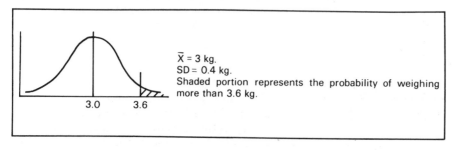

$\bar{X}$ = 3 kg.
SD = 0.4 kg.
Shaded portion represents the probability of weighing more than 3.6 kg.

3.0    3.6

**FIG. 25–4.** Diagrammatic representation of the percentage of a group of rabbits weighing more than 3.6 kg. when the group has a mean weight of 3 kg. and a standard deviation of 0.4 kg.

**Table 25-9. A Portion of the Standard Normal Table Showing the Area above a Selected Z-score**

| Z | 0.00 | 0.01 | 0.02 |
|-----|--------|--------|--------|
| 0.0 | 0.5000 | 0.4960 | 0.4920 |
| 0.1 | 0.4602 | 0.4562 | 0.4522 |
| 1.0 | 0.1587 | 0.1562 | 0.1539 |
| 1.5 | 0.0668 | 0.0655 | 0.0643 |

for which data is available, weighing more than 3.6 kg. would be 0.0668.

Similarly, it is possible to determine the proportion of rabbits that weigh between 3.0 and 3.6 kg. (the unshaded portion to the right of the mean (3.0) in Fig. 25-4). Since the total area under the standard normal curve is 1.0, each half is 0.5. Hence the area (proportion) between the mean and 3.6 kg. is

$$0.5 - 0.0668 = 0.4332$$

To determine an area between two variates, one of which is to the left of the mean and the other to the right, the Z-score of each variate is computed. The area between the two standardized normal deviates is simply 1.0 minus the sum of their respective proportions derived from the standard normal table. Thus it is possible to determine the area (or relative infrequency of the variates) that occurs between any two values of variates from a normally distributed variable if they are transformed to standardized normal deviates.

Using the same example of 100 rabbits with normally distributed weights, with a mean weight of 3.0 kg. and a standard deviation of 0.4 kg., what is the probability of a rabbit which weighs less than 2 kg. being in the group?

The procedure of analysis is as follows:

1. Determine the Z-score.

$$Z = \frac{2 - 3.0}{0.4} = \frac{-1.0}{0.4} = -2.5$$

This indicates that a weight of 2 kg. is 2.5 standard deviations *below* the mean. The negative sign for the Z-score indicates that the weight is below the mean, rather than above it.

2. The picture of the distribution of weights and the shaded area is illustrated in Fig. 25-5.

3. Since the normal distribution is symmetrical, the area above a Z of 2.50 is equivalent to the area below a Z of −2.50; consequently, the Z table (Appendix 2-1) is used to determine the area *greater* than a Z of +2.50. The table indicates that this value is 0.0062, which means that the probability of a weight being less than 2 kg. is very low, 0.0062.

## DISTRIBUTIONS OTHER THAN THE "NORMAL"

A given set of data may not be bell-shaped and normally distributed, but may instead be skewed to one side, or all class frequencies may be of uniform height on a histogram. There may be other formulas available to describe the shape of any given distribution. The binomial, hypergeometric, and Poisson distribution often apply when the data are discrete variates. Some data which initially lacks a normal distribution may become normally distributed if the data is converted to logarithms (income of patients is a good example). Most researchers find it too time-consuming to determine whether their distribution is of a

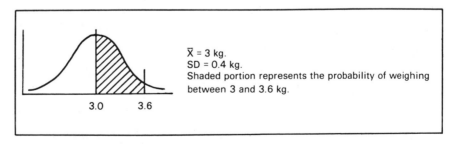

$\bar{X}$ = 3 kg.
SD = 0.4 kg.
Shaded portion represents the probability of weighing between 3 and 3.6 kg.

3.0    3.6

**FIG. 25-5.** Diagrammatic representation of the percentage of a group of rabbits weighing between 3 and 3.6 kg. when the group has a mean of 3 kg. and a standard deviation of 0.4 kg.

particular known form. In this case, a statistician could be consulted, or the data can be reported either in the form of a histogram, or, alternatively, in a summary statement of the percentage of observations which fall below or above a specified number. For example, the depressed clinic manager could use the data in Table 25–1 to report that 13 per cent of his patients were older than 31 years and 10 per cent younger than 19 years.

When no distribution is stated and only the mean and standard deviation are given, all that is known, from mathematical studies that have previously been done, is that at least 75 per cent of the observations for a variable lie within 2 standard deviations (2 above and 2 below) of the mean. When the range covered by ± 2 standard deviations is large in comparison to the mean, a more precise description of the distribution's shape can be presented by noting the percentage of the observations falling above, below, or between any two variates. It is always best to show the histogram, if space is available. As stated earlier, the median should always be presented along with the mean.

Table 25–10 presents the summary descriptive statistics for the three sample data sets, treating each as representing a population or sample, as indicated. Other statistical concepts are available for describing data sets; however, the most frequently reported are the total number of observations; the proportion having a certain characteristic when the data is nominal; the mean, median, and standard deviation, and a brief description of the *shape* of the distribution, if the variable is measured at the interval or ratio level. Descriptive statistics can be calculated for any numerical data, provided the measurement level is adequate for the statistic selected. Only those statistics that are meaningful should be reported. For example, the rabbit data in Table 25–10 are summarized in terms of all the rabbits used in the experiment. Although this collective description is correct, it is not a useful description, given the nature of the experiment. In this case, the researcher should provide descriptive statistics for each experimental group, based on drug dosage.

As for the Crystal-Ball Gazer data, since the data is a time-series (i.e., each observation comes from a different quarter of different years in the past), the change over the course of time may be more interesting than the average, as will be shown in the section about time-series analysis in Chapter 27. If there is no trend, upward or downward, over the

## Table 25–10. Descriptive Statistics for Data in Examples

| Item | N | Proportion w/ characteristic | Mean | Median | Std. dev. | 75% of observations are below: |
|---|---|---|---|---|---|---|
| *Case of depressed clinic mgr.* *(sample)* | | | | | | |
| Drop out (proportion) | 30 | 0.50 | | | | |
| Desired no. of additional children upon admission | 30 | | 1.27 | 1.00 | 1.53 | 2.00 |
| Knowledge score | 30 | | 74.50 | 82.50 | 21.99 | 90.00 |
| On the pill | 30 | 0.50 | | | | |
| On IUD | 30 | 0.17 | | | | |
| On foam and condom | 30 | 0.33 | | | | |
| Has hypertension | 30 | 0.20 | | | | |
| Age at entry | 30 | | 24.00 | 25.00 | 4.73 | 27.00 |
| Parity | 30 | | 1.20 | 1.00 | 0.85 | 2.00 |
| *Case of the high rabbits (sample)* | | | | | | |
| Weight (kg.) | 30 | | 3.08 | 3.00 | 0.36 | 3.40 |
| Drug dose | 30 | | 0.93 | 0.61 | 0.90 | 1.25 |
| Postcoital LH | 30 | | 16.40 | 17.50 | 16.27 | 29.00 |
| Proportion ovulating | | 0.53 | | | | |
| No. of corpora lutea per animal | 30 | | 5.00 | 7.00 | 4.91 | 9.00 |
| No. of implantations per animal | 30 | | 4.43 | 6.00 | 4.38 | 9.00 |
| *Case of crystal-ball gazer* | | | | | | |
| Quarterly no. of visits *(population)* | 40 | | 106.00 | 110.00 | 35.95 | 140.00 |

years, then it would be appropriate to show the average. However, the average is reported here only as an example of the reporting of a data set.

A review of the Depressed Manager data about the desired number of additional children, summarized in Table 25-9, indicates that the distribution is somewhat skewed to the right (i.e., the hump is to the left, and the tail extends to the right), since the mean is higher than the median. This indicates that one or two women wanted an extremely high number of additional children, but that most wanted only 1 more child. A look back at Table 25-1 reveals that one person did want 8 more children. She was young (age 15), cur-

rently had no children, and had high knowledge of family planning. Also, since the standard deviation was high (higher than the mean, giving a large coefficient of variation), the mean is not a good indicator of the central tendency of the group. This discussion is an example of what a reader can learn from a relatively small set of numbers—the mean, median, and standard deviation.

## REFERENCES

1. Nie NH, Hull CH, Jenkins JG, Steinbrenner K, Bent DH: Statistical Package for the Social Sciences, 2nd ed. New York, McGraw-Hill, 1975
2. Stevens SS: On the theory of scales of measurement. Science 103:677, 1946

# 26

# Statistical Inference: Confidence Intervals, Sample Size, and Hypothesis Testing

**Harold D. Dickson**
**Rebecca A. Lane**

Describing the population distribution of a variable in a few summary measures, such as proportions, means, and standard deviations, reduces data sets to manageable proportions. When such measures are estimated using data from a sample of the population, they may be used to infer the properties of the population from which the sample is derived. This process is called *statistical inference,* and is based directly on probability theory; however, mathematical proofs for statistical inference will not be considered here. Consequently, many statements in this explanation must be accepted on faith, so that we may proceed to useful applications of sample statistics.

The chapter focuses on the following aspects of statistical inference:

1. Establishing a *confidence interval* (or range of possible values) for a population mean, given a sample mean and standard deviation.

2. Determining the sample size required to enable one to state as narrow a confidence interval as possible for a population parameter.

3. Determining the extent to which a previously observed or suspected population mean, proportion, difference between two means, or difference between two proportions has changed, after reviewing the results of a sample—the concept of *hypothesis testing.*

The underlying theoretical basis for conducting the statistical inferences indicated above is the *central limit theorem.* This will be discussed in terms of the distribution of sample means, prior to the detailed description of the procedures.

As an example of the confidence interval, assume that a sample of females, aged 15–44, in the community is taken to determine the desired age of their first pregnancy. First, assume that the sample was random (see Appendix 2-6 for a random number table and the related discussion of how to use it), and contained 100 women. Also assume that the mean of first pregnancy was 25, with a standard deviation of 10. The following statement would be a 95 per cent confidence interval statement: "Unless an error (5% chance) has occurred, the mean desired age of first pregnancy for all women age 15–44 in the entire community is between 23.04 years and 26.96 years of age." Alternatively, "We are 95 per cent confident that the true mean desired age is

$$25 \pm 1.96 \, \frac{10}{(\sqrt{10})}."$$

## THE SAMPLING DISTRIBUTION OF MEANS

Decisions about the effects of new policies or treatments on a population of interest can be made on the basis of a single sample size *n* (number of observations in the sample) from that population. Even if, in practice, only a single sample is chosen, the procedure of choosing a sample and then making an inference about the larger population can be justified by considering a theoretical situation in which *repeated random samples* of size *n* are taken from the same population. When taking repeated samples of size *n* from a known population, different sample means could result each time. Each of the repeated samples of size *n* will give an estimate of the population mean, *μ*, based on the sample mean; the plot of the distribution of these *sample means* approximates a normal curve.

It is important to note that three distinct distributions are involved in this discussion: *1*) The *population distribution,* which is the distribution of variates within the population; *2*) the *sample distribution,* which is the distribution of variates within a single sample, and *3*) the *sampling distribution,* which uses the independent sample *means* as variates. While the sample distribution is plotted from the set of variates in an actual sample that has been collected, the population distribution is generally not known (otherwise a sample would not be needed), and the sampling distribution is theoretical. The following theorem (the *central limit theorem*) expresses the relationship among these three distributions:

If repeated samples of size *n* are drawn from a population with any shape of distribution, then the distribution of sample means will be approximately normal (*t* = distribution when *n* is less than 30) with a mean $\mu_{\bar{X}} = \mu$, and standard deviation $\sigma_{\bar{X}} = \sigma/\sqrt{n}$.

Each of the three distributions has a mean and standard deviation. The standard deviation of the distribution of sample means is called the *standard error of the mean.* By using the properties of the sampling distribution, it is possible to use probability theory to make statements about the population, based on estimates from a single sample. For example, it is known that 95 per cent of the means of samples drawn from a population will fall within 1.96 standard errors of the population mean.

The smaller the standard error of the mean, the less variability of the sample means around the true mean; therefore, the greater the probability that a sample mean from a single sample closely approximates the population mean. By examining the formula for the standard error of the mean, it can be seen that as sample size *n* increases, the standard error decreases; therefore, the sample mean is more likely to approximate the population mean when the sample size is large.

## CONFIDENCE INTERVALS

### BASIC CONCEPTS

Confidence intervals may be viewed as probability statements concerning the likelihood of particular sample results. The *estimate* of the descriptive parameter is called a *statistic.* The term, in this sense, represents an estimator of a population parameter, not a number. It is bracketed by an interval, the width of which is a multiple of the *standard error* of the estimate. As an example, suppose that the average age of the *sample* of 30 women shown in Data Set 1 (Chap. 25) was 24, with a sample standard deviation of 4.73 years. The 99 per cent confidence interval statement would be that with 99 per cent certainty, the true mean age (of all women enrolling in the clinic) is somewhere between 21.6 and 26.4 years of age. Another example would be that, based on the *sample* of 30 women in Data Set 1, where 0.5 of the 30 patients dropped out of the clinic after 2 years, the true proportion (that proportion which would be obtained if the dropout rate of *all* women enrolled were measured) is somewhere between 0.32 and 0.68, with 95 per cent confidence.

The actual procedure used to obtain an interval estimate or confidence interval for a mean or a proportion involves no new concepts. The interval is obtained by proceeding in both directions from the sample mean or proportion a certain multiple of standard errors corresponding to the areas under a normal curve (Chap. 25), or *t*-distribution. The area selected is interpreted as a confidence *level.* In Chapter 25, *Z*-scores were used to determine the probability associated with the selection of a single variate from a population. The standardized normal deviate, or *Z*, was defined as

$$Z = \frac{X_i - \mu}{\sigma} \qquad (1)$$

In the construction of confidence intervals, rather than determing the probability associated with a single variate, it is necessary to determine the probability of selecting a particular sample mean. Therefore the standardized normal deviate ($Z$) must be changed to

$$Z = \frac{\bar{X} - \mu}{\sigma_{\bar{X}}} \qquad (2)$$

This modification of $Z$ can be used to find areas contained under specific portions of the normal curve, since the normal curve also represents the distribution of the sample means. The Standard Normal Table is included in Appendix 2. It may be recalled that 95 per cent of all variates in a normal distribution fall within 1.96 standard deviations (plus or minus) of the mean. Thus to obtain the range of sample *means* within which the population mean is included 95 per cent of the time, the observed sample mean is used, and the interval is simply the mean, plus or minus 1.96 *standard errors* from the mean:

$$\mu = \bar{X} \pm 1.96 \, \sigma_{\bar{X}} = \bar{X} \pm 1.96 \, (\sigma/\sqrt{n})$$

A word of caution should be said regarding the interpretation of confidence levels. As in any case of statistical inference, the "confidence" is in the accuracy of the method, not in any particular sample result. For the case at hand, it must be remembered that the population mean ($\mu$) is *fixed,* and that intervals *vary* from sample to sample. The confidence level merely indicates the percentage of repeated samples from the same population in which intervals obtained by this procedure would include the population parameter.

As is discussed in the next section, it is possible to determine the *risk* of computing an interval that does not contain the true mean at any level desired by obtaining the proper multiple of the standard error. To reduce this risk, the width of the interval is increased, or the sample size is increased.

## CONFIDENCE INTERVALS FOR PROPORTIONS

The use of Formulas 1 or 2 above assumes that the standard deviation of the population is known. This is usually not the case, so a $t$-distribution is generally used, and the standard error computed as $\left(\frac{s}{\sqrt{n}}\right)$, where $s$ = the sample standard deviation. This will be discussed

later. However, the $Z$-distribution is used when the sample statistic is a proportion, rather than a mean. In this case, it is necessary to provide the *best guess* of the true population proportion. The confidence interval for a proportion is simply

Sample Proportion $\pm\ Z$ (Standard Error of a Proportion)

The computation procedure involves, first, the selection of the confidence level (percentage of confidence) desired. The $Z$ associated with the selected level is obtained from the Standard Normal Table. The confidence interval is

$$P = \frac{X}{n} \pm Z \left( \sqrt{\frac{P\,(1-P)}{n}} \right) \qquad (3)$$

where $X$ is the number of observations having the characteristic of interest,
$n$ is the number of observations,
and $P$ is the best guess of the true population proportion.

For example, the sample porportion discontinuing clinic use (Data Set 1, Chap. 25) was 0.5 of 30 patients. (Be aware, in constructing confidence intervals for a proportion, that the sample size $n$ must be for $n$ independent subjects. In this case, the 30 patients in the sample were 30 different patients, so a confidence interval is appropriate. If the 30 patients had 100 visits, half in which a doctor was seen, a confidence interval on the proportion seeing the doctor would not be appropriate, because there are only 30 patients in the 100 "visits," and the 100 visits are not independent.) To construct a 95 per cent confidence interval for this sample proportion, the $Z$ associated with 95 per cent of the area under a normal curve must be obtained. The Standard Normal Table (Appendix 2) presents areas *above* a selected $Z$ value. For the $Z$-distribution, 2.5 per cent lies above the $Z$ of 1.96, and 2.5 per cent lies below a $Z$ of $-1.96$; this means that 95 per cent of the distribution lies within 1.96 standard errors of the mean. Therefore 0.025 must be located in the Standard Normal Table. The location of 0.025 is the intersection of two columns of $Z$ scores: the $Z$ score given to the nearest tenth is in the first column, and the $Z$ score given for the nearest hundredth is read across the top of the table. The two coordinates are added together. For 0.025, the $Z$ score is 1.9 plus 0.06, or a $Z$ score of 1.96.

Using Formula 3, the 95 per cent confidence interval for the sample proportion can be calculated as

$$P = \frac{15}{30} \pm 1.96 \left( \sqrt{\frac{0.5\,(1 - 0.5)}{30}} \right)$$

$$P = 0.5 \pm 1.96\,(0.09)$$

$$P = 0.05 \pm 0.1789$$

and the interval can be written as

$$(0.5 - 0.1789) < P < (0.5 + 0.1789)$$

or

$$0.3211 < P < 0.6789.$$

This interval means that based on one sample of 30 women who began clinic services on a certain date, between 32 per cent and 68 per cent of all the patients will drop out after 2 years. Unless an error with a 5 per cent chance of happening has occurred, the true proportion is between 32 per cent and 68 per cent.

In the example, the sample proportion is taken as the *best guess* of the population proportion. This procedure is often adopted. Occasionally, however, previous experience suggests values for the population proportion different from the sample proportion. For example, assume that clinics nationwide experienced a 75 per cent dropout rate: 0.75 could be taken as the best guess of the population proportion. In this case, the confidence interval would be

$$P = 0.5 \pm 1.96 \left( \sqrt{\frac{0.75\,(1 - 0.75)}{30}} \right)$$

$$0.3450 < P < 0.6550.$$

In either case, the clinic manager should probably not be depressed: his dropout rate, somewhere between 0.32 and 0.68, obtained when the population proportion was assumed to be 0.5, is definitely lower than the national experience. An assumed true population proportion of 0.5 is the most conservative estimate, since the widest possible confidence interval is thereby obtained. Any other value (such as 0.6, 0.3) will give a smaller standard error.

## CONFIDENCE INTERVAL FOR A MEAN

Confidence intervals for sample means are probability statements about a mean selected from the theoretical distribution of means (the sampling distribution) of samples of size $n$. To

find the probability of selecting a particular sample mean, $Z$ was modified, in Formula 2 above. In comparing Formulas 1 and 2, note that in Formula 2 the sample mean $\bar{X}$ has been substituted for the original variates $X_i$ and that the standard error of the mean $(\sigma_{\bar{X}} = \sigma/\sqrt{n})$ has been substituted for the standard deviation of the population $(\sigma)$. Calculation of confidence intervals for the mean depend on whether $\sigma$ is known or unknown. When $\sigma$ is known, the standard normal curve $(Z)$ is used to determine multiples of the standard error. When $\sigma$ is unknown, a special distribution, called the *t-distribution*, must be used. When $\sigma$ is unknown, as is the usual case, the standard error $\sigma_{\bar{X}}$ must be estimated from the sample data; that is, the standard error becomes a statistic. The best estimate of the standard error of the mean is

$$S_{\bar{X}} = \frac{S_X}{\sqrt{n}} \qquad (4)$$

If this estimate is substituted for $\sigma_{\bar{X}}$, in Formula 2, the result is called $t$:

$$t = \frac{\bar{X} - \mu}{S_{\bar{X}}} \qquad (5)$$

Whereas the distribution of $Z$ is a normal curve, there are many distributions of $t$, depending on sample size $n$; however, all of these distributions are symmetrical. As $n$ increases, the distribution of $t$ tends toward normality. For samples of $n = 30$ or more, the normal distribution and the $t$-distribution are nearly identical.

The use of the $t$-distribution allows confidence intervals for $\mu$ to be constructed when $\sigma$ is unknown. The interval is simply

$$\mu = \bar{X} \pm t\,S_{\bar{X}} \qquad (6)$$

The $t$-distribution is a symmetrical distribution, and the various areas (probabilities) contained under the distribution of $t$ have been tabulated (see Appendix 2-2). However, since any given $t$ is dependent on sample size, use of the table also depends on sample size. The use of the $t$ table in Appendix 2-2 is discussed below.

### DEGREES OF FREEDOM

Any given sample compared with the $t$-distribution is restricted by a condition: namely, the sample variates must have a mean of $\bar{X}$. Every sample has $n$ variates, but since they must have a mean of $\bar{X}$, not all of the variates are free to vary independently of one another. The concept of the number of independently varying quantities is called the *degrees of freedom (df)*. Since there is one condition imposed on the sample variates compared to the *t*-distribution, the degrees of freedom is equal to $(n - 1)$ for the confidence interval of a single mean.

### USE OF THE T-TABLE

The table for the *t*-distribution is organized somewhat differently from the Standard Normal Table ($Z$). In the $Z$ table, the area for $Z$ values above a selected $Z$ was shown inside the table. The table for the *t*-distribution is also organized for the area of *t* values above a selected *t*, but the area is shown at the top of the column and the *t* is inside the table. Areas in the upper tail of the distribution are indicated by $\alpha$ (alpha) located across the top of the table. Use of the table requires knowing only two quantities—the $\alpha$ area and the degrees of freedom. For example, it is easy to locate the *t*-value needed to compute a 99 per cent confidence interval for a sample size of 30. To determine $\alpha$, it must be remembered that the percentage of the distribution beyond the confidence level (either direction) is simply 100 per cent, minus the confidence level. Stated in proportions, computation of $\alpha$ is simply $1.00 - 0.99 = 0.01$, which is then divided by 2 to determine the area in each tail: $0.01/2 = 0.005$. This value of $\alpha$ is located at the top of the *t* table. For a sample size of 30, the degrees of freedom is equal lo $(n - 1)$, or 29. The row and column intersect of $\alpha = 0.005$ and $df = 29$ yields a *t*-value of 2.756. Therefore, a 99 per cent confidence interval for a mean estimated from a sample size of 30 will be 2.756 standard errors from the sample mean. Until hypothesis testing is discussed, assume that $\alpha$ should be spread through both tails.

### EXAMPLES OF COMPUTATIONS

a. Compute a 99 percent confidence interval for the mean age of clinic attenders, based on the sample of 30 women in the clinic (Data Set 1, Chap. 25).

- Sample size $(n) = 30$
- Degrees of freedom $(df) = (n - 1) = 29$
- Area in each tail, $\alpha/2 = 0.005$

- Sample mean $(\bar{X}) = 24.0$ years
- Sample standard deviation $(S) = 4.73$ years

The confidence interval is

$$\mu = \bar{X} \pm t \, (s/\sqrt{n}) \tag{7}$$
$$\mu = 24.0 \pm 2.756 \, (4.73/\sqrt{30})$$
$$\mu = 24.0 \pm 2.37$$
$$21.63 < \mu < 26.37$$

b. Compute a 95 percent confidence interval for the same data.

$$\frac{\alpha}{2} = \frac{1.0 - 0.95}{2} = 0.025$$
$$t = 2.045$$
$$\mu = 24.0 \pm 2.045 \, (4.73/\sqrt{30})$$
$$22.24 < \mu < 25.76$$

Notice that the more confidence desired (99%, versus 95%), the wider the interval, and the better the chance of bracketing the true mean. This characteristic leads to the statement, "The surer you want to be, the less you have to be sure of!" The process of determining when to use $Z$ or $t$ can be assisted by the flowchart shown later in this chapter. In practice, when working a single mean or porportion, the rule of thumb is always to use $t$ when the statistic is a mean, and $Z$ when the statistic is a proportion.

### FINITE POPULATION CORRECTION

In all the cases of confidence interval statements, the confidence interval should be made narrower if the sample is large in comparison to the population size. If the population is, for example, 200 persons given the IUD as a method during a given year, then a sample of 50 of those persons would represent a sizable part of the population. To narrow the confidence interval in the formulas given, the *standard error* is adjusted by multiplying it by the "finite population correction factor" of

$$\sqrt{\frac{N - n}{N - 1}}$$

where $N =$ the population size and $n =$ the sample size

In the example given, the standard error would be multiplied by

$$\sqrt{\frac{200 - 50}{200 - 1}} = \sqrt{\frac{150}{199}} = \sqrt{0.754} = 0.868.$$

## THE DIFFERENCES BETWEEN TWO SAMPLE STATISTICS

### CONFIDENCE INTERVALS OF THE DIFFERENCE BETWEEN TWO INDEPENDENT POPULATION MEANS BASED ON TWO SAMPLES

Confidence intervals for the difference between two means may be computed; however, a distinction must be made between independent means and correlated means. If means are computed from two different sets of subjects, they are independent. Two means computed from a single set of subjects are termed *correlated means,* and are discussed in the section on "Confidence Intervals for the Difference between Correlated Means."

Confidence intervals for the difference between independent (uncorrelated) means can be easily determined, because of the following theorem:

If independent samples of size $n_1$ and $n_2$ are taken from populations 1 and 2, with means of $\mu_1$ and $\mu_2$ and variances of $\sigma_1^2$ and $\sigma_2^2$, then the sampling distribution of the difference between two samples means $(\bar{X}_1 - \bar{X}_2)$ *will be approximately normally distributed, with a mean of* $(\mu_1 - \mu_2)$ *and a variance of* $\left(\dfrac{\sigma_1^2}{n_1} + \dfrac{\sigma_2^2}{n_2}\right)$.

The confidence interval for the difference between independent sample means $\bar{X}_1$ and $\bar{X}_2$ is

$$\mu_1 - \mu_2 = (\bar{X}_1 - \bar{X}_2) \pm M \sigma_{\bar{X}_1 - \bar{X}_2} \quad (8)$$

where $M$ is the appropriate multiple of the standard error $(\sigma_{\bar{X}_1 - \bar{X}_2})$. The multiple used depends on whether $Z$ or $t$ is appropriate and on the degree of confidence desired.

The computation of standard error of the difference between two means when the population variances are unknown (which is generally the case) depends upon assumptions about the equality of the two population variances. The population variances are assumed to be unequal if the largest sample variance is divided by the smallest sample variance, and the result is greater than 4. If this ratio is less than 4, the population variances are assumed to be equal.

1. If the population variances are assumed to be *unequal,* then the standard error is written as

$$S_{\bar{X}_1 - \bar{X}_2} = \sqrt{\frac{S_1^2}{n_1} + \frac{S_2^2}{n_2}} \quad (9)$$

where $S_1^2$ and $S_2^2$ are the sample variances, and the degrees of freedom for the $t$-distribution is estimated as follows:

$$df = \frac{(W + V)^2}{\left[\dfrac{W^2}{(n_1 - 1)} + \dfrac{V^2}{(n_2 - 1)}\right]} \quad (10)$$

where $W = \dfrac{S_1^2}{n_1}$

$V = \dfrac{S_2^2}{n_2}$

The confidence interval for $(\mu_1 - \mu_2)$ is

$$\mu_1 - \mu_2 = (\bar{X}_1 - \bar{X}_2) \pm t \sqrt{\left(\frac{S_{pooled}^2}{n_1} + \frac{S_{pooled}^2}{n_2}\right)} \quad (11)$$

where $t$ is determined from the table (Appendix 2) based on the confidence level selected $(1 - \alpha)$, and the degrees of freedom is computed as in Formula 11.

2. If the population variances are *equal,* then the population variance can be estimated by a "pooled" variance, which is a weighted average of the two sample variances, according to the following formula:

$$S_{pooled}^2 = \frac{(n_1 - 1)S_1^2 + (n_2 - 1)S_2^2}{(n_1 + n_2 - 2)}$$

and then the standard error of the difference between two means is given as

$$\sqrt{\frac{S_{pooled}^2}{n_1} + \frac{S_{pooled}^2}{n_2}} \quad (12)$$

where $S_1^2$ and $S_2^2$ are the sample variances, and degrees of freedom for the $t$-distribution is $n_1 + n_2 - 2$.

As an example of a confidence interval for the difference between two means, suppose that in the depressed manager's clinic, ages of 15 dropouts and 15 continuing clinic patients were compared. The dropouts averaged 25.2 years of age, with a standard deviation of 4.38. The continuing patients averaged 22.8 years of age, with a standard deviation of 4.9.

Since the ratio of the two variances ($[4.90]^2 / [4.38]^2$) is less than 4, the Standard Error would be computed as follows:

$$S^2_{pooled} = \frac{(14)(4.38)^2 + 14(4.9)^2}{(15 + 15 - 2)} = 21.597$$

$$S_{\bar{X}_1} - \bar{x}_2 = \sqrt{\frac{21.597}{15} + \frac{21.597}{15}} = 1.697$$

and the degrees of freedom computed as (0.15 + 15 − 2) = 28 degrees of freedom. Therefore the 95 per cent confidence level for the differences between the mean age of patients who drop out and patients who continue would be as follows:

$$(\bar{X}_1 - \bar{X}_2) \pm t \; (S.E.)$$
$$(25.2 - 22.8) \pm (2.048)(1.697)$$
$$2.4 \pm 3.475$$
$$-1.075 < \mu_1 - \mu_2 < 5.875$$

## THE DIFFERENCE BETWEEN TWO PROPORTIONS

A distinction between independent and correlated proportions depends on which subjects are in each of the two samples. If the two sample proportions are derived from the same set of subjects, they are correlated. This is discussed in the section on "The Difference between Correlated Proportions."

A confidence interval for the difference between proportions estimated from two *independent* samples (in which the subjects in each group are different) is shown below:

$$P_1 - P_2 =$$
$$\left( \frac{X_1}{n_1} - \frac{X_2}{n_2} \right) \pm Z \qquad (13)$$
$$\left( \sqrt{\frac{pp(1-pp)}{n_1} + \frac{pp(1-pp)}{n_2}} \right)$$

where $X_1$ = no. in sample of group 1 with desired characteristic

$X_2$ = no. in sample of group 2 with desired characteristic

$n_1$ = sample size in group 1

$n_2$ = sample size in group 2

$pp = \frac{X_1 + X_2}{n_1 + n_2}$

As an example of a 95 per cent confidence interval for the difference between two proportions, suppose that a comparison is being made of the methods of contraception originally chosen by the dropouts and the clinic continuation group in the depressed man-

ager's clinic. Of 15 dropouts, 6 were on the pill (0.4), and of 15 continuing patients, 9 were on the pill (0.6). There is a 0.2 difference in the two proportions. According to the formula, the *pp* is computed as $(6 + 9)/(15 + 15)$, and is applied in the formulas as follows:

$$P_1 - P_2 =$$
$$(0.6 - 0.4) \pm 1.96$$
$$\left( \sqrt{\frac{0.5\,(1-0.5)}{15} + \frac{0.5.\,(1-0.5)}{15}} \right)$$
$$P_1 - P_2 = 0.2 \pm 1.96 \sqrt{(0.0333)}$$
$$P_1 - P_2 = 0.2 \pm 1.96 \times 0.1826$$
$$P_1 - P_2 = 0.2 \pm 0.358$$

The 95 per cent confidence interval for the true difference is

$$-0.158 < (P_1 - P_2) < 0.558$$

Since this interval contains zero, the true difference cannot be proven to be different from zero, although the sample proportion is different by 0.2. When a sample difference is large but not statistically significant (that is, zero is in the interval), it may be prudent to increase the sample size before concluding that the choice of methods was not related to the dropout rate. However, if the confidence interval had been *narrow* and had not included zero, more investigation into why the pill patient behaved differently would have been appropriate.

## CONFIDENCE INTERVALS FOR THE DIFFERENCE BETWEEN CORRELATED MEANS

When a variable is repeatedly measured from the same sample of subjects (before and after "treatment," for example), a confidence interval is constructed based on the difference between the variates obtained for each member of the sample. A confidence interval is then constructed for the mean of the differences, rather than for the difference between two means.

The "before-treatment" variable measured in a sample may be represented as $X_1, X_2, X_3, \ldots X_n$. After treatment, the variable is measured again, using the same individuals, and may be represented as $X'_1, X'_2, X'_3 \ldots X'_n$. The difference between variates for each member of the sample is $X'_1 - X_1, X'_2 - X_2, X'_3 - X_3 \ldots X'_n - X_n$. The mean and standard

**Table 26-1. Data Example for Correlated Means and Proportions**

| Person | Question 1 | Question 2 | Question 3 (years) | Question 4 (years) |
|--------|------------|------------|--------------------|--------------------|
| 1 | Y | Y | 1 | 1 |
| 2 | Y | Y | 1 | 1 |
| 3 | N | Y | 5 | 1 |
| 4 | N | Y | 6 | 1 |
| 5 | N | Y | 7 | 1 |
| 6 | N | N | 6 | 3 |
| 7 | N | N | 6 | 3 |
| 8 | N | N | 5 | 3 |
| 9 | N | N | 7 | 2 |
| 10 | N | N | 8 | 3 |

Y = Yes
N = No
The table reflects answers to a questionnaire given to ten multiparous women (age 15–44) to questions about tubal ligation. The questions were:
Question 1: Would you consider a tubal ligation within 1 year of when you have achieved your desired family size?
Question 2: Would you consider a tubal ligation within 1 year of when you have achieved your desired family size if the ligation had a 95 per cent chance of being reversible?
Question 3: If tubal ligations are not reversible, how many years would you wait to have one after your last desired child? Assumed difference between age 44 and age at birth of last child is shown if they do not want a ligation.
Question 4: If tubal ligations are 95 per cent reversible, how many years would you wait to have one after your last desired child?

deviation of the *differences* is computed, and the confidence interval is constructed as in Formula 7.

As an example, suppose that a sample of 10 women were asked how many years they would wait after their last desired child until having a tubal ligation. The results are shown in Table 26-1, questions 3 and 4. The mean number of years for a nonreversible ligation (question 3) is 5.2 and the mean number of years with availability of a reversible sterilization is 1.9 years. To determine the confidence interval for the difference between 5.2 and 1.9 years, one is tempted to construct a confidence interval of the difference between two means, as described in a previous section, but since the two means are computed from the same set of subjects, they are considered correlated means. Therefore, the methodology is to subtract the question 4 responses from the question 3 responses to get the set of *differences* (0, 0, 4, 5, 6, 3, 3, 2, 5, 5) which has a mean of 3.3 and a standard deviation of 2.11. The 95 per cent confidence interval for the mean difference would then be:

$$\mu_{(X - X')} = \bar{X}_{(X - X')} \pm \left(t_{n\frac{}{df}1}\right)\left(\frac{S_{(X - X')}}{\sqrt{n}}\right)$$

$$= 3.3 \pm 2.262\left(\frac{2.11}{\sqrt{10}}\right)$$

$$= 3.3 \pm 1.51$$

$$1.79 < \mu_{(X - X')} < 4.81 \text{ years}$$

This could also be called the "confidence interval for differences."

## THE DIFFERENCE BETWEEN CORRELATED PROPORTIONS—USE OF MCNEMAR'S TEST

The McNemar test for the significance of changes is appropriate for "before and after treatment" designs in which variates are obtained from the same individuals and are measured on either the nominal or ordinal scale. One example of the type of data for these is in questions 1 and 2 of the data in Table 26-1. The method involves hypothesis testing, and is discussed in the section entitled "McNemar's Test for Significance of Changes."

## DETERMINATION OF SAMPLE SIZE

In planning research, it is helpful to consider sample size in advance of data collection. A sample which is too small may lead to confidence intervals that are too wide to be useful as estimates of parameters. However, the arbitrary adoption of a large sample size may be unreasonable because of limited time and resources. In order to determine the sample size ($n$) other quantities must be known or estimated. It is then possible to use these values in various equations to calculate the most appropriate sample size.

Determination of appropriate sample size requires:

1. Selection of the confidence level (generally 90%, 95%, or 99%)
2. Determination of the degree of accuracy within which the parameter is to be estimated (i.e., how far off the sample statistic should be, at maximum, from the population parameter)
3. Estimates of the values of any statistics or parameters that appear in the formula, such as standard deviation or population proportion.

Selection of the confidence level is necessary so that the appropriate $Z$- or $t$-value may be looked up in the $Z$ or $t$ table. The degree of accuracy is called the *maximum allowable error* ($E$). The error selected is the maximum distance that the upper confidence limit should be from the sample mean or proportion. For example, if the desired confidence interval were ($0.2 < p < 0.3$), then $E$ would be 0.05, or half the distance between the high and low confidence limits.

Estimates of the values of needed statistics or parameters may be based on earlier studies. When these are not available, it is still possible to provide guesses. If a proportion must be estimated, the most conservative guess is 0.5 for $P$. If a mean is to be estimated, a guess of the standard deviation can be made, if the likely range of variates is known. Since 6 standard deviations generally encompass 99 percent of all variates, a good first estimate of the standard deviation is the reasonable range for 99 per cent of the potential variates divided by 6. For example, if the variates were estimated to be between 25 and 45, the standard deviation may be estimated as

$$\text{estimated } S = \frac{\text{range}}{6}$$

$$\text{estimated } S = \frac{45-25}{6} = \frac{20}{6} = 3.33$$

### SAMPLE SIZE FORMULAS FOR A MEAN, A PROPORTION, AND DIFFERENCES

Several formulas which may be used to estimate sample sizes are now presented.

1. *A single proportion:*

$$n = \frac{P(1-P) Z^2}{E^2} \tag{14}$$

If the true population proportion ($P$) were estimated as 0.7, and a 95 per cent confidence level were desired, when the sample proportion was to be no more than 0.04 from the true proportion (the value $E$), the sample size would be

$$n = \frac{(0.7)(0.3)(1.96)^2}{(0.05)^2}$$

$$n = 504$$

The $Z$ of 1.96 was used because the 95 per cent confidence interval was desired. The $E$ of 0.04 was used because we wanted to come within 0.04 of the true proportion.

2. *A single mean:*

$$n = \frac{(S^2)(t^2)}{E^2} \text{ if } \sigma^2 \text{ is unknown.} \tag{15}$$

Since a $t$-distribution requires the degrees of freedom and therefore a known $n$, an estimate of $n$ must be used initially, or $Z$ could be employed instead of $t$. As a better notion of the appropriate sample size is obtained, the $t$ can be revised and the formula recomputed. As an illustration, suppose that a test will be given on family planning knowledge that has a potential score of 0 to 50 for most of the participants. A 95 per cent confidence interval is desired, and the sample mean should be within 5 points of the true mean. The initial estimate is:

$$n = \frac{\left[\dfrac{50-0}{6}\right]^2 (1.96)^2}{(5)^2}$$

$$n = \frac{(8.33)^2 (1.96)^2}{25} = 11$$

The final estimate (after replacing the $Z$ of 1.96 with a $t$ with 10 degrees of freedom) is:

$$n = \frac{(8.33)^2 \ (t_{10df})^2}{E^2} = \frac{(8.33)^2 \ (2.33)^2}{(5)^2} = 15.$$

3. *The difference between two proportions:*

$$n_i = \frac{2 \ (Z^2) \ [pp \ (1-pp)]}{E^2} \qquad (16)$$

Where $n_i$ is the number in *each* sample and $pp$ is a guess of the combined proportion (see Formula 13), and $E$ is the distance desired between the sample difference between the two proportions and the upper confidence limit on the difference.

As an example, refer back to the example following Formula 13. In that example, the 95 per cent confidence interval for the difference between the proportion of clinic continuers and the clinic dropouts who were on the pill was:

$$\pm \left( 1.96 \ \sqrt{\dfrac{\dfrac{(0.6 - 0.4)}{0.5 \ (1 - 0.5)}}{15} + \dfrac{0.5 \ (1 - 0.5)}{0.5}} \right)$$

$$0.2 \quad \pm \ (1.96 \times 0.1826)$$
$$0.2 \quad \pm \ 0.358$$
$$- \ 0.158 < (P_1 - P_2) < 0.558$$

In this example the error ($E$) was 0.358 because the confidence interval statement indicated that the sample difference was within 0.358 of the true difference.

Assume that for practical use, this interval was too wide to be meaningful. In this case a lower $E$ of 0.1 is sought. What would be the required sample size? According to Formula 16, it would be computed as:

$$n_i = \frac{2 \ (1.96)^2 \ (0.5) \ (1 - 0.5)}{(0.1)^2} = \frac{1.9208}{0.01} \cong 192$$

This says that approximately 192 observations are needed of clinic dropouts and 192 of clinic continuing patients, with a total of (192 + 192) 384 patients. The 384 do not have to be divided absolutely equally between the two groups as the formula indicates, but the closer to equal division the better.

4. *The difference between 2 means.* The sample size for each group would be:

$$n_i = \frac{(Z^2) \ (S_1^2 + S_2^2)}{E^2}$$

where $S_1 =$ the estimate of the standard deviation for group 1 and $S_2 =$ the estimate of the standard deviation for group 2

The $Z$ could be replaced by a $t$-value based on the degrees of freedom implied by the sample size calculated in the first estimate of $n_i$ obtained when utilizing the $Z$. The $E$ is the distance desired between the sample difference between the 2 means and the upper confidence limit.

As an example, refer to the example associated with Formula 12. In that example, the 95 per cent confidence interval for the difference between the mean age of clinic continuers and clinic dropouts was given as:

$$\mu_1 - \mu_2$$

$$= (25.2 - 22.8) \pm 2.048 \ \sqrt{\frac{21.597}{15} + \frac{21.597}{15}}$$

$$= 2.4 \pm 2.048 \ (1.697)$$
$$= 2.4 \pm 3.48$$

or

$$- \ 1.08 < (\mu_1 - \mu_2) < 5.88$$

In this example, the error ($E$) was 3.48, because the sample difference was 2.4 years, and this was a maximum of 3.48 years away from the true mean. Suppose that it was desired to have this error only 1.5 years. Then the sample size for *each* group would be 1589, calculated as follows:

$$n_i = \frac{(1.96)^2 \ (4.38^2 + 4.9^2)}{(1.5)^2} = \frac{165.87}{2.25} \cong 74$$

Sample size formulas are somewhat different when a finite population is involved, and are given here:

5. *A single proportion (small and known population being sampled).* Earlier in the chapter it was stated that a confidence interval for a proportion would become more narrow (closer to the true mean) for a given sample size if the sample was large in comparison to the total population being studied, rather than very small in comparison to the population. The interval was narrowed by multiplying the standard error by $\sqrt{(N-n)/(N-1)}$ where $N$ was the population size. If the population size is known, and below 1000, the following formula will give the sample size required to estimate population proportion within an error $E$:

$$n = \frac{Z^2 p \,(1 - p)\, N}{(N - 1)\, E^2 + Z^2 p \,(1 - p)} \qquad (18)$$

where $N$ is the total population size.

6. *A single mean in a small and known population.* If a sample is large, relative to the size of the population from which the sample was drawn, the confidence interval for a *mean* will be narrower for a given sample size than if the population were large in comparison to the sample size. For this reason, when population has less than 1000 variates, the sample size required for a confidence level of a given level and error can be smaller than if the population size is greater than 1000, or unknown. The resulting sample size formulas for a single mean is as follows:

$$n = \frac{Z^2 S^2 N}{(N - 1)\, E^2 + Z^2 S^2} \qquad (19)$$

Once a sample has been taken, confidence intervals can be stated and/or hypotheses about the nature of the population being studied can be tested. Hypothesis testing is discussed in the next section.

## HYPOTHESIS TESTING

### CONFIDENCE INTERVALS AS TESTS OF HYPOTHESES

The hypotheses which we are concerned with are statements about the parameters which describe populations. When constructing confidence intervals, specific hypotheses are usually not stated, but are implied. That is, in a confidence interval, there is an implicit test for every value of $\mu$ or $P$ that might be hypothesized. For example, in the questionnaire of Table 26-1, it may be hypothesized that in the population of all women age 15–44 the mean difference between the years that they would wait after their last desired child until having a reversible, or a nonreversible, tubal ligation was zero (no difference, or a mean difference of zero). Notice that in the example the 95 per cent confidence interval was

$$1.79 < \mu_{(X - X')} < 4.81$$

This means that unless an error has been made (only 5% chance of such an error), then the true mean difference falls somewhere between 1.79 and 4.81 years. Since the hypothesized value of zero is not in the interval, the hy-

pothesis of "no difference between" must be rejected. It is concluded that a true difference (at least 1.79 years) does exist. If the confidence interval had been wider and had included zero within the interval, the hypothesis of no difference would have been accepted. Since confidence intervals are implicit tests of hypotheses, their use provides one approach to hypothesis testing. The approach is to first state a "null hypothesis" of no difference from a hypothesized value (which is generally a situation of the status quo). Also, state an alternate hypothesis which will lead to an *action* being taken. Then construct a confidence interval. If the null hypothesis value falls within the interval, accept the null hypothesis, and conclude that no action is required. In the example above, the null hypothesis was that reversibility of tubal ligation would make no difference in the years that a woman would wait (after her last child) before getting a ligation. If the difference were greater than zero, action might be taken to stimulate research into perfecting methods of tubal ligation. The 'status quo' assumption (that tubal ligation would make no difference), however, is assumed to be true until *proven* false. The proof of a change in the population mean difference is a confidence interval for a sample mean difference which does *not* include the null-hypothesized value.

This method of using confidence intervals to test hypotheses about population means, proportions, differences between two means, difference between two proportions, and mean differences is used in the hypothesis test flowchart presented later in the chapter. If the flowchart is followed, accurate confidence intervals will be constructed for the situation under which the test is being conducted.

There are two other approaches to hypothesis testing which give identical results. One could be called the *calculated statistic* approach and the other, which can be derived from the same approach, is called the *P-value* approach. The calculated statistic approach is more commonly used, because it facilitates understanding. This approach will be discussed in the following paragraphs.

Hypothesis testing using the calculated statistic approach involves several steps:

1. Statement of statistical hypotheses
2. Selection of a statistical model for determination of the relevant sampling distribution

3. Computation of the calculated test statistic
4. Making the statistical decision by comparing the test statistic with a table value
5. Statement of the decision in nonstatistical terms

The first three steps are accomplished without reference to the variate values obtained in a sample. A general discussion of these three steps will provide a basic understanding of hypothesis testing. A numerical example utilizing all six steps will also be presented. (A number of statistical models are available for both interval and ordinal data, and the reader is encouraged to consult a statistical text in order to obtain a broad perspective on the available possibilities.)

## STATEMENT OF STATISTICAL HYPOTHESES

Research propositions can be translated into specific statistical statements and contrasted with a "null hypothesis" designated as $H_0$. In general, the null hypothesis is the statistical hypothesis which one wishes to disprove. This is the case when research objectives involve establishing relationships that were previously unrecognized. The null hypothesis may take the form of equivalence between the parameters of two populations. Suppose that group $A$ is the group of females using a particular oral contraceptive and group $B$ is a group of females using the IUD, and $\mu$ is the mean number of desired additional children. The null hypothesis may state that the means of two populations, $A$ and $B$, are identical:

$$H_0 : \mu_A - \mu_B = 0$$
or
$$\mu_A = \mu_B$$

Since many decision-makers are reluctant to make unnecessary changes, and favor the status quo until it has been proven, with data, that a change is needed, statisticians assume that the null hypothesis (one of no difference) is true until data is accumulated to prove it false. The alternative statistical hypothesis asserts that $H_0$ is false. Alternative hypotheses to the null hypotheses above may be written as

$$H_1 : \mu_A - \mu_B \neq 0$$
or
$$\mu_A \neq \mu_B$$

These forms of alternative hypotheses are *non-directional*, since $H_0$ can be negated if $\mu_A > \mu_B$ or $\mu_A < \mu_B$. As will become evident in defining the critical region in step 3, tests of nondirectional hypotheses require a two-tailed test.

Research objectives may involve establishing interpopulation relationships which are *directional*. For example, if one is only interested in negating the null hypothesis of $H_0 : \mu_A = \mu_B$, if $\mu_A < \mu_B$, the alternative hypothesis is written as $H_1 : \mu_A < \mu_B$. Tests of directional hypotheses utilize a one-tailed test in defining the critical region in step 3.

Hypotheses may involve specific values for a parameter. For example, a null hypothesis may be $H_0 : \mu = 60$ and the alternative may be $H_1 : \mu_1 < 60$.

The determination of whether to use a directional (one-tailed) or a nondirectional (two-tailed) alternate hypothesis depends upon what change will key an *action* to be taken. In quality control, any deviation from a norm is considered bad, but in most managerial and research decisions, action will only be taken if there has been a change in the positive direction, so one-tailed tests are most common.

## SELECTION OF A STATISTICAL MODEL

Selection of a statistical model permits computation of probability statements for testing statistical hypotheses. The probability statements are based on the sampling distribution of the statistical model selected. Sampling distributions have been compiled and are available in table form. Quantities called calculated *test statistics* may be computed from the sample data and compared with those in the table. Two sampling distributions already described are $Z$ and $t$, and both are based on the conceptual model of the normal distribution of sample means, proportions, differences between 2 means, or differences between 2 proportions.

Selection of a model requires the acceptance of assumptions regarding the distribution of the sample statistics being considered, because sample statistics could take on many different values and still be close to the population parameter being used as the null hypothesis, due to sampling error alone. The researcher must be willing to assume that the conditions of the model selected hold for the conditions at hand. For example, the use of the normal distribution assumes a symmetrical distribution, with the maximum height at the mean and asymptotic tails (the tails of the distribution never touch the $X$-axis). The normal ($Z$) distribution is often selected as the statistical model because the sampling distribution of means approximates a normal distribution as the size of the sample gets larger, according to the central limit theorem. That is, even if variates are not normally distributed, the means of samples from these variates do tend toward normality (see "The Sampling Distribution of Means," in this chapter). A number of statistical models are available, and great care should be exercise in the selection of an appropriate model for particular data if fewer than ten observations are available, or if the proportion statistic is smaller than 0.01. For purposes of this general discussion, consideration is limited to the normal distribution.

Once an appropriate statistical model is selected, the model, in conjunction with the null hypothesis, constitutes a decision-making apparatus. As already mentioned, the null hypothesis is always assumed to be true until proven false. Empirical data are compared to expectations provided by the model and the null hypothesis. If the sample fails to agree with these expectations and the statistical model selected is appropriate, then the only conclusion possible is that the null hypothesis is an incorrect assumption, and it is *rejected*. That is, one *could* take a sample and get a result different from the null hypothesis just due to chance sampling error (as shown by the sampling distribution), but if the sample result is *drastically* different from the hypothesized value, it is assumed that the difference was due to more than just chance.

## SIGNIFICANCE LEVELS

Rejection or acceptance of a null hypothesis is a statistical decision. Since the decision must be based on inference from a sample, the potential for unavoidable errors in making the decision exists. There are two possibilities for making a correct decision, and two possibilities for making an incorrect one. If $H_0$ is true in the entire population (this could be discovered by a 100% sample), then a correct decision is made whenever $H_0$ is retained, based on a sample result. If $H_0$ is false (as could be discovered in a 100% sample of the population), then a correct decision is made whenever $H_0$ is re-

**Table 26–2. Outcomes of Possible Statistical Decisions**

| Statistical decision | The null hypothesis is actually: | |
|---|---|---|
| | True | False |
| Reject $H_0$ | Error I ($\alpha$) | Correct |
| Accept $H_0$ | Correct | Error II ($\beta$) |

jected. However, if $H_0$ is true and the decision is made, based on a single sample, to reject it, an error is made. Similarly, if $H_0$ is false and the decision is made to retain it, an error has occurred. These four possible outcomes are summarized in Table 26-2.

The incorrect rejection of a true $H_0$ is termed a Type I error, and the probability of its being committed is denoted by the symbol $\alpha$ (alpha). The confidence level selected in confidence interval estimates was 1, minus the probability of committing a Type I error. The incorrect acceptance of a false $H_0$ is called a Type II error, and the probability of its occurrence is denoted by the symbol $\beta$ (beta). For a given sample size $n$, the probabilities of $\alpha$ and $\beta$ are inversely related. Therefore, if one decreases the probability of incorrectly rejecting a true null hypothesis (decrease $\alpha$), the probability of accepting a false $H_0$ increases.

The actual nature of the situation being studied may dictate which type of error is more serious. This is often the case in medical research, for example, when consideration must be given to both the potential benefits of a newly proposed drug and possible dangerous side effects. In management decisions, the two types of errors inherent in statistical decisions may have financial implications. For example, suppose a clinic is financed by a foundation, provided its 2-year dropout rate does not exceed 40 per cent. The manager of the clinic constantly evaluates performance to ensure this standard. When a higher proportion of dropouts is detected, the manager conducts additional studies, so that action can be taken to conform to the standard. From a study of 30 patients, the sample proportoin of dropouts was 0.5 (Data Set 1, Chap. 25). Even though the sample proportion exceeded the standard, the manager must decide if the population of the entire clinic meets the required standard. The proposition may be stated in statistical terms for these proportions:

$$H_0: P \leq 0.4$$
and
$$H_1: P > 0.4$$

Note that the alternate hypothesis is directional, because action will only be taken if $P > 0.4$. To test this hypothesis the manager can construct a confidence interval. In choosing the significance level of the interval he must consider the two types of possible error:

- Error I: The erroneous conclusion that the population value is outside the interval surrounding the null-hypothesized value. In the example above, this would mean that he would decide that the dropout rate was greater than 40 per cent when it really wasn't. This is the Type I error of rejecting a null hypothesis when it is true.
- Error II: Erroneous conclusion that the population value is inside the interval. In the example above, this would mean that he would decide that the dropout rate was less than 40 per cent when it really was greater. This is the Type II error of accepting the null hypothesis when it is false.

Given these errors, the manager must consider the consequences of committing them, because the higher the probability of one of the errors, the lower the probability of the other, for a given sample size. If a true null hypothesis were rejected (Type I error), the manager would conduct further studies to try to determine the factors contributing to the apparently excessive dropout rate. This would be a waste of time, since the dropout rate of the entire population would be close to 0.4. However, if the manager incorrectly accepts the $H_0$ (Type II error), he would conclude that his clinic does not exceed the rate allowed. Thus he would be in a state of blissful ignorance until the foundation evaluation revealed the clinic to be out of compliance, and might be fired for not taking action. Therefore the manager concludes that the consequences of Type II error are more serious, and acts to minimize the probability of committing it, even though such a decision increases the probability of committing the Type I error.

To minimize the probability of committing a Type II error, the manager constructs a very narrow confidence interval. A 70 per cent confidence interval based on the sample proportion of 0.5 is

$$P = 0.5 \pm 0.09$$
$$0.41 < P < 0.59$$

The standard of 0.4 is not within this interval; therefore, $H_0$ is rejected; the manager concludes that the dropout rate is too high, and begins additional studies. The probability of committing a Type I error ($\alpha$) is 100 per cent minus the confidence level, or 30 per cent, in this example. That is, in minimizing the probability of a Type II error, the probability of rejecting a true null hypothesis (Type I error) is quite large. Nevertheless, in terms of the *consequences* of the errors, the manager was willing to increase the chance of committing a Type I error.

Researchers generally focus on $\alpha$, the probability of a Type I error. The probability of a Type I error is called the *level of statistical significance*. If research objectives are the absolute establishment of previously unrecognized relationships among certain factors, then it is desirable to minimize $\alpha$; that is, to minimize the probability of rejecting a true null hypothesis. This is statistical conservatism; decision-makers would be changing direction constantly if it were easy to prove new relationships. The $\alpha$ is generally set in the range of 0.10 to 0.01, with the rule of conservatism resulting in choices of 0.05 or 0.01. As already mentioned, however, this could result in a serious error for certain types of decision-making. For example, if a researcher doing a pilot study is looking for even a remote possibility of an effect of a new drug or procedure, than an $\alpha$ of 0.2 or even 0.3 may be appropriate.

## CRITICAL REGIONS

The link between sample results and a statistical model is the sampling distribution. From a knowledge of a sampling distribution it is possible to define "unlikely outcomes," which are referred to as the *critical region, or the region of rejection*. Definition of the critical region provides the operational criteria needed to test hypotheses. The critical region includes all possible empirical values (means or proportions) in the sampling distribution which are incompatible with a true null hypothesis, given the level of significance selected. This is analogous to a null-hypothesized mean or proportion that is outside the confidence interval. The level of significance ($\alpha$) is simply the sum of the probabilities of each of the

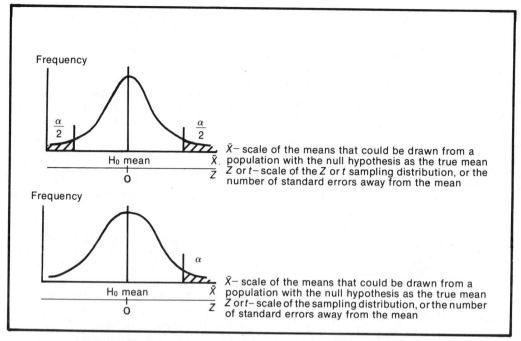

Frequency

$\frac{\alpha}{2}$          $\frac{\alpha}{2}$

$\bar{X}$– scale of the means that could be drawn from a
H₀ mean          $\bar{X}$. population with the null hypothesis as the true mean
0          Z          $Z$ or $t$– scale of the $Z$ or $t$ sampling distribution, or the
number of standard errors away from the mean

Frequency

$\alpha$

$\bar{X}$– scale of the means that could be drawn from a
H₀ mean          $\bar{X}$. population with the null hypothesis as the true mean
0          Z          $Z$ or $t$– scale of the sampling distribution, or the number
of standard errors away from the mean

**FIG. 26–1.** Location of $\alpha$ as affected by the direction of difference.

outcomes within the critical region of the sampling distribution.

When the alternative hypothesis is non-directional, the critical region is located in both tails of the sampling distribution. When the alternative hypothesis is directional, which is usually the case in administrative decision-making, the critical region is located in only one tail of the sampling distribution. Figure 26-1 illustrates these regions. Calculated statistics (number of standard errors that a hypothesized value falls from the null-hypothesized parameter) which fall within the critical region result in rejection of the null hypothesis, while calculated statistics which fall outside the critical region (or close to the null-hypothesis parameter) result in acceptance of the null hypothesis. The critical region is defined by the sampling distribution of the selected statistical model, and by alpha.

To summarize, special quantities can be calculated that are called test statistics; that is, they have a sampling distribution. Based on probability, the way test statistics vary in repeated sampling from the same population is given by their sampling distribution. Thus a computed value of a test statistic (obtained by subtracting the null-hypothesized value from the sample values and dividing the result by the standard error of the sample statistic) can be compared with its sampling distribution, and a decision can be made on the basis of the probability of its occurrence. In the following section, a numerical example is presented to clarify the the concepts involved in hypothesis testing.

## AN EXAMPLE OF HYPOTHESIS TESTING

The clinic manager in Data Set 1 (Chap. 25) was concerned that his dropout rate might exceed that allowed by the supporting foundation and wanted to understand the factors affecting the dropout rate. He suspected that there might be a difference in the mean *ages* of those who dropped out and those who continued. If there is a difference, he might need to alter the staffing, or hours of clinic operation, or at least conduct age-related studies, in order to deal with the dropout problem.

**Step 1.** State the statistical hypotheses. The null hypothesis states that the mean age of dropouts ($D$) and continuing clients ($C$) is the same.

$$H_0 : \mu_D = \mu_C$$
$$\text{or}$$
$$H_0 : \mu_D - \mu_C = 0$$

The manager has no basis for suspecting that dropouts may be older or younger than continuing clients. Therefore, the alternative hypothesis is nondirectional:

$$H_1 : \mu_D \neq \mu_C$$
or
$$H_0 : \mu_D - \mu_C \neq 0$$

If he had suspected that teenagers were dropping out, he would have stated that $\mu_D < \mu$, or $\mu_D - \mu_C < 0$).

**Step 2.** Select the statistical model and obtain the sampling distribution. The manager selects the $t$-distribution as the sampling distribution, since means (rather than proportions) are involved, the population's standard deviation is unknown, and the total sample size is less than 30. The decision to select a $t$-distribution can be made by following the hypothesis test flowchart through items B, E, and so forth (Fig. 26-2). After item I, the flowchart indicates that a $t$ table is necessary, and tells how to look up the critical value of $t$. The flowchart also reflects, after item E, how to compute the *standard error* which will be used in the calculated $t$-statistic. Use of the $t$-distribution requires calculating the degrees of freedom. Calculation of the degrees of freedom depends on whether $\sigma_D = \sigma_C$ or $\sigma_D \neq \sigma_C$. The manager assumes that the standard deviations for both populations are equal, and that the degrees of freedom is $(n_1 + n_2 - 2)$, where $n_1$ is the number of variates in the sample of dropouts and $n_2$ is the number of variates in the sample of continuing patients. When this assumption cannot be made, the degrees of freedom must be estimated, as discussed previously (in the discussion of confidence intervals for the difference between two means). The present example is intended as an illustration of the *concepts* involved in hypothesis testing, but the flowchart should be consulted for the precise determination of whether it can be assumed that $\sigma_1 = \sigma_2$. This is done in the flowchart in computing $(S^2_{largest} \div S^2_{smallest})$ and comparing that ratio to 4. If the ratio is greater than 4, it can be assumed that $\sigma_1 \neq \sigma_2$.

**Step 3.** Select the significance level and define the critical region. The manager wishes to avoid rejecting a true null hypothesis, since he does not want to waste time dealing with age-related problems when other factors may

be more important. Therefore a small alpha, such as 0.05, is selected. Since the alternative hypothesis is nondirectional, a two-tailed test is used. This means that the region of rejection will be defined in each tail of the sampling distribution. The critical region comprises the highest and lowest 2.5 per cent (for a total of 5%) of the $t$-distribution which contains unacceptable deviations from the null hypothesis. Half of alpha, or 0.025, will be to the right of the mean, and half to the left of the null-hypothesized mean, as illustrated in Figure 26-1.

The sampling distribution table for $t$ (Appendix 2-2) gives the empirical value of $t$ at the selected significance level when the degrees of freedom are known. The combined sample size of dropouts and continuing clients is 30, so the degrees of freedom is 28. From the distribution of $t$, the manager finds a value of $t = 2.048$ for $\alpha = 0.05$, and the degrees of freedom $= 28$ for a two-tailed test. This means that due to for routine sampling variation, it is likely that a sample result could be obtained that was up to 2.048 standard errors from the mean.

The manager will calculate a value of $t$ based on the sample (the test statistic, $t$). If the value calculated is greater than the table value of $t$, found as 2.048, the null hypothesis of no difference between the mean ages of dropouts and continuing clients will be rejected, because the difference is more than 2.048 standard errors away from the hypothesized value of zero, and therefore probably not due to chance or sampling variation.

**Step 4.** Compute the test statistic. The $t$-statistic for the difference between two means is

$$t = \frac{(\bar{X}_1 - \bar{X}_2) - 0}{S_{\bar{X}_1 - \bar{X}_2}}$$

where $S_{(\bar{X}_1 - \bar{X}_2)}$ is the standard error of the difference between two means and could be computed as $S_{(\bar{X}_1 - \bar{X}_2)} = SE =$

$$\sqrt{\frac{S^2_{pooled}}{n_1} + \frac{S^2_{pooled}}{n_2}}$$

This $t$-statistic is computed from the sample data. The denominator, which is the standard error of the estimate, is calculated in different ways, depending on the assumptions made regarding population variances. The reader should refer to the flowchart presented later in the chapter for computational details (see after item E).

The sample of dropouts had a mean age of 25.2 years. The sample of continuing clients had a mean age of 22.8 years, giving a difference of 2.4 years. Assuming that a standard error is computed from a set of data of 1.69, the manager calculates a $t$ for the difference betweeen these means as 1.42.

**Step 5.** Make the statistical decision. Since the calculated $t$ of 1.42 is less than the table $t$ of 2.048, the calculated statistic does not fall into the critical region, and the statistical decision is to accept $H_0$. Another way to word this is that the difference of 2.4 years in the sample was only 1.42 standard errors (standard error of a difference) away from the hypothesized difference of zero. This difference was not sufficient to reject the null hypothesis, because the alpha criteria required a difference of 2.048 standard errors from a mean difference of zero before the manager would be convinced that the sample was showing a true difference. If an $\alpha$ of 0.20 is selected, the critical $t$-statistic would be 1.313. Since the sample difference is greater than 1.313 standard errors from the hypothesized difference, the null hypothesis would be rejected. That $\alpha$ at which the null hypothesis would just barely be rejected is called the *P-value*. A report could then say that "there was a statistically significant difference ($P<0.19$)." Such a statement would indicate that at any alpha-level chosen that was above 0.19, the null hypothesis would be rejected. The "*P-value*" approach is an alternate way to report about a calculated $t$- or $Z$-statistic. One looks up the *calculated t* or $Z$ in the appropriate table in Appendix 2 and finds what level of $\alpha$ this value of $t$ or $Z$ would represent. Once the $P$-value is determined in this way, if the $P$-value is less than $\alpha$ the null hypothesis would be accepted.

**Step 6.** State the statistical decision in nonstatistical terms. The manager's sample did not allow rejection of the null hypothesis of equivalent age distributions for dropouts and continuing clients at $\alpha = 0.05$. This means there was not enough evidence to require consideration of attrition rates on the basis of the age of clients at the 5 per cent level of significance.

## HYPOTHESIS TEST FLOWCHART

A hypothesis test flowchart is presented in Figure 26-2 to assist the researcher in selecting an approach under various assumptions. The flowchart uses confidence intervals as tests of hypotheses, rather than considering the computation of test statistics. The chart can also be used for computing a calculated test statistic because the chart gives the appropriate sampling distribution and the standard error ($SE$). The calculated test statistic can then be computed by dividing the difference between a sample result and a hypothesized result by the standard error.

The chart includes more detail than has been considered in general discussion and is a convenient summary of information and computations needed to make statistical decisions. As in any flowchart, the diamonds contain the decisions that must be made prior to calculation. The lines from each diamond indicate the path to follow on the basis of the decision. Circled letters are continuation identifications and indicate the next position to follow in the chart.

If the flowchart technique were used for the example given in the preceding paragraphs, the steps would be as follows: since $\alpha = 0.05$, the 95 per cent confidence interval is required. Since it is a two-tailed test, due to the nondirectionality of the alternate hypothesis, the $(n_1 + n_2 - 2)$ is less than 30, and the sample standard deviations can be assumed to be equal (since the sample variance of the largest standard deviation is less than four times the sample variance of the smallest of the two sample standard deviations); therefore the standard error of the difference is:

$$SE = \sqrt{\frac{S_{pool}^2}{n_1} + \frac{S_{pool}^2}{n_2}} = \sqrt{\frac{21.59}{15} + \frac{21.59}{15}}$$

$$SE = 1.697$$

Where $S_{pool}^2 = \dfrac{(n_1 - 1)S_1^2 + (n_2 - 1)S_1^2}{n_1 + n_2 - 2}$

If the test is two-tailed, the table value of $t$ would be 2.048. The confidence interval is then:

$$(\bar{X}_1 - \bar{X}_2) \pm t\,(SE)$$

$$2.4 \pm (2.048)(1.697)$$

$$-1.075 < (\mu_1 - \mu_2) < 5.875$$

Since the null-hypothesized difference is in the interval, it is concluded that no statistical difference exists.

## HYPOTHESIS TESTING INVOLVING MORE THAN TWO MEANS OR PROPORTIONS: ANALYSIS OF VARIANCE AND CHI-SQUARE

Tests of hypotheses regarding the relationship between two populations can be handled easily by constructing confidence intervals; test statistics may also be computed from samples and compared to a defined critical region of the sampling distribution. It is this second approach that is used to test for differences among the means or proportions of more than two samples.

The present section introduces two test statistics: chi-square $(\chi^2)$ and $F$. The $F$ is the statistic computed in Analysis of Variance (abbreviated ANOVA) when multiple means are involved. Chi-square is used when more than two sample proportions are involved.

### CHI-SQUARE

The chi-square test is frequently used, since with its use variables need only be measured on a nominal scale. The chi-square is a measure of the difference between observed and expected frequencies. A common use of the test involves contingency problems; that is, it is used to determine whether the relationship evident among cross-classified variables is due to chance. For example, in the "high rabbit" case (Data Set 2, Chap. 25) a variable called "occurrence of ovulation" is measured at the nominal level: individual rabbits either did or did not ovulate. The researcher wishes to know if the proportion ovulating was related to dosage-level of THC, a variable presented as categories. These data are summarized in Table 26-3. A contingency table which cross-classifies individual rabbits in terms of ovulation and dosage level is presented in Table 26-4. Notice in Table 26-4 that for each dosage level, the number of total rabbits shown in the row totals is divided into the two components of the *number* ovulating and the *number not* ovulating. Chi-square (or contingency) tables show *frequencies,* or number count. The row and column totals are called *marginal* totals.

The number of rabbits expected in each "cell" of the table can be computed, given the

marginal totals. That is, the expected number is contingent upon the marginal totals. The expected frequency for a given cell is its column total times its row total, divided by the grand total. For example, the number of rabbits that received a high dosage and did ovulate is expected to be $[(16 \times 12)/30] = 6.4$ rabbits. Conceptually speaking, the expected values are the frequencies that would be expected under the circumstance that the proportion ovulating were the same for all of the groups. The overall proportion ovulating (16/30) is applied to each *row total* to get the expected number ovulating in the three columns. The overall proportion not ovulating (14/30) is multiplied by each row total to get the expected value for the proportion not ovulating. The expected frequency for each cell is indicated in parentheses in the contingency table. In Table 26-4A, it is shown that in several cells the expected frequencies are less than 5. With expected frequencies less than 5, the chi-square test will be more accurately performed if the medium-, low-, and no-dosage groups are recombined, as shown in Table 26-4B. The expected frequencies are the numerical statement of the null hypothesis that there are no differences in ovulation among

**Table 26-3. Proportion of Rabbits Ovulating per Dosage-level Group**

| Dosage | No. of rabbits | No. ovulating | Proportion of rabbits ovulating |
|---|---|---|---|
| High | 12 | 1 | 0.083 |
| Medium to low | 12 | 9 | 0.750 |
| None | 6 | 6 | 1.000 |

**Table 26-4. Contingency Table for Rabbits Cross-classified by Ovulation and Dosage Level**

A. Original Table*

| Dosage | Ovulation | | Row total |
|---|---|---|---|
| | Did | Did not | |
| High | 1 (6.4) | 11 (5.6) | 12 |
| Medium to low | 9 (6.4) | 3 (5.6) | 12 |
| None | 6 (3.2) | 0 (2.8) | 6 |
| Total | 16 | 14 | 30 |

B. Reduced Table*

| Dosage | Ovulation | | Row total |
|---|---|---|---|
| | Did | Did not | |
| High | 1 (6.4) | 11 (5.6) | 12 |
| Medium to none | 15 (9.6) | 3 (8.4) | 18 |
| Total | 16 | 14 | 30 |

* Expected frequencies in parentheses

dosage-level groups. If there are no differences, rabbits should be distributed according to these expected frequencies.

The sampling distribution for chi-square is presented in Appendix 2-3. Distributions differ according to the degrees of freedom involved. For contingency problems, the degrees of freedom do not depend on the number of cases sampled but instead on the number of cells in the contingency table. The degrees of freedom for a contingency table is computed as

$$df = (\text{no. of rows} - 1)(\text{no. of columns} - 1) \tag{20}$$

Thus the degrees of freedom for the contingency table constructed in part A of Table 26-4 would be $(3 - 1)(2 - 1) = 4$, but it would be $(2 - 1)(2 - 1) = 1$ for the table shown in part B.

The test statistic is defined as

$$\chi^2 = \sum_{i=1}^{n} \frac{(O_i - E_i)^2}{E_i} \tag{21}$$

where $O_i$ is the observed frequency in cell $i$ and $E_i$ is the expected frequency in cell $i$. The square of the difference between observed and expected frequencies is divided by the expected frequency, and the sum of these nonnegative quantities for all cells is the value of the calculated test statistics, chi-square. The larger the differences between observed and expected frequencies, the larger the value of chi-square. In the example, the calculated $X^2$ would be (from the data in Table 26-4B)

$$\chi^2 = \frac{(1 - 6.4)^2}{6.4} + \frac{(11 - 5.6)^2}{5.6} + \frac{(15 - 9.6)^2}{9.6} + \frac{(3 - 8.4)^2}{8.4}$$

$$= 4.56 + 5.21 + 3.04 + 3.47$$

$$= 16.28$$

To test a null hypothesis, it is necessary to select the significance level and define the critical region of the sampling distribution. A comparison of the test statistic with the sampling distribution indicates whether the test statistic is larger than would be expected by chance. The test statistic is calculated as squares of deviations, and cannot be negative: it is insensitive to the direction of relationships. The null hypothesis involved in a chi-square test is as follows:

$$H_0 : P_1 = P_2 = P_3 = P_4 = \ldots P_n$$

The alternate hypothesis is that *any* two proportions are *different*. This is a nondirectional hypothesis that applies when the chi-square statistic is computed for a contingecy table that has more than 2 rows or 2 columns. In this case, the chi-square test is a "screening" test to determine whether any differences exist. If chi-square indicates a difference, additional analyses (2-by-2 chi-square tables, or tests of the differences between two proportions) must be used to decide the location of the differences. In a 2-by-2 (i.e., 2 rows and 2 columns) chi-square contingency table, it is possible to state the alternate hypothesis in *directional* terms. When an alternate hypothesis is stated in directional terms, the significance level of a one-tailed test is half the significance level given in the chi-square table. That is, if it is stated that one proportion is greater than another, then the $\alpha$ used in looking in Appendix 2-3 would be twice that ordinarily chosen. Also, when either two-by-two chi-square or $t$ tests of two proportions are used *after* the chi-square has been used to reject the null hypothesis that *more than* two proportions are equal, then the $t$ test or chi-square alpha that is looked up in the Appendix 2 tables is the regular alpha divided by the number of proportions involved in all of the comparisons.

One further aspect of chi-square use should be stressed. The test statistic approximates the sampling distribution only when $n$, the sample size, is large. A general rule used to determine whether the number of cases is sufficiently large is based on the expected frequencies in each cell. If any of the expected frequencies is 5 or less, the row in which it occurs should be combined with another row. In the present example, the expected frequencies of rabbits who did and did not ovulate when receiving no THC are less than 5. Therefore the "none" category was combined with the "medium to low" category, resulting in the contingency table presented in Table 26-4B.

It is now possible to state and test the statistical hypotheses for the example. The null hypothesis is that there is no difference in ovulation between different dosage groups. The alternative hypothesis inherent in a 2-by-2 table which represents a purposeful experiment is that high-dosage rabbits ovulate less than medium-to-zero-dosage rabbits. To minimize the probability of a Type I error (rejection of a true null hypothesis), the significance level is selected as 0.01. This value is chosen because, in the researcher's opinion, it would be worse to indicate an effect of THC that *was not* truly there (Type I error) than to conclude that no effect existed, when in fact it did. Since the alternate hypothesis predicts a directional difference, the test will be one-tailed.

In order to define the critical region of the sampling distribution, the degrees of freedom are determined as $(2 - 1)(2 - 1) = 1$. From the table in Appendix 2-3, a chi-square for 1 *df* corresponding to $\alpha = 0.01$ for a one-tailed test (located at $\alpha = 0.02$ in the table) is 5.412. This means that values of chi-square $\geq 5.412$ have a probability associated with their occurrence of 0.01 or less. If the test statistic equals or exceeds this value, the null hypothesis will be rejected.

The test statistic is calculated as 16.28; therefore the null hypothesis is rejected. The probability of obtaining a test statistic of 16.28 is much less than 0.01 if the differences are due to chance. Thus there is sufficient evidence of a relationship between dosage level and reduced ovulation to warrant further investigation.

### MCNEMAR'S TEST FOR SIGNIFICANCE OF CHANGES

Differences between correlated proportions can be evaluated by McNemar's test. For example, back in Table 26-1, 10 women were asked (question 1) if they would consider undergoing a tubal ligation if it were nonreversible and (question 2) if they would do so if there was a 95 per cent chance of reversibility. Only 20 per cent responded positively for nonreversible tubal ligation, but 50 per cent responded positively for the reversible procedure. To determine the influence of reversibility on acceptability of tubal ligation, a four-fold table of frequencies is constructed, as in Table 26-5. Those individuals who responded differently to the first and second questions appear in cells *c* and *b*.

Since $c + b$ represents the total number who changed, the expectation under the null hypothesis of no change would be that $\frac{1}{2}(b + c)$ cases changed in one direction and $\frac{1}{2}(b + c)$ cases changed in the other direction.

Chi-square with one degree of freedom can be used as the sampling distribution for $\chi^2$ computed as

$$\chi^2 = \frac{(b - c)^2}{b + c} \qquad (22)$$

In Table 26-5 example, the calculated chi-square is:

$$\chi^2 = \frac{(0 - 3)^2}{3} = \frac{9}{3} = 3$$

which is the result of the sum of the observed frequencies minus the expected frequencies, for cells *b* and *c*. The null hypothesis for those who change is simply that the probability that any woman will change a response from no to yes (that is, cell *c*) is equal to the probability that she will change from yes to no (cell *b*), and each probability is equal to $\frac{1}{2}$. The alternate hypothesis is that the probability of changing from no on question 1 to yes on question 2 is greater than the probability of changing from yes to no.

The sampling distribution of $\chi^2$ computed by Formula 22 is approximated by the chi-square distribution with $df = 1$. Since the alternate hypothesis is directional, the region of rejection is one-tailed. In the example, the chi-square table value for $\alpha = 0.05$ is 2.71 since $2\alpha = 0.1$ for a one-tailed test. The calculated chi-square is less than the table value, and therefore the null hypothesis cannot be rejected; the sample size was too small to make a definitive statement.

### Table 26–5. Example of Data Table for McNemar's Test (Data from Table 26–1)

|  |  | Question 2: Tubal ligation if reversible | |
|---|---|---|---|
|  |  | Yes | No |
| Question 1: Tubal ligation if nonreversible | Yes | a = number saying yes to both questions<br>Total: 2 | b = number saying yes to Q. 1, but no to Q. 2<br>Total: 0 |
|  | No | c = number saying no to Q. 1, but yes to Q. 2<br>Total: 3 | d = number saying no to both questions<br>Total: 5 |

## ANALYSIS OF VARIANCE (ANOVA)

ANOVA can be used to test for the existence of differences among the means of more than two samples. In fact the *t*-distribution used for testing the difference between two means is a special case of the *F*-distribution used in ANOVA. ANOVA can indicate whether more detailed testing of pairs of means is necessary. In this respect it is like a chi-square, since it is a *screening* test which may be used to determine whether *any* two means are different, in a situation where the null hypothesis is stated as follows:

$$H_0 : \mu_1 = \mu_2 = \mu_3 = \mu_4 = \ldots \mu_n$$

As implied by its name, ANOVA is based on sample variances, rather than on means and standard errors, although means are being compared. The present discussion can only serve as an introduction to this powerful statistical method. A thorough understanding of the method is fundamental to experimental design and provides insight into the nature of variation. Readers interested in experimental research are encouraged to pursue this method in detail.

## BASIC CONCEPTS

The data in Table 26-6 are the weights of rabbits in the five experimental groups from Data Set 2. The calculated means look somewhat different, but the researcher wants to test whether any of these means are significantly different, statistically. The "analysis of variance" will conclude that *any two* are different if the variability of the means is *substantially* greater than the variability of the individual observations from which the means were computed. The ratio of these two variabilities is the calculated *F*-ratio, and whether or not

the ratio is "substantial" is determined by comparing the results to the *F* table of Appendix 2-4. The theory and method of this determination is discussed below. Actually, the *F*-ratio is the ratio of two population variances which, if they are equal, will be close to a value of 1.0.

If it is assumed that all populations from which these samples are derived have the same variance, it is possible to derive *two* independent estimates of this common variance. One estimate is based on a weighted average of the variances within each of the separate samples. That is, each sample variance is computed separately, and the estimate of the common variance is a weighted average of the separate variances. This is called the *variance within groups*. The second estimate of the common variance is based on the variance of the separate sample means treated as individual variates. This is called the *variance between or among groups* multiple by the sample size. Since $SE = \sigma_{\bar{X}} = \dfrac{\sigma_X}{\sqrt{n}}$, then $n\sigma_{\bar{X}}^2$ would give an estimate of the common variance, $\sigma_X$, the numerator of the *F* formula.

The basic question in ANOVA is whether these two independent estimates of the common variance are, in fact, estimates of the same parameter. If the within-group and between-group variances are both estimating the same parameter, a ratio in the form of

$$\frac{\text{between-group variance}}{\text{within-group variance}}$$

should be approximately unity, or one. If the between-group variance is large, due to differences between the means, the ratio will be greater than one. This ratio is a statistic called *F*, and its sampling distribution (i.e., the theoretical probability distribution) has been worked out, and is presented as the *F*-distribution in Appendix 2-4.

**Table 26–6. Weights of Rabbits per Dosage-level Group**

| Group 1 (2.5 mg./kg. THC) | Group 2 (1.25 mg./kg. THC) | Group 3 (0.612 mg./kg. THC) | Group 4 (0.306 mg./kg. THC) | Group 5 (Control) |
|---|---|---|---|---|
| 2.9 | 3.0 | 3.8 | 3.9 | 2.6 |
| 3.2 | 2.9 | 2.8 | 3.4 | 3.0 |
| 3.5 | 2.8 | 2.9 | 3.5 | 2.6 |
| 2.8 | 3.6 | 3.0 | 2.8 | 2.9 |
| 2.7 | 3.4 | 3.1 | 3.7 | 3.0 |
| 3.0 | 3.1 | 2.6 | 2.9 | 3.1 |
| Mean: 3.01 | 3.13 | 3.03 | 3.36 | 2.87 |
| Grand   mean: 3.08 | | | | |

## THE *F*-DISTRIBUTION

The shape of the *F*-distribution is determined by *two* values for the degrees of freedom, designated as $V_1$ and $V_2$. For every possible combination of these two degrees of freedom, each of which can range from one to infinity, there is a separate *F*-distribution. The degrees of freedom pertain to the numerator and denominator of the variance ratio. Thus in ANOVA, $V_1$ is the degrees of freedom for the between-group variance and $V_2$ is the degrees of freedom for the within-group variance.

The degrees of freedom for variation between groups depends only on the number of groups. If the number of groups (samples) is designated as *k*, the *df* among (between) groups is simply $(k - 1)$. The degrees of freedom *within* groups depend on both the number of groups and their sample size (*n*). The *df* for within groups is $k(n - 1)$, if the sample size is equal for all groups.

## THE HYPOTHESES TESTED IN ANOVA

The null hypothesis in utilizing the *F*-statistic is that the two variances estimate the same parametric variance. This will show up as true in the *F* ratio if the population means are equal. The alternate hypothesis in ANOVA is always that the variance estimated among (between) groups is greater than the variance estimated within groups. This is expected, if random samples are derived from a population with unequal means.

Since the alternate hypothesis is directional in terms of between- and within-group variances, the test of the null hypothesis is one-tailed in ANOVA and the *F*-distribution, although the alternate hypothesis about the means is nondirectional.

## COMPUTATION OF *F*

Computation of *F* by hand is tedious, especially when sample sizes in each group differ. The reader should consult an analysis of variance text for computational formulas. *F* can be computed much more easily by the computer, and statistical programs for computer computation are readily available, so the present discussion will be limited to using the output from such programs.

*F* is the ratio between two independent estimates of variance; the estimates are based on the sum of squared deviations from the mean. The total variation of all variates can be expressed in terms of squared deviations from the grand mean; that is

$$\sum_{i=1}^{n} (X_i - \bar{X})^2$$

which is called the *total variation,* or *total sum of squares.* This total variation is divided into two parts. The sum of squared deviations of individual scores from their own group mean is the *within sum of squares.* A measure of variability among samples, involving the deviations of group means from the grand mean, is called the *between sum of squares.* These three sums of squares (total, between, and within) are included in an ANOVA table as output from statistical programs.

The variance estimated from within and between groups is based on the appropriate sum of squares divided by their respective degrees of freedom provided in the ANOVA table. The resulting estimates are not called variances in ANOVA: they are called *mean squares.* The sums of squares and mean squares are frequently abbreviated as *SS* and *MS,* respectively. The mean squares are the important numbers because the calculated *F*-statistic is the ratio

$$\frac{MS_{\text{between}}}{MS_{\text{within}}}$$

and is the value compared with a defined critical region of the *F*-distribution, with between degrees of freedom in the numerator and within degrees of freedom in the denominator.

## EXAMPLES

It is now possible to follow the steps for hypothesis testing. The first example is based on the data in Table 26-6. The researcher wants to test for differences in rabbits' weights among groups.

**Step 1.** The null hypothesis is that the population means are equal. As discussed, the alternate hypothesis for ANOVA is always that the parametric variance estimated by between-group variance is greater than that estimated by within-group variance. If the null hypothesis is rejected, groups cannot be considered samples from the same population. This indicates that any of the multiple means could be different.

**Table 26–7. Analysis-of-variance Table for Weights of Different Groups of Rabbits (from Data Set 2)**

| Effect | df | SS | MS |
|---|---|---|---|
| Between levels | 4 | 0.820000 | 0.205000 |
| Error, or "within" | 25 | 2.941667 | 0.117667 |
| Total | 29 | 3.761667 | |

F-ratio   1.742209632

**Table 26–8. Mean Number of Implantations per Dosage-level Group**

| Dosage | Mean implantations | Sample size |
|---|---|---|
| High (1.25–2.5 mg./kg.) (Group 1) | 0.83 | 12 |
| Medium (0.306–0.612 mg./kg.) (Group 2) | 6.42 | 12 |
| None (Group 3) | 7.67 | 6 |

**Step 2.** The statistical model assumes normal populations for each group, with equal population variances. In conjunction with the null hypothesis of equal population means, the method thus assumes that groups are from the same population. $F$ is the sampling distribution.

**Step 3.** In order to define the critical region, the degrees of freedom must be calculated for between- and within-group variances. Since the sample size in each group is equal, the within-$df$ is $5(6 - 1) = 25$ and the between-$df$ is $(5 - 1) = 4$. The significance level ($\alpha$) is selected as 0.05. The critical $F$ with 4 and 25 $df$ at the 0.05 level (written as $F_{0.05(4,25)}$) is obtained from the table (Appendix 2-4) as 2.76, although the number had to be interpolated with the information given in Appendix 2-4. This means that values of $F_{(4,25)} \geq 2.76$ have a probability associated with their occurrence of 0.05 or less.

**Step 4.** Table 26–7 presents the ANOVA table for the weights of the five groups of rabbits. The $F$-ratio is 1.74, which is less than the table $F$ of 2.76.

**Step 5.** The null hypothesis of equal sample means is accepted. Therefore the weights can be considered equivalent for the rabbits in each of the groups under study.

Another example illustrates the importance of ANOVA to experimental design. Experiments are performed when it is suspected that some treatment will have an effect on a variable. In terms of within- and between-roup variance, experiments are designed to deliberately inflate between-group variation. Inflation will result if there is increased variation between group means, due to treatment effects. The $F$-test is used to evaluate the statistical significance of treatment effects. For example, Table 26–8 gives the mean number of implantations for each of three dosage groups in Data Set 2. The question is whether the drug (the treatment) has resulted in shifting the mean number of implantations sufficiently so that the three groups can no longer be considered samples from the same population.

The ANOVA table for these data is presented in Table 26–9. The $F$-ratio is calculated as 12.28. From the $F$-distribution, the following values are obtained:

$$F_{0.05(2,27)} = 3.41; F_{0.01(2,27)} = 5.49$$

Thus the probability of obtaining a calculated $F$-statistic of 12.28 when the null hypothesis is true is less than 0.01. The large $F$-ratio indicates that at least one of the groups is different, but further analysis is necessary in order to determine which group or groups show the treatment effect. Such a test will be discussed in the next paragraph.

## A POSTERIORI TESTS

Additional analysis suggested by the result of a completed experiment is termed *a posteriori*, or *unplanned*. There are several methods for testing differences between two groups after ob-

**Table 26–9. Analysis-of-variance Table for Number of Implantations in Three Different Groups of Rabbits (from Data Set 2)**

| Effect | df | SS | MS |
|---|---|---|---|
| Between levels | 2 | 265.443270 | 132.721635 |
| Error | 27 | 291.910983 | 10.811518 |
| Total | 29 | 557.354253 | |

F-ratio   12.27594832

The table value of $F$ for computung FSD = 3.41

Means 1 and 2 differ by −5.583; Scheffe's *FSD* is 3.500; *t*-test is −4.159*

Means 1 and 3 differ by −6.833; Scheffe's *FSD* is 4.287; *t*-test is −4.156*

Means 2 and 3 differ by −1.250; Scheffe's *FSD* is 4.287; *t*-test is −0.760

* Significant

taining a significant $F$ in ANOVA. One method is Scheffe's Fully Significant Difference (*FSD*). The *FSD* between the means of groups $i$ and $j$ is

$$FSD = \left( \sqrt{(\text{Between } df) \times F_{\text{within } df}^{\text{between } df}} \right) \times \left( \sqrt{MSE \times (1/n_i + 1/n_j)} \right) \quad (23)$$

where $n_i$ = number of observations in group $i$ and

$n_j$ = number of observations in group $j$ and

$MSE = MS_{\text{within}}$

This *FSD* is the difference between means $i$ and $j$ that would give a statistical difference. The $F$-value for a selected significance level ($\alpha$) with the between and within $df$ given in the ANOVA table is obtained from the $F$-distribution. The $df$-between and $MS$-within (mean square within) are also obtained from the ANOVA table. The mean square within is sometimes called the *mean-square error,* and abbreviated as *MSE*. The number of variates ($n$) for groups $i$ and $j$ is obtained from the original data.

Each group mean is compared with every other group mean in terms of the *absolute difference between means*. If the absolute difference between two means is *greater* than the *FSD* for the two groups, the two means are statistically different at the alpha level selected for $F$.

To examine which groups showed a treatment effect in Table 26-9, the group-1 mean is compared to the group-2 mean, the group-1 mean is compared to the group-3 mean, and the group-2 mean is compared to the group-3 mean. The absolute differences between the means and the *FSD* for each comparison are given in Table 26-9, along with the analysis-of-variance table. There it can be seen that groups 2 and 3 are very similar, but group 1 is

definitely different from groups 2 or 3. Apparently the dosage of THC above 1.25 mg./kg. has a definite impact on reducing the number of implantations of corpora lutea in rabbits. Scheffe's is a very conservative test. If it indicates a difference, then, a true difference assuredly exists. Table 26-9 also has the regular $t$ test results, which agree with the conclusions of Scheffe's test in this instance. At times, however, the $t$ test may show a difference when Scheffe's does not. In that circumstance it is best to report both results. If the routine $t$ test of the difference between two means is used for comparisons, the desired level of alpha should be divided by the *between*-levels degrees of freedom, with the $t$ table degrees of freedom the same as the within or error degrees of freedom in the ANOVA table.

Many other types of useful ANOVA procedures are available. When two different factors are possibly related to the level of a measurement of a variable, a two-way analysis of variance can be performed to determine which factor has the greatest influence on the variable under disussion. When more than two factors are involved, $N$-way analysis of variance can help to determine *interactions* that can occur between the various levels of the factors. For example, if the number of implantations in a rabbit were affected by both weight and level of THC dosage given experimentally, it *may* be possible that the relationship is particularly strong, or even in the opposite direction, when a selected dosage is given to an animal of a certain weight. If this were the case, it is said that *interaction* has occurred.

These other methods of ANOVA are not discussed in detail here because the authors feel that many of the applications that are done with ANOVA can be done equally well with regression analysis, which is the topic of the next chapter.

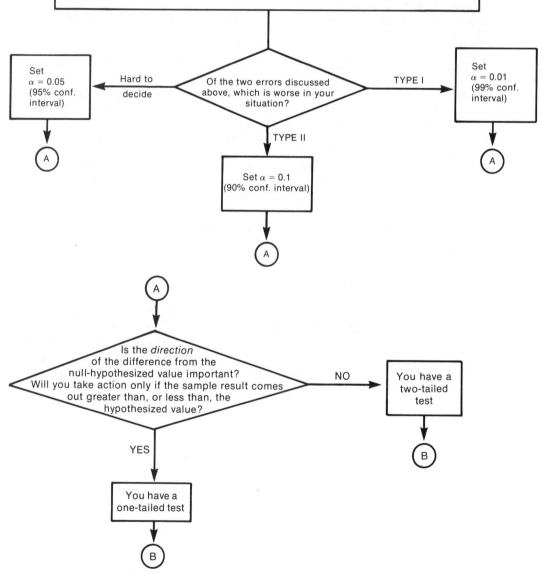

**FIG. 26-2.** Hypothesis test flowchart (using confidence intervals).

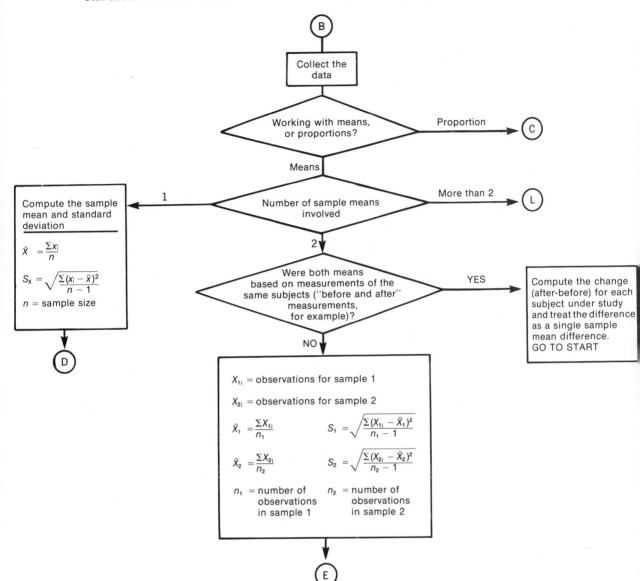

**FIG. 26–2.** (*Continued*)

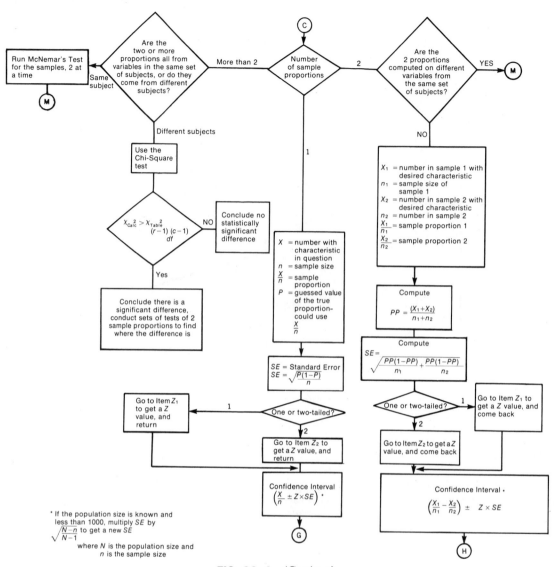

FIG. 26–2. (*Continued*)

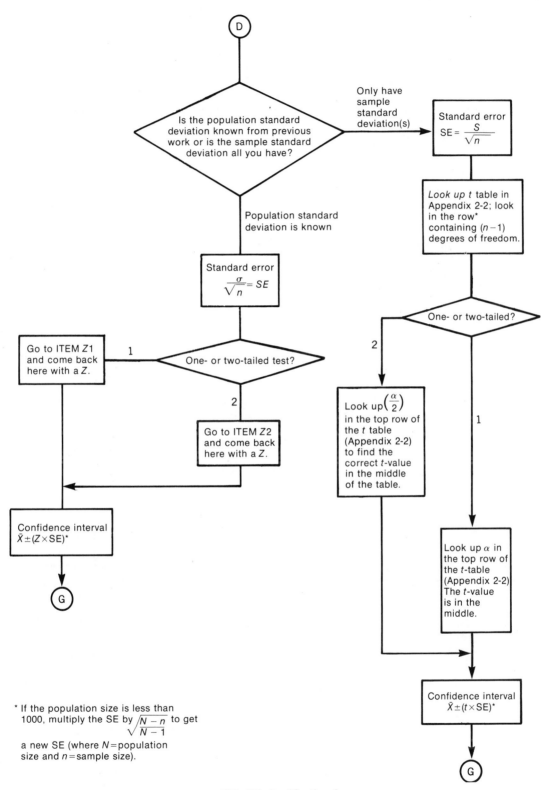

**FIG. 26–2.** (*Continued*)

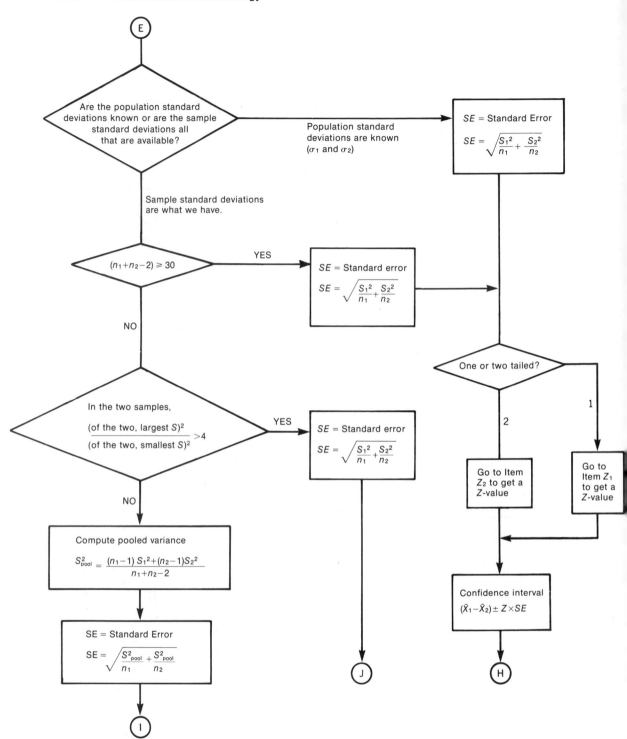

**FIG. 26–2.** (*Continued*)

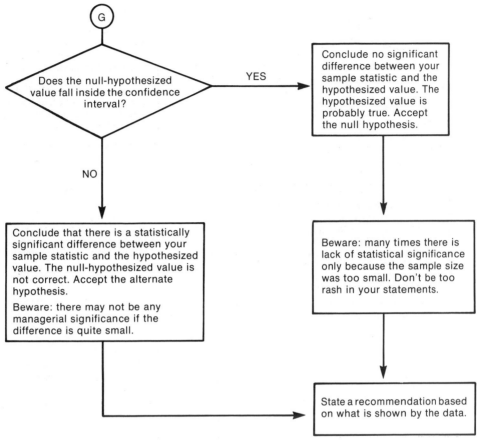

**FIG. 26–2.** (*Continued*)

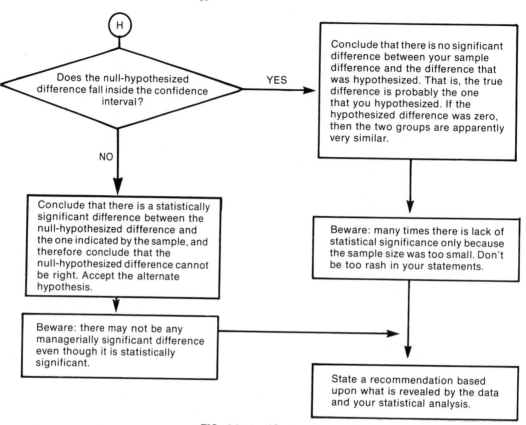

FIG. 26-2. (*Continued*)

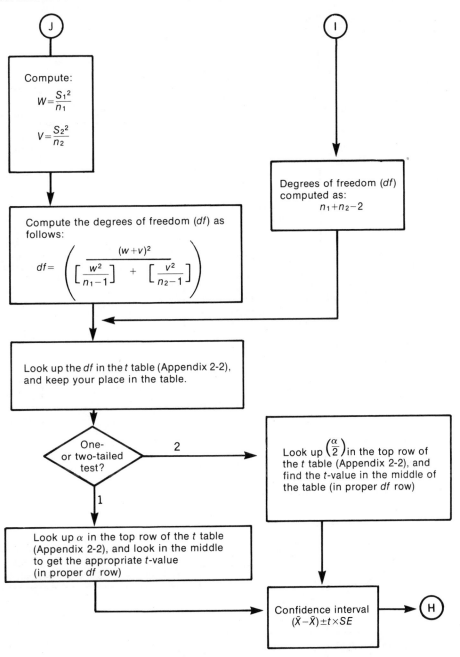

**FIG. 26-2.** (*Continued*)

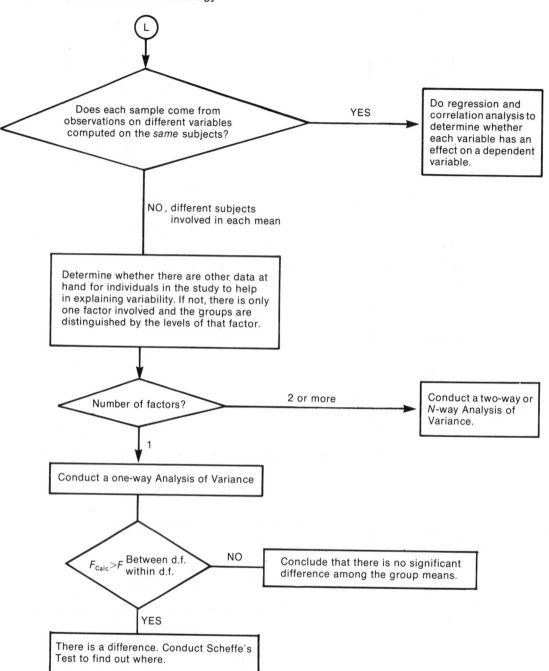

**FIG. 26–2.** (*Continued*)

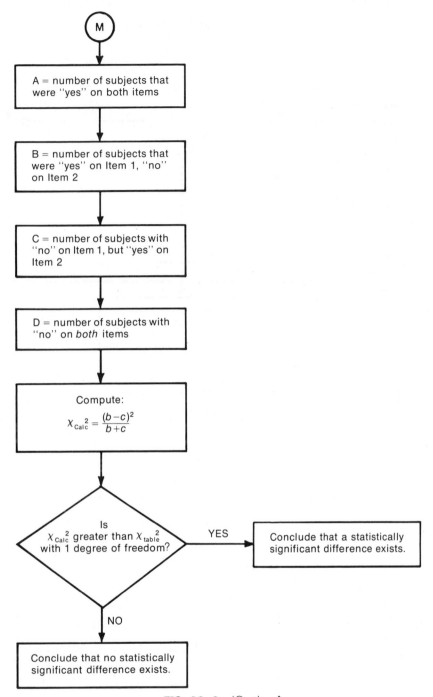

**FIG. 26–2.** (*Continued*)

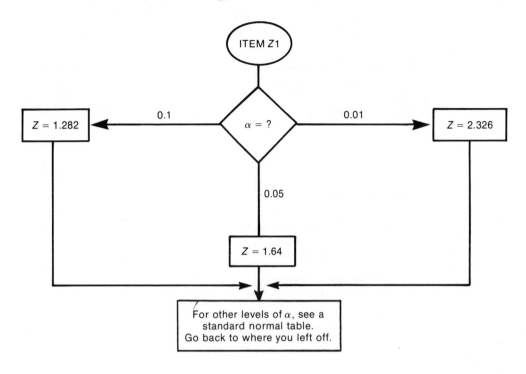

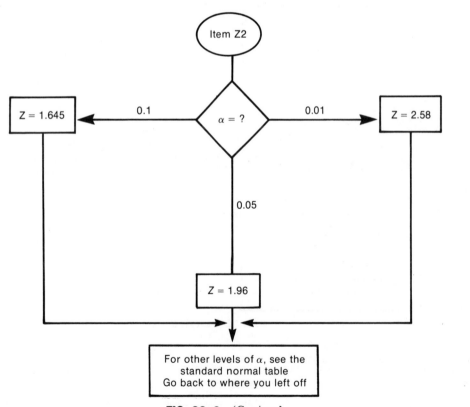

**FIG. 26–2.** (*Continued*)

# 27

# Regression and
# Time Series Analysis

## Harold D. Dickson

This chapter provides the methods for answering the following two questions posed in Chapter 25:

1. How can the independent impact of several variables potentially affecting experimental results be determined with the use of multiple regression analysis?

2. How can future family planning clinic activity be predicted from historical data with the use of *time series analysis* (sometimes called *trend analysis*)?

Most business statistics textbooks discuss the theory of these two procedures in detail, and the reader should refer to such texts for the theoretical explanations. This chapter will emphasize the step-by-step application to family planning problems. The general concept of correlations and regression is presented first, followed by a generalized discussion of the detailed steps which are taken when working with a set of data and utilizing a computer program which will calculate correlation and regression coefficients. Some readers may prefer to begin with the section entitled "Examples of Multiple Linear Regression" (p. 389). The generalized discussion does not contain examples, because a reader with a set of data can easily follow the steps and obtain assistance with the interpretation of the data without having to read all of the examples.

## REGRESSION ANALYSIS

The variable being studied, or outcome variable (such as number of implantations or cor-

pora lutea in rabbits) is called the *dependent variable (DV)*; other variables that may be related to implantations are called the *experimental* or *independent variables (IV)*.

Many factors besides the variable being experimentally varied can affect the outcome of an experiment. In the laboratory, those factors are controlled to the maximum extent possible. However, because it is not always possible to exert full control, mathematical methods are utilized to determine the extent to which the factors of interest affect the outcome variable. For example, a researcher may want to determine how the number of implantations of corpora lutea (the outcome variable in Data Set 2, Chap. 25) could be related to several other factors, such as the rabbit's weight, room temperature, dosage level of a drug given to the rabbit prior to mating, etc. In this case, the appropriate data should be collected for each animal, and a multiple-regression computer program utilized.

In general, regression analysis is used when a dependent variable could be affected by several factors, and a change in any of the latter could result in change in that dependent variable. Once the factors are identified, an equation is developed through which the impact of changing the level of a single independent variable can be assessed. For example, assume that income per capita, fertility rate, and charges per clinic visit may affect number of monthly visits, and that a given clinic is considering raising fees. Under these circumstances it would be advisable to first establish the impact of fees on clinic use, including the actual decrease in visits resulting from increased charges, if income per capita remained constant.

For this type of problem, i.e., one in which the variable of interest is potentially affected by several factors simultaneously, there are two reasons why regression analysis is preferable to individual significance tests between means. First, if there are many sources of variability a true difference in the *DV* caused by a particular *IV* may be obscured in a simple *t*-test because of high, unexplained variation of the *DV* values. Second, the regression will provide an equation which relates values of the *IV* to the values of the *DV*.

Regression is related to correlation (which is discussed in more detail later in the chapter) in the following way: correlation indicates that two variables are related, and the strength of that relationship, whereas regression provides an equation describing the relationship. For example:

clinic visits per month = 100 − 1.5 (charge per visit)

The equation is more difficult to compute than the correlation. If a correlation indicates that no relationship exists, then the need for obtaining the equation is eliminated.

The existence of a linear relationship or association may not imply causation. For example, knowledge that clinic visits are highest during odd months (hypothetically) may help predict future monthly visits. This, however, does not mean that month number *causes* changes in clinic use. Questions of causality cannot be solved by statistical methods alone.

Before proceeding to simple and multiple regression, it is also necessary to differentiate such methods from *discriminant function analysis.* When the dependent variable is nominal data rather than measurement data, the appropriate technique is *classification analysis,* as opposed to regression analysis. In classification analysis, the effort is to determine ways to classify subjects into two or more groups, based on various *IVs,* but in regression analysis a specific value of the *DV* is predicted, using the formula and a knowledge of the value of the *IV*. A subset of classification analysis, *discriminant function analysis,* is used when the dependent variable has only two categories, as in the depressed clinic manager case (Data Set 1, Chap. 25). Here each patient either continued or discontinued the clinic after a certain period. Although this variable could be transformed into measurement data by collecting new observations indicating the length of time a patient received services, the data in question is nominal. When only two categories are present, discriminant function analysis is the appropriate technique to distinguish the dropouts from the continuing patients. As will be described later, this technique can be approximated with the use of multiple regression analysis.

## BASIC CONCEPTS AND DEFINITIONS

The concept and method of simple and multiple linear regression will be discussed and will then be illustrated with the sample data sets. Because regression programs are readily available, computational formulas are not presented.

### SIMPLE LINEAR REGRESSION

A set of data collected on two different variables from the same set of subjects can be plotted on a graph, as shown in Figure 27-1. If the dots (each dot represents each subject in the study) can be connected with a straight line, it is called a perfect linear relationship. Establishing such a relationship is useful because a formula can easily be produced, so that other values of the independent variable could be translated with great certainty into a predicted value of the dependent variable. Also, in a linear relationship a one-unit increase of the independent variable will cause the same change in the dependent variable, irrespective of the value of the independent variable. The amount of this change is reflected in the slope, or steepness, of the straight line.

The concept of a linear relationship (or straight line) can best be explained by considering a situation with a single independent variable. The concept of a *simple* (single independent variable) linear equation is that of a *straight*-line graph illustrating the relationship between a dependent and an independent variable. The *simple linear* equation, as graphically illustrated in Figure 27-1, has the following components:

1. A *dependent* variable which is shown graphically as the vertical axis. This is labeled *Y*.
2. An *independent* variable which is shown graphically as the horizontal axis. This is termed *X*.
3. The *Y intercept,* denoted as *a,* the value of

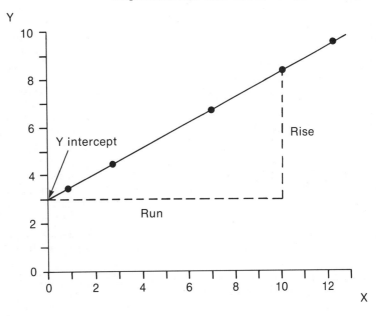

**FIG. 27-1.** The graph of a simple linear relationship.

which is the location of the line on the $Y$ axis when $X = 0$.

4. A *slope*, denoted as *b*, which indicates the extent to which the dependent variable $Y$ would rise when the independent variable, $X$, increases by one unit.

The slope is a measure of the steepness of a straight-line relationship. If both the vertical and horizontal axes were identically scaled (same units), a slope of 1 would indicate a line with a 45° angle passing through the point where $X$ and $Y$ both equal zero.

Given a straight-line graph, the slope can be determined by starting at the $Y$ intercept, and running a dotted line to the right which is parallel to the horizontal axis. The dotted line can be extended any distance to the right, but for ease of computation, 10 units (on the horizontal axis) is suggested (see Fig. 27-1). The dotted line is then extended upward (if the relationship is positive) until it touches the line indicating the slope. The distance the line was extended upward or downward is determined in terms of the units on the $Y$, or vertical, axis. This distance is called the *rise*. The distance extended to the right from the $Y$ intercept is called the *run*. The slope is then computed as the rise over the run, or *rise/run*. If the graph line slopes downward, the rise would be negative, and the slope therefore negative, because

as you run out to the right, you must *fall* to hit the graph. A fall is the same as a negative rise.

In the graph in Figure 27-1, the run is 10 units, the rise is 5 units, and the slope is $5/10 = 0.5$. Since the $Y$ intercept is 3, the linear equation for the line graphed is:

$$Y = a + bX$$
$$Y = 3 + 0.5X$$

This means that when $X$ is 0, $Y$ is 3, and every unit increase in the value of variable $X$ would be associated with a 0.5 unit increase in the variable $Y$. It also means that if any value of the variable $X$ is inserted into the formula, the predicted value of the variable $Y$ could be computed by multiplying the chosen value of $X$ by 0.5 and adding that result to the number 3.

If the coordinates of the dots shown on the straight line were input data for a computer regression program, the printout would provide the $Y$ intercept and the slope as the "regression coefficients." Ordinarily, however, the data collected from a research experiment or operating clinic, when plotted on an $X, Y$ axis does not form a perfectly straight line. It appears more like the *scatter diagram* shown in Figure 27-2. In this case, the regression program would provide the intercept and slope for a straight line which passes through the

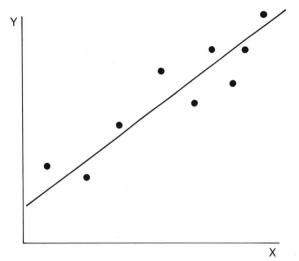

**FIG. 27–2.** Scatter diagram in which the *X, Y* dots do not form a straight line.

dots in such a way that the vertical distances between the dots and the line are minimized (see Fig. 27-2). More accurately, the sum of the squared differences betweeen the dots and the line is minimized; therefore, regression is called the *method of least squares*. When the dots are scattered and do not form a straight line, a measure of the extent to which there is something close to a linear relationship is needed. The correlation coefficient and the coefficient of determination discussed later in this chapter fulfill this need.

**MULTIPLE LINEAR REGRESSION**

In general, multiple linear regression provides equations when there is more than one independent variable, each of which is related in a linear fashion to the dependent variable. The following equation with 2 independent variables is an example of a multiple regression equation:

$$Y = a + (bX) + (cZ)$$

where *Y* is the dependent variable and *X* and *Z* are the independent variables. Any number of independent variables can be included, provided there are at least 3 times as many observations per variable as there are variables.

    *a* is the *Y* intercept (a number to be estimated by the regression equation). Sometimes this is called the *constant*.

*b* and *c* represent the regression coefficients (numbers that will be computed by the regression program in the computer).

The coefficient *b* is the change in variable *Y* that would be associated with a one-unit change in variable *X*, other things (namely, variable *Z*) considered and held constant. This allows analysis of the independent impact of a selected independent variable. The coefficient *c* is the change in variable *Y* that would be associated with a one-unit change in variable *Z*, when variable *X* is held constant.

The general form shown above is *linear*. The equation with multiple independent variables, such as *X* and *Z*, is developed in such a way that if the original *X* and *Z* values were put into the formula, the *Y* values predicted by the formula $(\hat{Y})$ would closely approximate the original *Y* values in the data set. As in the case of simple linear regression, the sum of the squared deviations of the actual values minus the predicted values for each subject in the original data set are minimized. The data for the *independent variables* may be either interval measurements or nominal categories. If the data are nominal, the variable is converted to a set of zeroes and ones, and called *dummy variables*. For further discussion, see the section entitled "Dummy Variables."

**STEP-BY-STEP PROCEDURES FOR COMPUTER ANALYSIS**

Given a dependent variable and associated independent variables for each subject in the study, the following steps are taken:

**STEP 1**

The data are obtained and prepared in a format acceptable for the computer program being used. The data for a regression must contain variability, so that a meaningful mathematical relationship may be derived. Such variability can be obtained in a *cross-sectional* manner by examining different persons, experimental animals, or different clinics at a given point in time or *longitudinally* (using the *timeseries* approach) by examining the same facility, person, or animal over a period of time, with the differing years, months, or days, etc., providing the variability. In the "high" rabbit study of Chapter 25, the data are cross-sectional, since each observation represents a different animal; the crystal-ball gazer study of Chapter 25 presents timeseries data, since each observation is the number of clinic visits for each succeeding quarter of the year.

The dependent variable, such as number of implantations per rabbit, may be stored in any order. The observations, or variates (individual measurements) are obtained for independent variables that are assumed to be involved. When these variates are stored, they are entered as an array of data in the same order as their corresponding dependent variate. If values for independent variates are missing, there are two possibilities:

1. If less than 20 per cent of the observations are missing, the average of the other variates for that variable is inserted for the missing data.
2. If more than 20 per cent are missing, the independent variable generally cannot be used in estimating a regression equation. However, where a large number (such as eight times the number of independent variables) of observations are available for all variables, but more than 20 per cent are missing from a specific variable, the individual cases with missing data can be eliminated, and the program run, as long as the eliminated cases were not biased in some regard.

**STEP 2**

A *correlation matrix,* with all the variables (dependent and independent) listed both down the side and (in the same order) across the top, is obtained which contains coefficients showing the correlation between any two variables under consideration. This helps in preselecting the independent variables to be utilized in a regression equation. An example of such a matrix is shown in Table 27-5.

A *correlation coefficient* is a statistic which measures the strength of the linear relationship between two variables. A correlation coefficient of +1.0 indicates a perfectly positive linear relationship between two variables. That is, whenever the value of one variable increases, the value of the other *always* increases by a specified amount. A correlation coefficient of −1.0 indicates a perfectly inverse linear relationship. Whenever the value of one variable increases, the value of the other always declines by a specified amount. A coefficient of zero indicates no linear relationship. A correlation coefficient that is close to zero but greater than zero by an amount that is statistically significant indicates a relationship that is less well supported by the data (see Appendix 2-5 for a table of significant correlations, given the sample size). The graphs in Figure 27-3 illustrate the scatter diagram for each of the correlations mentioned above.

A *correlation matrix* contains the correlation coefficients for all the variables in the study, compared two at a time (see Table 27-5 for the example). It is advisable to construct the matrix so that the dependent variable is in the top row and first column and the independent variables are in the other rows and columns. The matrix format assists the researcher to determine which independent variables are most highly correlated with the dependent variable and thus most appropriately used in the equation. This avoids inserting data unrelated to the dependent variable into a regression equation. Table 27-1 contains the format of such a matrix, but the correlation values are replaced by small letters to facilitate discussion and generalize the results.

The variables in Table 27-1 appear in the same order in the rows (down the left-hand side) as in the columns (across the top). The correlation coefficients on the diagonal are 1.0, because they represent the correlation of a variable to itself. Since the rows and columns have the same variables, the correlation coefficients are repeated above and below the diagonal. Some matrices, therefore, only provide the coefficients that are above the diagonal of ones.

In Table 27-1 the dependent variable ($DV$) is in the first row and column. The matrix is used as explained in the following steps, but the explanation is given in very general terms. Reading with a precise example in mind (such as Table 27-5) will help in understanding the process. The purpose of steps 1 and 2 is to select, from a large list of possible independent variables, those that should be used in a regression equation. The concept is to select independent variables which relate strongly to the dependent variable, but do not correlate strongly with each other.

1. The correlations (one variable at a time) of each of the independent variables ($IV$) to the dependent variable ($DV$) are reviewed.

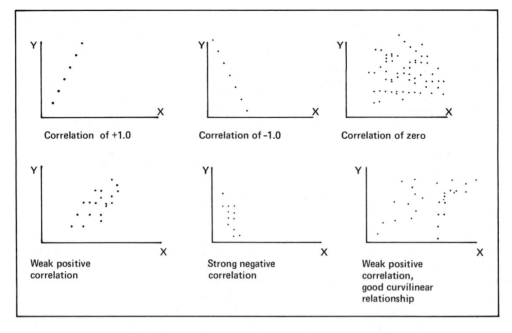

**FIG. 27–3.** Scatter diagram for various correlation coefficients.

These correlations are represented in Table 27-1 by *b*, *c*, and *d.* If any of the *IV*s are weakly correlated (closer to zero than +1 or −1) with the *DV*, they should be dropped from consideration, because they probably have very little impact on the dependent variable. The correlation can be considered low if it does not pass the statistical tests for correlation shown in Appendix 2-5. The values in the appendix show the correlation coefficients needed, given the number of observations in any one variable, to be statistically greater than zero. Generally, an

absolute value of 0.4, or higher, is desired. However, if there are more than 200 observations per variable, a 0.2 may be statistically greater than zero (but still low). In the discussion that follows, the absolute value of the correlation is considered, regardless of sign. All that the sign indicates is whether the linear relationship is positive (upsloping) or negative (inverse, or downsloping).

2. After determining which *IV*s are highly correlated with the *DV*, independent variables are reviewed for correlation with one another. These correlations are represented in Table 27-1 by *e, f,* and *g.* Those which are highly intercorrelated are eventually eliminated. To do this, the two independent variables which are most highly correlated with the dependent variable are first compared. If the correlation *between the two IVs* is equal to, or greater than the correlation of either *IV* to the *DV*, the *IV* with the lowest correlation to the *DV* should be deleted. If the correlation of the two *IV*s is within 0.1 correlation units of the correlation of either *IV* with the *DV*, the deletion of that *IV* with the lowest correlation to the *DV* should be seriously considered.

**Table 27–1. Generalized Correlation Matrix For Use in Explaining the Selection of Independent Variables in Regression Analysis**

|      | DV  | IV1 | IV2 | IV3 |
| ---- | --- | --- | --- | --- |
| DV   | 1.0 | b   | c   | d   |
| IV1  | b   | 1.0 | e   | f   |
| IV2  | c   | e   | 1.0 | g   |
| IV3  | d   | f   | g   | 1.0 |

Key:

DV = The dependent variable
IV1 = The 1st independent variable
IV2 = The 2nd independent variable
IV3 = The 3rd independent variable

If the intercorrelation between the two *IV*s is more than 0.1 correlation units lower than the correlation of either *IV* with the *DV*, then both *IV*s can enter the equation. This process is continued until every pair of *IV*s is compared.

In the generalized correlation matrix of Table 27-1, assume that correlations *b* and *c* were high (with *b* highest), but *d* was very low. Variable *IV3* would be dropped immediately, since *d* is very low (0.01, for example). Before considering both *IV1* and *IV2* as independent variables, intercorrelation *e* should be checked. If *e* is low, both *IV1* and *IV2* should be considered as independent variables, and if *e* is higher than either *b* or *c*, then *IV2* would definitely be dropped from further consideration, since the correlation of *DV* and *IV2* was assumed to be highest of *b* and *c*. However, if *e* is close (within 0.1 units) to *b* or *c*, then the procedure is less clear; in this case it is suggested that *IV2* be dropped from consideration.

The use of intercorrelated independent variables in the regression equations is discouraged, because it is impossible to determine the independent impact of either one. However, rather than deleting two intercorrelated variables completely, it is possible to add or multiply them, and include them in the equation as a composite variable. This completes the process of selecting the independent variables to be included in the analysis.

### STEP 3

The regression program is used. In order to do so, the following information must be provided:

The *number of observations*. This refers to the number of observations (also called cases, or variates) in each variable. The case is the unit of analysis which provides the variability among the numbers in the variable.

The *number of independent variables*. This refers to the count of all the *IV*s that will be entered (as determined through analyzing the correlation matrix).

## INTERPRETATION OF REGRESSION RESULTS

The output of the computer program should include the following information:

### REGRESSION COEFFICIENTS

Regression coefficients are the number values (either positive or negative) of *a*, *b*, and *c* in the formula $DV = a + (b\ IV1) + (c\ IV2)$. Sometimes the intercept (*a*) is provided in a separate location on the printout. Regression coefficients (*b* and *c*) are each multiplied by their respective *IV*. Each coefficient indicates the amount of change (positive or negative) in the *DV*, associated with a 1-unit increase in the *IV*, holding other *IV*s constant.

### STATISTICS

The calculated *t*-statistics are provided with the regression coefficients. They represent the number of standard errors the regression coefficient is away from zero. A regression coefficient of zero would indicate the lack of a relationship between that *IV* and the *DV* of interest. When the absolute value of this number (the calculated *t*, or "*t* calc") is greater than 1.6, it is concluded that the associated *IV* has a definite impact on the *DV*, regardless of the level of the other independent variables. The rule of thumb for a good *IV* is that the absolute value of *t* calc should be greater than 2. More precise criteria can be found in the *t*-table in Appendix 2-2 for a selected alpha (generally 0.05) and *n–k* degrees of freedom, where $n =$ number of observations per variable and $k =$ total number of variables in the equation, including the dependent variable.

If a *t* calc is less than 1.6, the *IV* associated with that *t* should be dropped from the equation, and the regression formula rerun without the associated *IV*. Some computer outputs provide only the standard error of the regression coefficients. In that case, the *t*-statistic can be computed by dividing the regression coefficient by the standard error. Often the *t* for the intercept will be low. This implies that the regression coefficient stated as the intercept is not statistically reliable, and, in fact, is probably zero. Most regression programs readily available on computers do not allow forcing of the intercept through the origin (zero), i.e., do not allow the researcher to solve the equation with intercept $a = 0$. Therefore, a low *t*-value for the intercept is ignored as long as there are good *t*-values for the rest of the *IV*s, and the intercept given is utilized to predict values, using the equation.

## THE COEFFICIENT OF DETERMINATION OR R² (R SQUARED)

The $R^2$, or coefficient of determination, indicates how well the formula fits the data. It is the proportion of variability in the $DV$ that is explained by the equation containing the $IVs$ under consideration. Most statisticians would consider the following grading scale for $R^2$:

$$0.90 \text{ and above} = A$$
$$0.80 \text{ through } 0.89 = B$$
$$0.70 \text{ through } 0.79 = C$$
$$0.60 \text{ through } 0.69 = D$$
$$\text{Below } 0.6 = F$$

In practice, in most social science research, a $R^2$ of 0.5 may be considered good. If $R^2$ is low, additional $IVs$ are needed to account for the variability of the $DV$. However, if $R^2$ is low but the $t$-values are good, the $IVs$, as a group, affect the $DV$, but the formula as a whole does not adequately explain any one individual observation or allow accurate prediction for any one case.

$R^2$ is computed by the following steps:

1. The standard deviation of the $DV$ is computed and squared to obtain the variance of the $DV$.
2. The *regression formula* is used to *predict DV* values, utilizing the same values of the $IV$ that were in the original data set.
3. The predicted values of the $DV$ are subtracted from the original data values. This set of number is called the *deviations*.
4. The deviations are squared to obtain the variance of the deviations.
5. The variance of the deviations is divided by the variance of the $DV$'s original values obtained in Step 1 above. This result is named the *proportion of unexplained variation*.
6. The proportion of unexplained variation is subtracted from 1 to obtain $R^2$.

The following formula illustrates the preceding steps, where $DV_i$ indicates an original observation of a dependent variable, $DVP_i$ indicates the predicted value of an observation of the dependent variable, $\overline{DV}$ is the average of all the observations in the dependent variable, and $DVP$ is the average of the predicted values:

$$R^2 = 1 - \frac{\sum_{i=1}^{n}(DV_i - DVP_i)^2}{\sum_{i=1}^{n}(DV_i - \overline{DV})^2}$$

### F-STATISTIC

Finally, the $F$-statistic is presented, to ensure that the $R^2$ is statistically reliable. If there are 10 observations and 10 $IVs$, an $R^2$ of 1.0 will result, but the formula is not reliable because the sample size available for each independent variable is too small for population inferences. An $F$-statistic, or "$F$ calc," is computed, to determine if $R^2$ is statistically greater than 0. $F$ calc is computed as follows:

$$F_{calc} = \frac{\left(\dfrac{R^2}{k-1}\right)}{\left(\dfrac{1-R^2}{n-k}\right)}$$

where n = number of observations per variable

k = number of variables in equation, including the $DV$

As a rule of thumb, when the $F$ is greater than 4, the sample size is assumed to be sufficiently large to substantiate that $R^2$ is truly greater than zero, given the number of $IVs$ in the equation. More precisely, the $F$ calc should be greater than $F$-table values with $k - 1$ and $n - k$ degrees of freedom (see Appendix 2-4), where $n$ = number of observations per variable and $k$ = total number of dependent and independent variables.

In summary, after deriving the regression equation, the following conditions should prevail to ensure a good equation:

1. $F_{calc} > 4$
2. $R^2$ high as possible ($> 0.9$ is optimal)
3. The absolute value of the $t$-statistics should be greater than 1.6, and preferably greater than 2.
4. If $F_{calc}$ is less than 4, more observations for each variable should be sought before a statistically reliable $R^2$ can be obtained, or, alternatively, some of the independent variables should be dropped.
5. If $R^2$ is low (0.5 and below), additional variables are needed before predictions can be made about specific individuals. How-

**Table 27-2. Example of the Creation of Dummy Variables**

| Person number | Code for contraceptive method used* | Dummy variables Oral contraceptives (OC) | IUD | Other (OT) |
|---|---|---|---|---|
| 1 | 1 | 1 | 0 | 0 |
| 2 | 1 | 1 | 0 | 0 |
| 3 | 2 | 0 | 1 | 0 |
| 4 | 3 | 0 | 0 | 1 |
| 5 | 2 | 0 | 1 | 0 |
| 6 | 3 | 0 | 0 | 1 |
| 7 | 3 | 0 | 0 | 1 |
| 8 | 1 | 1 | 0 | 0 |
| 9 | 2 | 0 | 1 | 0 |
| 10 | 1 | 1 | 0 | 0 |

* 1 = Oral contraceptive
2 = IUD
3 = Other

ever, if the $t_{calc}$ for each independent variable is greater than 1.6, then each of those independent variables does have an impact on the dependent variable. It's just that some other variable, currently unmeasured, may have a greater impact.

Before turning to examples, three other topics will be presented: dummy variables, discriminant analysis through regression, and curvilinear regression.

## DUMMY VARIABLES

When the data for one of the *IV*s is nominal, dummy variables should be created and used. A dummy variable is created by considering each possible category of a classification as a separate variable. When an individual unit of study (person, clinic, or animal) has the characteristic of the category, a one is inserted as the observation. When the unit of study does not have the characteristic, a zero is inserted; therefore, the observations for that *IV* consist only of zeros and ones. For example, in a hypothetical study of 10 persons using various contraceptive methods, the methods used were coded as: 1 = oral contraceptive, 2 = IUD, and 3 = other. If the coded observations were arrayed in a column, they would appear as illustrated in Table 27-2. The table indicates that the first two persons on the list are using oral contraceptives, the third is using an IUD, etc.

Table 27-2 illustrates that each of the dummy variables is comprised of zeros and ones. The set of dummy variables, rather than the original codes, is used as *IV*s in regression analysis. However, if there are *M* categories in the original variable, only $(M - 1)$ dummy variables need to be inserted in the regression equation. For example, the variable "method of contraception" would require two dummy variables, OC and IUD, or OC and OT, or IUD and OT. The effect of the nonselected category is provided by the regression equation intercept.

In a hypothetical study, the number of clinic visits (abbreviated CV) per person per year is the dependent variable. The independent variables include years of age (coded as AGE), which is a measurement variable, and two dummy variables indicating the family planning method (OC and IUD). In the regression equation [CV = 2 + 0.05 (AGE) + 1.5 (OC) − 0.2 (IUD)] the value of the $Y$ intercept of 2.0 would represent the number of visits if the value of all the independent variables were zero. Age would never be zero in a family planning clinic. If the average age (24) is considered, the average number of visits when OC and IUD are zero (which means that OT or "other" is the contraceptive method used, since it is the only dummy variable for *method* that has not been included in the equation), would be 2 + 0.05 (24) = 3.2 visits. Therefore persons using *other* methods of birth control have the formula [CV = 2 + 0.05 (AGE)], and when a person using *other* methods of birth control is of average age, the visits per year average 3.2.

Continuing with the equation [CV = 2.0 + 0.05 (AGE) + 1.5 (OC) − 0.2 (IUD)], it can be seen that a one-year increase in age means 0.05 more visits per year, other things being equal, because of the regression coefficient 0.05 along with the independent variable of age. Therefore persons who are 10 years older would have an average of 0.5 more visits per year, regardless of their contraceptive method.

The equation also shows that women using oral contraceptives (OC) have 1.5 more visits per year than those using other methods, and that persons who are using the IUD have an average of 0.2 fewer visits per year than those using methods other than the IUD.

## DISCRIMINANT ANALYSIS USING REGRESSION

Regression analysis may be used to predict into which of two groups an individual case will fall. When the *DV* is nominal, with a 2-category classification, a special type of dummy variable is created as the *DV*. Instead of zeros and ones, the observations become either $(+\frac{1}{n_1})$ or $(-\frac{1}{n_2})$, where $n_1$ is the number of persons in the data set having characteristic 1, and $n_2$ is the number of persons having characteristic 2. If the individual case has characteristic 1, the value for the *DV* becomes $(+\frac{1}{n_1})$ for that person. When the individual case has characteristic 2, the *DV* value becomes $(-\frac{1}{n_2})$. This differentiation may appear arbitrary, but discussion of its theoretical base is beyond the scope of this chapter. However, empirically, it has been shown to exert the maximum amount of discrimination. Multiple regression is conducted as already described. Those *IVs* with good *t*-statistics are the ones which help to distinguish between those units of analysis having characteristic 1 and characteristic 2. As an example, to determine the factors which independently distinguish clinic-continuing patients from those who drop out, characteristic 1 would be continuing, and characteristic 2, dropping out. Further, if 15 patients continued and 20 dropped out, the dependent variable would be constructed by inserting $(+\frac{1}{15})$ for every person who continued and a $(-\frac{1}{20})$ for every individual who dropped out.

The formula derived can be used in a predictive way to classify other individuals, provided the values of the relevant *IVs* (possibly age, ethnicity, etc.) for that individual are known. When used in this manner, the values of the *IV* are inserted in the formula and the predicted value of the *DV* computed. If the predicted value is higher than that value which is half the distance between $(+\frac{1}{n_1})$ and $(-\frac{1}{n_2})$ then that unit of analysis (person, clinic, animal) would be predicted to fall in Group 1. If lower, it would be predicted to fall in Group 2. Applying the formula to each unit in the original study would provide a set of predicted classifications. Those can be compared to the actual classifications to determine the equation's validity. A measure called *classification power* is computed by dividing the number of correct classifications provided by the formula by the total number of observations. To continue the previous example of continuing patients and dropouts, assume that the following formula were developed, based on 35 persons, (15 who continue and 20 who discontinue):

$$\begin{pmatrix} \text{Drop} \\ \text{or} \\ \text{Cont.} \end{pmatrix} = 0.05 + 0.001\,(\text{Age}) - 0.1 \begin{pmatrix} \text{Eth-} \\ \text{nicity} \end{pmatrix} - 0.003 \begin{pmatrix} \text{Ann.} \\ \text{Inc.} \end{pmatrix}$$

The data for age, ethnicity (a dummy variable where 1 = Anglo; 0 = other), and income for each person who dropped out are inserted into the formula, and a dropout or continuing value computed. If the result for that person is less than + 0.0085 (the number halfway between +1/15 or + 0.067 and −1/20 or − 0.05), then that person is *classified* as a dropout. The same procedure is completed for all those indi-

**Table 27–3. Example of Computing the Classification Power of a Discriminant Formula**

| Group the subject was actually in | Classification according to the formula | | Total in actual group |
|---|---|---|---|
| | Continuing patient | Dropped out | |
| Continuing patient | 10 | 5 | 15 |
| Dropped out | 8 | 12 | 20 |
| Total classified by formula to be in the group | 18 | 17 | 35 |

Classification power = percentage correctly classified
= [(10 + 12) ÷ 35] × 100% = 63%.

viduals who dropped out, to determine the formula's predictive accuracy. The results could be shown as depicted in Table 27-3. The classification power would then be

$$[(10 + 12) \div (35)] \times 100 = \frac{22}{35} \times 100 = 63\%$$

That is, individuals are correctly classified 63 per cent of the time, using the equation. This percentage of correct classifications can be compared to the expected correct classifications based on observed continuing and discontinuing patients in the sample. Since 15/35, or 43 per cent, continued and 20/35, or 57 per cent, discontinued, the expected correct classification by chance is

$$\frac{(0.43)(15) + (0.57)(20)}{35} \times 100\% = 51.1\%$$

Since 63 per cent correct classification by the regression equation is better than 51 per cent classification by chance, use of the equation is preferred.

## CURVILINEAR REGRESSION

Two variables may be related in a *curvilinear* manner, but the *linear* correlation or regression may appear very low (see Fig. 27-4). It is wise to plot a scatter diagram of the variables to explore the possibility of curvilinear relationships. If it seems likely that a curve is involved, the usual regression packages can still be employed.

There are three common formulas which can approximate a curve when there is a single independent variable. The first is

$$DV = a + b\,IV1 + c\,IV1^2 \qquad (1)$$

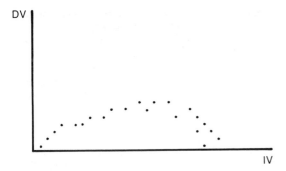

**FIG. 27–4.** Illustration of a good curvilinear relationship which would have a poor linear correlation.

This is a second-degree polynomial, and can be obtained by inserting two independent variables in the regression program. The second *IV* is the squared value of each observation of *IV1*. Coefficients *a*, *b*, and *c* are provided in the computer output.

The second equation is:

$$DV = a\,IV^b \qquad (2)$$

In order to determine the values of *a* and *b*, the natural logarithms of each observation of the *DV* must be calculated and entered as a new *DV* (*NDV*) for the regression program. Also the natural logarithms of the *IV* are computed (*NIV*) and entered into the regression. The results of the regression will be a formula, such as $NDV = A + b\,NIV$ or $(Ln\,DV = (Ln\,a) + b\,(Ln\,IV)$. The value of the regression coefficient (*b*) for *NIV* is used as the power in the original formula, $DV = a\,IV^b$. The intercept from this regression is the natural logarithm of the *a* in the formula $DV = a \times IV^b$. Since the computer regression program provides the value for the logarithm of *a*, *a* can be computed by taking the antilog of that intercept A.

The third equation is:

$$DV = a \times b^{IV} \qquad (3)$$

Determination of *a* and *b* is similar to that described for equation number 2, discussed above. The dependent variable inserted into the regression program is actually the natural logarithm of the original data, and the independent variable is the original data.

The computer output provides an intercept and another coefficient. The antilog of the intercept will provide the *a*, and the antilog of the other coefficient the *b*, for the formula shown above.

The technique with which to determine the best equation involves trying each one (including the linear equation [$DV = a + b\,IV$]) and selecting the one providing the highest $R^2$, consistent with good *t*-values (absolute value higher than 2) for the coefficients and an *F*-statistic higher than 4.

## EXAMPLES OF MULTIPLE LINEAR REGRESSION

### REGRESSION EXAMPLE 1: "HIGH" RABBIT DATA

The first example utilizes Data Set 2 from Chapter 25. The data included for the present analysis, concerning the effect of marihuana

### Table 27-4. Rabbit Data

| Weight (WGT) | Dosage of THC (THC) | Postcoital LH level (PCLH) | Ovulation 1 = yes 0 = no (OVUL) | Number of corpora lutea (NOCL) | Number of implantations (NOIM) |
|---|---|---|---|---|---|
| 2.9 | 2.500 | 00.5 | 1 | 0 | 0 |
| 3.2 | 2.500 | 00.5 | 1 | 0 | 0 |
| 3.5 | 2.500 | 00.5 | 1 | 0 | 0 |
| 2.8 | 2.500 | 00.5 | 1 | 0 | 0 |
| 2.7 | 2.500 | 00.5 | 1 | 0 | 0 |
| 3.0 | 2.500 | 00.5 | 1 | 0 | 0 |
| 3.0 | 1.250 | 00.5 | 1 | 0 | 0 |
| 2.9 | 1.250 | 00.5 | 1 | 0 | 0 |
| 2.8 | 1.250 | 00.5 | 1 | 0 | 0 |
| 3.6 | 1.250 | 00.5 | 1 | 0 | 0 |
| 3.4 | 1.250 | 00.5 | 1 | 0 | 0 |
| 3.1 | 1.250 | 38.0 | 1 | 10 | 10 |
| 3.8 | 0.612 | 00.5 | 0 | 0 | 0 |
| 2.8 | 0.612 | 00.5 | 0 | 0 | 0 |
| 2.9 | 0.612 | 00.5 | 0 | 0 | 0 |
| 3.0 | 0.612 | 30.0 | 1 | 10 | 10 |
| 3.1 | 0.612 | 29.0 | 1 | 9 | 8 |
| 2.6 | 0.612 | 42.0 | 1 | 8 | 7 |
| 3.9 | 0.306 | 50.0 | 1 | 9 | 7 |
| 3.4 | 0.306 | 18.0 | 1 | 10 | 9 |
| 3.5 | 0.306 | 29.0 | 1 | 12 | 10 |
| 2.8 | 0.306 | 28.0 | 1 | 13 | 11 |
| 3.7 | 0.306 | 31.0 | 1 | 8 | 8 |
| 2.9 | 0.306 | 28.0 | 1 | 7 | 7 |
| 2.6 | 0.000 | 45.0 | 1 | 9 | 9 |
| 3.0 | 0.000 | 25.0 | 1 | 10 | 9 |
| 2.6 | 0.000 | 23.0 | 1 | 8 | 6 |
| 2.9 | 0.000 | 29.0 | 1 | 9 | 6 |
| 3.0 | 0.000 | 33.0 | 1 | 11 | 10 |
| 3.1 | 0.000 | 17.0 | 1 | 7 | 6 |

on number of implantations, is shown in Table 27-4. The correlation matrix is provided in Table 27-5. When "number of implantations" (coded as the variable NOIM) is the dependent variable, the independent variable should be the dosage of THC (see Chap. 25 for definition). The correlation of NOIM and THC is − 0.7025. Appendix 2-5 indicates that with 30 observations (29 degrees of freedom) a 0.35 correlation (positive or negative) is required for statistical reliability. The correlation of NOIM and weight (WGT) is too low (at a value of − 0.01) to pass this test, so weight is excluded as an independent variable. The postcoital LH level (PCLH) is dropped from direct consideration as an independent variable because it is *also* affected by the THC dosage and is evidently part of the mechanism for reducing the number of implantations. The *correlation* of − 0.7025 between NOIM and THC provides evidence *that* a linear relationship *exists* between NOIM and THC dosage. The *regression* equation indicates *what* the rela-

tionship is. The computer printout in Figure 27-5 illustrates the regression program output. The resulting equation is shown as follows:

$$NOIM = 7.62 − 3.42 \ (THC)$$

The regression coefficient of 7.62 indicates that even if THC were zero, the average num-

### Table 27-5. Correlation Matrix for the Rabbit-Marihuana Analysis

| | NOIM | THC | WGT | PCLH* |
|---|---|---|---|---|
| NOIM | 1.0000 | −0.7025 | −0.0106 | 0.9066 |
| THC | −0.7025 | 1.0000 | −0.0307 | −0.6639 |
| WGT | −0.0106 | −0.0307 | 1.0000 | 0.0303 |
| PCLH* | 0.9066 | −0.6639 | 0.0303 | 1.0000 |

NOIM = number of implantations
THC = dosage of THC
WGT = weight of the rabbit
PCLH = postcoital LH level

* The PCLH is included to get an idea of the mechanism at work, rather than as an independent variable for the initial analysis. In the initial analysis, ignore the PCLH row and column.

→            DREG
NO. OBSERV PER VAR
□:
→           30
NO. INDEP VARS
□:
→           1
ENTER DEPENDENT VARIABLE
□:
→           NOIM
DATA FOR INDEP VAR 1
□:
→           THC
REGRESSION COEFF (INTERCEPT FIRST) 7.624830233 -3.418484254

T-STATISTIC FOR COEFFICIENTS  9.052115041  -5.22277683

R-SQUARED = 0.4934638549 FCALC = 27.27739782 WITH 1 AND 28 D.F.
OTHER SPECIAL INFO ? TYPE Y OR N
Y
DURBIN-WATSON ? Y OR N
N
WANT COV MATRIX ? Y OR N
N
WANT OBSERVED, PREDICTED, AND DEVIATIONS? Y OR N
Y

| OBSERVED | PREDICTED | DEVIATIONS |
|---|---|---|
| 0 | -0.9213804026 | 0.9213804026 |
| 0 | -0.9213804026 | 0.9213804026 |
| 0 | -0.9213804026 | 0.9213804026 |
| 0 | -0.9213804026 | 0.9213804026 |
| 0 | -0.9213804026 | 0.9213804026 |
| 0 | -0.9213804026 | 0.9213804026 |
| 0 | 3.351724915 | -3.351724915 |
| 0 | 3.351724915 | -3.351724915 |
| 0 | 3.351724915 | -3.351724915 |
| 0 | 3.351724915 | -3.351724915 |
| 0 | 3.351724915 | -3.351724915 |
| 10 | 3.351724915 | 6.648275085 |
| 0 | 5.53271787 | -5.53271787 |
| 0 | 5.53271787 | -5.53271787 |
| 0 | 5.53271787 | -5.53271787 |
| 10 | 5.53271787 | 4.46728213 |
| 8 | 5.53271787 | 2.46728213 |
| 7 | 5.53271787 | 1.46728213 |
| 7 | 4.578774051 | 0.4212259487 |
| 9 | 6.578774051 | 2.421225949 |
| 10 | 6.578774051 | 3.421225949 |
| 11 | 6.578774051 | 4.421225949 |
| 8 | 6.578774051 | 1.421225949 |
| 7 | 6.578774051 | 0.4212259487 |
| 9 | 7.624830233 | 1.375169767 |
| 9 | 7.624830233 | 1.375169767 |
| 6 | 7.624830233 | -1.624830233 |
| 6 | 7.624830233 | -1.624830233 |
| 10 | 7.624830233 | 2.375169767 |
| 6 | 7.624830233 | -1.624830233 |

WANT HELP IN INTERPRETATION ? Y OR N
→ Y
COEFFICIENTS (EXCEPT FOR CONSTANT) INDICATES THE CHANGE IN
   THE DEPENDENT VARIABLE RESULTING FROM
   A ONE UNIT CHANGE IN THE INDEPENDENT VARIABLE ASSOCIATED
     WITH THE COEFFICIENT

IT VALUES! < 2, THEN THINK ABOUT DELETING THE VARIABLE AND
   RERUNNING THE REGRESSION

IF FCALC IS LESS THAN 4, THEN DO SOMETHING DIFFERENT BECAUSE
   THE EQUATION IS NO GOOD. PERHAPS DELETE VARIABLES OR GET
   NEW ONES

R SQUARED OF .9 OR ABOVE IS AN 'A'

PREDICTED VALUES THE FORMULA WOULD GIVE FOR THE GIVEN
VALUES OF THE INDEPENDENT VARIABLES ARE STORED IN PRED

   PLEASED TO BE OF SERVICE

**FIG. 27–5.** Computer printout for regression analysis of the
"high" rabbit data (*arrow* indicates items typed on a terminal
by the user).

ber of implantations would be 7.62. The coefficient −3.42 means that as the THC increases by 1 unit (mg./kg.), the number of implantations decreases by 3.42. The *t*-statistics are good, since both are greater than 2. The *F* calc is much higher than 4, indicating the $R^2$ is significantly greater than zero. The $R^2$ of 0.49 means that 49 per cent of the variability in the number of implantations from animal to animal is explained by the varying levels of THC. This $R^2$ is somewhat low; therefore it would be wise to seek more data (new variables) that may be related to implantation number. However, since so many rabbits had zero implantations, it may be difficult to produce a much higher $R^2$ without expanding the number of variates (rabbits) in the study. The high incidence of zero implantations is probably due to the effect of the high THC dosage.

The formula can be used to predict the number of implantations for a given rabbit if the THC dosage is known. For example, a dosage of 0.5 mg./kg. would provide a predicted number of implantations of 5.91, according to the following calculation:

$$\text{NOIM} = 7.62 - 3.42(0.5) = 5.91$$

If such predictions are made for each animal in the original experiment, using the THC level actually given, there would be predicted values for NOIM as shown in Figure 27-5, toward the bottom of the printout. A review of the deviations may reveal patterns useful to the researcher. Cases with large deviations should be reviewed carefully to uncover measurement error, coding error, or unique characteristics in the particular experimental subject (rabbit, in this instance). If a rabbit had a deviation (observed-predicted) of 15 or 20, then the case should be carefully studied and perhaps dropped from the data set.

Figure 27-6 is included to illustrate what the regression would have looked like if weight (WGT) had been included as an independent variable. Notice that the equation would have been written as:

$$\text{NOIM} = 8.83 - 3.42(\text{THC}) - 0.39(\text{WGT})$$

Although the $R^2$ is slightly higher in this equation than in the previous one, the calculated *F* is considerably lower. Since the absolute value of the *t*-statistic for the regression coefficient for WGT is less than 1.6, the equation is not as good as the previous one. If the *t*

```
        ➤           DREG
          NO. OBSERV PER VAR
          □:
        ➤             30
          NO. INDEP VARS
          □:
        ➤             2
          ENTER DEPENDENT VARIABLE
          □:
        ➤           NOIM
          DATA FOR INDEP VAR 1
          □:
        ➤           THC
          DATA FOR INDEP VAR 2
          □:
        ➤           WGT
          REGRESSION COEFF (INTERCEPT FIRST)
                  8.834717227     -3.423274768     -0.3909452662

          T-STATISTIC FOR COEFFICIENTS
                  1.689989073     -5.138668985     -0.2346121024

          R-SQUARED = 0.4944943906   FCALC = 13.20593511 WITH 2 AND 27 D.F.
          OTHER SPECIAL INFO ? TYPE Y OR N
        ➤ N
          PREDICTED VALUES THE FORMULA WOULD GIVE FOR THE GIVEN
          VALUES OF THE INDEPENDENT VARIABLES ARE STORED IN PRED

          PLEASED TO BE OF SERVICE
```

**FIG. 27–6.** Example of multiple regression, using the "high" rabbit data.

**Table 27-6. Data Required for Multiple Regression Equation to Conduct a Modified Discriminant Analysis Using the Depressed Manager's Case**

| Drop or continue variable (DCGN) | Desired number of additional children (DESC) | Family planning knowledge score (KNOW) | Age of program entry (EAGE) | Parity at entry (PAR) | Method dummy variables | | | Hypertension dummy variables | |
|---|---|---|---|---|---|---|---|---|---|
| | | | | | Oral contraceptive (OC) | IUD (IUD) | Foam and condom (FC) | Has hypertension (DHYP) | No hypertension (DNHYP) |
| 0.067 | 2 | 100 | 25 | 1 | 1 | 0 | 0 | 1 | 0 |
| −0.067 | 0 | 50 | 30 | 3 | 0 | 1 | 0 | 0 | 1 |
| −0.067 | 1 | 30 | 25 | 1 | 1 | 0 | 0 | 1 | 0 |
| 0.067 | 0 | 75 | 32 | 2 | 0 | 0 | 1 | 0 | 1 |
| 0.067 | 1 | 55 | 27 | 1 | 1 | 0 | 0 | 0 | 1 |
| −0.067 | 1 | 60 | 22 | 2 | 0 | 1 | 0 | 0 | 1 |
| −0.067 | 2 | 30 | 20 | 0 | 0 | 1 | 0 | 1 | 0 |
| 0.067 | 3 | 25 | 18 | 0 | 0 | 0 | 1 | 0 | 1 |
| 0.067 | 1 | 80 | 22 | 2 | 0 | 0 | 1 | 0 | 1 |
| −0.067 | 2 | 85 | 15 | 0 | 1 | 0 | 0 | 0 | 1 |
| −0.067 | 0 | 100 | 31 | 2 | 0 | 0 | 1 | 0 | 1 |
| 0.067 | 0 | 85 | 32 | 2 | 0 | 0 | 1 | 1 | 0 |
| 0.067 | 1 | 99 | 26 | 1 | 1 | 0 | 0 | 0 | 1 |
| −0.067 | 0 | 85 | 27 | 2 | 0 | 1 | 0 | 0 | 1 |
| −0.067 | 0 | 95 | 25 | 0 | 1 | 0 | 0 | 0 | 1 |
| 0.067 | 1 | 60 | 27 | 1 | 1 | 0 | 0 | 0 | 1 |
| 0.067 | 2 | 50 | 21 | 1 | 0 | 1 | 0 | 0 | 1 |
| 0.067 | 1 | 50 | 20 | 1 | 0 | 0 | 1 | 1 | 0 |
| −0.067 | 2 | 65 | 16 | 1 | 0 | 0 | 1 | 0 | 1 |
| −0.067 | 1 | 75 | 25 | 1 | 1 | 0 | 0 | 0 | 1 |
| 0.067 | 0 | 90 | 28 | 2 | 0 | 0 | 1 | 0 | 1 |
| −0.067 | 1 | 88 | 23 | 2 | 1 | 0 | 0 | 0 | 1 |
| 0.067 | 0 | 76 | 29 | 2 | 0 | 0 | 1 | 1 | 0 |
| −0.067 | 2 | 84 | 21 | 0 | 1 | 0 | 0 | 0 | 1 |
| 0.067 | 1 | 96 | 23 | 1 | 1 | 0 | 0 | 0 | 1 |
| 0.067 | 2 | 91 | 20 | 0 | 1 | 0 | 0 | 0 | 1 |
| 0.067 | 0 | 98 | 28 | 2 | 0 | 0 | 1 | 0 | 1 |
| −0.067 | 8 | 90 | 15 | 0 | 1 | 0 | 0 | 0 | 1 |
| −0.067 | 2 | 81 | 22 | 1 | 1 | 0 | 0 | 0 | 1 |
| −0.067 | 1 | 87 | 25 | 2 | 1 | 0 | 0 | 0 | 1 |

for WGT had been greater than 1.6, then the regression coefficient shown in Figure 27-6, − 0.39, would have meant that holding THC constant, an increase in weight of 1 kg. would have *decreased* (due to the negative sign for the coefficient) implantations by 0.39 per animal.

**REGRESSION EXAMPLE 2: THE DEPRESSED CLINIC MANAGER DATA (DISCRIMINANT FUNCTION)**

This example utilizes Data Set 1 in Chapter 25 and provides an application of *discriminant function analysis* performed through the multiple regression approach. The data set prepared for the analysis is provided in Table 27-6. Notice that the family planning methods are coded as 3 dummy variables (OC, IUD, FC) and the hypertensive patients as 2 dummy variables (DHYP and DNHYP). Since the dependent variable, DCGN (dropping out), is

nominal, it was recoded to have a $(+\frac{1}{15})$ or + 0.067, for each dropout and $(-\frac{1}{15})$, or − 0.067, for each continuing patient. The correlation matrix is shown in Table 27-7. The asterisks in the matrix indicate a number too small to print in the existing space. The best independent variable, according to the correlation matrix, is FC, indicating that the foam and condom users were most likely to discontinue services. No other correlations exceeded the standard, 0.35, set forth in Appendix 2-5. However, if the level of significance (0.05) were relaxed, age of the patient at time of entry into the program (EAGE) should be considered, since it correlates at 0.2582 with the dependent variable (DCGN). Use of the IUD method should also be considered, since it correlates at − 0.26 with the dependent vari-

**Table 27-7. Correlation Matrix for Depressed Clinic Manager Data**

| | Drop or continue (DCGN) | Additional desired number children (DESC) | Family plan knowledge score (KNOW) | Age at entry (EAGE) | Parity (PAR) | Oral contraceptive (OC) | IUD (IUD) | Foam and condom (FC) | Hyper-tensive (DHYP) | Not hyper-tensive (DNHYP) |
|---|---|---|---|---|---|---|---|---|---|---|
| DCGN | 1.0000 | -0.1773 | 0.0385 | 0.2582 | 0.0801 | -0.2000 | -0.2683 | 0.4243 | 0.1667 | -0.1667 |
| DESC | -0.1773 | 1.0000 | -0.0861 | -0.7296 | -0.6015 | 0.3103 | -0.0793 | -0.2664 | -0.0886 | 0.0886 |
| KNOW | 0.0385 | -0.0861 | 1.0000 | 0.2123 | 0.1426 | 0.3037 | -0.4033 | -0.0033 | -0.2929 | 0.2929 |
| EAGE | 0.2582 | -0.7296 | 0.2133 | 1.0000 | 0.6977 | -0.2295 | ***** | 0.2434 | 0.1255 | -0.1255 |
| PAR | 0.0801 | -0.6015 | 0.1426 | 0.6977 | 1.0000 | -0.4804 | 0.2148 | 0.3397 | -0.0200 | 0.0200 |
| OC | -0.2000 | 0.3103 | 0.3037 | -0.2295 | -0.4804 | 1.0000 | -0.4472 | -0.7071 | -0.1667 | 0.1667 |
| IUD | -0.2683 | -0.0793 | -0.4033 | ***** | 0.2148 | -0.4472 | 1.0000 | -0.3162 | ***** | 0.0000 |
| FC | 0.4243 | -0.2664 | -0.0033 | 0.2434 | 0.3397 | -0.7071 | -0.3162 | 1.0000 | 0.1768 | -0.1768 |
| DHYP | 0.1667 | -0.0886 | -0.2929 | 0.1255 | -0.0200 | -0.1667 | ***** | 0.1768 | 1.0000 | -1.0000 |
| DNHYP | -0.1667 | 0.0886 | 0.2929 | -0.1255 | 0.0200 | 0.1667 | 0.0000 | -0.1768 | -1.0000 | 1.0000 |

***** Asterisks indicate a correlation smaller than 0.0001

able. However, IUD and FC have an inter-correlation of $-0.3162$. The absolute value is higher than the correlation of either to the dependent variable. Therefore only one of the two variables (IUD or FC) should be entered into the equation. Since IUDs correlation to the dependent variable is lower, IUD should be dropped from consideration as an *independent* variable. The correlation of FC with EAGE is 0.2434, which is very close to the correlation of EAGE to the dependent variable. Therefore only FC *should* be considered as an independent variable. However, to illustrate the effect of retaining EAGE in the equation, a regression was performed, with the following results:

$$DCGN = -0.075 + 0.0024 \,(EAGE) + 0.0546(FC)$$
(*t*-statistics) $(-1.236)$ $(0.9311)$ $(2.1722)$
$$R^2 = 0.21$$
$$F^2_{27} = 3.49$$

Notice that *F* calc is low. This indicates that the $R^2$ is barely significantly different from zero. According to Appendix 2-4, the *F*-table or criterion value for $F^2_{27}$ ($\alpha = 0.05$) is 3.32. The $R^2$ of 0.21 is low, indicating that only 21 per cent of the variability of the dependent variable can be explained by the independent variables, EAGE and FC. The *t*-statistic for EAGE is also too low; therefore, the coefficient 0.0024 is deemed not statistically significantly greater than zero, and the variable is deleted. The regression is rerun (Figure 27-7), and the new equation appears as follows:

$$DCGN = -0.0201 + 0.0603(FC)$$
(*t*-statistics) $(-1.4314)$ $(2.4792)$
$$R^2 = 0.18$$
$$F^1_{28} = 6.15$$

The $R^2$ is low, indicating that additional independent variables should be sought (new data) to obtain a better equation. The *F* calc has improved, because there is one less variable, with the same number of observations per variable. The *t*-statistic for FC is above 2, and therefore indicates that foam and condom users are different with respect to dropping out. They discontinue more, as shown by the fact that the coefficient is *positive,* indicating that when FC increases (goes from 0 to 1, since it is a dummy variable), DCGN increases.

The formula could be used to predict a dropout in the following way. An FC of *1*

would be the code for someone using foam and condom, so *1* is plugged into the formula as follows:

$$DCGN = -0.0201 + 0.0603(1)$$
$$DCGN = -0.0402$$

Since this value is greater than zero (the zero is established as the criterion because it is halfway between 0.067 and $-0.067$, the two values used to code the dependent variable), the person is predicted to drop out.

If a zero is plugged into the formula, the result is:

$$DCGN = -0.0201 + 0.0603(0)$$
$$DCGN = -0.0201$$

Since the resulting $-0.02$ is below the zero criterion, that person would be predicted to *continue.*

Applying this formula to each of the original observations in the data set provides the *predicted* situation for each person already in the data set. These values can be compared to the actual situation to measure the formula's usefulness. At the bottom of the computer printout (Fig. 27-7), columns entitled "observed" and "predicted" appear. The "observed" represents the original values of the dependent variable. The "predicted" represents results obtained from using the formula to predict the dependent variable for each case. A star has been inserted by each prediction that would have been *inaccurate.* There were 9 erroneous classifications. Since there were 30 observations, 21 of 30 were accurate. The classification power is then $\frac{21}{30} = 70\%$. This is preferable to flipping a coin to determine who will discontinue; however, not all users of foam and condoms will drop out, although the formula indicates that they would. The *classification matrix* is considered from the observed and predicted values (Table 27-8). More of the continuing patients were correctly predicted $(\frac{13}{15} = 0.87)$ than were the actual dropouts $(\frac{8}{15} = 0.53)$.

**REGRESSION EXAMPLE: THE CRYSTAL-BALL GAZER'S DATA**

This example uses Data Set 3 in Chapter 25 and provides an example of curvilinear regression analysis.

```
        )COPY ASOP4 DREG
SAVED 13.40.30 06/02/78
              DREG
NO. OBSERV PER VAR
□:
              30
NO. INDEP VARS
□:
              1
ENTER DEPENDENT VARIABLE
□:
              DCGN
DATA FOR INDEP VAR 1
□:
              FC
REGRESSION COEFF (INTERCEPT FIRST) -0.0201  0.0603

T-STATISTIC FOR COEFFICIENTS -1.431356171  2.479181612

R-SQUARED = 0.18   FCALC = 6.146341463 WITH 1 AND 28 D.F.
OTHER SPECIAL INFO ? TYPE Y OR N
Y
DURBIN-WATSON ? Y OR N
N
WANT COV MATRIX ? Y OR N
N
WANT OBSERVED, PREDICTED, AND DEVIATIONS? Y OR N
Y
```

| OBSERVED | PREDICTED | DEVIATIONS |
|---|---|---|
| 0.067 | -0.0201 * | 0.0871 |
| -0.067 | -0.0201 | -0.0469 |
| -0.067 | -0.0201 | -0.0469 |
| 0.067 | 0.0402 | 0.0268 |
| 0.067 | -0.0201 * | 0.0871 |
| -0.067 | -0.0201 | -0.0469 |
| -0.067 | -0.0201 | -0.0469 |
| 0.067 | 0.0402 * | 0.0268 |
| 0.067 | 0.0402 | 0.0268 |
| -0.067 | -0.0201 * | -0.0469 |
| -0.067 | 0.0402 | -0.1072 |
| 0.067 | 0.0402 | 0.0268 |
| 0.067 | -0.0201 | 0.0871 |
| -0.067 | -0.0201 | -0.0469 |
| -0.067 | -0.0201 | -0.0469 |
| 0.067 | -0.0201 * | 0.0871 |
| 0.067 | -0.0201 * | 0.0871 |
| 0.067 | 0.0402 | 0.0268 |
| -0.067 | 0.0402 * | -0.1072 |
| -0.067 | -0.0201 | -0.0469 |
| 0.067 | 0.0402 | 0.0268 |
| -0.067 | -0.0201 | -0.0469 |
| 0.067 | 0.0402 | 0.0268 |
| -0.067 | -0.0201 | -0.0469 |
| 0.067 | -0.0201 * | 0.0871 |
| 0.067 | -0.0201 * | 0.0871 |
| 0.067 | 0.0402 | 0.0268 |
| -0.067 | -0.0201 | -0.0469 |
| -0.067 | -0.0201 | -0.0469 |
| -0.067 | -0.0201 | -0.0469 |

```
WANT HELP IN INTERPRETATION ? Y OR N
N
     PREDICTED VALUES THE FORMULA WOULD GIVE FOR THE GIVEN
     VALUES OF THE INDEPENDENT VARIABLES ARE STORED IN PRED
```

**FIG. 27–7.**  Regression printout for predicting dropout from a family planning clinic.

**Table 27-8. Classification Matrix Example for the Clinic Dropout Prediction Using Discriminant Function Analysis**

| | | Prediction by formula | | |
|---|---|---|---|---|
| | | Drop | Continue | Total actual |
| Actual | Drop | 8 | 7 | 15 |
| experience | Continue | 2 | 13 | 15 |
| | Total predicted: | 10 | 20 | 30 |

The dependent variable $(DV)$ is the number of visits per quarter, and the independent variable $(IV)$ is one created to represent time in quarters from a given date. Therefore the sequence of numbers 1 through 30 is used. The original data set is shown in Chapter 25. Plotting the observations indicates that the data set is nearly linear over time, but may have a curve; therefore the curvilinear formulas are employed initially. The expanded data set required for these formulas is shown in Table

27-9 and includes the time squared and the natural logarithm of each variable.

The formulas are shown below in Table 27-10. In the linear equation, Visits = 59.5 + 2.26 × Time, with $t$ values > 5, and an $R^2$ of 0.52; the curvilinear equation with the highest $R^2$ (0.53) has $t$-calculated values of less than 1.6. Consequently, the linear equation is preferable.

Among the three curvilinear equations, the semilog form is the best because it has the highest $R^2$ consistent with a good $F$ calc and good $t$-calculated values. Since the $R^2$ for the linear equation is higher (0.53 versus 0.519), it is chosen.

## PREDICTING FUTURE ACTIVITY ON THE BASIS OF HISTORICAL DATA

The method used for forecasting monthly or quarterly levels of activity in a clinic is called *timeseries analysis*. The formulas needed for this form of analysis are found in most business

**Table 27-9. Data for the Number of Visits to a Clinic and the Quarter (Time Period), in Preparation for Calculating a Curvilinear Regression Formula**

| Visits | Time | $Log_e$ time | $Log_e$ visits | Time$^2$ |
|---|---|---|---|---|
| 50 | 1 | 0 | 3.912 | 1 |
| 80 | 2 | 0.6931 | 4.382 | 4 |
| 70 | 3 | 1.099 | 4.248 | 9 |
| 75 | 4 | 1.386 | 4.317 | 16 |
| 100 | 5 | 1.609 | 4.605 | 25 |
| 110 | 6 | 1.792 | 4.7 | 36 |
| 90 | 7 | 1.946 | 4.5 | 49 |
| 60 | 8 | 2.079 | 4.094 | 64 |
| 60 | 9 | 2.197 | 4.094 | 81 |
| 80 | 10 | 2.303 | 4.382 | 100 |
| 50 | 11 | 2.398 | 3.912 | 121 |
| 70 | 12 | 2.485 | 4.248 | 144 |
| 50 | 13 | 2.565 | 3.912 | 169 |
| 70 | 14 | 2.639 | 4.248 | 196 |
| 70 | 15 | 2.708 | 4.248 | 225 |
| 80 | 16 | 2.773 | 4.382 | 256 |
| 110 | 17 | 2.833 | 4.7 | 289 |
| 130 | 18 | 2.89 | 4.868 | 324 |
| 120 | 19 | 2.944 | 4.787 | 361 |
| 110 | 20 | 2.996 | 4.7 | 400 |
| 140 | 21 | 3.045 | 4.942 | 441 |
| 160 | 22 | 3.091 | 5.075 | 484 |
| 120 | 23 | 3.135 | 4.787 | 529 |
| 110 | 24 | 3.178 | 4.7 | 576 |
| 120 | 25 | 3.219 | 4.787 | 625 |
| 110 | 26 | 3.258 | 4.7 | 676 |
| 90 | 27 | 3.296 | 4.5 | 729 |
| 80 | 28 | 3.332 | 4.382 | 784 |
| 160 | 29 | 3.367 | 5.075 | 841 |
| 110 | 30 | 3.401 | 4.7 | 900 |

**Table 27-10. Curvilinear Regression Formulas for Crystal-Ball Gazer Trend Data**

| | Log-log | Semilog | 2nd degree polynominal |
|---|---|---|---|
| Regression equation (t-values) | $(Ln\ Visits) = 3.857 + 0.27\ (Ln\ Time)$<br>$(26.38)\quad (5.33)$ | $(Ln\ Visits) = 4.147 + 0.022\ (Time)$<br>$(50.88)\quad (6.42)$ | $Visits = 65.32 + 1.44\ Time + 0.02\ Time^2$<br>$(5.13)\quad (1.005)\quad (0.59)$ |
| $R^2$ | 0.428 | 0.519 | 0.534 |
| $F_{38}^1$ | 28.5 | 41.2 | $F_{37}^2 = 21.2$ |
| Antilogs | Antilog of 3.86 = 46.99 | Antilog of 4.147 = 63.23<br>Antilog of 0.022 = 1.022 | |
| Final formula | $Visits = 46.99\ Time^{0.27}$ | $Visits = 63.23 \times 1.022^{Time}$ | $Visits = 65.32 + 1.44\ Time + 0.02\ Time^2$ |

statistics books. This section will summarize one method and illustrate its use, employing the crystal-ball gazer data set.

In the method of timeseries analysis used here, all observations (or level of activity) for a given month (or quarter) are conceived to have four multiplicative components: Trend ($T$), Seasonal ($S$), Cyclical ($C$), and Irregular ($I$). It is necessary to isolate each component, determine that component's future direction, and then multiply the four components to obtain a prediction. Each component and the method for determining its future direction are discussed in the following paragraphs. An example of a computer printout used by the author to perform the analysis is then presented.

## TREND

The broad, long-range (beyond 1 or 2 years) movement of a set of observations through time is the *trend*. It can be characterized by terms such as *steady, slowly rising, slowly falling,* and *rapidly falling*. The future values of the trend, using only the single data set, are determined by performing curvilinear regression analysis, as discussed in the previous section. The best formula is selected, and predictions are made for selected time periods (month by month) in the future. If the time periods are indicated by the numbers 1 through 60 for the previous 60 months of data, a formula is obtained which relates the *DV* to time, as measured by the numbers 1 through 60. If the next 5 months are to be predicted, then the numbers 61, 62, 63, 64, and 65 are inserted in the time variable of the trend equation. In this way a prediction of the trend component of the timeseries data is obtained. For example, a regression equation in which the dependent variable is the number of monthly clinic visits for each of 60 months (CV) and the independent variable is the corresponding months, i.e., numbers 1 through 60 (coded as TIME), may appear as follows:

$$CV = 300 + 2(TIME)$$

This equation would indicate that with the passage of time, the trend grows by two visits per month. If the last month of available data were coded as 60, the trend prediction for the following month would use a time value of $(60 + 1) = 61$, as follows:

$$CV = 300 + 2(61) = 300 + 122 = 422 \text{ visits}$$

Predicting the trend component of monthly visits 1 year hence requires using a time value of $(60 + 13) = 73$, as follows:

$$CV = 300 + 2(73) = 300 + 146 = 446 \text{ visits}$$

## SEASONAL

The within-year patterns which normally repeat themselves annually are called *seasonals*. For example, if January is always characterized by fewer family planning visits, the January seasonal index would be low. A seasonal index for January of 0.8 means that the typical January has a value which is 80 per cent of the trend (or is 20 per cent below the trend). A seasonal index of 1.5 for March means that the typical March has a value which is 150 per cent of the trend (or 50 per cent above the trend).

The concept of computing a seasonal index is discussed here. Computational formulas can be found in a business statistics text. A "specific seasonal" is computed for each observation in the original data series by starting at a specific month (or quarter, if the data is quarterly) of a specific year and averaging the monthly values for the preceding and following 6 months (called a *moving average*). That moving average is then divided into the original value for the month of interest. Dividing the moving average into the original observation eliminates the trend and cyclical components, leaving the seasonals and irregulars. "Irregulars" are unpredictable fluctuations in the data, such as low monthly visits due to extremely bad weather. This may be represented as:

$$\frac{\text{(actual value)}}{\text{(smoothed trend and cyclical)}} = \frac{T \times C \times S \times I}{T \times C} = S \times I$$

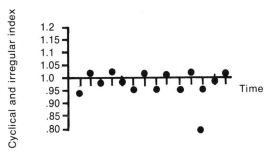

**FIG. 27-8.** Plot of cyclical and irregular components.

Data were already stored as "VISITS"

```
      )COPY 40896 ASOP6 DTIME
SAVED 17.35.55 12/05/77
              NTIMER
TIMER HERE
FIRST TIME? Y OR N
N


TYPE  A  DESCRIPTION  OF  YOUR
          DATA SET
```
➨ VISITS PER QUARTER TO CLINIC
```
TYPE IN THE DESCRIPTION OF THE STARTING DATE
```
➨ QUARTER1 1969
```
ENTER NUMBER OF PERIODS PER YEAR
□:
```
➨          4
```
ENTER DATA
□:
```
➨              VISITS
```
WANT  TO  SEE  THE  CORRELATION  MATRIX  FOR  LOG  TREND
EQUATIONS?? TYPE Y OR N
```
➨ N
```
FOR VISITS PER QUARTER TO CLINIC
WHERE TIME PERIOD 1 IS QUARTER1 1969
AND THE MOST RECENT DATA PERIOD IS 40
THE TREND EQUATION IS Y = A + BxT
WITH A AND B GIVEN BY 59.53846154 2.26641651
AND T-STATISTICS OF   7.301432492  6.538964862

R-SQUARED FOR TREND ALONE IS 10.52945874

WANT TO RUN YOUR OWN LINEAR OR POLYNOMIAL TREND EQUATION?
TYPE Y OR N
```
➨ N
```
WANT A PLOT OF DATA AND TREND? Y OR N
```
➨ Y
```
PLOT OF VISITS PER QUARTER TO CLINIC GIVEN TIME
   WHERE PERIOD 1 IS QUARTER1 1969

   WHEN READY FOR PLOT TYPE Y
   I.E. ALLOW PAGE OR SCOPE TO LINE UP
Y
```

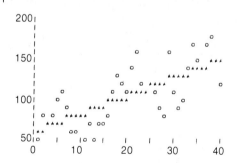

**FIG. 27–9.** Sample computer printout of a time-series analysis of clinic visits. (Data were already stored as "visits.")

```
ENTER THE PERIOD OF THE YEAR OF THE FIRST OBSERVATION IN YOUR
DATA, FOR EXAMPLE, IF IT IS MARCH, PUT IN A 3
        OR IF THE THIRD QUARTER, PUT IN A 3
    □:
→               1
FOR VISITS PER QUARTER TO CLINIC
THE FIRST DATA OF WHICH IS QUARTER1 1969
THE SEASONAL INDEX FOR EACH PERIOD OF THE TYPICAL YEAR IS
GIVEN BELOW
    IF YOU ENTERED THE CORRECT STARTING VALUE, THEN THE PERIOD 1
        BELOW REPRESENTS JANUARY IF THE DATA IS MONTHLY OR FIRST
        QUARTER IF QUARTERLY


PERIOD OF THE YEAR          SEASONAL INDEX
        1                   1.065891972
        2                   1.136808984
        3                   0.9187447171
        4                   0.878554327


0.6526369026
R-SQUARED WITH SEASONALS APPLIED IS 0.6526369026
SEASONALS HELP R-SQUARED. BE SURE TO USE
THEY ARE STORED UNDER THE NAME SEAS
CYCLICALS ARE STORED AS CYC
WANT A PLOT OF THEM? Y OR N
→ Y
GET PAGE OR SCOPE READY FOR PLOT
WHEN READY TYPE Y
→ Y
```

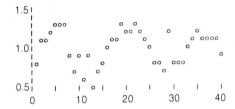

```
PLEASED TO BE OF SERVICE
```

**FIG. 27–9.** (*Continued*)

A data set containing several years of monthly specific seasonals would contain several specific seasonal and irregular $(S \times I)$ values for every month derived from each year of data. For example, 5 years of data would contain 5 seasonals for January, February, March, etc. Taking the median of the $(S \times I)$ values for every month eliminates the irregular component. The median figure is thus equivalent to the monthly seasonal index.

To obtain a prediction which includes the seasonal aspect, the trend prediction is multiplied by the seasonal index for the part of the year (month or quarter) under consideration.

## CYCLICALS AND IRREGULARS

The cyclical component is that pattern of movement through time which remains after accounting for the trend and seasonal. A true cycle has a fluctuating pattern through time which repeats every 2 or 3 years. However, in health care applications at the clinic management level, true cycles are seldom observed.

*Cyclicals* are used to plot the cyclical component through time and estimate its future direction. If no clear patterns are indicated in the data, the plot provides an index of the variation that has not been explained by trend and seasonal components. If the plot resembled the one in Figure 27-8, the actual outcome would be predicted to be between 1.05 and 0.98 of the value computed by the trend and seasonal components. The trend and seasonal prediction could be adjusted through multiplication by 1.05 to obtain the upper estimate, or by 0.98 to obtain the lower estimated level of clinic activity.

In Figure 27-8, a dot appears on the index as 0.8. This was a unique event which could not have been predicted, and is called an *irregular*. This component is not used in the prediction because it probably cannot be predicted to occur at any particular time in the future.

Cyclicals are computed by using the trend equation and seasonal index to *predict* values for each time period for which the original data was available. These predictions are divided into the original observations for the corresponding time period. The mathematical reasoning is shown below:

$$\frac{\text{(actual value)}}{\begin{array}{c}\text{(predicted values}\\ \text{of trend and season)}\end{array}} = \frac{T \times S \times C \times I}{T \times S} = C \times I$$

Timeseries analysis of Data Set 3, using a program written in APL (A Programming Language) by the author, is shown in Figure 27-9. In this program, the arrows point to input data requested by the interactive computer terminal and entered by the author. The remainder of the data was provided by the computer.

The trend equation is linear:

$$\text{Trend} = 59.5 + 2.27 \text{ (Time)}$$

The trend prediction for two quarters following the last period of actual available data would be

$$T = 59.5 + 2.27 \text{ (41)} = 152.6$$
$$T = 59.5 + 2.27 \text{ (42)} = 154.8$$

The seasonal index for each quarter is:

Quarter I—1.066
Quarter II—1.137
Quarter III—0.919
Quarter IV—0.879

Since Quarters I and II are to be predicted, the trend values are multiplied by the appropriate seasonal index values of 1.066 and 1.137, respectively. The resulting equation is:

$$T \times S = 152.6 \times 1.066 = 162.7;$$
$$T \times S = 154.8 \times 1.137 = 176.0$$

The plot of the cyclicals for the 40 quarters shown in the second part of Figure 27-9 is used, by viewing only, to predict values of 0.8 and 0.7 for Quarters 41 and 42. Applying these cyclicals to the trend and seasonal projections results in the following equation:

$$T \times S \times C = 152.6 \times 1.066 \times 0.8 = 130$$
$$\text{and}$$
$$T \times S \times C = 154.8 \times 1.137 \times 0.7 = 123$$

This means that the best prediction of visits for quarters 41 and 42 would be 130 and 123, respectively.

If the cycle had not been so clear, it could have been observed that the cyclicals varied from 0.7 to 1.2 during most of the past periods. A range for each quarter could then have been given. For example, the trend and seasonal for time-period 41 was 162.7 visits. However, a range of 114 (= 162.7 × 0.7) to 195 (= 192.7 × 1.2) may be reported as possible low and high values for that quarter.

The timeseries projection should be considered as the starting point for further analysis. It is based only on historical experience. A clinic manager may have knowledge of certain policy changes that could greatly affect the forecast. It may be possible to obtain a better prediction of the trend and cyclical components by introducing other data regarding weather, various funding programs, business activity, income, etc., that may relate to clinic visits. Once such a relationship is found, however, the independent variables must be known in advance, in order to be useful in predicting future activity.

# Appendixes

| Region or country | Population estimate mid-1978 (millions) | Birth rate (per 1,000) | Death rate (per 1,000) | Rate of natural increase (percentage) | Number of years to double population | Population projection to 2000 (millions) | Infant mortality rate (per 1,000 live births) | Population under 15 years (percentage) | Population over 64 years (percentage) | Life expectancy at birth (years) | Urban population (percentage) | Projected labor force increase 1978–2000 (millions) | Per-capita gross national product (US$) |
|---|---|---|---|---|---|---|---|---|---|---|---|---|---|
| AFRICA | 436 | 46 | 19 | 2.7 | 26 | 813 | 147 | 44 | 3 | 46 | 25 | 121 | 440 |
| NORTHERN AFRICA | 103 | 43 | 14 | 2.9 | 24 | 184 | 128 | 44 | 3 | 52 | 40 | 25 | 650 |
| Algeria | 18.4 | 48 | 14 | 3.4 | 20 | 36.4 | 145 | 48 | 3 | 53 | 52 | 4.7 | 990 |
| Egypt | 39.6 | 38 | 12 | 2.5 | 28 | 63.5 | 108 | 41 | 3 | 53 | 44 | 7.4 | 280 |
| Libya | 2.8 | 48 | 9 | 3.9 | 18 | 5.3 | 130 | 49 | 4 | 53 | 30 | 0.6 | 6,310 |
| Morocco | 18.9 | 45 | 14 | 3.1 | 22 | 35.4 | 133 | 46 | 2 | 53 | 38 | 5.3 | 540 |
| Sudan | 17.1 | 48 | 16 | 3.1 | 22 | 33.3 | 141 | 45 | 3 | 49 | 20 | 5.8 | 290 |
| Tunisia | 6.0 | 36 | 13 | 2.3 | 30 | 10.5 | 135 | 45 | 4 | 55 | 50 | 1.3 | 840 |
| WESTERN AFRICA | 128 | 49 | 22 | 2.7 | 26 | 243 | 158 | 45 | 3 | 42 | 19 | 36 | 350 |
| Benin | 3.4 | 49 | 22 | 2.7 | 26 | 6.0 | 149 | 46 | 4 | 41 | 14 | 1.1 | 130 |
| Cape Verde | 0.3 | 28 | 9 | 1.8 | 38 | 0.4 | 105 | 48 | 5 | 50 | 8 | — | 260 |
| Gambia | 0.6 | 43 | 23 | 2.0 | 35 | 0.9 | 165 | 41 | 2 | 40 | 16 | 0.1 | 180 |
| Ghana | 10.9 | 40 | 20 | 2.9 | 24 | 21.4 | 115 | 47 | 4 | 49 | 31 | 3.5 | 580 |
| Guinea | 4.8 | 46 | 21 | 2.5 | 28 | 8.4 | 175 | 43 | 3 | 41 | 20 | 1.3 | 150 |
| Guinea-Bissau | 0.6 | 41 | 24 | 1.7 | 41 | 0.8 | 208 | 37 | 4 | 39 | 23 | 0.1 | 140 |
| Ivory Coast | 7.2 | 45 | 19 | 2.6 | 27 | 13.2 | 154 | 43 | 3 | 44 | 20 | 1.7 | 610 |
| Liberia | 1.7 | 50 | 21 | 2.9 | 24 | 3.0 | 159 | 42 | 3 | 45 | 28 | 0.4 | 450 |
| Mali | 6.3 | 50 | 25 | 2.5 | 28 | 11.5 | 188 | 49 | 2 | 38 | 13 | 2.2 | 100 |
| Mauritania | 1.5 | 45 | 24 | 2.1 | 33 | 2.6 | 187 | 42 | 6 | 39 | 23 | 0.2 | 340 |
| Niger | 5.0 | 52 | 24 | 2.7 | 26 | 9.6 | 200 | 43 | 3 | 39 | 9 | 1.3 | 160 |
| Nigeria | 68.4 | 49 | 21 | 2.8 | 25 | 134.8 | 157 | 45 | 2 | 41 | 18 | 19.4 | 380 |
| Senegal | 5.4 | 47 | 23 | 2.4 | 29 | 9.2 | 159 | 43 | 3 | 40 | 32 | 1.1 | 390 |
| Sierra Leone | 3.3 | 44 | 19 | 2.5 | 28 | 5.8 | 136 | 43 | 3 | 44 | 15 | 0.7 | 200 |
| Togo | 2.4 | 50 | 22 | 2.8 | 25 | 4.5 | 163 | 46 | 3 | 41 | 15 | 0.7 | 260 |
| Upper Volta | 6.5 | 48 | 25 | 2.3 | 30 | 11.1 | 182 | 43 | 3 | 38 | 4 | 2.0 | 110 |
| EASTERN AFRICA | 124 | 47 | 20 | 2.7 | 26 | 238 | 146 | 45 | 3 | 45 | 12 | 39 | 210 |
| Burundi | 4.0 | 48 | 22 | 2.5 | 28 | 72 | 150 | 44 | 2 | 42 | 2 | 1.2 | 120 |
| Comoros | 0.3 | 45 | 20 | 2.5 | 28 | 0.5 | 160 | 43 | 3 | 46 | 10 | 0.1 | 180 |
| Djibouti | 0.1 | 48 | 24 | 2.4 | 29 | 0.2 | — | — | — | — | 70 | — | 1,940 |
| Ethiopia | 30.2 | 49 | 25 | 2.4 | 29 | 53.9 | 162 | 44 | 3 | 42 | 12 | 8.0 | 100 |
| Kenya | 14.8 | 48 | 15 | 3.3 | 21 | 31.3 | 119 | 46 | 3 | 50 | 10 | 5.0 | 240 |
| Madagascar | 8.0 | 47 | 22 | 2.5 | 28 | 16.3 | 102 | 45 | 3 | 44 | 16 | 3.5 | 200 |
| Malawi | 5.4 | 50 | 26 | 2.4 | 29 | 9.8 | 142 | 45 | 3 | 43 | 10 | 1.5 | 140 |
| Mauritius | 0.9 | 26 | 8 | 1.8 | 38 | 1.2 | 40 | 38 | 4 | 63 | 44 | 0.2 | 680 |
| Mozambique | 9.9 | 42 | 19 | 2.3 | 30 | 17.7 | 140 | 43 | 3 | 44 | 6 | 2.1 | 170 |
| Reunion | 0.5 | 28 | 7 | 2.1 | 33 | 0.7 | 44 | 43 | 4 | 63 | 51 | 0.1 | 1,920 |
| Rhodesia | 7.0 | 48 | 13 | 3.5 | 20 | 15.2 | 122 | 48 | 2 | 52 | 19 | 2.2 | 550 |
| Rwanda | 4.5 | 51 | 22 | 2.8 | 25 | 8.6 | 133 | 44 | 3 | 41 | 4 | 2.0 | 110 |
| Seychelles | 0.1 | 28 | 8 | 2.0 | 35 | 0.1 | 35 | 43 | 6 | 65 | 26 | — | 580 |
| Somalia | 3.4 | 48 | 21 | 2.7 | 26 | 6.5 | 177 | 45 | 2 | 41 | 28 | 0.9 | 110 |
| Tanzania, United Rep. of | 16.5 | 47 | 22 | 2.5 | 28 | 33.1 | 167 | 47 | 2 | 44 | 7 | 5.7 | 180 |
| Uganda | 12.7 | 45 | 15 | 3.0 | 23 | 24.8 | 160 | 44 | 3 | 50 | 7 | 4.1 | 240 |
| Zambia | 5.5 | 50 | 19 | 3.1 | 22 | 11.5 | 159 | 46 | 3 | 44 | 36 | 1.7 | 440 |
| MIDDLE AFRICA | 50 | 44 | 20 | 2.4 | 29 | 90 | 164 | 43 | 3 | 42 | 27 | 12 | 230 |
| Angola | 6.4 | 47 | 23 | 2.4 | 29 | 11.7 | 203 | 42 | 3 | 38 | 18 | 1.3 | 330 |
| Cameroon, United Rep. of | 8.0 | 41 | 21 | 2.0 | 35 | 13.7 | 137 | 40 | 3 | 41 | 29 | 1.5 | 290 |
| Central Africa Empire | 1.9 | 43 | 21 | 2.2 | 32 | 3.4 | 190 | 42 | 3 | 41 | 36 | 0.6 | 230 |
| Chad | 4.3 | 44 | 23 | 2.1 | 33 | 6.9 | 160 | 40 | 3 | 38 | 14 | 0.8 | 120 |
| Congo, People's Rep. of | 1.5 | 45 | 19 | 2.6 | 27 | 2.8 | 180 | 42 | 3 | 44 | 40 | 0.4 | 520 |
| Equatorial Guinea | 0.3 | 36 | 18 | 1.7 | 41 | 0.5 | 165 | 37 | 3 | 44 | 45 | 0.1 | 330 |
| Gabon | 0.5 | 29 | 21 | 0.8 | 87 | 0.7 | 178 | 32 | 4 | 41 | 32 | — | 2,590 |
| Sao Tome and Principe | 0.1 | 40 | 13 | 2.7 | 26 | 0.1 | 75 | — | — | 53 | 16 | — | 490 |
| Zaire | 26.7 | 45 | 18 | 2.7 | 26 | 49.9 | 160 | 44 | 3 | 44 | 29 | 7.1 | 140 |
| SOUTHERN AFRICA | 31 | 41 | 16 | 2.5 | 28 | 57 | 119 | 42 | 4 | 52 | 44 | 10 | 1,240 |
| Botswana | 0.7 | 47 | 21 | 2.6 | 27 | 1.4 | 97 | 48 | 6 | 56 | 12 | 0.3 | 410 |
| Lesotho | 1.3 | 40 | 18 | 2.1 | 33 | 2.1 | 114 | 40 | 4 | 46 | 3 | 0.3 | 170 |
| Namibia | 1.0 | 45 | 16 | 2.9 | 24 | 1.9 | 177 | 41 | 4 | 49 | 32 | 0.2 | 980 |
| South Africa | 27.5 | 40 | 15 | 2.5 | 28 | 51.0 | 117 | 41 | 4 | 52 | 48 | 8.5 | 1,340 |
| Swaziland | 0.5 | 49 | 20 | 2.9 | 24 | 1.0 | 168 | 48 | 3 | 44 | 8 | 0.2 | 470 |

## Population Data for Asia, 1978

| Region or country | Population estimate mid-1978 (millions) | Birth rate (per 1,000) | Death rate (per 1,000) | Rate of natural increase (percentage) | Number of years to double population | Population projection to 2000 (millions) | Infant mortality rate (per 1,000 live births) | Population under 15 years (percentage) | Population over 64 years (percentage) | Life expectancy at birth (years) | Urban population (percentage) | Projected labor force increase 1978–2000 (millions) | Per-capita gross national product (US$) |
|---|---|---|---|---|---|---|---|---|---|---|---|---|---|
| ASIA | 2,433 | 30 | 12 | 1.9 | 36 | 3,656 | 105 | 38 | 4 | 58 | 26 | 509 | 610 |
| SOUTHWEST ASIA | 92 | 40 | 13 | 2.7 | 26 | 166 | 117 | 43 | 4 | 55 | 45 | 25 | 1,730 |
| Bahrain | 0.3 | 43 | 8 | 3.5 | 20 | 0.6 | 78 | 44 | 3 | 63 | 78 | — | 2,410 |
| Cyprus | 0.6 | 20 | 10 | 1.0 | 69 | 0.8 | 27 | 28 | 10 | 71 | 42 | 0.1 | 1,480 |
| Gaza | 0.4 | 49 | 16 | 3.3 | 21 | 0.9 | — | 53 | 5 | 52 | 87 | — | — |
| Irag | 12.2 | 48 | 14 | 3.4 | 20 | 24.2 | 104 | 48 | 3 | 53 | 65 | 3.1 | 1,390 |
| Israel | 3.7 | 28 | 7 | 2.1 | 33 | 5.6 | 20 | 33 | 8 | 73 | 86 | 0.9 | 3,920 |
| Jordan | 2.9 | 48 | 13 | 3.4 | 20 | 5.8 | 97 | 48 | 3 | 53 | 42 | 0.7 | 610 |
| Kuwait | 1.1 | 43 | 5 | 3.9 | 18 | 2.8 | 44 | 44 | 2 | 69 | 56 | 0.4 | 15,480 |
| Lebanon | 2.9 | 40 | 9 | 3.1 | 22 | 5.6 | 59 | 41 | 5 | 64 | 60 | 0.9 | — |
| Oman | 0.8 | 49 | 18 | 3.2 | 22 | 1.6 | 138 | — | — | — | 5 | — | 2,680 |
| Qatar | 0.1 | 44 | 14 | 3.0 | 23 | 0.2 | 138 | — | — | — | 69 | — | 11,400 |
| Saudi Arabia | 7.8 | 49 | 19 | 3.0 | 23 | 14.9 | 152 | 45 | 3 | 45 | 21 | 2.1 | 4,480 |
| Syria | 8.1 | 45 | 14 | 3.1 | 22 | 16.0 | 114 | 48 | 3 | 57 | 47 | 2.1 | 780 |
| Turkey | 48.2 | 34 | 11 | 2.3 | 30 | 71.1 | 119 | 40 | 4 | 57 | 45 | 12.3 | 990 |
| United Arab Emirates | 0.8 | 44 | 14 | 3.0 | 23 | 1.6 | 138 | — | — | — | 52 | — | 13,990 |
| Yemen | 5.8 | 49 | 19 | 3.0 | 23 | 10.9 | 155 | 45 | 3 | 45 | 9 | 1.7 | 250 |
| Yemen, Democratic | 1.9 | 49 | 19 | 3.0 | 23 | 3.5 | 155 | 48 | 4 | 45 | 33 | 0.4 | 280 |
| MIDDLE SOUTH ASIA | 879 | 37 | 15 | 2.2 | 32 | 1,459 | 133 | 41 | 3 | 49 | 21 | 222 | 220 |
| Afghanistan | 17.8 | 48 | 22 | 2.6 | 27 | 31.2 | 190 | 44 | 3 | 40 | 15 | 5.4 | 160 |
| Bangladesh | 85.0 | 47 | 20 | 2.7 | 26 | 153.5 | 153 | 43 | 3 | 46 | 9 | 22.8 | 110 |
| Bhutan | 1.3 | 43 | 19 | 2.4 | 29 | 2.1 | — | 42 | 3 | 44 | 3 | 0.4 | 70 |
| India | 634.7 | 34 | 14 | 2.0 | 35 | 1,017.7 | 129 | 40 | 3 | 49 | 21 | 156.6 | 150 |
| Iran | 35.5 | 45 | 14 | 3.1 | 22 | 65.4 | 104 | 47 | 3 | 57 | 47 | 9.8 | 1,930 |
| Maldives | 0.1 | 50 | 23 | 2.7 | 26 | 0.2 | — | 44 | 2 | — | 11 | — | 110 |
| Nepal | 13.4 | 44 | 20 | 2.3 | 30 | 23.0 | 152 | 40 | 3 | 44 | 4 | 4.4 | 120 |
| Pakistan | 76.8 | 44 | 14 | 3.0 | 23 | 145.1 | 139 | 46 | 3 | 51 | 26 | 20.4 | 170 |
| Sri Lanka | 14.2 | 26 | 9 | 1.7 | 41 | 20.4 | 47 | 39 | 4 | 68 | 22 | 3.0 | 200 |
| SOUTHEAST ASIA | 341 | 37 | 13 | 2.4 | 29 | 574 | 118 | 43 | 3 | 52 | 21 | 94 | 330 |
| Burma | 32.2 | 38 | 15 | 2.4 | 29 | 52.7 | 140 | 40 | 4 | 50 | 22 | 7.6 | 120 |
| Dem. Kampuchea (Cambodia) | 8.2 | 47 | 18 | 2.9 | 24 | 14.7 | 150 | 45 | 3 | 45 | 12 | 2.6 | — |
| East Timor | 0.8 | 44 | 22 | 2.3 | 30 | 1.2 | 175 | 42 | 3 | 40 | 11 | 0.1 | — |
| Indonesia | 140.2 | 38 | 14 | 2.4 | 29 | 226.4 | 137 | 44 | 2 | 48 | 18 | 33.7 | 240 |
| Lao People's Dem. Rep. | 3.6 | 44 | 21 | 2.4 | 29 | 5.8 | 175 | 42 | 3 | 40 | 15 | 0.9 | 90 |
| Malaysia | 13.0 | 31 | 6 | 2.5 | 28 | 21.7 | 41 | 43 | 3 | 68 | 27 | 4.1 | 860 |
| Philippines | 46.3 | 35 | 10 | 2.5 | 28 | 84.7 | 80 | 43 | 3 | 58 | 32 | 15.7 | 410 |
| Singapore | 2.3 | 19 | 5 | 1.4 | 50 | 3.1 | 12 | 32 | 4 | 71 | 100 | 0.4 | 2,700 |
| Thailand | 45.1 | 33 | 10 | 2.3 | 30 | 83.3 | 89 | 45 | 3 | 61 | 13 | 17.8 | 380 |
| Vietnam | 49.2 | 41 | 19 | 2.2 | 32 | 80.3 | 115 | 41 | 4 | 48 | 22 | 11.4 | — |
| EAST ASIA | 1,122 | 22 | 8 | 1.4 | 50 | 1,457 | 59 | 33 | 6 | 66 | 31 | 167 | 900 |
| China, People's Rep. of | 930 | 22 | 8 | 1.4 | 50 | 1,213 | 65 | 33 | 6 | 65 | 24 | 136.9 | 410 |
| Hong Kong | 4.5 | 18 | 5 | 1.3 | 53 | 5.8 | 14 | 30 | 6 | 72 | 92 | 0.7 | 2,110 |
| Japan | 114.4 | 16 | 6 | 1.0 | 69 | 132.1 | 9 | 24 | 8 | 74 | 76 | 12.0 | 4,910 |
| Korea, Dem. People's Rep. of | 17.1 | 34 | 9 | 2.5 | 28 | 27.4 | 70 | 42 | 4 | 61 | 43 | 6.1 | 470 |
| Korea, Rep. of | 37.1 | 24 | 7 | 1.7 | 41 | 53.5 | 47 | 39 | 4 | 65 | 48 | 8.3 | 670 |
| Macao | 0.3 | 25 | 7 | 1.8 | 38 | 0.4 | 78 | 38 | 5 | — | 97 | — | 780 |
| Mongolia | 1.6 | 35 | 8 | 2.7 | 26 | 2.7 | 70 | 44 | 3 | 61 | 46 | 0.5 | 860 |
| Taiwan (Rep. of China) | 16.9 | 26 | 5 | 2.1 | 33 | 22.1 | 25 | 35 | 4 | 70 | 64 | 2.7 | 1,070 |

**Population Data for Latin America, 1978**

| Region or country | Population estimate mid-1978 (millions) | Birth rate (per 1,000) | Death rate (per 1,000) | Rate of natural increase (percentage) | Number of years to double population | Population projection to 2000 (millions) | Infant mortality rate (per 1,000 live births) | Population under 15 years (percentage) | Population over 64 years (percentage) | Life expectancy at birth (years) | Urban population (percentage) | Projected labor force increase 1978–2000 (millions) | Per-capita gross national product (US$) |
|---|---|---|---|---|---|---|---|---|---|---|---|---|---|
| LATIN AMERICA | 344 | 36 | 9 | 2.7 | 26 | 606 | 84 | 42 | 4 | 62 | 61 | 96 | 1,100 |
| MIDDLE AMERICA | 87 | 42 | 8 | 3.3 | 21 | 174 | 68 | 46 | 3 | 63 | 58 | 28 | 1,000 |
| Costa Rica | 2.1 | 29 | 5 | 2.4 | 29 | 3.6 | 38 | 44 | 4 | 68 | 41 | 0.6 | 1,040 |
| El Salvador | 4.4 | 40 | 8 | 3.3 | 21 | 8.5 | 55 | 46 | 3 | 58 | 39 | 1.5 | 490 |
| Guatemala | 6.6 | 43 | 12 | 3.1 | 22 | 12.2 | 75 | 45 | 3 | 53 | 36 | 1.8 | 630 |
| Honduras | 3.0 | 47 | 13 | 3.5 | 20 | 6.1 | 103 | 47 | 2 | 55 | 31 | 1.1 | 390 |
| Mexico | 66.9 | 42 | 8 | 3.4 | 20 | 135.6 | 66 | 46 | 3 | 65 | 64 | 21.4 | 1,090 |
| Nicaragua | 2.4 | 47 | 13 | 3.4 | 20 | 4.8 | 110 | 48 | 3 | 53 | 49 | 0.9 | 750 |
| Panama | 1.8 | 32 | 7 | 2.6 | 27 | 3.2 | 47 | 43 | 4 | 66 | 50 | 0.5 | 1,310 |
| CARIBBEAN | 28 | 29 | 8 | 2.0 | 35 | 44 | 64 | 41 | 5 | 64 | 48 | 6 | 1,060 |
| Bahamas | 0.2 | 20 | 5 | 1.4 | 50 | 0.3 | 35 | 44 | 3 | 66 | 58 | — | 3,310 |
| Barbados | 0.3 | 19 | 9 | 0.9 | 77 | 0.3 | 28 | 34 | 9 | 69 | 44 | — | 1,550 |
| Cuba | 9.7 | 21 | 5 | 1.5 | 46 | 14.7 | 27 | 37 | 6 | 70 | 60 | 2.1 | 860 |
| Dominican Republic | 5.1 | 39 | 9 | 3.0 | 23 | 10.6 | 96 | 48 | 3 | 58 | 47 | 1.7 | 780 |
| Grenada | 0.1 | 27 | 6 | 2.2 | 32 | 0.1 | 24 | — | — | 63 | 15 | — | 420 |
| Guadeloupe | 0.3 | 28 | 7 | 2.1 | 33 | 0.4 | 35 | 40 | 5 | 65 | 48 | 0.1 | 1,500 |
| Haiti | 4.8 | 39 | 17 | 2.2 | 32 | 7.1 | 115 | 42 | 4 | 50 | 23 | 1.0 | 200 |
| Jamaica | 2.1 | 30 | 7 | 2.3 | 30 | 2.8 | 20 | 46 | 6 | 68 | 41 | 0.5 | 1,070 |
| Martinique | 0.3 | 22 | 7 | 1.6 | 43 | 0.4 | 32 | 41 | 5 | 65 | 50 | 0.1 | 2,350 |
| Netherlands Antilles | 0.3 | 28 | 7 | 2.1 | 33 | 0.4 | 28 | 38 | 5 | 62 | 48 | — | 1,680 |
| Puerto Rico | 3.4 | 24 | 6 | 1.7 | 41 | 4.2 | 21 | 35 | 7 | 72 | 62 | 0.4 | 2,430 |
| Trinidad and Tobago | 1.1 | 23 | 6 | 1.6 | 43 | 1.4 | 31 | 39 | 4 | 66 | 49 | 0.2 | 2,240 |
| TROP. SOUTH AMERICA | 188 | 37 | 9 | 2.8 | 25 | 337 | 98 | 43 | 3 | 61 | 60 | 57 | 1,090 |
| Bolivia | 4.9 | 47 | 18 | 2.9 | 24 | 8.7 | 157 | 42 | 4 | 48 | 34 | 1.5 | 390 |
| Brazil | 115.4 | 36 | 8 | 2.8 | 25 | 205.2 | 109 | 42 | 3 | 61 | 60 | 33.5 | 1,140 |
| Colombia | 25.8 | 33 | 9 | 2.4 | 29 | 46.7 | 90 | 44 | 3 | 61 | 64 | 8.7 | 630 |
| Ecuador | 7.8 | 40 | 9 | 3.2 | 22 | 14.8 | 66 | 45 | 4 | 60 | 41 | 2.7 | 640 |
| Guyana | 0.8 | 27 | 7 | 2.0 | 35 | 1.2 | 50 | 44 | 3 | 68 | 40 | 0.2 | 540 |
| Paraguay | 2.9 | 39 | 8 | 3.1 | 22 | 5.3 | 65 | 45 | 3 | 62 | 37 | 0.9 | 640 |
| Peru | 17.1 | 40 | 11 | 2.9 | 24 | 31.2 | 80 | 45 | 3 | 56 | 55 | 5.1 | 800 |
| Surinam | 0.5 | 37 | 7 | 3.0 | 23 | 0.9 | 30 | 50 | 4 | 66 | 50 | 0.2 | 1,370 |
| Venezuela | 13.1 | 36 | 7 | 3.0 | 23 | 23.2 | 49 | 45 | 3 | 65 | 75 | 4.1 | 2,570 |
| TEMP. SOUTH AMERICA | 40 | 23 | 9 | 1.4 | 50 | 52 | 57 | 30 | 7 | 66 | 80 | 5 | 1,400 |
| Argentina | 26.4 | 23 | 9 | 1.3 | 53 | 32.9 | 59 | 29 | 8 | 68 | 80 | 2.7 | 1,550 |
| Chile | 10.8 | 25 | 7 | 1.8 | 38 | 15.4 | 56 | 35 | 5 | 63 | 79 | 2.1 | 1,050 |
| Uruguay | 2.8 | 21 | 10 | 1.1 | 63 | 3.4 | 49 | 28 | 9 | 69 | 83 | 0.3 | 1,390 |

## Population Data for the Developed World, 1978

| Region or country | Population estimate mid-1978 (millions) | Birth rate (per 1,000) | Death rate (per 1,000) | Rate of natural increase (percentage) | Number of years to double population | Population projection to 2000 (millions) | Infant mortality rate (per 1,000 live births) | Population under 15 years (percentage) | Population over 64 years (percentage) | Life expectancy at birth (years) | Urban population (percentage) | Projected labor force increase 1978–2000 (millions) | Per-capita gross national product (US$) |
|---|---|---|---|---|---|---|---|---|---|---|---|---|---|
| EUROPE | 480 | 15 | 10 | 0.4 | 173 | 538 | 20 | 24 | 12 | 71 | 65 | 30 | 4,420 |
| NORTHERN EUROPE | 82 | 13 | 12 | 0.1 | 693 | 90 | 13 | 23 | 14 | 72 | 73 | 5 | 4,910 |
| Denmark | 5.1 | 13 | 11 | 0.2 | 347 | 5.4 | 10 | 23 | 13 | 74 | 67 | 0.2 | 7,450 |
| Finland | 4.8 | 14 | 9 | 0.5 | 139 | 4.8 | 10 | 22 | 10 | 71 | 59 | 0.1 | 5,620 |
| Iceland | 0.2 | 19 | 6 | 1.3 | 53 | 0.3 | 8 | 30 | 9 | 75 | 87 | — | 6,100 |
| Ireland | 3.2 | 22 | 10 | 1.1 | 63 | 4.0 | 15 | 31 | 11 | 71 | 52 | 0.4 | 2,560 |
| Norway | 4.1 | 13 | 10 | 0.3 | 231 | 4.5 | 10 | 24 | 14 | 75 | 45 | 0.3 | 7,420 |
| Sweden | 8.3 | 12 | 11 | 0.1 | 693 | 9.2 | 9 | 21 | 15 | 75 | 83 | 0.6 | 8,670 |
| United Kingdom | 56.0 | 12 | 12 | 0.0 | — | 61.6 | 14 | 23 | 14 | 72 | 76 | 3.5 | 4,020 |
| WESTERN EUROPE | 153 | 12 | 11 | 0.1 | 693 | 169 | 14 | 23 | 14 | 72 | 79 | 9 | 6,900 |
| Austria | 7.5 | 12 | 13 | −0.1 | — | 8.0 | 18 | 23 | 15 | 71 | 52 | 0.5 | 5,330 |
| Belgium | 9.9 | 12 | 12 | 0.0 | — | 10.7 | 14 | 23 | 14 | 71 | 87 | 0.4 | 6,780 |
| France | 53.4 | 14 | 10 | 0.3 | 231 | 61.2 | 13 | 24 | 14 | 73 | 70 | 4.9 | 6,550 |
| Germany, Federal Rep. of | 61.3 | 10 | 12 | −0.2 | — | 65.6 | 17 | 21 | 15 | 71 | 92 | 2.1 | 7,380 |
| Luxembourg | 0.4 | 11 | 13 | −0.2 | — | 0.4 | 18 | 20 | 13 | 70 | 69 | — | 6,460 |
| Netherlands | 13.9 | 13 | 8 | 0.5 | 139 | 16.0 | 11 | 25 | 11 | 74 | 76 | 1.0 | 6,200 |
| Switzerland | 6.2 | 12 | 9 | 0.3 | 231 | 6.9 | 11 | 22 | 13 | 73 | 55 | 0.4 | 8,800 |
| EASTERN EUROPE | 108 | 18 | 11 | 0.7 | 99 | 122 | 25 | 23 | 11 | 70 | 58 | 8 | 2,820 |
| Bulgaria | 8.8 | 16 | 10 | 0.6 | 116 | 9.9 | 23 | 22 | 11 | 71 | 58 | 0.3 | 2,310 |
| Czechoslovakia | 15.2 | 19 | 11 | 0.8 | 87 | 17.0 | 21 | 23 | 12 | 70 | 67 | 1.0 | 3,840 |
| German Democratic Rep. | 16.7 | 12 | 14 | −0.2 | — | 17.4 | 14 | 21 | 16 | 72 | 76 | 0.9 | 4,220 |
| Hungary | 10.7 | 18 | 12 | 0.5 | 139 | 11.1 | 30 | 20 | 13 | 69 | 50 | 0.2 | 2,280 |
| Poland | 35.1 | 20 | 9 | 1.1 | 63 | 40.2 | 24 | 24 | 9 | 71 | 55 | 3.5 | 2,860 |
| Romania | 21.9 | 20 | 10 | 1.0 | 69 | 26.0 | 31 | 25 | 10 | 70 | 48 | 1.9 | 1,450 |
| SOUTHERN EUROPE | 137 | 17 | 9 | 0.8 | 87 | 158 | 24 | 26 | 11 | 71 | 51 | 8 | 2,620 |
| Albania | 2.6 | 32 | 8 | 2.4 | 29 | 4.1 | 87 | 40 | 5 | 68 | 34 | 0.9 | 540 |
| Greece | 9.3 | 16 | 8 | 0.8 | 87 | 9.9 | 23 | 24 | 12 | 72 | 65 | 0.2 | 2,590 |
| Italy | 56.7 | 14 | 10 | 0.4 | 173 | 61.8 | 19 | 24 | 12 | 72 | 53 | 2.1 | 3,050 |
| Malta | 0.3 | 19 | 10 | 0.9 | 77 | 0.3 | 14 | 26 | 9 | 70 | 94 | — | 1,390 |
| Portugal | 9.7 | 19 | 10 | 0.9 | 77 | 10.8 | 39 | 27 | 10 | 69 | 26 | 0.4 | 1,690 |
| Spain | 36.8 | 18 | 8 | 1.0 | 69 | 45.3 | 11 | 28 | 10 | 72 | 61 | 2.8 | 2,920 |
| Yugoslavia | 22.0 | 18 | 8 | 1.0 | 69 | 25.6 | 36 | 26 | 8 | 68 | 39 | 1.7 | 1,680 |
| USSR | 261 | 18 | 9 | 0.9 | 77 | 313 | 28 | 25 | 9 | 69 | 62 | 20 | 2,760 |
| NORTH AMERICA | 242 | 15 | 9 | 0.6 | 116 | 292 | 15 | 25 | 10 | 73 | 74 | 30 | 7,850 |
| Canada | 23.6 | 16 | 7 | 0.9 | 77 | 31.3 | 14 | 26 | 8 | 73 | 76 | 3.7 | 7,510 |
| United States | 218.4 | 15 | 9 | 0.6 | 116 | 260.4 | 15 | 24 | 11 | 73 | 74 | 26.6 | 7,890 |
| AUSTRALIA AND NEW ZEALAND | 17.5 | 17 | 8 | 0.9 | — | 24.2 | 14 | 28 | 8 | 72 | 85 | 3.2 | 5,762 |
| JAPAN | 114.4 | 16 | 6 | 1.0 | 69 | 132.1 | 9 | 24 | 8 | 74 | 76 | 12.0 | 4,910 |

(Source: World Population Data Sheet, 1978, Population Reference Bureau, Washington, D.C.)

Appendix 2-1

Standard Normal, Cumulative Probability in Right-Hand Tail
(For Negative Values of $z$, Areas are Found by Symmetry)

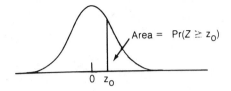

Area = $\Pr(Z \geq z_0)$

0  $z_0$

| | | | | | Second Decimal Place of $z_0$ | | | | | |
|---|---|---|---|---|---|---|---|---|---|---|
| $z_0$ | .00 | .01 | .02 | .03 | .04 | .05 | .06 | .07 | .08 | .09 |
| 0.0 | .5000 | .4960 | .4920 | .4880 | .4840 | .4801 | .4761 | .4721 | .4681 | .4641 |
| 0.1 | .4602 | .4562 | .4522 | .4483 | .4443 | .4404 | .4364 | .4325 | .4286 | .4247 |
| 0.2 | .4207 | .4168 | .4129 | .4090 | .4052 | .4013 | .3974 | .3936 | .3897 | .3859 |
| 0.3 | .3821 | .3783 | .3745 | .3707 | .3669 | .3632 | .3594 | .3557 | .3520 | .3483 |
| 0.4 | .3446 | .3409 | .3372 | .3336 | .3300 | .3264 | .3228 | .3192 | .3156 | .3121 |
| 0.5 | .3085 | .3050 | .3015 | .2981 | .2946 | .2912 | .2877 | .2843 | .2810 | .2776 |
| 0.6 | .2743 | .2709 | .2676 | .2643 | .2611 | .2578 | .2546 | .2514 | .2483 | .2451 |
| 0.7 | .2420 | .2389 | .2358 | .2327 | .2296 | .2266 | .2236 | .2206 | .2177 | .2148 |
| 0.8 | .2119 | .2090 | .2061 | .2033 | .2005 | .1977 | .1949 | .1922 | .1894 | .1867 |
| 0.9 | .1841 | .1814 | .1788 | .1762 | .1736 | .1711 | .1685 | .1660 | .1635 | .1611 |
| 1.0 | .1587 | .1562 | .1539 | .1515 | .1492 | .1469 | .1446 | .1423 | .1401 | .1379 |
| 1.1 | .1357 | .1335 | .1314 | .1292 | .1271 | .1251 | .1230 | .1210 | .1190 | .1170 |
| 1.2 | .1151 | .1131 | .1112 | .1093 | .1075 | .1056 | .1038 | .1020 | .1003 | .0985 |
| 1.3 | .0968 | .0951 | .0934 | .0918 | .0901 | .0885 | .0869 | .0853 | .0838 | .0823 |
| 1.4 | .0808 | .0793 | .0778 | .0764 | .0749 | .0735 | .0722 | .0708 | .0694 | .0681 |
| 1.5 | .0668 | .0655 | .0643 | .0630 | .0618 | .0606 | .0594 | .0582 | .0571 | .0559 |
| 1.6 | .0548 | .0537 | .0526 | .0516 | .0505 | .0495 | .0485 | .0475 | .0465 | .0455 |
| 1.7 | .0446 | .0436 | .0427 | .0418 | .0409 | .0401 | .0392 | .0384 | .0375 | .0367 |
| 1.8 | .0359 | .0352 | .0344 | .0336 | .0329 | .0322 | .0314 | .0307 | .0301 | .0294 |
| 1.9 | .0287 | .0281 | .0274 | .0268 | .0262 | .0256 | .0250 | .0244 | .0239 | .0233 |
| 2.0 | .0228 | .0222 | .0217 | .0212 | .0207 | .0202 | .0197 | .0192 | .0188 | .0183 |
| 2.1 | .0179 | .0174 | .0170 | .0166 | .0162 | .0158 | .0154 | .0150 | .0146 | .0143 |
| 2.2 | .0139 | .0136 | .0132 | .0129 | .0125 | .0122 | .0119 | .0116 | .0113 | .0110 |
| 2.3 | .0107 | .0104 | .0102 | .0099 | .0096 | .0094 | .0091 | .0089 | .0087 | .0084 |
| 2.4 | .0082 | .0080 | .0078 | .0075 | .0073 | .0071 | .0069 | .0068 | .0066 | .0064 |
| 2.5 | .0062 | .0060 | .0059 | .0057 | .0055 | .0054 | .0052 | .0051 | .0049 | .0048 |
| 2.6 | .0047 | .0045 | .0044 | .0043 | .0041 | .0040 | .0039 | .0038 | .0037 | .0036 |
| 2.7 | .0035 | .0034 | .0033 | .0032 | .0031 | .0030 | .0029 | .0028 | .0027 | .0026 |
| 2.8 | .0026 | .0025 | .0024 | .0023 | .0023 | .0022 | .0021 | .0021 | .0020 | .0019 |
| 2.9 | .0019 | .0018 | .0017 | .0017 | .0016 | .0016 | .0015 | .0015 | .0014 | .0014 |

(Wonnacott T, Wonnacott R: Introductory for Statistics for Business and Economics, 2nd ed. New York, John Wiley & Sons, 1977)

Appendix 2-2

Student's *t* Critical Points

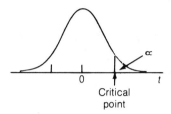

Critical
point

| df \ ∝ | .25 | .10 | .05 | .025 | .010 | .005 | .0025 | .0010 | .0005 |
|---|---|---|---|---|---|---|---|---|---|
| 1 | 1.000 | 3.078 | 6.314 | 12.706 | 31.821 | 63.637 | 127.32 | 318.31 | 636.62 |
| 2 | .816 | 1.886 | 2.920 | 4.303 | 6.965 | 9.925 | 14.089 | 22.326 | 31.598 |
| 3 | .765 | 1.638 | 2.353 | 3.182 | 4.541 | 5.841 | 7.453 | 10.213 | 12.924 |
| 4 | .741 | 1.533 | 2.132 | 2.776 | 3.747 | 4.604 | 5.598 | 7.173 | 8.610 |
| 5 | .727 | 1.476 | 2.015 | 2.571 | 3.365 | 4.032 | 4.773 | 5.893 | 6.869 |
| 6 | .718 | 1.440 | 1.943 | 2.447 | 3.143 | 3.707 | 4.317 | 5.208 | 5.959 |
| 7 | .711 | 1.415 | 1.895 | 2.365 | 2.998 | 3.499 | 4.020 | 4.785 | 5.408 |
| 8 | .706 | 1.397 | 1.860 | 2.306 | 2.896 | 3.355 | 3.833 | 4.501 | 5.041 |
| 9 | .703 | 1.383 | 1.833 | 2.262 | 2.821 | 3.250 | 3.690 | 4.297 | 4.781 |
| 10 | .700 | 1.372 | 1.812 | 2.228 | 2.764 | 3.169 | 3.581 | 4.144 | 4.537 |
| 11 | .697 | 1.363 | 1.796 | 2.201 | 2.718 | 3.106 | 3.497 | 4.025 | 4.437 |
| 12 | .695 | 1.356 | 1.782 | 2.179 | 2.681 | 3.055 | 3.428 | 3.930 | 4.318 |
| 13 | .694 | 1.350 | 1.771 | 2.160 | 2.650 | 3.012 | 3.372 | 3.852 | 4.221 |
| 14 | .692 | 1.345 | 1.761 | 2.145 | 2.624 | 2.977 | 3.326 | 3.787 | 4.140 |
| 15 | .691 | 1.341 | 1.753 | 2.131 | 2.602 | 2.947 | 3.286 | 3.733 | 4.073 |
| 16 | .690 | 1.337 | 1.746 | 2.120 | 2.583 | 2.921 | 3.252 | 3.686 | 4.015 |
| 17 | .689 | 1.333 | 1.740 | 2.110 | 2.567 | 2.898 | 3.222 | 3.646 | 3.965 |
| 18 | .688 | 1.330 | 1.734 | 2.101 | 2.552 | 2.878 | 3.197 | 3.610 | 3.922 |
| 19 | .688 | 1.328 | 1.729 | 2.093 | 2.539 | 2.861 | 3.174 | 3.579 | 3.883 |
| 20 | .687 | 1.325 | 1.725 | 2.086 | 2.528 | 2.845 | 3.153 | 3.552 | 3.850 |
| 21 | .686 | 1.323 | 1.721 | 2.080 | 2.518 | 2.831 | 3.135 | 3.257 | 3.189 |
| 22 | .686 | 1.321 | 1.717 | 2.074 | 2.508 | 2.819 | 3.119 | 3.505 | 3.792 |
| 23 | .685 | 1.319 | 1.714 | 2.069 | 2.500 | 2.807 | 3.104 | 3.485 | 3.767 |
| 24 | .685 | 1.318 | 1.711 | 2.064 | 2.492 | 2.797 | 3.091 | 3.467 | 3.745 |
| 25 | .684 | 1.316 | 1.708 | 2.060 | 2.485 | 2.787 | 3.078 | 3.450 | 3.725 |
| 26 | .684 | 1.315 | 1.706 | 2.056 | 2.479 | 2.779 | 3.067 | 3.435 | 3.707 |
| 27 | .684 | 1.314 | 1.703 | 2.052 | 2.473 | 2.771 | 3.057 | 3.421 | 3.690 |
| 28 | .683 | 1.313 | 1.701 | 2.048 | 2.467 | 2.763 | 3.047 | 3.408 | 3.674 |
| 29 | .683 | 1.311 | 1.699 | 2.045 | 2.462 | 2.756 | 3.038 | 3.396 | 3.659 |
| 30 | .683 | 1.310 | 1.697 | 2.042 | 2.457 | 2.750 | 3.030 | 3.385 | 3.646 |
| 40 | .681 | 1.303 | 1.684 | 2.021 | 2.423 | 2.704 | 2.971 | 3.307 | 3.551 |
| 60 | .679 | 1.296 | 1.671 | 2.000 | 2.390 | 2.660 | 2.915 | 3.232 | 3.460 |
| 120 | .677 | 1.289 | 1.658 | 1.980 | 2.358 | 2.617 | 2.860 | 3.160 | 3.373 |
| ∞ | .674 | 1.282 | 1.645 | 1.960 | 2.326 | 2.576 | 2.807 | 3.090 | 3.291 |

Appendix 2-3

$X^2$ Critical Points

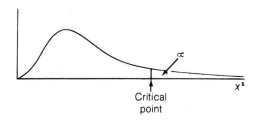

Critical
point

| oc \\ d f | .250 | .100 | .050 | .025 | .010 | .005 | .001 |
|---|---|---|---|---|---|---|---|
| 1 | 1.32 | 2.71 | 3.84 | 5.02 | 6.63 | 7.88 | 10.8 |
| 2 | 2.77 | 4.61 | 5.99 | 7.38 | 9.21 | 10.6 | 13.8 |
| 3 | 4.11 | 6.25 | 7.81 | 9.35 | 11.3 | 12.8 | 16.3 |
| 4 | 5.39 | 7.78 | 9.49 | 11.1 | 13.3 | 14.9 | 18.5 |
| 5 | 6.63 | 9.24 | 11.1 | 12.8 | 15.1 | 16.7 | 20.5 |
| 6 | 7.84 | 10.6 | 12.6 | 14.4 | 16.8 | 18.5 | 22.5 |
| 7 | 9.04 | 12.0 | 14.1 | 16.0 | 18.5 | 20.3 | 24.3 |
| 8 | 10.2 | 13.4 | 15.5 | 17.5 | 20.1 | 22.0 | 26.1 |
| 9 | 11.4 | 14.7 | 16.9 | 19.0 | 21.7 | 23.6 | 27.9 |
| 10 | 12.5 | 16.0 | 18.3 | 20.5 | 23.2 | 25.2 | 29.6 |
| 11 | 13.7 | 17.3 | 19.7 | 21.9 | 24.7 | 26.8 | 31.3 |
| 12 | 14.8 | 18.5 | 21.0 | 23.3 | 26.2 | 28.3 | 32.9 |
| 13 | 16.0 | 19.8 | 22.4 | 24.7 | 27.7 | 29.8 | 34.5 |
| 14 | 17.1 | 21.1 | 23.7 | 26.1 | 29.1 | 31.3 | 36.1 |
| 15 | 18.2 | 22.3 | 25.0 | 27.5 | 30.6 | 32.8 | 37.7 |
| 16 | 19.4 | 23.5 | 26.3 | 28.8 | 32.0 | 34.3 | 39.3 |
| 17 | 20.5 | 24.8 | 27.6 | 30.2 | 33.4 | 35.7 | 40.8 |
| 18 | 21.6 | 26.0 | 28.9 | 31.5 | 34.8 | 37.2 | 42.3 |
| 19 | 22.7 | 27.2 | 30.1 | 32.9 | 36.2 | 38.6 | 32.8 |
| 20 | 23.8 | 28.4 | 31.4 | 34.2 | 37.6 | 40.0 | 45.3 |
| 21 | 24.9 | 29.6 | 32.7 | 35.5 | 38.9 | 41.4 | 46.8 |
| 22 | 26.0 | 30.8 | 33.9 | 36.8 | 40.3 | 42.8 | 48.3 |
| 23 | 27.1 | 32.0 | 35.2 | 38.1 | 41.6 | 44.2 | 49.7 |
| 24 | 28.2 | 33.2 | 36.4 | 39.4 | 32.0 | 45.6 | 51.2 |
| 25 | 29.3 | 34.4 | 37.7 | 40.6 | 44.3 | 46.9 | 52.6 |
| 26 | 30.4 | 35.6 | 38.9 | 41.9 | 45.6 | 48.3 | 54.1 |
| 27 | 31.5 | 36.7 | 40.1 | 43.2 | 47.0 | 49.6 | 55.5 |
| 28 | 32.6 | 37.9 | 41.3 | 44.5 | 48.3 | 51.0 | 56.9 |
| 29 | 33.7 | 39.1 | 42.6 | 45.7 | 49.6 | 52.3 | 58.3 |
| 30 | 34.8 | 40.3 | 43.8 | 47.0 | 50.9 | 53.7 | 59.7 |
| 40 | 45.6 | 51.8 | 55.8 | 59.3 | 63.7 | 66.8 | 73.4 |
| 50 | 56.3 | 63.2 | 67.5 | 71.4 | 76.2 | 79.5 | 86.7 |
| 60 | 67.0 | 74.4 | 79.1 | 83.3 | 88.4 | 92.0 | 99.6 |
| 70 | 77.6 | 85.5 | 90.5 | 95.0 | 100 | 104 | 112 |
| 80 | 88.1 | 96.6 | 102 | 107 | 112 | 116 | 125 |
| 90 | 98.6 | 108 | 113 | 118 | 124 | 128 | 137 |
| 100 | 109 | 118 | 124 | 130 | 136 | 140 | 149 |

(Wonnacott T, Wonnacott R: Introductory for Statistics for Business and Economics, 2nd ed. New York, John Wiley & Sons, 1977)

# Appendix 2-4

## F Critical Points

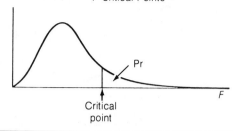

Critical
point

| | | | | | | | Degrees of freedom for numerator | | | | | |
|---|---|---|---|---|---|---|---|---|---|---|---|---|---|
| | ∝ | 1 | 2 | 3 | 4 | 5 | 6 | 8 | 10 | 20 | 40 | ∝ |
| **1** .25 | | 5.83 | 7.50 | 8.20 | 8.58 | 8.82 | 8.98 | 9.19 | 9.32 | 9.58 | 9.71 | 9.85 |
| .10 | | 39.9 | 49.5 | 53.6 | 55.8 | 57.2 | 58.2 | 59.4 | 60.2 | 61.7 | 62.5 | 63.3 |
| .05 | | 161 | 200 | 216 | 225 | 230 | 234 | 239 | 242 | 248 | 251 | 254 |
| **2** .25 | | 2.57 | 3.00 | 3.15 | 3.23 | 3.28 | 3.31 | 3.35 | 3.38 | 3.43 | 3.45 | 3.48 |
| .10 | | 8.53 | 9.00 | 9.16 | 9.24 | 9.29 | 9.33 | 9.37 | 9.39 | 9.44 | 9.47 | 9.49 |
| .05 | | 18.5 | 19.0 | 19.2 | 19.2 | 19.3 | 19.3 | 19.4 | 19.4 | 19.4 | 19.5 | 19.5 |
| .01 | | 98.5 | 99.0 | 99.2 | 99.2 | 99.3 | 99.3 | 99.4 | 99.4 | 99.4 | 99.5 | 99.5 |
| .001 | | 998 | 999 | 999 | 999 | 999 | 999 | 999 | 999 | 999 | 999 | 999 |
| **3** .25 | | 2.02 | 2.28 | 2.36 | 2.39 | 2.41 | 2.42 | 2.44 | 2.44 | 2.46 | 2.47 | 2.47 |
| .10 | | 5.54 | 5.46 | 5.39 | 5.34 | 5.31 | 5.28 | 5.25 | 5.23 | 5.18 | 5.16 | 5.13 |
| .05 | | 10.1 | 9.55 | 9.28 | 9.12 | 9.10 | 8.94 | 8.85 | 8.79 | 8.66 | 8.59 | 8.53 |
| .01 | | 34.1 | 30.8 | 29.5 | 28.7 | 28.2 | 27.9 | 27.5 | 27.2 | 26.7 | 26.4 | 26.1 |
| .001 | | 167 | 149 | 141 | 137 | 135 | 133 | 131 | 129 | 126 | 125 | 124 |
| **4** .25 | | 1.81 | 2.00 | 2.05 | 2.06 | 2.07 | 2.08 | 2.08 | 2.08 | 2.08 | 2.08 | 2.08 |
| .10 | | 4.54 | 4.32 | 4.19 | 4.11 | 4.05 | 4.01 | 3.95 | 3.92 | 3.84 | 3.80 | 3.76 |
| .05 | | 7.71 | 6.94 | 6.59 | 6.39 | 6.26 | 6.16 | 6.04 | 5.96 | 5.80 | 5.72 | 5.63 |
| .01 | | 21.2 | 18.0 | 16.7 | 16.0 | 15.5 | 15.2 | 14.8 | 14.5 | 14.0 | 13.7 | 13.5 |
| .001 | | 74.1 | 61.3 | 56.2 | 53.4 | 51.7 | 50.5 | 49.0 | 48.1 | 46.1 | 45.1 | 44.1 |
| **5** .25 | | 1.69 | 1.85 | 1.88 | 1.89 | 1.89 | 1.89 | 1.89 | 1.89 | 1.88 | 1.88 | 1.87 |
| .10 | | 4.06 | 3.78 | 3.62 | 3.52 | 3.45 | 3.40 | 3.34 | 3.30 | 3.21 | 3.16 | 3.10 |
| .05 | | 6.61 | 5.79 | 5.41 | 5.19 | 5.05 | 4.95 | 4.82 | 4.74 | 4.56 | 4.46 | 4.36 |
| .01 | | 16.3 | 13.3 | 12.1 | 11.4 | 11.0 | 10.7 | 10.3 | 10.1 | 9.55 | 9.29 | 9.02 |
| .001 | | 47.2 | 37.1 | 33.2 | 31.1 | 29.8 | 28.8 | 27.6 | 26.9 | 25.4 | 24.6 | 23.8 |
| **6** .25 | | 1.62 | 1.76 | 1.78 | 1.79 | 1.79 | 1.78 | 1.77 | 1.77 | 1.76 | 1.75 | 1.74 |
| .10 | | 3.78 | 3.46 | 3.29 | 3.18 | 3.11 | 3.05 | 2.98 | 2.94 | 2.84 | 2.78 | 2.72 |
| .05 | | 5.99 | 5.14 | 4.76 | 4.53 | 4.39 | 4.28 | 4.15 | 4.06 | 3.87 | 3.77 | 3.67 |
| .01 | | 13.7 | 10.9 | 9.78 | 9.15 | 8.75 | 8.47 | 8.10 | 7.87 | 7.40 | 7.14 | 6.88 |
| .001 | | 35.5 | 27.0 | 23.7 | 21.9 | 20.8 | 20.0 | 19.0 | 18.4 | 17.1 | 16.4 | 15.8 |
| **7** .25 | | 1.57 | 1.70 | 1.72 | 1.72 | 1.71 | 1.71 | 1.70 | 1.69 | 1.67 | 1.66 | 1.65 |
| .10 | | 3.59 | 3.26 | 3.07 | 2.96 | 2.88 | 2.83 | 2.75 | 2.70 | 2.59 | 2.54 | 2.47 |
| .05 | | 5.59 | 4.74 | 4.35 | 4.12 | 3.97 | 3.87 | 3.73 | 3.64 | 3.44 | 3.34 | 3.23 |
| .01 | | 12.2 | 9.55 | 8.45 | 7.85 | 7.46 | 7.19 | 6.84 | 6.62 | 6.16 | 5.91 | 5.65 |
| .001 | | 29.3 | 21.7 | 18.8 | 17.2 | 16.2 | 15.5 | 14.6 | 14.1 | 12.9 | 12.3 | 11.7 |
| **8** .25 | | 1.54 | 1.66 | 1.67 | 1.66 | 1.66 | 1.65 | 1.64 | 1.63 | 1.61 | 1.59 | 1.58 |
| .10 | | 3.46 | 3.11 | 2.92 | 2.81 | 2.73 | 2.67 | 2.59 | 2.54 | 2.42 | 2.36 | 2.29 |
| .05 | | 5.32 | 4.46 | 4.07 | 3.84 | 3.69 | 3.58 | 3.44 | 3.35 | 3.15 | 3.04 | 2.93 |
| .01 | | 11.3 | 8.65 | 7.59 | 7.01 | 6.63 | 6.37 | 6.03 | 5.81 | 5.36 | 5.12 | 4.86 |
| .001 | | 25.4 | 18.5 | 15.8 | 14.4 | 13.5 | 12.9 | 12.0 | 11.5 | 10.5 | 9.92 | 9.33 |
| **9** .25 | | 1.51 | 1.62 | 1.63 | 1.63 | 1.62 | 1.61 | 1.60 | 1.59 | 1.56 | 1.55 | 1.53 |
| .10 | | 3.36 | 3.01 | 2.81 | 2.69 | 2.61 | 2.55 | 2.47 | 2.42 | 2.30 | 2.23 | 2.16 |
| .05 | | 5.12 | 4.26 | 3.86 | 3.63 | 3.48 | 3.37 | 3.23 | 3.14 | 2.94 | 2.83 | 2.71 |
| .01 | | 10.6 | 8.02 | 6.99 | 6.42 | 6.06 | 5.80 | 5.47 | 5.26 | 4.81 | 4.57 | 4.31 |
| .001 | | 22.9 | 16.4 | 13.9 | 12.6 | 11.7 | 11.1 | 10.4 | 9.89 | 8.90 | 8.37 | 7.81 |

(Continued)

| | | | | | Degrees of freedom for numerator | | | | | | | |
|---|---|---|---|---|---|---|---|---|---|---|---|---|
| | ∞ | 1 | 2 | 3 | 4 | 5 | 6 | 8 | 10 | 20 | 40 | ∞ |
| 10 | .25 | 1.49 | 1.60 | 1.60 | 1.59 | 1.59 | 1.58 | 1.56 | 1.55 | 1.52 | 1.51 | 1.48 |
| | .10 | 3.28 | 2.92 | 2.73 | 2.61 | 2.52 | 2.46 | 2.38 | 2.32 | 2.20 | 2.13 | 2.06 |
| | .05 | 4.96 | 4.10 | 3.71 | 3.48 | 3.33 | 3.22 | 3.07 | 2.98 | 2.77 | 2.66 | 2.54 |
| | .01 | 10.0 | 7.56 | 6.55 | 5.99 | 5.64 | 5.39 | 5.06 | 4.85 | 4.41 | 4.17 | 3.91 |
| | .001 | 21.0 | 14.9 | 12.6 | 11.3 | 10.5 | 9.92 | 9.20 | 8.75 | 7.80 | 7.30 | 6.76 |
| 12 | .25 | 1.56 | 1.56 | 1.56 | 1.55 | 1.54 | 1.53 | 1.51 | 1.50 | 1.47 | 1.45 | 1.42 |
| | .10 | 3.18 | 2.81 | 2.61 | 2.48 | 2.39 | 2.33 | 2.24 | 2.19 | 2.06 | 1.99 | 1.90 |
| | .05 | 4.75 | 3.89 | 3.49 | 3.26 | 3.11 | 3.00 | 2.85 | 2.75 | 2.54 | 2.43 | 2.30 |
| | .01 | 9.33 | 6.93 | 5.95 | 5.41 | 5.06 | 4.82 | 4.50 | 4.30 | 3.86 | 3.62 | 3.36 |
| | .001 | 18.6 | 13.0 | 10.8 | 9.63 | 8.89 | 8.38 | 7.71 | 7.29 | 6.40 | 5.93 | 5.42 |
| 14 | .25 | 1.44 | 1.53 | 1.53 | 1.52 | 1.51 | 1.50 | 1.48 | 1.46 | 1.43 | 1.41 | 1.38 |
| | .10 | 3.10 | 2.73 | 2.52 | 2.39 | 2.31 | 2.24 | 2.15 | 2.10 | 1.96 | 1.89 | 1.80 |
| | .05 | 4.60 | 3.74 | 3.34 | 3.11 | 2.96 | 2.85 | 2.70 | 2.60 | 2.39 | 2.27 | 2.13 |
| | .01 | 8.86 | 5.51 | 5.56 | 5.04 | 4.69 | 4.46 | 4.14 | 3.94 | 3.51 | 3.27 | 3.00 |
| | .001 | 17.1 | 11.8 | 9.73 | 8.62 | 7.92 | 7.43 | 6.80 | 6.40 | 5.56 | 5.10 | 4.60 |
| 16 | .25 | 1.42 | 1.51 | 1.51 | 1.50 | 1.48 | 1.48 | 1.46 | 1.45 | 1.40 | 1.37 | 1.34 |
| | .10 | 3.05 | 2.67 | 2.46 | 2.33 | 2.24 | 2.18 | 2.09 | 2.03 | 1.89 | 1.81 | 1.72 |
| | .05 | 4.49 | 3.63 | 3.24 | 3.01 | 2.85 | 2.74 | 2.59 | 2.49 | 2.28 | 2.15 | 2.01 |
| | .01 | 8.53 | 6.23 | 5.29 | 4.77 | 4.44 | 4.20 | 3.89 | 3.69 | 3.26 | 3.02 | 2.75 |
| | .001 | 16.1 | 11.0 | 9.00 | 7.94 | 7.27 | 6.81 | 6.19 | 5.81 | 4.99 | 4.54 | 4.06 |
| 18 | .25 | 1.41 | 1.50 | 1.49 | 1.48 | 1.46 | 1.45 | 1.43 | 1.42 | 1.38 | 1.35 | 1.32 |
| | .10 | 3.01 | 2.62 | 2.42 | 2.29 | 2.20 | 2.13 | 2.04 | 1.98 | 1.84 | 1.75 | 1.66 |
| | .05 | 4.41 | 3.55 | 3.16 | 2.93 | 2.77 | 2.66 | 2.51 | 2.41 | 2.19 | 2.06 | 1.92 |
| | .01 | 8.29 | 6.01 | 5.09 | 4.58 | 4.25 | 4.01 | 3.71 | 3.51 | 3.08 | 2.84 | 2.57 |
| | .001 | 15.4 | 10.4 | 8.49 | 7.46 | 6.81 | 6.35 | 5.76 | 5.39 | 4.59 | 4.15 | 3.67 |
| 20 | .25 | 1.40 | 1.49 | 1.48 | 1.46 | 1.45 | 1.44 | 1.42 | 1.40 | 1.36 | 1.33 | 1.29 |
| | .10 | 2.97 | 2.59 | 2.38 | 2.25 | 2.16 | 2.09 | 2.00 | 1.94 | 1.79 | 1.71 | 1.61 |
| | .05 | 4.35 | 3.49 | 3.10 | 2.87 | 2.71 | 2.60 | 2.45 | 2.35 | 2.12 | 1.99 | 1.84 |
| | .01 | 8.10 | 5.85 | 4.94 | 4.43 | 4.10 | 3.87 | 3.56 | 3.37 | 2.94 | 2.69 | 2.42 |
| | .001 | 14.8 | 9.95 | 8.10 | 7.10 | 6.46 | 6.02 | 5.44 | 5.08 | 4.29 | 3.86 | 3.38 |
| 30 | .25 | 1.38 | 1.45 | 1.44 | 1.42 | 1.41 | 1.39 | 1.37 | 1.35 | 1.30 | 1.27 | 1.23 |
| | .10 | 2.88 | 2.49 | 2.28 | 2.14 | 2.05 | 1.98 | 1.88 | 1.82 | 1.67 | 1.57 | 1.46 |
| | .05 | 4.17 | 3.32 | 2.92 | 2.69 | 2.53 | 2.42 | 2.27 | 2.16 | 1.93 | 1.79 | 1.62 |
| | .01 | 7.56 | 5.39 | 4.51 | 4.02 | 3.70 | 3.47 | 3.17 | 2.98 | 2.55 | 2.30 | 2.01 |
| | .001 | 13.3 | 8.77 | 7.05 | 6.12 | 5.53 | 5.12 | 4.58 | 4.24 | 3.49 | 3.07 | 2.59 |
| 40 | .25 | 1.36 | 1.44 | 1.42 | 1.40 | 1.39 | 1.37 | 1.35 | 1.33 | 1.28 | 1.24 | 1.19 |
| | .10 | 2.84 | 2.44 | 2.23 | 2.09 | 2.00 | 1.93 | 1.83 | 1.76 | 1.61 | 1.51 | 1.38 |
| | .05 | 4.08 | 3.23 | 2.84 | 2.61 | 2.45 | 2.34 | 2.18 | 2.08 | 1.84 | 1.69 | 1.51 |
| | .01 | 7.31 | 5.18 | 4.31 | 3.83 | 3.51 | 3.29 | 2.99 | 2.80 | 2.37 | 2.11 | 1.80 |
| | .001 | 12.6 | 8.25 | 6.60 | 5.70 | 5.13 | 4.73 | 4.21 | 3.87 | 3.15 | 2.73 | 2.23 |
| 60 | .25 | 1.35 | 1.42 | 1.41 | 1.38 | 1.37 | 1.35 | 1.32 | 1.30 | 1.25 | 1.21 | 1.15 |
| | .10 | 2.79 | 2.39 | 2.18 | 2.04 | 1.95 | 1.87 | 1.77 | 1.71 | 1.54 | 1.44 | 1.29 |
| | .05 | 4.00 | 3.15 | 2.76 | 2.53 | 2.37 | 2.25 | 2.10 | 1.99 | 1.75 | 1.59 | 1.39 |
| | .01 | 7.08 | 4.98 | 4.13 | 3.65 | 3.34 | 3.12 | 2.82 | 2.63 | 2.20 | 1.94 | 1.60 |
| | .001 | 12.0 | 7.76 | 6.17 | 5.31 | 4.76 | 4.37 | 3.87 | 3.54 | 2.83 | 2.41 | 1.89 |
| 120 | .25 | 1.34 | 1.40 | 1.39 | 1.37 | 1.35 | 1.33 | 1.30 | 1.28 | 1.22 | 1.18 | 1.10 |
| | .10 | 2.75 | 2.35 | 2.13 | 1.99 | 1.90 | 1.82 | 1.72 | 1.65 | 1.48 | 1.37 | 1.19 |
| | .05 | 3.92 | 3.07 | 2.68 | 2.45 | 2.29 | 2.17 | 2.02 | 1.91 | 1.66 | 1.50 | 1.25 |
| | .01 | 6.85 | 4.79 | 3.95 | 3.48 | 3.17 | 2.96 | 2.66 | 2.47 | 2.03 | 1.76 | 1.38 |
| | .001 | 11.4 | 7.32 | 5.79 | 4.95 | 4.42 | 4.04 | 3.55 | 3.24 | 2.53 | 2.11 | 1.54 |
| ∞ | .25 | 1.32 | 1.39 | 1.37 | 1.35 | 1.33 | 1.31 | 1.28 | 1.25 | 1.19 | 1.14 | 1.00 |
| | .10 | 2.71 | 2.30 | 2.08 | 1.94 | 1.85 | 1.77 | 1.67 | 1.60 | 1.42 | 1.30 | 1.00 |
| | .05 | 3.84 | 3.00 | 2.60 | 2.37 | 2.21 | 2.10 | 1.94 | 1.83 | 1.57 | 1.39 | 1.00 |
| | .01 | 6.63 | 4.61 | 3.78 | 3.32 | 3.02 | 2.80 | 2.51 | 2.32 | 1.88 | 1.59 | 1.00 |
| | .001 | 10.8 | 6.91 | 5.42 | 4.62 | 4.10 | 3.74 | 3.27 | 2.96 | 2.27 | 1.84 | 1.00 |

Degrees of freedom for denominator

(Wonnacott T, Wonnacott R: Introductory Statistics for Business and Economics, 2nd ed. New York, John Wiley & Sons, 1977).

Appendix 2-5

Values of the Correlation Coefficient
for Different Levels of Significance

The absolute value of a calculation correlation must be greater than this number in the table to be significantly different from zero.

| | ∝ | | |
|---|---|---|---|
| (n-k)* | .05 | .02 | .01 |
| 1 | .996917 | .9995066 | .9998766 |
| 2 | .95000 | .98000 | .990000 |
| 3 | .8783 | .93433 | .95873 |
| 4 | .8114 | .8822 | .91720 |
| 5 | .7545 | .8329 | .8745 |
| 6 | .7067 | .7887 | .8343 |
| 7 | .6664 | .7498 | .7977 |
| 8 | .6319 | .7155 | .7646 |
| 9 | .6021 | .6851 | .7348 |
| 10 | .5760 | .6581 | .7079 |
| 11 | .5529 | .6339 | .6835 |
| 12 | .5324 | .6120 | .6614 |
| 13 | .5139 | .5923 | .6411 |
| 14 | .4973 | .5742 | .6226 |
| 15 | .4821 | .5577 | .6055 |
| 16 | .4683 | .5425 | .5897 |
| 17 | .4555 | .5285 | .5751 |
| 18 | .4438 | .5155 | .5614 |
| 19 | .4329 | .5034 | .5487 |
| 20 | .4227 | .4921 | .5368 |
| 25 | .3809 | .4451 | .4869 |
| 30 | .3494 | .4093 | .4487 |
| 35 | .3246 | .3810 | .4182 |
| 40 | .3044 | .3578 | .3932 |
| 45 | .2875 | .3284 | .3721 |
| 50 | .2732 | .3218 | .3541 |
| 60 | .2500 | .2948 | .3248 |
| 70 | .2319 | .2737 | .3017 |
| 80 | .2172 | .2565 | .2830 |
| 90 | .2050 | .2422 | .2673 |
| 100 | .1946 | .2301 | .2540 |

*The degrees of freedom are the number of observations in any one variable in the correlation minus the number of variables being considered. In a regular correlation matrix, a correlation coefficient represents a correlation between two variables.

Partial correlation is the correlation between two variables holding other variable or variables constant. In this case *k* is the total number of variables involved.

(Clark C, Schkade L: Statistical Analysis for Administrative Decisions, 2nd ed. Dallas, South-Western Publishing Co., 1974)

## General Notes

*Sources of data:* Aside from population estimates and projections (see footnotes 2 and 6), number of years to double population (footnote 5), projected labor force increase (footnote 10), and per capita Gross National Product (footnote 11), most of the data in this table were reported in the following United Nations (UN) publications: *Demographic Yearbook,* 1975 and 1976 editions; *Population and Vital Statistics Report, Data Available as of 1 January 1978,* Statistical Papers, Series A, Vol. XXX, No. 1; *Selected World Demographic Indicators by Countries, 1950-2000,* ESA/P/WP.55, 28 May 1975; and *Single-Year Population Estimates and Projections for Major Areas, Regions, and Countries of the World, 1950-2000,* ESA/P/WP.56, 6 October 1975. A few figures shown were from other sources, including draft materials for the forthcoming U.S. Bureau of the Census report, *World Population: 1977;* unpublished materials and reports of the Census Bureau's Foreign Demographic Analysis Division; D. Nortman and E. Hofstatter, *Population and Family Planning Programs: A Factbook,* 9th edition, The Population Council, forthcoming May 1978; various analytical studies; and official data reported by individual countries. The source for any figure shown on the *Data Sheet* may be obtained by writing or telephoning the Population Reference Bureau.

*Figures for the regions and the world:* Population totals take into account small areas not listed on the *Data Sheet.* Totals may also not equal the sums of their parts because of independent rounding. All other data are weighted averages for countries for which data are available.

Dashes indicate data are unavailable.

## Footnotes

[1] The *Data Sheet* lists all UN members and all geopolitical entities with a population larger than 200,000.

[2] Except for the People's Republic of China, based on a population total from a very recent census or on the most recent official country or UN estimate; for almost all countries the estimate was for mid-1976. Each estimate was updated by the Population Reference Bureau to mid-1978 by applying the same rate of growth as indicated by population change during part or all of the period since 1970.

[3] Annual number of births or deaths per 1,000 population. For the more developed countries with complete or nearly complete registration of births and deaths, nearly all the rates shown pertain to 1975 or 1976. For most developing countries with incomplete registration, the rates refer to 1976 and were obtained by interpolating the 1970-75 and 1975-80 estimates of the UN to 1976. The 1970-75 and 1975-80 rates were used in the medium variant estimates and projections as assessed by the UN in 1973 (UN, *Selected World Demographic Indicators . . .*). The interpolated figures should be considered as rough approximations only.

[4] Birth rate minus the death rate. Since the rates were based on unrounded birth and death rates, some rates do not exactly equal the difference between the birth and death rates shown because of rounding.

[5] Based on the rate of natural increase shown and assuming no change in the rate.

[6] Except for the United States, estimated by the Population Reference Bureau by applying the percentage increase in the population 1978-2000 implied by the UN medium variant projections to the population total as estimated for mid-1978. For the United States, the figure shown is the Series II projection given in the U.S. Bureau of the Census, *Projections of the Population of the United States: 1977 to 2050,* P-25, No. 704, July 1977.

[7] Annual number of deaths to infants under one year of age per 1,000 live births. For countries with complete or nearly complete registration of births and deaths, nearly all rates pertain to 1975 or 1976. For many developing countries with incomplete registration, rates are the latest available estimates generally obtained from the UN sources noted above; from World Health Organization, *World Health Statistics Report,* Vol. 29, No. 11, 1976; or from U.S. Bureau of the Census, *World Population: 1975,* and draft materials of the forthcoming *World Population: 1977.*

[8] The "age dependency ratio" for each country or region can be derived by adding the percentages under 15 years and over 64 years and dividing by the complement. For the world as a whole, for example, 36% + 6% ÷ 58% gives a figure of 72 persons in the "dependent ages" for each 100 persons in the "working ages" of 15 to 64.

[9] The percentage of the total population living in areas defined as urban by each country.

[10] An asterisk (*) denotes a labor force increase of less than 50,000. Except for the People's Republic of China and Taiwan, the source for all figures is *Labour Force Estimates and Projections, 1950-2000,* 2nd edition, International Labour Office (ILO), Geneva, 1977. These labor force projections are based on estimated and projected age-sex specific activity rates for each country and the UN medium variant projections of the total population of each country. The 1978 labor force figure was obtained by interpolating the ILO figures for 1975 and 1980. Figures for the People's Republic of China and Taiwan were obtained by applying the ILO's projected activity rates for China (including Taiwan) for 1978 (interpolated from 1975 and 1980 rates) and 2000 to the PRB's population totals for these dates. It was assumed that the activity rates for Taiwan would be the same as for the People's Republic of China.

[11] Data refer to 1976 except for 12 of the smaller countries for which the data refer to 1975. All data for the individual countries are from the *World Bank Atlas: Population, Per Capita Product and Growth Rates,* World Bank, 1977.

[12] Recent reports of provincial population totals announced through Chinese radio and newspapers during the 1975-77 period indicate that the population of the People's Republic of China is much higher than previous estimates have shown. Consequently, most estimates of the PRC's population have been revised upward to take into account these higher provincial totals. Recent reports of the PRC's successful efforts in

family planning and health care have also led to downward revisions in the estimated levels of fertility and mortality. After evaluating estimates from a variety of sources, the Population Reference Bureau considers the estimates shown here to be reasonable.

[13] The UN does not show figures for Taiwan. These figures were separately estimated on the basis of official Taiwan data. The population was assumed to increase to 2000 at the same rate as that of the People's Republic of China.

# Glossary

## Robert Jansen

**Abortifacient.** Agent used to induce *abortion.*

**Abortion.** Termination of pregnancy, generally before the 20th week; either unintentional (spontaneous) or intentional (therapeutic).

**Acidophilic.** Possessing an affinity for acid histologic stains—e.g., cell cytoplasm, collagen.

**Acrosome.** Cap or envelope over the head of a *spermatozoon,* important in penetration of the *ovum* during *fertilization.*

**Adenohypophysis.** Anterior pituitary gland, which is composed of glandular tissue that secretes, among other hormones, *follicle-stimulating hormone, luteinizing hormone,* and *prolactin;* see also *hypothalamus.*

**Adhesions.** Postinflammatory connective tissue bands or webs between viscera and/or body wall resulting from surgery, trauma, or infection.

**Adnexa.** Accessory structures; particularly, the *fallopian tubes* and *ovaries* in relation to the uterus.

**Adrenergic.** Pertaining to *epinephrine.*

**Albuginea.** See *tunica albuginea.*

**Alkali.** Organic substance with basic (as opposed to acid) properties; neutralizes acid; see also *pH.*

**Alkaloid.** Nitrogen-containing, alkaline organic substances extracted from plants, with powerful pharmacologic properties.

**Alpha subunit.** See *gonadotropin.*

**Alveoli.** Tiny saclike spaces for gas exchange in the lung, lined by blood capillaries.

**Amenorrhea.** Prolonged absence of menstruation.

**Amino acid.** Organic substance bearing two special groups, an amino group and a carboxylic acid group, through which a bond may form (peptide bond) to link successive amino acids into a *polypeptide* chain.

**Amniocentesis.** Insertion of a needle through the abdomen into the amniotic cavity either to withdraw fluid for testing purposes or to instill an *abortifacient.*

**Amniotic.** Related to the amnion, the innermost embryonic membrane forming a fluid-filled sac, the amniotic cavity, which protects the fetus during intrauterine life.

**AMP.** Adenosine monophosphate; depleted form of *ATP;* see also *cyclic AMP.*

**Anabolic.** Tending to cause growth and weight gain; in particular, the response to testosterone normally seen in adolescent males, consisting of increasing height, and increasing bone and muscle mass.

**Analog.** Synthetic chemical substance structurally or functionally related to a natural biological entity; for example see *progestin.*

**Analogous.** Of similar function, but not necessarily of similar origin.

**Androgen.** Male sex hormone—for example, testosterone.

**Androgen binding globulin.** See *sex hormone binding globulin.*

**Androstane.** A *steroid* chemically related to *testosterone.*

**Androstenedione.** Weak *androgen;* precursor for *testosterone* and *estrone* synthesis.

**Anovulation.** Absence of ovulation.

**Antenatal.** See *antepartum* (synonym).

**Antepartum.** Occurring before childbirth.

**Anterior.** Front side of erect animals, such as humans.

**Anterior pituitary gland.** See *adenohypophysis*.

**Antibody.** Natural protein capable of a specific immunological reaction with an *antigen*.

**Antigen.** Chemical substance, usually foreign to the body, capable of eliciting the formation of *antibodies*.

**Antinatalist.** Favoring low fertility.

**Antiserum.** Specially prepared blood serum that contains at least one specific *antibody*.

**Arcuate nucleus.** Cluster of nerve cell bodies in the medial *hypothalamus*; important associations with the *adenohypophysis*.

**Aromatization.** Chemical desaturation of a six-carbon ring component of a molecule to the configuration of that of benzene; occurs in the conversion of an *androgen* to an *estrogen*.

**Arteriole.** Small branch of an artery.

**Astringent.** Shrinking, and driving the blood from, the tissues.

**ATP.** Adenosine triphosphate; molecule that stores energy inside cells.

**Atretic.** Characterized by atresia, the absence, or loss, of "hollowness" of an organ or tissue; follicular atresia is the cessation of further development and regression of a *follicle*, without ovulation.

**Attrition** (*special sense*). Dropping out of a study.

**Autosomal.** Pertaining to any of the 22 pairs of nonsex chromosomes.

**Autotransplantation.** Process of surgically removing an organ and replacing it in the same subject at its original, or a new, location.

**Azoospermia.** Absence of *spermatozoa* in the *semen*.

**Basalis.** Deepest layer of the *endometrium*; normally not shed at menstruation, and serves as the source for subsequent endometrial regeneration.

**Basophilic.** Possessing an affinity for basic histologic stains—e.g., cell nuclei.

**Beta subunit.** One of two *polypeptide* chains of pituitary glycoprotein hormones; provides the property of specificity of biological action to the whole hormone; see also *gonadotropin*; in practice, refers to a *radioimmunoassay* that distinguishes *chorionic gonadotropin* from *luteinizing hormone*.

**Biodegradable.** Capable of being broken down by biological processes; specifically, describes a synthetic matrix used as an implanted vehicle for the storage and release of drugs.

**Blastocyst.** Stage of embryo development subsequent to the *morula,* reached before *implantation;* hollow sphere, with an aggregation of cells at one pole destined to become the embryo proper; outer cells develop into the *trophoblast.*

**Blastocyst hatching.** Emergence of the developing mammalian embryo from its thick protective coat (the *zona pellucida*) just prior to implantation.

**Bolus.** Collection of food, secretion, or pharmaceutical preparation moving through a hollow organ or tissue.

**Bound hormone.** *Hormone* in the plasma bound to a plasma protein and so not immediately available to the tissues for biological activity; such binding is especially important for *steroid* hormones, which are otherwise only barely soluble in water; see also *free hormone.*

**Breakthrough bleeding.** Uterine bleeding between the times of normal menstruation, of sufficient degree normally to require sanitary protection; see also *spotting.*

**Brideprice.** Money, goods, or estate given to a woman or her kin by the bridegroom or his kin at marriage.

**Bromsulphalein.** Pharmacological marker substance used in liver function tests; the ability of the liver to clear BSP from the blood and secrete it into the bile is directly related to the health of the liver.

**Bronchiole.** Small duct in the lungs connecting, through several branches, the more major bronchi with the *alveoli.*

**Bulbourethral gland.** Paired genital glands at the proximal end of the penile urethra in the male.

**Cannula.** Tube designed to be inserted into a duct or cavity.

**Cauterization.** Use of heat, electric current, or caustic chemicals to destroy a tissue or tissue surface, causing a scar to form.

**Cephalad.** Towards the head end of the body.

**Cervix.** Literally, "neck"; the cervix of the *uterus* is that part that does not participate in the specific uterine changes that support a pregnancy; it is a firm cylindrical structure situated between the body (corpus) of the uterus and the vagina; dilates during labor prior to giving birth; its canal (the endocervix) is lined by *columnar epithelium,* which produces *mucus* that must be penetrated by *spermatazoa* before *fertilization* can take place; its vaginal surface (the ectocervix) is normally covered with *squamous epithelium;* cancers of the cervix usually occur at the junction between the endocervix and ectocervix, and so are detectable by taking a Papanicolaou ("Pap") smear from this region or by *colposcopy.*

**Cholesterol.** Chemical substance, fat-soluble, of wide occurrence; precursor for synthesis of all *steroid* hormones.

**Chorionic gonadotropin.** The *gonadotropin* of pregnancy, produced by the *trophoblast;* very similar in structure and function to *luteinizing hormone.*

**Chromosome.** Structures in the cell nucleus composed of *DNA* in tight combination with basic protein; divide prior to cell division in *mitosis; diploid* cells have 46 chromosome; *haploid* cells have 23.

**Cilia.** Submicroscopic, motile, threadlike structures on the apex of cells of some mucosal surfaces, capable of causing the transport of secretion over such surfaces; singular: cilium.

**Cleavage.** Repeated division by mitosis of the fertilized ovum.

**Clines** (*demography*). Gradients.

**Clinic continuation rate.** Rate at which clients seeking nonpermanent methods of contraception continue to return for services and supplies.

**Clitoris.** Small erectile organ in front of the urethra and vagina, homologous to the male *penis.*

**Coagulate.** To clot, as in blood; or to cauterize tissue, as in tubal sterilization.

**Cohort** (*demography*). Aggregate of individuals who experience important events in their life cycles at the same time.

**Coitus interruptus.** Form of contraception in which the penis is withdrawn from the vagina before ejaculation.

**Colposcopy.** Specialized visual examination of the surface of the uterine *cervix* and the vagina using magnification.

**Colpotomy.** Surgical incision of the wall of the vagina; in particular, such entry into the *cul-de-sac* for the purpose of *tubal ligation.*

**Columnar cell.** Tall, usually glandular, epithelial cell; the lining of the canal of the cervix is composed of columnar cells.

**Columnar epithelium.** *Epithelium* composed of a single layer of tall cells, as opposed to *squamous epithelium;* occurs in the female reproductive tract (among other sites) in the canal of the *cervix,* in the *endometrium* and in the *fallopian tubes*—in all of which sites two types of cells are generally found: those that produce secretion, and those that bear *cilia.*

**Compactum.** Superficial layer of the *endometrium.*

**Conceptus.** Product of conception, the early embryo.

**Condyloma acuminatum.** Wartlike growth in the genital area, caused by a virus normally transmitted venereally.

**Confidence interval** (*statistics*). Range of values for estimating a *parameter.*

**Conjugal.** Pertaining to marriage; marital.

**Connective tissue.** General term for tissue that is not covering a surface, i.e., that is not *epithelium;* many specializations occur, such as bone, cartilage, muscle, nervous tissue, and blood vessels, and so it is usual to restrict the term to the loose or dense fibrous tissue that exists between the more specialized tissues.

**Consensuality.** Acceptance, agreement.

**Contraindication.** Unfavorable aspect tending to dissuade the physician from the use of a procedure or drug, usually because the procedure or drug is potentially harmful in such a circumstance.

**Copolymer.** See *polymer.*

**Cornual recess.** Corner of the cavity of the *uterus* on each side, at the apex of which the *fallopian tube* is received; also known as the uterine angle.

**Corona radiata.** Layer of elongated follicle cells immediately surrounding the ovum at ovulation; see also *cumulus cells.*

**Corpus albicans.** Connective tissue scar in the substance of the ovary after regression of the *corpus luteum.*

**Corpus cavernosum.** See *penis;* also present in the *clitoris.*

**Corpus luteum.** Yellow colored glandular structure in the ovary, formed from the ruptured *graafian follicle;* secretes *progesterone,* the hormone that dominates the *luteal phase* of the menstrual cycle.

**Corpus spongiosum.** See *penis.*

**Correlation coefficient.** See *product moment correlation coefficient.*

**Cortical dominance.** Embryonic development of an organ such as the ovary, in which the principal adult elements are derived from the cortex, or outside, of the embryonic organ (in contradistinction to the testis, which develops through *medullary dominance*).

**Cosmesis.** Preservation or enhancement of normal or attractive appearance.

**Cross-reactivity** (*special sense*). Reaction between an antiserum and different but related antigens.

**Crypts.** Infoldings of an epithelial surface, particularly in the canal of the *cervix*.

**Cul-de-sac.** Downward extension of the pelvic peritoneal cavity between the cervix and upper vagina and the rectum.

**Culdoscopy.** Direct visualization of the female internal genital organs (the uterus, tubes, and ovaries) by means of an optical instrument (culdoscope) inserted through the posterior vagina into the cul-de-sac; see also *laparoscopy*.

**Cumulus cells.** Follicle cells attached to the ovum more loosely than the *corona radiata;* may assist ovum pickup by the fallopian tube.

**Curettage.** See *dilatation and curettage*.

**Cyclic AMP.** Special molecule formed inside cells from *ATP;* acts as a "second messenger" in response to action at the cell surface of a *hormone* or other substance and initiates protein synthesis within the cell; *gonadotropins,* but not steroid hormones, owe most of their actions to cyclic AMP.

**Cyclical** (*statistics*). In a time-series set of data, that pattern of movement through time that remains after removing the trend and seasonal component; a cyclical for a given month is computed by dividing the original data by the trend and seasonal amount estimated (from time-series analysis) for that month.

**Cystitis.** Inflammation of the urinary bladder.

**Cytology.** Microscopial examination of exfoliated cells, especially from the cervix or vagina.

**Cytoplasm.** Protoplasm of a cell, excluding the *nucleus*.

**Cytotoxic agent.** Substance that causes cell death.

**Dalton.** Unit of molecular mass.

**Daughter cell.** Cell produced by the division of another cell.

**Decapeptide.** *Polypeptide* compound of ten *amino acids*.

**Decidua.** Thickening of the endometrium that occurs in pregnancy, largely through hypertrophy of *stromal* cells; mostly lost at birth with separation of the *placenta*.

**Degrees of freedom** (*statistical sense*). Number of independently varying quantities.

**Dehydroepiandrosterone (DHA** or **DHEA).** Very weak *androgen,* precursor to *androstenedione*.

**Demethylation.** Chemical reaction involving the removal of a single carbon atom from a molecule.

**Demic diffusion.** Dispersion of individuals from a local population or deme (composed of individuals who mate most frequently with one another, and hence tend to resemble one another more closely than individuals in adjacent demes).

**Deoxyribonucleic acid.** See *DNA*.

**Dependent** (*special sense*). Hanging down, inferiorly situated in relation to another structure anatomically.

**Depot-medroxyprogesterone acetate.** A long-acting *progestin* given by injection.

**Diachronic.** Existing at different times; opposite: *synchronic*.

**Differentiation.** Process of growth and specialization.

**Dihydrotestosterone.** Reduced, more potent, metabolic product of *testosterone*.

**Dilatation and curettage.** Surgical procedure involving mechanical widening of the cervical canal (dilatation) to allow the uterine cavity and lining to be scraped out with a spoon-shaped instrument (curette); abbreviated "D & C."

**Diploid.** Having the number of chromosomes (46) normal to a somatic cell or primordial germ cell; twice the *haploid* number (23) characteristic of a mature germ cell.

**Distal.** Situated away from a central point of reference; opposite: *proximal*.

**DNA.** Deoxyribonucleic acid; complex organic substance consisting of two strands wound helically about each other; precise composition constitutes the code for genetic inheritance; contained mostly within the *chromosomes;* see also *RNA*.

**Dominant gene.** Gene that expresses itself in the *phenotype,* irrespective of whether there are one or two such genes in the *genotype;* see also *recessive gene*.

**Dopamine.** *Neurotransmitter* important in transmission of impulses between nerves, especially in the *hypothalamus;* the precursor for *norepinephrine* synthesis; the *inhibiting factor* that controls *prolactin* production from the *adenohypophysis.*

**Dorsal.** Situated at, or relatively nearer to, the back; opposite: *ventral.*

**Dowry.** Money, goods, or estate that the bride brings with her, or that is given to the groom or his family at the time of marriage.

**Ectoderm.** Epithelium covering the exterior surface of the body, particularly in the embryo.

**Ectopic.** Situated out of the normal position.

**Edema.** Presence, between cells, of abnormally large amounts of fluid in a tissue.

**Efferent ducts.** Very fine tubules carrying *spermatozoa* from the *seminiferous tubules* in the *testis* to the *epididymis.*

**Electrocautery.** Use of electric current to coagulate small blood vessels in surgery, or to coagulate tissue to close a *lumen,* as in tubal sterilization.

**Embolism.** Process of passage of an *embolus.*

**Embolus.** Abnormal material, such as blood clot, amniotic fluid, fat, or air, carried in the bloodstream from one site to another.

**Embryo.** Developmental stage from fertilization of an ovum to birth; in man, the term is not often used after 2 months of development (see *fetus*).

**Emmenagogue.** Substance that stimulates menstruation.

**Endocrine gland.** Ductless gland secreting one or more *hormones* into the bloodstream.

**Endocrinology.** Science concerned with the function of the *endocrine glands.*

**Endoderm.** Epithelium lining the gut, particularly in the embryo.

**Endometrium.** Glandular layer or *mucosa* that lines the cavity of the uterus; responds to *estrogen* with proliferation (growth) and to *progesterone* with secretion; partly shed at *menstruation.*

**Ependyma.** Epithelium that lines the *ventricles* of the brain; ependymal cells possess a brush border of *microvilli* and may be involved in transport of substances from cerebrospinal fluid to adjacent neurons.

**Epididymis.** Long, coiled, fine tube adjacent to the testis; receives the *efferent ducts* and leads to the *vas deferens;* maturation of *spermatozoa* is completed in the epididymis.

**Epididymitis.** Inflammation of the *epididymis.*

**Epinephrine.** Neurotransmitter of the *sympathetic nervous system;* also called adrenalin.

**Epithelium.** Coherent and adherent sheet of cells covering external or internal surfaces of the body, and the glandular tissues connected to or derived from such surfaces; see also *columnar epithelium, squamous epithelium.*

**Estradiol.** Potent *estrogen;* derived from *testosterone* or from *estrone;* secreted principally by the developing *graafian follicle,* but also by the *corpus luteum;* produces growth of the *endometrium.*

**Estrogen.** Female sex hormone—e.g., *estradiol, estrone,* and various synthetic analogs.

**Estrogen-primed.** Status of having been subjected to the action of an estrogen.

**Estrone.** *Estrogen,* less potent than *estradiol;* the main estrogen produced after the menopause.

**Ever-married** (*demography*). Either currently or previously married.

**Exogenous.** Produced from without.

**Extended family.** Family unit containing more than two generations.

**Fallopian tubes.** Paired organs situated on each side of the uterus, connecting it to the ovaries; receives ovulated eggs from the ovary and transmits sperm from the cavity of the uterus; the site of *fertilization;* see also *uterus.*

**Family of orientation.** Family in which one is born and raised, as opposed to the conjugal family one forms at marriage.

**Fascia.** Sheet of *connective tissue.*

**Fecundity.** Ability to produce children.

**Fenestrated.** Bearing one or more openings, or "windows."

**Fertility.** Ability to produce children; in demography, the term is restricted to the demonstrated production of children.

**Fertilization.** Union of a *spermatozoon* and an *ovum* to produce a *zygote;* see also *syngamy.*

**Fetus.** Stage of further development of the *embryo* subsequent to attainment of the main features recognizable as those of full development; i.e., from the 3rd through the 9th month of intrauterine development.

**Fibrils.**   Minute fibers or filaments, usually arranged as bundles or groups to form larger, more complex fibers.

**Fiscal.**   Of, or related to, finance or financial matters.

**Fistula.**   Abnormal passage through a tissue connecting two body cavities, or connecting a body cavity with the exterior.

**Five alpha reductase.**   Enzyme that converts *testosterone* to *dihydrotestosterone*.

**Flushing** (for sperm).   Introduction and recovery of fluid from the female reproductive tract or peritoneal cavity for subsequent examination in order to determine the presence or absence of spermatozoa.

**Follicle (ovarian).**   Functional unit of the ovary, composed of an *ovum* surrounded by (*a*) a nest of specialized follicle cells (granulosa cells), which increase in number as the follicle grows, and (*b*) by a condensation of ovarian connective tissue, the inner layer of which is specialized and is called the *theca interna;* the source of *estradiol* production prior to ovulation in the menstrual cycle; multiple follicles at various stages of development are always present throughout reproductive life; see also *graafian follicle, atretic.*

**Follicle cell.**   See *follicle.*

**Follicle-stimulating hormone (FSH).**   *Glycoprotein* hormone produced by the *adenohypophysis,* responsible for the stimulation of (*a*) development of the *follicle,* in the ovary, and (*b*) *spermatogenesis,* in the testis.

**Follicular phase.**   Phase of the *menstrual cycle* before *ovulation,* as opposed to the *luteal phase* after ovulation.

**Formulary.**   Listing of medicinal substances and formulas.

**Free hormone.**   Proportion of *hormone* in the blood not bound to plasma transport proteins and so immediately available for biological activity; in equilibrium with *bound hormone,* so that as free hormone leaves the blood to exert its activity, it is quickly replaced.

**FSH.**   See *follicle-stimulating hormone.*

**Fundus.**   Bottom or base, part of a hollow organ farthest from its mouth.

**Gamete.**   Mature sex cells, *haploid* in number of chromosomes; female gamete is the *ovum,* male gamete is the *spermatozoon.*

**Gametogenesis.**   Development of germ cells or gametes.

**Genital folds.**   Folds on either side of the developing external genitalia of the embryo; form the urethra of the male and the *labia minora* of the female.

**Genital ridge.**   See *urogenital ridge.*

**Genital swellings.**   Pair of folds in the embryo outside, and wider than, the *genital folds;* they form the *scrotum* in the male and the *labia majora* in the female.

**Genital tubercle.**   Swelling towards the front of the developing genitalia in the embryo; subsequently forms the *clitoris* in females and the *penis* in males.

**Genitalia.**   External and/or internal reproductive organs.

**Genotype.**   Genetic makeup of an individual, as opposed to physical appearance (see *phenotype*).

**Germ cells.**   See *gamete;* term includes also the *diploid* precursors of the gametes, the primordial germ cells.

**Germinal epithelium.**   Epithelium of the *seminiferous tubule;* contains male germ cells; term also (loosely) applied to the thin epithelial covering of the ovary.

**Gestation.**   Pregnancy.

**Gestation period.**   Period from conception to birth.

**Globulins.**   Group of proteins, roughly spherical in shape, soluble in blood plasma.

**Glomerulonephritis.**   Inflammation of the small blood-filtering bodies (the glomeruli) of the kidney.

**Glucuronide.**   Molecule esterified with glucuronic acid; such conjugates of *steroid hormones* are biologically inactive, but greatly increase water solubility and so allow excretion into the urine.

**Glycoprotein.**   Protein molecule with an added carbohydrate component.

**Gonad.**   General term for the female *ovary* and the male *testis.*

**Gonadotrope** (also called **gonadotroph**).   Cell of the *adenohypophysis* that produces one or more *gonadotropins.*

**Gonadotropin** (also called **gonadotrophins**).   Hormone capable of stimulating the *gonads* (ovaries and testes); includes follicle-stimulating hormone, luteinizing hormone, and chorionic gonadotropin, all of which are *glycoprotein* hormones composed of two polypeptide chains or subunits: a common alpha chain that is the same for each hormone, and a beta chain that is different.

**Gonococcal.**  Pertaining to the bacterium that causes gonorrhea, *Neisseria gonorrheae.*

**Graafian follicle.**  Large, maturing ovàrian *follicle* that is destined to *ovulate.*

**Granuloma.**  Tumor-like mass of fibrous tissue caused by chronic inflammation.

**Granulosa cells.**  Follicle cells (see *follicle*).

**Gravid.**  Pregnant.

**Guanethidine.**  An antihypertensive drug that works by blocking the adrenergic nervous system.

**Habitus.**  Physique, physical appearance.

**Halogenated.**  Chemical substance that includes a halogen element: fluorine, chlorine, bromine, or iodine.

**Haploid.**  Having half the (*diploid*) number of chromosomes normal to a somatic cell, as in mature germ cells after *meiosis.*

**hCG.**  Human chorionic gonadotropin (see *chorionic gonadotropin*).

**Hematocrit.**  Volume percentage of red blood cells in whole blood.

**Hematoma.**  Bruising; infiltration of blood into the tissues after rupture of a blood vessel, usually leading to a swelling.

**Hematopoietic.**  Pertaining to, or affecting, the formation of blood cells.

**Hepatotoxicity.**  Property of a chemical substance injurious to the liver.

**Heterologous.**  Relating to different types of species; opposite: *homologous.*

**Heuristic.**  Serving to stimulate investigation.

**Homologous.**  Relating to the same type or species, opposed to *heterologous;* also, of similar embryonic origin, opposed to *analogous.*

**Hormone.**  Substance secreted in minute amount from one part of the body (see *endocrine gland*) and carried in the blood to another part, where it stimulates or inhibits biological activity.

**Huntington's chorea.**  Hereditary disease of the central nervous system manifesting after the attaining of reproductive age, and characterized by tremor and progressive deterioration of intellect terminating in dementia; usually fatal within 15 years of the onset of symptoms; inherited through a *dominant gene.*

**H-Y antigen.**  A substance (detected immunologically) closely related to the gene responsible for the development of the embryo into a male; the most sensitive indicator known of male genetic sex.

**Hyaline.**  Glassy and translucent.

**Hydrophilic.**  Possessing an affinity for water.

**Hydrophobic.**  Possessing an affinity for fatty substances, rather than for water and for water-soluble substances.

**Hydroxylation.**  Chemical addition of a hydroxyl (alcohol) group to a molecule; tends to make *steroids* more water soluble.

**Hyperfunctional.**  Exhibiting increased physiological function.

**Hyperplastic growth.**  Growth by hyperplasia (increase in cell numbers), as opposed to *hypertrophic growth.*

**Hypertonic.**  Having in a solution a higher content of osmotically active substances (such as ions) than is normal in most body fluids.

**Hypertrophic growth.**  Growth by hypertrophy (increase in cell size), as opposed to *hyperplastic growth.*

**Hypofunctional.**  Exhibiting decreased physiological function.

**Hypophysiotropic agent.**  Substance, normally from the *hypothalmus,* capable of stimulating or inhibiting secretion from the *adenohypophysis;* see also *releasing factor, inhibiting factor.*

**Hypothalamus.**  Part of the base of the brain immediately above, and connected to, the pituitary gland; in addition to regulation of the pituitary gland, concerned with emotions and with temperature control.

**Hypothalamo-hypophyseal portal system.**  A system of blood vessels running between the hypothalamus and the pituitary gland, transporting *release* and *inhibiting factors.*

**Hypothyroidism.**  Insufficient production of thyroid hormone by the thyroid gland; main clinical features result from slowing down of the body's metabolism, and include cold intolerance, weight gain, brittleness of the hair and, eventually, mental dullness.

**Hysterectomy.**  Surgical removal of the uterus.

**Hysteroscopy.**  Visual examination of the cavity of the uterus and also the cervical canal; often gives information complementary to that gained by *laparoscopy,* but it is unrelated to *colposcopy.*

**Immotile.**  See (opposite) *motile.*

**Implantation.**  Attachment of the developing *embryo* to the *endometrium;* normally takes place

1 week after ovulation and fertilization; see also *trophoblast*.

**Incubation.** Furnishing conditions, especially heat, necessary for growth and development.

**Infra-** (*prefix*). Below.

**Infundibular stalk.** Narrow connection between hypothalamus and pituitary containing neurosecretory neurons to the *neurohypophysis*, and the *hypothalamo-hypophyseal portal vessels* to the *adenohypophysis*.

**Inguinal.** Of the groin.

**Inhibiting factor (hypothalamic).** Hypothalamic hormone that prevents synthesis or release of hormones in the adenohypophysis.

**Innervation.** System of nerves supplying, and present in, an organ.

**In situ** (*Latin*). In place in the body; when used to describe a nonanatomical object, such as an I.U.D., means that the object is where it ought to be, namely in the uterus.

**Intercrural.** Situated between crescent-shaped ligamentous folds (crura), particularly those of the external inguinal ring at the base of the scrotum.

**Interstitial cell.** Cell lying between follicles in the ovary, or between seminiferous tubules in the testis; may secrete *androgens*, particularly in the testis, where they are especially well developed (*Leydig cells*) and secrete testosterone.

**Interstitial tissue.** Connective tissue between follicles in the ovary, or between seminiferous tubules in the testis; see also *interstitial cell*.

**Intramural.** Within the walls or boundaries of an organ.

**Intromission.** Insertion, particularly of the penis into the vagina.

**In vitro** (*Latin*). Literally, "within glass", so, observable in a test tube; or used to describe all artificial conditions in which, to facilitate scientific observation, physiological processes are studied in the laboratory rather than in the body (*in vivo*).

**In vivo** (*Latin*). In the living state, within the body.

**Ion.** An atom or molecule carrying a positive or negative charge.

**Ionic balance.** Balance between positively and negatively charged *ions*.

**Ischemia.** Insufficient blood supply.

**I.U.D.** Intrauterine (contraceptive) device.

**Kinase.** Enzyme that activates other enzymes.

**KOH wet mount.** Screening test for women who have suspected monilia.

**Labia.** Lateral epithelial folds at the vaginal orifice, homologous to the *scrotum; labia majora* are relatively wide and contain subcutaneous fat; *labia minora* are relatively thin, lie inside the labia majora, and contain no fat.

**Labioscrotal fold.** See *genital swelling*.

**Lagged regression** (*statistics*). Technique for predicting a dependent variable from independent variables that have been chronologically lagged, i.e., observed for a time period prior to the time period observed for the dependent variable.

**Laparoscopy.** Visualization of the abdominal and pelvic viscera with a thin optical device (a laparoscope), which is inserted through a small abdominal wound, usually immediately below the umbilicus.

**Laparotomy.** Surgical operation involving incision into the abdominal cavity.

**Latent period** (*special sense*). Period of sexual inactivity.

**Leydig cell.** Specialized *interstitial cell* of the testis responsible for the secretion of *testosterone*.

**LH.** See *luteinizing hormone*.

**Ligament.** Connective tissue attachment between bones or soft tissues, usually providing structural support.

**Lobule (alveolar).** Subdivision of lung tissue containing *alveoli* and their ducts, and supplied by a single *bronchiole*.

**Lumen.** Channel, passage, or cavity, in a hollow organ such as the fallopian tube, or a hollow tissue such as a blood vessel.

**Luteal.** Relating to the *corpus luteum*.

**Luteal phase.** Phase of the *menstrual cycle* after ovulation up to the time of menstruation, as opposed to the *follicular phase*, before ovulation; see also *corpus luteum*.

**Luteinize.** Literally, render a yellow appearance to; in endocrinology refers to the promotion in a tissue of the ability to synthesize *steroid hormones* (which, when present to a marked degree, causes the tissue to have a yellow color); see also *corpus luteum, luteinizing hormone*.

**Luteinizing hormone.** *Glycoprotein* hormone produced by the *adenohypophysis*, responsible for (a) *ovulation* and *corpus luteum* formation in the ovary, and (b) *testosterone* production in the testis.

**Luteolytic agent.** Substance that causes the *corpus luteum* to decrease or stop its progesterone production.

**Luteotropic** (also called **luteotrophic**). Capable of stimulating *progesterone* production from the *corpus luteum*.

**Lymphoma.** A neoplastic tumor of lymphoid tissue.

**Lysis.** The dissolving of tissue or cells; in surgery, the division or letting loose of adhesions.

**Macrodynamic** (*demography*). Involving processes of change that can be identified at the aggregate level; opposed to *microdynamic*.

**Mean** (*statistics*). Average value.

**Median eminence.** Medial and inferior part of the *hypothalamus* from which the *infundibular stalk* arises; immediately below the *arcuate nucleus;* contains neural tissue of the *tuberal hypothalamus*, and vascular elements connected to the *hypothalamico-hypophyseal portal system;* the site at which hypothalamic *releasing* and *inhibiting factors* are secreted.

**Medulla.** Central part of any organ.

**Medulla oblongata.** Lower part of the brain stem, continuous with the spinal cord.

**Medullary dominance.** Embryonic development of an organ such as the testis, in which the principal adult elements are derived from the *medulla* of the embryonic organ (in contradistinction to the ovary, which develops through *cortical dominance*).

**Meiosis.** Division of *diploid* cells such that there is a reduction in the number of chromosomes to the *haploid* number; occurs in the formation of *gametes*.

**Menarche.** First episode of menstrual bleeding; normally occurs between the ages of 9 and 16 years.

**Menopause.** Last episode of menstrual bleeding; normally occurs between the ages of 40 and 55 years.

**Menstrual cycle.** The interval associated with successive episodes of *menstruation*, and divided into two phases: *follicular phase*, and *luteal phase;* timed from the first day of menstruation to the first day of the next menstruation; average cycle length is 28 days, but may be up to 35 days in normal women, and is often shorter than 28 days in older women; tends to be irregular at the beginning and end of reproductive life.

**Menstruation.** Periodic bleeding from the uterus through the vagina, associated with partial shedding of the *endometrium;* see also *menstrual cycle, progesterone*.

**Mesenchymal cell.** Cell of the mesenchyme, or undifferentiated *connective tissue* of the *embryo*.

**Mesentery.** Double layer of *peritoneum* suspending an organ or part of an organ from the wall of the *peritoneal cavity*.

**Mesoderm.** Epithelium in the embryo lining those body cavities that contain the abdominal organs, the lungs, and the heart.

**Mesonephric duct.** See *mesonephros*.

**Mesonephros.** Embryonic kidney that develops before the metanephros (which ultimately gives rise to the definitive kidney of the fetus and adult); reabsorption and loss of function occur, except for its duct in the male (see *Wolffian duct*).

**Mesosalpinx.** *Mesentery* suspending the *fallopian tube*.

**Messenger RNA.** Type of ribonucleic acid (*RNA*) formed in the *nucleus* of a cell from *DNA;* carries in its precise composition instructions for protein synthesis from amino acids, which takes place in *ribosomes*.

**Metabolite.** Substance produced by metabolism.

**Metaphase.** Second stage of *mitosis* or *meiosis*.

**Microdynamic** (*demography*). Involving processes of change that can be identified at the individual level; opposed to *macrodynamic*.

**Micronized.** Particles reduced in size to about one micron (1/1000 millimeter) diameter.

**Microsurgery.** Surgery performed with the aid of optical magnification, using special instruments, fine suture material and needles, and meticulous handling of tissue.

**Microvilli.** Very small cytoplasmic extensions at the surface of a cell that increase surface area, and so (for example) aid exchange of materials across the cell membrane.

**Mitosis.** Cell division without any reduction in the (*diploid*) number of chromosomes in the daughter cells.

**Monoamine.** Chemical substance with a single amino group, frequently of considerable biological importance; includes catecholamine *neurotransmitters.*

**Mons pubis.**    Pubic mound; superficial pad of fat in the female overlying the *pubic symphysis.*

**Monte Carlo simulation model** (*demography, statistics*).    Probability of occurrences of events applied to individuals randomly, as opposed to individuals in categories.

**Morbidity rate.**    Proportion of patients who experience injury, disease, or other defined complications, usually as a result of a surgical or medical procedure.

**Morula.**    Early stage of embryo development; solid ball of cells prior to the formation of the hollow center that characterizes the *blastocyst.*

**Motile** (*special sense*).    Possessing the quality of propulsive movement: used of either a single moving cell such as a *spermatozoon,* or the *cilia* of a ciliated epithelial cell; opposite: *immotile.*

**Mucosa.**    Epithelial surface (and underlying connective tissue), kept moist by *mucus* (see also *epithelium*).

**Mucous membrane.**    Surface of *mucosa.*

**Mucus.**    Secretion containing high-molecular-weight, carbohydrate-rich *glycoproteins;* often, but not always, found in association with ciliated epithelium; see also *cervix.*

**Müllerian duct.**    Duct that forms in the embryo beside the *mesonephric duct,* but which persists in females and, by joining with the duct from the opposite side before making connection with the developing vagina, ultimately produces the *fallopian tubes,* the *uterus* and *cervix,* and the upper part of the *vagina.*

**Multiple regression** (*statistics*).    A strategy for predicting a single dependent variable from two or more independent variables.

**Multivariate regression.**    See *multiple regression.*

**Mutagenic.**    Capable of causing genetic mutation.

**Myocardial infarction.**    *Necrosis* of heart muscle tissue from sudden loss of adequate blood supply to it ("coronary occlusion"; "heart attack").

**Myometrium.**    Muscular component of the wall of the uterus; constitutes the main mass of the uterus; see also *endometrium.*

**N** (*statistics*).    Total number of observations in a population.

**n** (*statistics*).    Number of observations in a sample of a population.

**Natality** (*demography and anthropology*).    Birth rate.

**Natriuresis.**    Excretion of excessive sodium in the urine.

**Necrosis.**    Death of a portion of a tissue.

**Neolithic.**    Period in the cultural evolution of man later than the *paleolithic;* characterized by domestication of animals and cultivation of grains.

**Neonatal.**    Pertaining to the newborn infant, up to the age of 4 weeks.

**Neoplastic.**    Literally, "new growth"; usually a tumor, either benign or malignant.

**Neurohypophysis.**    Posterior pituitary gland; composed of a neural downgrowth from the *hypothalmus;* secretes two hormones: oxytocin (which stimulates contraction of the uterus), and vasopressin (which prevents dehydration).

**Neurotransmitter.**    Chemical substance released by a nerve ending, capable of stimulating an adjacent nerve.

**Noradrenergic.**    Pertaining to *norepinephrine.*

**Norepinephrine.**    Neurotransmitter; precursor for the synthesis of *epinephrine;* more important than epinephrine as a neurotransmitter in the brain.

**Norethisterone oenanthate.**    Synthetic progestin suitable for use in long-term injectable preparations.

**Norgestrel.**    Potent synthetic progestin; see also *racemic mixture.*

**Nuclear family.**    Unit composed of husband, wife, and their children.

**Nucleolus.**    Small body inside the cell nucleus; contains *RNA,* and is the site of synthesis of *ribosomal RNA.*

**Nucleus.**    More or less central body in the cell, surrounded by the *cytoplasm* and containing the *chromosomes.*

**Nulliparous.**    State of never having borne children.

**Occlude.**    Close off or block.

**Oligomenorrhea.**    Infrequent menstruation; menstruation at intervals of more than 35 days.

**Oligospermia.**    Reduced numbers of *spermatozoa* in the *semen;* often contributes to infertility.

**Oocyte.**    Ovum before completion of *meiosis;* ova in *follicles* are oocytes, and meiosis is normally not completed until *ovulation* and *fertilization* occur.

**Oogenesis.** Formulation of ova in the ovary; female equivalent of *spermatogenesis;* the process takes place only in the fetus, and after birth no new ova are produced.

**Oogonium.** Primordial female *germ cell* present in the fetal ovary; produces *oocytes* by *mitosis.*

**Optic neuritis.** Inflammation of the optic nerve, frequently causes blindness.

**Orchitis.** Inflammation of the *testis.*

**Os.** Opening; in particular, the opening of the canal of the uterine *cervix* into the vagina (external os) and into the uterus (internal os).

**Ostium.** Opening; in particular, the opening of the *fallopian tube* into the peritoneal cavity next to the ovary, through which the ovum passes into the tube after *ovulation.*

**Ovariectomy.** Surgical excision of the ovary.

**Ovary.** Paired internal reproductive organ of the female situated on each side of the pelvis; produces female germ cells, or *ova,* during reproductive life, as well as the female sex hormones, the most important of which are the *estrogens.*

**Oviduct.** See *fallopian tube.*

**Ovulation.** Extrusion of the ovum from its follicle; normally takes place about 14 days before menstruation, if fertilization does not occur.

**Ovum.** Female germ cell; egg; plural, ova.

**Oxytocin.** Polypeptide hormone secreted by the *neurohypophysis;* acts (*a*) on the *myometrium,* to cause contraction of the pregnant uterus, and (*b*) during breast feeding on muscular cells in the substance of the breast, to cause milk ejection ("let down") in response to nipple stimulation; available commercially in synthetic form.

**pH.** Symbol for the logarithm of the reciprocal of the hydrogen ion concentration of a solution; values range from 1 for a strong *acid,* through 7 for a neutral solution, to 14 for a strong *alkali* (weaker acids and alkalis have intermediate values).

**Paleolithic.** Early period in the cultural evolution of man; characterized by the use of the earliest tools, which were made by chipping or flaking stone; see also *neolithic.*

**Pandemic.** Widespread epidemic.

**Para-aortic lymph node dissection.** Surgical procedure involving dissection and removal of lymph nodes in the vicinity of the abdominal aorta, usually used in the treatment of cancer.

**Paramesonephric duct.** See *Müllerian duct.*

**Parameter** (*statistics*). Number used to describe a characteristic of a population set of data (examples are the *mean* and the *standard deviation*), as distinguished from estimates of these characteristics, based on samples (see *statistic*).

**Parenchyma.** Functional epithelial component of a tissue; opposed to the supporting component (the *stroma*).

**Path analysis.** Statistical strategy for dealing with two or more regression equations, in which influence of independent variables on other independent variables may be ordered chronologically.

**Pelvic relaxation.** Loss of strength of the supporting tissues of the pelvis in women, with consequent sagging and perhaps prolapse of the pelvic organs; predisposed to most frequently by childbirth.

**Penis.** Male reproductive organ used to introduce *semen* into the *vagina;* becomes rigid and erect with sexual arousal, owing to congestion with blood in specialized tissues, the *corpora cavernosa* (right and left, dorsal to the *urethra*) and the *corpus spongiosum* (surrounding the urethra).

**Peptide.** See *polypeptide.*

**Peptide bond.** See *amino acid.*

**Perinatal.** Occurring around the time of birth, when this is after 20 weeks' gestation, and including the *neonatal* period; "perinatal mortality" therefore includes stillbirths and deaths in the neonatal period.

**Periovulatory.** Occurring around the time of ovulation.

**Peristalsis.** Propagated waves of contraction in a muscular, tubular organ, normally resulting in transport of its contents.

**Peritoneal cavity.** Abdominal–pelvic cavity containing the abdominal organs and internal reproductive organs; a closed cavity in the male, but potentially continuous with the outside via the fallopian tubes, uterus, and vagina in the female.

**Peritoneum.** Membrane lining the *peritoneal cavity* and enveloping the contained *viscera.*

**Periventricular nuclei.** Clusters of nerve cell bodies of the *hypothalamus* adjacent to the third *ventricle.*

**Pessary.** Vaginal suppository; may be used to provide support in cases of *pelvic relaxation,* or to deliver drugs that act on, or are absorbed through, the vagina.

**Phagocyte.**　Cell capable of ingesting cellular or noncellular material.

**Phenotype.**　Physical makeup or constitution of an individual; results from the expression of the *genotype* and the interaction of this expression with the environment.

**Pituitary gland.**　Small but extremely important *endocrine gland* situated behind the nose at the base of the brain under the *hypothalamus;* composed of anterior and posterior parts known respectively as the *adenohypophysis* and *neurohypophysis.*

**Placenta.**　Vascular organ of respiration, nutrition, and excretion for the fetus, which is attached to it by the umbilical cord; composed largely of *trophoblast,* which comes into intimate contact with maternal blood in the endometrium after implantation; produces several hormones important to pregnancy; shed after birth (therefore known as the "afterbirth").

**Pleistocene.**　Geologically defined prehistoric time during which human evolution began.

**Plexus.**　Complex network of interconnecting nerves or blood vessels.

**Polar body.**　Extraneous, highly condensed nuclear material made redundant during *meiosis* in the female.

**Polyandry.**　Marriage of a woman to more than one man; see also *polygyny.*

**Polyethylene.**　*Polymer* composed of ethylene units; a plastic with wide application in medicine because of its tendency not to cause inflammation when placed in the body.

**Polygamy.**　That form of marriage consisting of one male and more than one female (*polygyny*), or one female and more than one male (*polyandry*).

**Polygyny.**　Marriage of a man to more than one woman; see also *polyandry.*

**Polylactide.**　*Polymer* of lactide units; flexible material used for absorbable suture material; biodegradable; used as a dissolving matrix for the implantation of contraceptive steroid hormones under the skin.

**Polymer.**　Any large molecule formed by the chemical union of five or more identical combining molecules.

**Polypeptide.**　Large molecule consisting of a chain of *amino acids;* proteins are composed of one or more polypeptide chains.

**Polypropylene.**　*Polymer* of propylene units; flexible plastic used for nonabsorbable suture material; not biodegradable; similar to polyethylene.

**Pons.**　Part of the brainstem interposed between the *medulla oblongata* and the midbrain.

**Portal vessels.**　Blood vessels so placed that they lead from one system of capillaries to another (other than the capillaries of the lung); see also *hypothalamo-hypophyseal portal system.*

**Posterior fornix.**　Area of the vagina behind the cervix.

**Posterior pituitary gland.**　See *neurohypophysis.*

**Postnatal.**　Occurring after the time of birth; see also *puerperium.*

**Pregnenolone.**　Steroid precursor of (among others) progesterone, testosterone, and the estrogens.

**Presumptive** (*special sense*).　Indicative of immaturity, incomplete development, or potentiality.

**Primary spermatocyte.**　See *spermatocyte.*

**Primogeniture.**　Exclusive right of inheritance belonging to the firstborn.

**Primordium.**　Cell mass constituting the first trace of an organ part; rudiment.

**Probability sampling.**　Techniques of subject selection that are based on the principle that every unit or subject has an equal chance of being chosen; normally involves random selection.

**Product moment correlation coefficient (*r*).**　Measure of the degree of linear relationship between an independent variable and a dependent variable.

**Progesterone.**　Female hormone responsible for the preparation for and maintenance of pregnancy; produced during the menstrual cycle after ovulation by the *corpus luteum;* causes the endometrium to secrete and to become receptive to *implantation* of an early embryo, if fertilization has taken place; if implantation does not take place, progesterone production ceases, and withdrawal of its support of the endometrium results in *menstruation;* in pregnancy the corpus luteum continues to produce progesterone for several weeks, after which the *placenta* becomes the main source; see also *luteal phase.*

**Progestin.**　Synthetic steroid hormone capable of some or all of the actions of *progesterone.*

**Progestogen.**　See *progestin* (synonym).

**Prolactin.**　Protein hormone produced by the *adenohypophysis* under the control of an inhibiting factor (*dopamine*) from the *hypothalamus;* responsible for lactation after pregnancy, and may have other reproductive functions that are not completely understood.

**Proliferative phase.**　Alternative term for the *fol-*

*licular phase* of the menstrual cycle, based on the proliferation of *endometrium* that takes place during this phase.

**Pronatalist.** Favoring high fertility.

**Pronucleus.** *Haploid* nucleus of an *ovum* or a *spermatozoon* after penetration of the ovum by the fertilizing spermatozoon; the female and male pronuclei then fuse to form the *diploid* nucleus of the fertilized egg or *zygote.*

**Prophase.** First stage of *mitosis* or *meiosis.*

**Prospective study.** Experimental study planned in advance, to observe events that have not already taken place; generally yields more reliable information than a *retrospective study*, because, if planned properly, is less likely to be biased.

**Prostaglandin.** Class of substances with great biological activity; widely distributed in body tissues, as well as in semen; biological activity is usually confined to the immediate vicinity of the site of production, unless administered therapeutically and systemically.

**Prostaglandin E.** Subclass of *prostaglandins;* in the termination of pregnancy, prostaglandin $E_2$ causes the cervix to soften, as well as stimulating uterine contractions.

**Prostaglandin $F_{2\alpha}$.** Important *prostaglandin* produced in several sites in the reproductive tract; stimulates uterine contractions, both during menstruation and during labor, and also after therapeutic administration to induce abortion or labor.

**Prostate.** Accessory sex gland in the male situated below the bladder; contributes secretion that is a component of *semen.*

**Prostatitis.** Inflammation of the prostate.

**Proximal.** Situated towards a central point of reference; opposite to *distal.*

**Puerperium.** *Postnatal* period that dates from the delivery of the *placenta,* and lasts until the reproductive organs have returned to their normal nonpregnant state; lasts about 6 weeks.

**Racemic mixture.** Mixture composed of two isomeric forms of the same chemical substance, distinguishable as *dextro-* (*d-*) or *levo-* (*l-*) according to the direction in which the isomer in its pure form rotates light; confusingly, the convention for description has changed recently, and similar designations are now based on the architecture of the substance's molecular structure; usually only one of the two isomers is biologically active, and so, for instance, the substance *levo*—norgestrel (pre-

viously "*d*-norgestrel") has twice the potency of the racemic mixture *d,l*-norgestrel.

**Radioimmunoassay.** Highly sensitive and specific assay, frequently used to detect very small quantities of steroid, glycoprotein, or polypeptide hormones (among others); depends on immunological recognition of part of the structure of the hormone being assayed, by a label that is measurable through being radioactive.

**Radioreceptor assay.** Highly sensitive and specific assay that is faster to perform in the laboratory than a *radioimmunoassay,* though not so widely available; depends on the biologically active part of the hormone being assayed.

**Reanastomosis.** See *tubal reanastomosis.*

**Receptor.** Molecule or molecular complex on a cell membrane or within the cell cytoplasm that binds a hormone or drug with high affinity and specificity, and is then capable of initiating a cellular action; probably all hormone actions require binding to a receptor, and it is the presence of receptors that confers hormone sensitivity on a tissue.

**Recessive gene.** Gene that is not expressed in the *phenotype* unless the *genotype* contains two such genes; see also *dominant gene.*

**Rectum.** Terminal part of the bowel directly connected to the anus.

**Releasing factor (hypothalamic).** Hypothalamic hormone that elicits synthesis and release of hormones in the anterior pituitary gland.

**Renal disease.** Kidney disease.

**Renin-angiotensin system.** Hormone-enzyme system exerting control on blood pressure and fluid balance in response to changes in blood volume and salt content.

**Resection.** Excision of a portion of an organ or other structure.

**Retinal thrombosis.** Occlusion by blood clot of one or more veins draining the retina.

**Retrospective study.** Experimental study conducted after the events to be studied have already taken place; generally much easier and cheaper to perform than a *prospective study.*

**Ribonucleic acid.** See *RNA.*

**Ribosomal RNA.** Type of *RNA* present in *ribosomes;* synthesized in the *nucleolus.*

**Ribosome.** Particle in the cell cytoplasm important for the synthesis of *polypeptides* from *amino acids;* contains *ribosomal RNA* and protein.

**RNA.** Ribonucleic acid; complex organic substance of similar structure to *DNA;* exists in several forms: *messenger RNA* (mRNA), *ribosomal RNA* (rRNA), and *transfer RNA* (tRNA).

**Rugosity.**    Characterized by wrinkles and ridges.

**Sacrum.**    Fused group of lower vertebrae constituting the back wall of the bony pelvis.

**Saline.**    Salt (sodium chloride) solution; "physiological saline" has the same osmotic pressure as body fluid, and has a concentration of 0.9 per cent.

**Sampling distribution** (*statistics*).    Theoretical probability distribution of a statistic.

**Sampling error.**    Estimate of the probable magnitude of error when reliance is placed on data from only a sample of a total population.

**Sclerosis.**    Hardening.

**Scrotum.**    Pouch of skin containing the testes, which are consequently kept at a temperature somewhat lower than general body temperature.

**Seasonals** (*statistics*).    Within-year patterns that are annually repetitive.

**Sebaceous glands.**    Skin glands producing fatty secretion (*sebum*).

**Sebum.**    See *sebaceous glands*.

**Secondary analysis.**    Study conducted with data originally obtained for another purpose, e.g., hospital patient records.

**Secondary spermatocyte.**    See *spermatocyte*.

**Secretory phase.**    Alternative term for the *luteal phase* of the menstrual cycle, so named because of the secretion that takes place in the *endometrium* during this phase.

**Semen.**    Fluid ejaculated by the male after sexual stimulation; contains *spermatozoa* and secretions, chiefly from the *seminal vesicles* and *prostate;* the semen volume may be normal even in the absence of spermatozoa.

**Semen analysis.**    See *spermogram*.

**Seminal plasma.**    Liquid portion of the *semen,* not including *spermatozoa*.

**Seminiferous tubules.**    Tissue of the *testis* responsible for the production of *spermatozoa;* contains male germ cells in immature form (see *spermatogenesis*), as well as *Sertoli cells,* which together constitute the *seminiferous epithelium;* connect with (rather fewer) *efferent ducts*.

**Sepsis.**    Infection.

**Septum.**    Partition.

**Sertoli cell.**    Supporting and nursing cell for developing male germ cells (see *spermatogenesis*) in the seminiferous tubule.

**Seventeen-hydroxyprogesterone.**    Steroid precursor of testosterone and estrogens.

**Sex hormone binding globulin.**    Special plasma protein that binds testosterone and estradiol in the circulation.

**Sinus.**    Biological space or cavity; also a pathological defect in a tissue, similar to a *fistula,* but continuous with only one surface (onto which it discharges its contents).

**Social mobility.**    Change in status or occupation in either an upward or downward direction.

**Somatic.**    Pertaining to the body.

**Somatic cells.**    All cells of the body other than the *germ cells*.

**Somatic tissue.**    Tissue of the body wall or surrounding the body cavities, as opposed to *viscera*.

**Spermacide.**    Contraceptive substance that kills spermatozoa.

**Spermatid.**    *Haploid* developing male germ cell in the *seminiferous tubule;* matures into a *spermatozoon* without further cellular division.

**Spermatocyte.**    Male germ cells in the *seminiferous tubule* undergoing the process of *meiosis*.

**Spermatogenesis.**    Formation of *spermatozoa* in the testis; male equivalent of *oogenesis;* occurs throughout male reproductive life through *mitosis* of spermatogonia, *meiosis* of spermatocytes, and then maturation of spermatids; see also *epididymis*.

**Spermatogonium.**    Primordial male germ cell; produces spermatocytes by mitosis.

**Spermatozoon.**    Mature male germ cell; composed of (*a*) a head, which contains the highly condensed nucleus and over which is situated the *acrosome,* (*b*) a middle piece, which stores and produces the energy required for motility, and (*c*) a tail, or flagellum, which by beating causes the spermatozoon to move forwards; plural: spermatozoa.

**Spermogram.**    Analysis of the *semen* including quantitation of spermatozoa (their total number, the percentage that show normal and abnormal motility, and the percentage normal or abnormal in form); used as a diagnostic test in assessment of fertility; "sperm count."

**Sphincter.**    Ring or band of muscle fibers that constricts a natural orifice or closes off a passage area in a hollow organ.

**Spongiosum.**    Middle layer of endometrium, composed of less dense tissue than the deeper *basalis* or more superficial *compactum*.

**Spotting.** Slight uterine bleeding, usually of insufficient degree to require sanitary protection.

**Squamous epithelium.** *Epithelium* composed of flat cells, usually in multiple (stratified), as opposed to *columnar epithelium;* the vaginal surface of the cervix, as well as the lining of the vagina itself, is composed of squamous epithelium.

**Standard deviation** (*statistics*). Measure of dispersion in terms of deviation of variables from their *mean.*

**Standard error** (*statistics*). *Standard deviation* of the sampling distribution.

**Standard error of the mean** (*statistics*). The *standard deviation* of the distribution of sample *means.*

**Standardized partial regression coefficients** (*statistics*). Slopes in a multiple regression equation standardized through multiplication by the ratio of standard deviations of the independent variables to the dependent variable; also known as betas.

**Statistic.** Value calculated from a sample; used in conjunction with its sampling distribution to infer properties of the population.

**Sterilization.** Deliberate and usually irreversible total interference with fertility in the male or female, normally not accompanied by any change in the capacity to produce male or female sex hormones; see also *tubal ligation, vasectomy.*

**Steroid.** Diverse organic substances related chemically to *cholesterol,* from which many are derived.

**Steroid hormones.** Include *androgens, estrogens, progesterone,* and adrenal hormones; only barely soluble in water, but soluble in fat and so readily able to pass through cell membranes to exert biological activity; see also *glucuronide, bound hormone, receptor.*

**Steroidogenesis.** Production of steroid hormones.

**Stochastic.** Statistical description in terms of chance, or of probability or randomness.

**Stroma.** Supporting framework of a tissue, composed of connective tissue and including blood vessels and nerves; opposed to the functional, epithelial component (the *parenchyma*).

**Subcutaneous.** Under the skin.

**Subnuclear.** Smaller than, and residing within, the cell nucleus.

**Sulfate.** Chemical group that contains sulfur and oxygen; the addition of such a group to a *steroid* (sulfation; sulfate conjugation) greatly decreases biological activity by increasing water solubility and decreasing fat solubility.

**Supra-** (*prefix*). Above.

**Sympathetic nervous system.** Together with the parasympathetic nervous system, constitutes the autonomic, or involuntary, nervous system.

**Symphysis pubis.** Fibrocartilaginous junction and union of the pubic bones.

**Synapse.** Nerve junction; see also *neurotransmitter.*

**Synchronic.** Concurrence of existence in time; opposite: *diachronic.*

**Syncytiotrophoblast.** Tissue derived from the outermost layer of the *blastocyst;* invades the endometrium at *implantation* and eventually constitutes a large part of the *placenta.*

**Syncytium.** Composite cell consisting of many separate nuclei that share a common cytoplasm.

**Synergistic.** Working together toward a common goal; opposite to antagonistic.

**Syngamy.** Fusion of male and female *pronuclei* during *fertilization.*

**Ten-hydroxylated prostaglandins.** Biologically inactive metabolites of primary *prostaglandins.*

**Testis.** Paired reproductive organ of the male, situated in the scrotum; produces male germ cells or *spermatozoa,* as well as male sex hormones such as *testosterone.*

**Theca.** Tissue sheath or covering made of connective tissue; the term is used only in several restricted senses.

**Theca externa.** Unspecialized condensation of ovarian connective tissue around the *follicle,* external to the *theca interna.*

**Theca interna.** Specialized condensation of ovarian connective tissue immediately around the granulosa cells of the *follicle;* estrogen production by a growing follicle is through the production of precursor *androgens* supplied by the theca interna.

**Thromboembolus.** *Embolus* composed of a thrombus (blood clot).

**Thrombophlebitis.** Inflammation of a vein (phlebitis) with clotting of its contents.

**Thrombosis.** Clotting of blood inside an artery or vein, preventing blood flow to or from a tissue or organ.

**Thrombotic vascular accident.** See *thrombosis.*

**Tonic** (*special sense*).   Constant, steady.

**Transfer RNA.**   Type of ribonucleic acid (*RNA*) in the cell cytoplasm that transports *amino acids* to *ribosomes* for the synthesis of *polypeptides.*

**Transudation.**   Passage of components of blood plasma through a tissue.

**Transuterine sterilization.**   Sterilization accomplished by occluding the entrance of the fallopian tubes into the cavity of the uterus by a procedure performed through the canal of the uterine cervix; see also *hysteroscopy.*

**Trend** (*statistics*).   Broad, long-range movement of a set of observations over a period of time.

**Triglyceride.**   Fatty substance composed of three molecules of fatty acid and one molecule of glycerol; the usual storage form of fat.

**Tripeptide.**   Small peptide composed of three amino acids; see also *polypeptide.*

**Trophic.**   Giving nourishment.

**Trophoblast.**   Epithelial tissue derived from the outer part of the *blastocyst;* gives rise to the *placenta;* comprises *syncytiotrophoblast* and cytotrophoblast.

**Tropic.**   Able to cause switching from one functional state to another, or from a nonfunctional state to a functional one.

**Tubal ligation.**   Female sterilization operation in which, usually, a segment of the middle of the fallopian tube is removed surgically, cauterized, or occluded with a plastic ring or clip; depending largely on the exact site and length of the removed or damaged segment, the operation may be reversible surgically (see *tubal reanastomosis*).

**Tubal reanastomosis.**   Surgical operation in which an attempt is made to repair the fallopian tube after *tubal ligation.*

**Tuberal hypothalamus.**   Most inferior part of the *hypothalamus* (the tuber cinereum); see also *median eminence.*

**Tubercle.**   Anatomical nodule or prominence.

**Tunica albuginea.**   White-colored fibrous connective tissue covering of the ovary or testis.

**Urea.**   Main excretory substance in urine, produced in the body from the metabolism of proteins; can also be injected in high concentration into the amniotic cavity to terminate pregnancy in the middle trimester.

**Uremia.**   Accumulation of excessive urea in the blood, owing to renal failure.

**Ureter.**   Duct carrying urine from the kidney to the bladder.

**Urethra.**   Duct that carries urine from the bladder to the exterior, in both sexes; in males the urethra also transports the semen.

**Urethritis.**   Inflammation of the urethra; passing urine is painful, and there may be a discharge.

**Urogenital ridge.**   Ridge of tissue in the peritoneal cavity of the embryo in which the *mesonephros* and the *gonads* develop.

**Urogenital system.**   All organs involved in either the excretion of urine or in reproduction; there is considerable overlap among them, both embryologically, anatomically, and functionally.

**Uterine mucosa.**   See *uterus.*

**Uterotonic.**   Producing uterine contractions.

**Uterus.**   Single midline organ of reproduction in the female pelvis in which the embryo develops (the womb); composed of two anatomical parts: the body (corpus) or main bulk of the uterus, which receives on each side the *fallopian tubes* at the *fundus* of the uterus, and the neck (*cervix*), through which the cavity of the uterus communicates with the vagina; the wall of the uterus is composed of muscle (the *myometrium*), and is lined by a mucosal surface (the *endometrium*).

**Vacuole.**   Membrane-bound constituent of a cell that contains a substance thereby excluded from direct contact with the remaining cytoplasm; often contains material that is to be secreted (such as hormones, mucus, or enzymes) or stored (such as fat) by the cell.

**Vagina.**   Single midline organ of female reproduction that receives the penis during sexual intercourse, and through which the *uterus* communicates with the exterior; constitutes the major portion of the birth canal during childbirth.

**Vaginitis.**   Inflammation of the vagina; usually characterized by an abnormal vaginal discharge.

**Variates** (*statistics*).   Individual measurements.

**Varicocele.**   Abnormal dilatation of the veins that drain the *testes,* comparable to varicose veins in the legs; thought to increase the temperature within the *scrotum,* so interfering with *spermatogenesis* and contributing to infertility; treatable surgically by a relatively simple operation.

**Vas.**   Vessel or conduit; see *vas deferens.*

**Vas deferens.** Duct in the male that conveys spermatozoa from the *epididymis* to the *urethra*.

**Vasa efferentia.** See *efferent ducts*.

**Vasectomy.** Male sterilization operation in which, usually, a small portion of the *vas deferens* on each side is excised in the upper part of the *scrotum*, so preventing the passage of spermatozoa into the semen; depending largely on the length of the portion excised, the operation may be reversed with microsurgery.

**Vasoactive.** Able to exert a physiologic or pharmacologic effect on blood vessels.

**Vasovasostomy.** Operation for reversal of *vasectomy*.

**Venous.** Pertaining to veins, as opposed to arteries.

**Ventral.** Situated at, or relatively nearer to, the front of the body; opposite: *dorsal*.

**Ventricle.** Special term describing one of two types of body cavity: (*a*) in the brain, where there are four ventricles filled with cerebrospinal fluid, and (*b*) in the heart, where the two ventricles cause movement of the blood through the lungs and the body.

**Vestibule.** Antechamber or entrance to the *vagina*, bounded on each side by the *labia minora* and *labia majora*, and in front by the *clitoris*; the *urethra* also opens into it.

**Villi, chorionic.** Fingerlike projections of *trophoblast* containing embryonic blood vessels, which come into direct contact with maternal blood as the *placenta* develops.

**Viscera.** Internal organs of the body contained within, particularly, the abdominal and pelvic cavity, but also including the heart, the lungs, and the major blood vessels.

**Vitelline.** Pertaining to an egg, or *ovum*.

**Vitelline membrane.** Cell membrane of the ovum.

**Vitellus.** Nutrient store of an egg or embryo.

**Wolffian duct.** Duct of the embryonic *mesonephros*; disappears almost completely in females, but in males forms the *epididymis* and the *vas deferens*.

**Yolk sac.** Transient structure in the human *embryo* connected to the developing gut.

**Zero order release rate.** Constant release, as opposed to a rate of release that decreases with time.

**Zona pellucida.** Homogenous membrane around the *ovum*; needs to be penetrated by the fertilizing *spermatozoon*; the *blastocyst* must "hatch" through it before *implantation* can take place.

**Zygote.** Fertilized ovum before it divides; chromosome number is *diploid*.

---

## Acknowledgments

Grateful acknowledgment is made to David R. Archer for his assistance.

---

# Index

*A page number followed by* f *refers to a figure;* t *refers to a table.*